Signs and Symptoms
in Cardiology

Edited by

Lawrence D. Horwitz, M.D.

Professor of Medicine
Head, Division of Cardiology
University of Colorado Health Sciences Center
Denver, Colorado

and

Bertron M. Groves, M.D.

Associate Professor of Medicine, Division of Cardiology
Director, Cardiac Catheterization Laboratory
University of Colorado Health Sciences Center
Denver, Colorado

19 additional contributors

Signs and Symptoms in Cardiology

 J. B. Lippincott Company
Philadelphia

London Mexico City New York
St. Louis São Paulo Sydney

The authors and publisher have exerted every effort to ensure that drug selection and dosage set forth in this text are in accord with current recommendations and practice at the time of publication. However, in view of ongoing research, changes in government regulations, and the constant flow of information relating to drug therapy and drug reactions, the reader is urged to check the package insert for each drug for any change in indications and dosage and for added warnings and precautions. This is particularly important when the recommended agent is a new or infrequently employed drug.

Sponsoring Editor: Darlene D. Pedersen
Manuscript Editor: Patrick O'Kane
Indexer: Ruth Low
Art Director: Maria S. Karkucinski
Production Supervisor: J. Corey Gray
Production Coordinator: Charlene Catlett Squibb
Compositor: ICC
Printer/Binder: Murray Printing

        1   3   5   6   4   2

Library of Congress Cataloging in Publication Data
Main entry under title:

Signs and symptoms in cardiology.

    Includes index.
    1. Cardiovascular system—Diseases—Diagnosis.
2. Symptomatology. I. Horwitz, Lawrence D., 1939–
II. Groves, Bertron M., 1938–   . [DNLM: 1. Cardiovascular Diseases—diagnosis. 2. Cardiovascular Diseases
—physiopathology. WG 141 S578]
RC683.S53   1985   616.1'2075   84-7893
ISBN 0-397-50512-4

CONTRIBUTORS

Jonathan Abrams, M.D.
Professor of Medicine, Chief of Cardiology, University of New Mexico, Albuquerque, New Mexico

Joseph R. Benotti, M.D.
Assistant Professor of Medicine, Division of Cardiovascular Medicine, University of Massachusetts Medical School, Worcester, Massachusetts

Edward I. Curtiss, M.D.
Associate Professor of Medicine, University of Pittsburgh School of Medicine, Pittsburgh, Pennsylvania

James E. Dalen, M.D.
Professor and Chairman, Department of Medicine, University of Massachusetts Medical School, Worcester, Massachusetts

Antonio C. de Leon, Jr., M.D.
Medical Director, Cardiovascular Institute, St. John Medical Center, Tulsa, Oklahoma

Roy V. Ditchey, M.D.
Assistant Professor of Medicine, Division of Cardiology, University of Colorado Health Sciences Center, Denver, Colorado

Gordon A. Ewy, M.D.
Professor of Medicine, Chief of Cardiology, University of Arizona Health Sciences Center, University Hospital, Tucson, Arizona

E. Wayne Grogan, M.D.
Fellow in Cardiology, University of Colorado Health Sciences Center, Denver, Colorado

Bertron M. Groves, M.D.
Associate Professor of Medicine, Division of Cardiology, University of Colorado Health Sciences Center, Denver, Colorado

Lawrence D. Horwitz, M.D.
Professor of Medicine, Head, Division of Cardiology, University of Colorado Health Sciences Center, Denver, Colorado

Dennis L. Kirch, M.S.E.E.
Assistant Clinical Professor of Radiology, University of Colorado Health Sciences Center, Denver, Colorado

JoAnn Lindenfeld, M.D.
Assistant Professor of Medicine, Division of Cardiology, University of Colorado Health Sciences Center, Denver, Colorado

Suzanne Oparil, M.D.
Professor of Medicine, Associate Professor of Physiology and Biophysics, The University of Alabama in Birmingham, School of Medicine, Birmingham, Alabama

Joseph K. Perloff, M.D.
Streisand/American Heart Association Professor of Medicine and Pediatrics, University of California-Los Angeles School of Medicine, Los Angeles, California

P. Sudhakar Reddy, M.D.
Associate Professor of Medicine, University of Pittsburgh School of Medicine, Pittsburgh, Pennsylvania

John T. Reeves, M.D.
Professor of Medicine, Division of Cardiology, University of Colorado Health Sciences Center, Denver, Colorado

Nathaniel Reichek, M.D.
Associate Professor of Medicine, University of Pennsylvania School of Medicine, Philadelphia, Pennsylvania

Ralph Shabetai, M.D., F.R.C.P, Edin.
Chief of Cardiology, San Diego Veterans Administration Medical Center, San Diego, California

John F. Stapleton, M.D.
Professor of Medicine, Georgetown University School of Medicine, Washington, D.C.

Peter P. Steele, M.D.
Director of Nuclear Cardiology, Valley View Hospital, Thornton, Colorado

John V. Weil, M.D.
Professor of Medicine, Director, Cardiovascular Pulmonary Research Laboratory, Division of Cardiology, University of Colorado Health Sciences Center, Denver, Colorado

PREFACE

The purpose of *Signs and Symptoms in Cardiology* is to provide comprehensive discussions of the pathophysiology and clinical characteristics of signs and symptoms commonly encountered by physicians who care for patients with cardiac diseases. Although the emphasis is on adults, many chapters are highly relevant to children with cardiac disorders. The mechanisms and physiologic basis of the various findings are reviewed in depth. The discussions of clinical interpretation should have practical value for practicing physicians. In addition to individual signs and symptoms, groups of findings associated with clinical syndromes such as heart failure, pulmonary hypertension, or cardiac tamponade are considered. We anticipate that *Signs and Symptoms in Cardiology* will be of interest to a wide spectrum of physicians, including general medical audiences and specialists in medical or surgical treatment of cardiac diseases.

LAWRENCE D. HORWITZ, M.D.
BERTRON M. GROVES, M.D.

CONTENTS

11 CONGESTIVE HEART FAILURE   261

Lawrence D. Horwitz, M.D., and E. Wayne Grogan, M.D.

12 PULMONARY EMBOLISM   277

Joseph R. Benotti, M.D., and James E. Dalen, M.D.

13 CARDIAC TAMPONADE AND CONSTRICTION   298

Ralph Shabetai, M.D., F.R.C.P., Edin

Signs and Symptoms
in Cardiology

1

CHEST PAIN

Lawrence D. Horwitz, M.D.

Definition

Although chest discomfort is the most common complaint of patients with coronary artery disease, it can be one of the most confusing and misleading of symptoms. The discomfort may involve such diverse entities as the sudden agony often encountered in acute myocardial infarction or aortic dissection, the recurrent pain of angina or esophagitis, or the varying degrees of pain of musculoskeletal origin—which may be disturbing to patients yet have no sinister implication of risk of imminent death.

Our purpose is to describe the pathophysiology and clinical presentation of pain due to cardiac disorders and to distinguish it from the myriad other causes of chest discomfort that can mimic it. Thus, we can define *chest pain* as an unpleasant sensation that is generally located, at least in part, in the thorax and is possibly due to a disease of the heart or great vessels. The most common type of heart disease that may signal its presence by chest pain is coronary artery disease. Other cardiovascular entities, however, such as aortic or pulmonic valve disease, obstructive or nonobstructive cardiomyopathy, pulmonary hypertension due to mitral stenosis or other causes, or disease of the aorta, may also cause chest discomfort. The recognition of chest pain caused by cardiovascular pathology and its differentiation from other causes, both harmful and harmless, are important aspects of medical care worthy of the attention of most physicians.

Physiology

PAIN AND ITS PERCEPTION

Pain consists of two components: the original sensation and the reaction to that sensation. The stimulus is usually an occurrence that injures or destroys, or threatens to injure or destroy, tissue. It may be due to chemical, mechanical, thermal, or electrical processes. It is believed that accumulation of irritating, endogenous biochemical products is the usual cause of cardiac pain, although mechanical factors may also be relevant. In all forms of pain, the perception of the original sensation induced by the stimulus is strongly influenced by psychological factors, autonomic nervous system activation, and somatic efferent nerve activation. Psychological factors include personality differences, age, sex, racial or cultural differences, previous experience, and anxiety levels. Because of the diverse nature of reactions to the original sensation, especially the psychological components, pain perception varies widely for approximately equal stimuli.[1]

Receptors in tissue are activated by noxious stimuli, and pain is then transmitted by afferent peripheral nerve fibers. Pain originating in deep visceral structures such as the heart is transmitted predominantly by unmyelinated C fibers and, to a lesser extent, by myelinated fibers. Visceral pain differs from cutaneous pain in both its neural transmission and its characteristics. Cutaneous pain tends to be sharp, to be rapidly perceived and rapidly extinguished by withdrawal of the stimulus, and to be accurately localized by the person. Visceral pain tends to be dull or aching in quality, to be slow in onset, to persist even after the stimulus is removed, to be poorly localized, and is often referred to locations distant from the site of origin. Myelinated nerve fibers, which are the most prevalent form of pain-transmitting fibers in the skin, are more rapidly responsive and allow more precise localization of stimuli than unmyelinated C nerve fibers. With either type of fiber, the intensity and the rate of stimulation are factors that determine whether pain occurs or not, although the various aspects of the reaction to the stimulation can often influence mechanisms of perception.[1,2]

Both C fibers and myelinated fibers capable of transmitting pain enter the spinal cord through the dorsal column system where the cell bodies are located and synapse in the substantia gelatinosa. From the substantia gelatinosa, pain impulses pass into the anterolateral columns of the opposite side, either directly through axons of cell bodies in the substantia gelatinosa or by way of intercalated neurons. The sensations are then transmitted to the thalamus and subsequently to the cerebral cortex.[1,2]

The nature of the nervous pathways that carry pain has been the subject of controversy. The "specificity theory" of pain transmission, which has been generally invoked, proposes that there are specific pain receptors and pain fibers that project to a specific pain center or centers in the brain.[3] There is evidence that some specialized pain fibers exist in peripheral nerves, but it is not clear that all fibers capable of transmitting pain respond exclusively to this specific sensation, nor is it clear that there are specialized pain centers in the brain.[3] Certain phenomena such as causalgia (a burning pain caused by partial lesions of peripheral nerves), peripheral neuralgias caused by nerve infection or degeneration, and the strong influence of psychological factors on pain perception are difficult to explain by the specificity theory.[3]

Melzak and his colleagues have proposed a "gate control" theory that may resolve these objections.[3] They propose that the cells in the substantia gelatinosa act as a gate that modulates synaptic transmission of pain-induced impulses from the tissue to central cells. They postulate that when impulses appear in large numbers, a negative feedback reduces their effects, whereas small numbers of impulses activate a positive feedback that accentuates their effects. Also, they propose that the brain can activate efferent fibers that influence afferent conduction by acting on the gate control system in the substantia gelatinosa. As a result of these influences on the gate system, the output into the central nervous system (CNS) may differ substantially from the input from peripheral fibers. Thus, the gate concept furnishes a means by which the influence of emotion, memory, or other CNS functions on the input of pain signals can be understood.

The degree to which central control can be exerted may depend on the magnitude and rate of rise in intensity of peripheral pain impulses. For example, an acute myocardial infarction may result in such a rapid, overwhelming increase in impulses in peripheral pain fibers that the gate control system is ineffective, so that negative feedback cannot occur. Less severe forms of cardiac pain, however, may be more susceptible to central modulation. Thus, a patient with coronary artery disease who does not perceive anginal pain, despite electrocardiographic evidence of ischemia during physical activity, may be effectively suppressing the input to the cerebral cortex through central modulation by means of the gate control system.

Other reactions to pain may modify human experience, particularly if the pain is severe. Autonomic reflexes in response to noxious stimuli are common. Sympathetic efferent activation may result in tachycardia, vasoconstriction or vasodilation, sweating, and dilation of the pupils.[2] Parasympathetic stimulation may result in bradycardia and hypotension.[2] Discomfort due to cardiovascular problems may result in either sympathetic or parasympathetic stimulation. Some forms of discomfort may result in reflex contraction of skeletal muscles through the activation of somatic efferent fibers. Splinting of the chest with certain extracardiac thoracic disorders or the guarding of abdominal muscles with acute abdominal disease are examples of this response.

Cardiac pain and pain from other visceral organs are often referred to other regions of the body, such as skin and skeletal muscle that share common segmental neural distributions with the organ involved. Thus, if sensory or motor fibers from a given region of the spinal cord are shared by a deep organ and a superficial nerve, pain originating in the deep organ may be perceived in a distant locus innervated by the superficial nerve.[1,2] Examples are cardiac pain that is referred to the left chest, left arm, neck, and jaw or pain originating in the central diaphragmatic pleura that is referred to the shoulder.

ORIGINS OF CARDIAC PAIN

By the early part of the 20th century it was well known that angina was due to obstructive disease of the coronary arteries.[4-7] The fact that ischemia, or deficiency in blood supply to the myocardium, and the resultant disparity between myocardial oxygen supply and oxygen need, was the basis of anginal pain was clearly expounded by Keefer and Resnik in 1928.[8] In 1932 Thomas Lewis proposed that pain was produced by the accumulation of a certain metabolite.[9] He postulated that hypoxic myocardial cells released a "P substance" that activated neural pain fibers. Although Lewis's theory of the cause of anginal pain is generally accepted, the identity of the pain-producing metabolite remains unknown. There is recent evidence to suggest that bradykinin or other kinins are the agents stimulating the pain fibers.[10] Changes in the kinogen–kinin system in the circulating blood have been demonstrated in animal and human subjects with myocardial infarction or ischemia.[10] Other substances that have been suggested as possible biochemical mediators are lactic, pyruvic succinic, and phosphoric acids, potassium ions, histamine, and serotonin.[10,11]

The usual cause of cardiac pain is ischemia or damage due to obstruction of the coronary arteries by atherosclerotic plaques. Myocardial ischemia or infarction can also occur in patients with variant, or Prinzmetal's, angina in which coronary artery spasm due to inappropriate vasoconstriction is severe enough to obstruct blood flow.[12-14] Such spasms may involve coronary vessels free of atherosclerosis or with lesions of varying severity.[12-14] Thrombosis of the coronary artery, the usual basis of myocardial infarction, generally occurs at the site of atherosclerotic plaques or coronary spasm, but may also occur where there are structural abnormalities due to aneurysm or achalasia. Other causes of ischemic cardiac pain are various congenital abnormalities of the coronary arteries. When a coronary artery has an anomalous origin in the pulmonary artery or when there is a coronary arteriovenous fistula, flow patterns of oxygenated blood to the myocardial cells are disturbed.[15,16] Abnormal flow rates may also occur as a result of coronary artery aneurysm or achalasia. Mechanical obstruction to coronary flow may occur in some cases of anomalous circumflex coronary artery and in some cases of aneurysm of the sinus of Valsalva.[17,18] Other acquired conditions, including coronary arteritis in collagen vascular disease, traumatic lesions, and emboli originating in the left side of the heart, can also obstruct the coronary arteries.

Cardiac pain could potentially be caused by excessive oxygen demand in the absence of problems with myocardial blood flow. In animals, infusion of massive dosages of catecholamines causes myocardial damage, presumably because increased myocardial oxygen need, due largely to tachycardia, exceeds the capacity of the normal coronary arterial bed to provide oxygenated blood.[19,20] Whether endogenous catecholamine release caused by emotional distress, extreme physical exertion, painful injury, or other factors can cause ischemia is still the subject of controversy. Tachyarrhythmias could result in chest pain because of a similar increase in myocardial oxygen demand, although such pain usually occurs in older patients in whom some coronary obstructive component is likely to be present. Increased oxygen demand due to a hypercontractile state and increased left ventricular (LV) pressure and afterload has been proposed as the major cause of the chest pain frequently experienced in obstructive cardiomyopathy (idiopathic hypertrophic subaortic stenosis).[21] Increased ventricular pressure and afterload due to hypertension of either the pulmonary or the systemic circulation, or to aortic or pulmonic valvular or supravalvular obstruction, could also, in part, cause chest pain by increasing myocardial oxygen demand in excess of supply. Hypertrophy of the myocardium may increase the discrepancy between oxygen supply and demand because of the increased diffusion distances from capillaries to myocardial cells and the possibly increased oxygen requirements of the enlarged cells.[22,23] The chest pain in nonobstructive forms of cardiomyopathy may be related to increased oxygen consumption due to hypertrophy and dilation of the ventricles, perhaps together with diminished coronary flow due to low cardiac output.

Although the release of a noxious biochemical substance in response to oxygen deficiency is probably the major cause of cardiac pain, in some circumstances other mechanisms may be at work. Wenckebach in 1924 proposed that sudden mechanical distention of vessels may stimulate nerve endings in the adventitia, causing pain.[24] This is not likely to be a mechanism of pain with coronary disease but may be a cause of the chest pain occasionally encountered with acute aortic or pulmonary hypertension in which nerves at the roots of the aorta or pulmonary artery are stimulated.[25,26] Direct mechanical deformation of vessels may also stimulate nerve endings and is probably the major cause of chest pain in dissection of the aorta and in chest pain associated with iatrogenic dissection of coronary arteries or traumatic damage to vessels. The atypical chest pain that very commonly occurs in patients with mitral valve prolapse does not seem to be related to a disturbance in myocardial oxygenation. In this condition mechanical traction by the valve structure on adjacent myocardium during valve prolapse may be the mechanism by which chest pain is induced.

NEURAL TRANSMISSION OF CARDIAC PAIN AND CARDIAC PAIN PATTERNS

Painful impulses originating in the heart begin in receptors at nerve endings in the adventitia of coronary vessels and the myocardium. The nerve fibers enter the superficial and deep cardiac plexuses and travel by way of the superior, middle, and inferior cardiac nerves to the cervical and upper thoracic ganglia of the sympathetic chain. The cell bodies for these afferent fibers are located in the dorsal roots of thoracic spinal segments T1–T5, and the fibers reach these sites by passing through the sympathetic chain to communications in the thoracic sympathetic ganglia.[1,27-29]

As noted previously, the heart shares with other viscera a propensity for referral of pain to skin or skeletal muscles that share nerve supplies from the same, or adjacent, spinal segments. In the case of the heart, such pain will commonly radiate to regions innervated by thoracic segments T1–T5 and also into regions innervated by adjacent cervical and thoracic segments. The regions of the body surface supplied by the first five thoracic segments include the anterior chest wall from just below the clavicles to approximately the region overlying the seventh rib, including the adjacent sternum; the posterior portions of the chest wall overlying the first through approximately the seventh rib and the scapula; and the interposed portions of the lateral chest walls.[30] T1 and T2 also supply the medial aspect of the arms. The eighth cervical segment (C8) supplies the ulnar aspects of the forearm, wrist, and hand, and C7 innervates the more central aspects of the arm, wrist, and hand. The next higher cervical segments (C3–C6) innervate the remaining portions of the arms, the shoulders, and portions of the neck. Adjacent thoracic segments (T6–T10) innervate the lower chest wall and portions of the abdomen.

Pain originating in the heart is commonly located in the distribution of segments T1–T5.[1,27–29] It may on occasion be referred to regions supplied by segments as high as C3 or as low as T10. Embryologically, the left side of the heart develops in association with the left side of the nervous system. As a result, pain from LV ischemia, the most common site in coronary disease, is transmitted predominantly to left sided locations. Thus, cardiac pain is most commonly located in the substernal area, on the left side of the chest, and in the medial aspect of the left arm. The pain, especially if it is very severe, may be referred more widely to other regions, including the neck; the ulnar aspects of the forearm, wrist, and hand; the right arm or chest; and the upper abdomen. Rarely, cardiac pain may radiate into the jaw, probably by spread of impulses into the upper cervical segments and the descending nucleus of the trigeminal nerve. Cardiac pain referred to the neck is generally relatively anterior and is not referred to the posterior neck muscles. It may relate to referral of pain to the nerves supplying the anterior or lateral vertebral muscles, which are in the distribution of the lower cervical segments of the spinal cord.

It is noteworthy that cardiac pain, like pain from other deep organs, has preferred pathways of referral within the spinal segments. Referred pain from any organ may involve only portions of a segment and need not be referred to the entire segment (cardiac pain referred to the body surface usually involves predominantly anterior portions of thoracic spinal segments, so that pain is commonly experienced in the anterior chest but infrequently in the back, despite the fact that both are innervated by the same segments). The tendency to involve the left arm and chest preferentially is probably due to the left-sided embryologic origin of the left heart chambers. Like other organs, the heart is more likely to refer pain to higher adjacent spinal segments than to lower ones, which explains why cardiac pain occurs more commonly in regions innervated by cervical segments than in the abdominal region innervated by lower thoracic segments. Even when only a portion, usually the anterior portion, of those segments (T1–T5) that directly innervate the heart is affected, referral is common.

TRANSMISSION OF CHEST PAIN OF PERICARDIAL AND NONCARDIAC ORIGIN

The visceral pericardium is not innervated. However, the phrenic nerve, which originates from spinal segments C3, C4, and C5, supplies the central diaphragmatic portion of the parietal pericardium, and the vagus and sympathetic nerves innervate the posterior portion.[1] Stimulation of the central diaphragmatic portion of the pericardium by inflammation or other causes frequently results in referral of pain to the region of the trapezius muscle in the shoulder and to the posterior portion of the neck, which share innervation by the C3 and C4 segments of the spinal cord.[1,29] The central diaphragmatic portion of the parietal pleura and the diaphragm itself have the same innervation, and stimuli in these areas may also result in referral to the trapezius region. The visceral pleura, like the visceral pericardium, has no nerve supply, but the parietal pleura, in addition to the phrenic nerve innervation, is well supplied by fibers in the intercostal nerves that enter the thoracic segments of the cord.[1] With the exception of the central diaphragmatic portion, stimulation of the pleura usually results in pain felt in the chest wall immediately overlying the site of stimulation. Most pericardial pain probably results from stimulation of nerves in contiguous pleura and also is felt directly over the site of irritation.[1,31]

Pain from the esophagus is frequently felt in the chest.[32] The esophagus is innervated by sensory fibers that originate in spinal segments C7–T12. Pain is commonly felt in the substernal region and may also be felt in other overlying areas of the chest anteriorly or posteriorly. Occasionally it may be referred to the arm.[1] Sensory fibers from T7–T9 innervate the stomach, pancreas, liver, and biliary tract. In some cases pain from these sites may be referred to the lower chest or epigastrium in a manner similar to cardiac pain.

Pain originating in the chest wall from costochondritis, muscle problems, or other causes will be perceived at its site of origin and will at times be confused with cardiac pain that could be referred to the same sites.[33] Pain due to arthritis or other causes in the cervical or thoracic vertebrae may be referred to the chest because of irritation of nerves entering these sites.[33]

Clinical Presentation

ANGINA PECTORIS

Typical Angina

No dissertation on coronary artery disease is complete without reference to the classic description of angina by William Heberden in his "Pectoris Dolor," first printed in 1772.[34]

> But there is a disorder of the breast marked with strong and peculiar symptoms, considerable for the kind of danger belonging to it, and not extremely rare, which deserves to be mentioned more at length. The seat of it, and sense of strangling, and anxiety with which it is attended, may make it not improperly be called angina pectoris.
>
> They who are afflicted with it, are seized while they are walking, (more especially if it be up hill, and soon after eating) with a painful and most disagreeable sensation in the breast, which seems as if it would extinguish life, if it were to increase or to continue; but the moment they stand still, all this uneasiness vanishes.

> In all other respects, the patients are, at the beginning of this disorder, perfectly well, and in particular have no shortness of breath, from which it is totally different. The pain is sometimes situated in the upper part, sometimes in the middle, sometimes at the bottom of the os sterni, and often more inclined to the left than to the right side. It likewise very frequently extends from the breast to the middle of the left arm. The pulse is, at least sometimes, not disturbed by this pain, as I have had opportunities of observing by feeling the pulse during the paroxysm. Males are most liable to this disease, especially such as have past their fiftieth year.

Heberden's description continues to survive the passage of time as a vivid picture of typical cases of angina due to obstructive atheromatous lesions of the coronary arteries. More that 200 years after it was written, only his exclusion of shortness of breath, which does sometimes occur in conjunction with angina, can be criticized.

Typical angina is precipitated by exertion and relieved by rest. During exercise the increased myocardial oxygen requirements cannot be met by an appropriate increase in blood flow through atherosclerotic coronary arteries. With cessation of exertion, heart rate and blood pressure decrease, myocardial oxygen requirements are reduced, and anginal pain subsides. Some patients will experience angina after walking a few yards whereas others will have it only with extreme degrees of physical activity. There is a tendency for angina to be highly reproducible at a given level of a specific type of physical activity.[35] This reflects the occurrence of angina when a specific level of myocardial oxygen consumption is reached, as can be estimated by an index such as the product of the heart rate and blood pressure.[36] The type of physical activity is highly relevant. Most people have more difficulty working with their arms than with their legs, and tasks done with the arms above the head are particularly poorly tolerated. Strenuous lifting tends to be a potent stimulus of angina. People who have been regularly using certain muscles for long periods may be able to achieve surprisingly high levels of physical work with their accustomed activities, yet experience angina that prevents relatively low performance levels with activities that use different muscle groups. Presumably, adaptations due to conditioning have occurred that permit work with frequently used muscles at relatively low myocardial oxygen cost compared with the oxygen cost of similar work to untrained people.

Emotional stress may be as potent a stimulus of angina as physical stress in many patients. A likely mechanism is the release of catecholamines, which cause tachycardia and increased myocardial oxygen consumption. While exertion or emotional stress are the commonest settings for angina, it may occur with other stimuli in many patients.[37] Cold weather may induce angina even with minimal activity, perhaps because of cold-induced coronary vasoconstriction.[38] Approximately an hour after eating a large meal patients may experience angina because vasodilation in the splanchnic vessels redistributes blood flow away from the coronary bed. Nocturnal angina that awakens patients from sleep is common and may in some cases be related to dream-induced catecholamine release.[39] Some patients have so little reserve capacity in their diseased coronary vessels that flow is barely adequate to meet myocardial oxygen requirements under basal conditions. They experience angina at rest without an apparent precipitating cause.

Most patients describe anginal pain as a pressurelike sensation, but some may also describe it as sharp, dull, or burning.[37] The intensity of discomfort varies widely from person to person. Almost all patients with angina experience pain in their chest.[37] Generally it is substernal, but it may be partially on the left side of the chest. Approximately 80% of patients with angina regularly have associated discomfort in their left arm during attacks. This may be only in the upper arm or may extend to the ulnar aspects of the forearm, wrist or hand. Anginal discomfort commonly radiates to the neck or throat and to the right arm (Fig. 1-1).[37] Rarely, it may radiate to the back, epigastrium, or jaw.[1,37]

Other symptoms commonly accompany angina (Table 1-1). Slightly more than half the victims of this disorder are short of breath during attacks. Sweating, weakness, nausea, and abdominal fullness or gas are quite common during angina. Palpitations during attacks are experienced by 12% of patients with this disorder.[37]

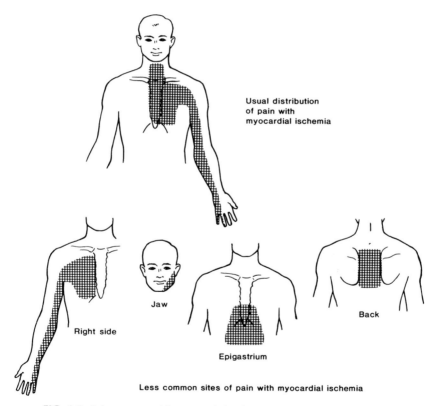

Usual distribution
of pain with
myocardial ischemia

Jaw

Right side

Epigastrium

Back

Less common sites of pain with myocardial ischemia

FIG. 1-1. Pain patterns with myocardial ischemia. The usual distribution is referral to all or part of the sternal region, the left side of the chest, the neck, and down the ulnar side of the left forearm and hand. With severe ischemic pain, the right chest and right arm are often involved as well, although isolated involvement of these areas is rare. Other sites sometimes involved, either alone or together with pain in other sites, are the jaw, epigastrium, and back.

Table 1–1. Summary of Findings in Cases of Coronary Artery Disease and Patients with Chest Pain of Unknown Etiology and Normal Angiograms

	Coronary Artery Disease Confirmed by Angiograms (n=49)	Normal Coronary Angiograms (n=23)
	No. of Cases (%)	No. of Cases (%)
Type of angina		
Exertional	46(94)	19(83)
Emotional	37(76)	17(74)
Cold-induced	22(45)	9(39)
Postprandial	18(37)	4(17)
Nocturnal	31(63)	12(52)
Rest-related	24(49)	14(61)
Location of pain		
Chest	49(100)	22(96)
Left arm	39(80)	13(57)
Right arm	17(35)	6(26)
Neck or throat	20(41)	7(30)
Epigastrium	3(6)	3(13)
Back	6(12)	6(26)
Quality of pain		
Sharp	14(29)	12(52)
Dull	12(24)	4(17)
Burning	10(20)	4(17)
Deep	36(73)	18(78)
Superficial	13(27)	5(22)
Pressure	37(76)	16(70)
Accompanying symptoms		
Sweating	24(49)	14(61)
Weakness	20(41)	19(83)
Nausea	13(27)	7(30)
Shortness of breath	30(61)	17(74)
Gas or abdominal fullness	22(45)	8(35)
Palpitations	6(12)	4(17)
Physical findings		
Fourth heart sound	45(92)	7(30)
Hypertension	11(22)	4(17)
Murmurs or clicks	13(27)	2(9)
Decreased peripheral pulses	4(8)	0(0)
Third heart sound	3(6)	0(0)
Ectopic lift	9(18)	0(0)
Cardiomegaly	4(8)	0(0)

(Horwitz, LD: The diagnostic significance of anginal symptoms. JAMA 229:1196, 1974. Copyright 1974, American Medical Association)

The duration of angina attacks tends to be between 30 seconds and 30 minutes.[39] Shorter episodes of pain are much more likely to have a musculo-skeletal than a cardiac origin. Pains of longer duration due to myocardial ischemia would generally result in myocardial infarction. Nitroglycerin is so effective in relieving angina that the response to this drug is of diagnostic value. Seventy-six percent of patients with angina have consistent total or almost total relief of their pain within 3 minutes of taking 0.3 mg to 0.6 mg of nitroglycerin sublingually.[40] Another 16% experience relief that is delayed beyond 3 minutes after the drug is taken.[40] Patients with delayed or absent responses to nitroglycerin usually are found to have more extensive disease at cardiac catheterization.[40]

Certain correlative evidence may be of value in distinguishing angina from other forms of chest pain. A thallium exercise test that is positive for reversible ischemia has a very high specificity for coronary artery disease, although negative tests may occur even when obstructive coronary lesions are present.[41] Evidence of ischemia on an exercise electrocardiogram (ECG) is less reliable because of the test's lower sensitivity and its high incidence of false positive results.[42] Evidence of an old myocardial infarction or of "ischemia" on a resting ECG is of limited value. Transient repolarization changes, however, particularly ST segment depression, during episodes of chest pain are strong evidence of angina. More than 90% of patients with angina due to coronary athero-sclerosis have a fourth heart sound, but this is too common in the general population to be of much value in diagnosis.[37] Evidence at rest of wall-motion abnormalities by palpation of ectopic lifts or by nuclear or ultrasound tests help demonstrate the presence of coronary artery disease but do not necessarily mean that chest pain is due to cardiac ischemia. A demonstration of the appearance of wall-motion abnormalities or a decrease in the ejection fraction by nuclear gated blood pool testing during exercise may be firmer evidence that concomitant chest pain is due to cardiac ischemia.[43] The Levine test, in which anginal chest pain is relieved by carotid massage, which slows the heart rate and abruptly lowers myocardial oxygen requirements, may be helpful on occasion.[44] The most reliable evidence of atherosclerotic coronary artery disease is coronary angiography. However, the presence of anatomical lesions is not a guarantee that a patient's chest pain is angina, and the significance of borderline coronary artery stenoses can be difficult to evaluate. Demonstration of hemodynamic deterioration, ECG changes, or abnormal coronary blood flow responses to tachycardia due to electrical pacing or isoproterenol infusion at cardiac cathetheterizations may be helpful in analyzing the physiological importance of coronary stenoses.[45,46]

Certain terminology is often applied to anginal chest pain. *Typical angina* is the classical form of angina alluded to in this section. *Atypical angina* is a general term referring to recurrent pain that is thought to be related to myocardial ischemia but that varies in some substantial manner from the classical pattern. Atypical angina may not have the usual clearcut relationship to physical exertion or to relief by rest, it may be associated with pain unusual in quality or location, or it may not respond in the usual manner to nitroglycerin. Many patients with atypical pain patterns do not have cardiac disease. Also, many atypical angina patients have obstructive atheromatous coronary disease but some unknown neural or humoral factor may be altering pain perception. Some patients with atypical angina are subject to coronary artery spasm.

Another common system of classification uses the concept of "stable" and "unstable" angina to divide patients. *Stable angina* is usually considered to be of at least two months' duration, reasonably well related in a predictable fashion to a given level of exertion or emotional stress, and fairly constant over a prolonged period in quality, location, intensity, and duration of pain under usual circumstances for a given patient. The underlying disease consists of atherosclerotic obstructions that have not progressed recently, and the implication is that the probability of an impending acute myocardial infarction is low. *Unstable angina* either is new in onset, has had a recent acceleration in pattern, or occurs at rest. Unstable angina has a high risk of acute myocardial infarction if effective surgical or medical treatment is not promptly instituted. Angina that has recently increased in frequency or intensity without a change in lifestyle has a particularly ominous prognosis if no intervention is made. Angina that regularly occurs at rest without obvious precipitating factors generally implies limited or no coronary reserve capacity and also has a poor short-term prognosis. The underlying disease process in unstable angina is either atherosclerotic coronary disease or coronary artery spasm. When atherosclerotic lesions are the cause, they have generally either progressed to cause more advanced obstruction recently or are very severe in nature, probably involving multiple vessels or either the main left coronary artery or the takeoff of the left anterior descending coronary artery. *Status anginosus* is a form of unstable angina that occurs almost continuously at rest. *Preinfarction angina* is a similar but more vague term than status anginosus. *Angina decubitus* is angina that occurs when the patient assumes a recumbent position and is often a form of unstable angina but may also refer to less severe forms of nocturnal angina.

Variant Angina

There is a substantial group of patients subject to transient chest pain due to myocardial ischemia whose discomfort is due primarily to coronary artery spasm rather than to fixed atherosclerotic obstructions.[12-14] Patients with this condition may have atherosclerotic lesions on which coronary artery spasm is superimposed or may have coronary arteries that appear to be normal angiographically between episodes of spasm. The chest pain experienced by these patients, whose condition is termed *variant angina* or *Prinzmetal's angina*, differs markedly from the classical form of angina due to atherosclerotic obstructions of the coronary arteries. In most of these patients, the occurrence of chest pain has no relationship to physical exertion or emotional stress.[12,14] Pain most commonly occurs at rest and may occur at the same time of day, particularly in the morning, in a recurrent pattern. Only a minority of patients with variant angina have pain during exertion. Palpitations are extremely common in variant angina, whereas in classical angina they are present during attacks in only 12% of patients.[14,37] The pain resembles classical angina in quality and location, although individual episodes of pain may be unusually severe and quite variable in duration. Like classical angina, variant angina may respond to nitroglycerin, although higher dosages may be needed and responses tend to be more variable and less complete.

Unlike classical angina, variant angina is usually not related to levels of myocardial oxygen consumption. Coronary artery spasm tends to be severe enough to create inadequate myocardial oxygen delivery even at rest, when myocardial oxygen needs are low. Thus, it is the occurrence of spasm rather than the level of myocardial oxygen consumption that causes an attack of variant angina. The cause of spasm and the circumstances that precipitate it are unknown. Ergonovine will induce attacks, and infusion of this drug has been used as a diagnostic test.[47] Ischemia in classical angina is usually predominantly subendocardial and characteristically causes transient depression of the ST segment on the ECG. Ischemia in variant angina tends to be transmural and characteristically causes transient elevation of the ST segment.[12] Arrhythmias during attacks are extremely common in variant angina.[14] Thus, pain that is of the same quality and location as classical angina but is unrelated to physical activity and is associated with ST segment elevation on the ECG, and often with arrhythmias as well, is the hallmark of variant angina due to coronary artery spasm.

ACUTE MYOCARDIAL INFARCTION

In most patients the pain of acute myocardial infarction has the same pressurelike or constricting quality as angina. However, it tends to be more severe and to last longer. Patients may describe the pain as a sensation of "being caught in a vise," "having someone sitting on my chest," or "being crushed under a heavy load." Burning, aching, or sharp pain may also be described. Typically, the pain lasts for at least an hour and it may last several hours; in a milder form, it may last for one or two days. The location is the same as in angina. Most commonly it is substernal, feels deep, and spreads laterally in the anterior chest, especially on the left. It may radiate to the arms, neck, throat, epigastrium, and back.

About half of the patients have prodromal symptoms, usually angina.[48] The pain of infarction will generally resemble previous angina but will also have certain differences apparent to the patient. The differences are usually greater severity, greater duration, and more extensive radiation of the pain.

In some cases, the pain is not severe and may be more of a dull, aching sensation or a numbness in locations typical of cardiac pain patterns. Often a distinctive feature of this discomfort is its persistence for at least an hour and usually longer, commonly accompanied by a feeling of weakness. At times pain may be less prominent in the chest than in peripheral locations such as the arms or wrists, particularly on the left side, or in the neck or the jaw. Pain in the jaw may be mistaken for a toothache.

In most cases, the pathogenesis of the pain of myocardial infarction resembles variant angina more closely than classical angina. That is, the disruption of the coronary circulation is so severe that the occurrence of an infarct is independent of the level of myocardial oxygen consumption at the time. Acute myocardial infarctions do occur during intercourse, high levels of physical exercise, or major emotional stress—settings in which myocardial oxygen consumption is high. In these cases, infarction may occur not because of acute disruption of the coronary bed but simply because myocardial oxygen need exceeds supply in the presence of a fixed atherosclerotic obstruction for a period long enough for myocardial necrosis to occur. The usual immediate reason for an acute myocardial infarction, however, is a coronary thrombosis that abruptly reduces regional myocardial blood flow below levels necessary to sustain cellular viability even at rest. In some cases, coronary spasm may be the initial cause of the reduction in flow, and, if it is sustained, infarction may occur whether or not a thrombus forms.[49] Whether the same pain-producing metabolite that is active in angina is responsible for the pain of infarction is unknown. Either this metabolite is produced in greater amounts with cell damage than with cellular ischemia, or a separate pain-producing metabolite that causes greater or more prolonged pain may be released.

Arrhythmias with or without palpitations are frequent with infarction. Profound weakness or a feeling of doom is often noted. Sweating and gaseous distention of the abdomen are extremely common. Nausea and vomiting may occur, possibly because of vagus stimulation. Dyspnea is frequently present, especially if the lungs become congested. Dizziness may be a complaint, because of either arrhythmias or low cardiac output. Rarely, inferior infarcts may present with hiccups from diaphragmatic irritation. In older patients, especially, symptoms and signs of a stroke related to an embolus or low output may be a prominent part of the presenting picture. Signs of hypotension hypertension, congestive heart failure, or shock all may be present.

In general, confirmation of myocardial infarction is readily obtained within 24 hours. Serial ECGs showing evolution of distinctive changes, elevation in serum creatine phosphokinase or other cardiac enzymes, and evidence of acute changes on nuclear cardiac studies are all reliable indications of acute cardiac damage.

PERICARDITIS

Acute pericarditis most often presents with precordial pain due to inflammatory irritation of the parietal pericardium and adjacent pleura. The pain is often located in some of the same sites as the pain related to myocardial ischemia or damage, and thus pericarditis is sometimes misdiagnosed as myocardial infarction.

There are, however, certain distinctive features of pericardial pain that generally allow it to be distinguished from myocardial pain. Pericardial pain usually has a pleuritic component that is characterized by worsening of the pain with a deep breath. Pericardial pain is position-sensitive—most commonly, it is relieved by leaning forward. Myocardial pain from infarction or ischemia does not vary with change of position, and alteration in chest pain with any change in body position should suggest pericarditis as a possible diagnosis. Pain from pericarditis is often referred to the region of the trapezius muscle at the back of the shoulder and neck.[1] This is due to referral of pain from the central diaphragmatic parietal pericardium in spinal segments C3–C5 through the phrenic nerve. Myocardial pain is only rarely referred this high in the spinal cord. On the other hand, pericardial pain virtually never radiates down the inside of the arms and to the ulnar sides of the forearm and hands, regions innervated by C8–T2 that are common sites of pain with myocardial ischemia or damage.

Dyspnea, orthopnea, and tachycardia with pericarditis are usually seen with tamponade due to pericardial fluid accumulation. Other symptoms depend on the cause of the pericarditis and may include sore throat preceding the illness, joint pain, skin abnormalities, fever, weakness, or uremic symptoms. A pericardial rub is suggestive of pericarditis but may occasionally be present with pericardial extension of a myocardial infarction. The ECG typically reveals diffuse ST segment elevations with later return to baseline, followed by diffuse T wave inversions. Pericardial fluid may be discernible on the echocardiogram.

MITRAL CLICK–MURMUR SYNDROME

A frequently encountered cause of recurrent chest pain is mitral valve prolapse, or the mitral click–murmur syndrome.[49,50] This syndrome is extremely common, occurring in perhaps 6% of the normal population.[51] It is often familial, inherited as an autosomal dominant. Myxomatous proliferation of the spongiosa of the mitral valve causes leaflets and chordae tendineae to become redundant.[52] The enlarged valve apparatus prolapses into the atrium during systole, resulting in a sharp, high-pitched click and often a murmur as well.[49]

The chest pain is usually not of the classical anginal type. It is poorly related to exertion, is often sharp rather than dull or pressurelike, and can be located anywhere in the chest but rarely radiates to the arms or neck. It often is experienced together with palpitations. The duration of the pain is quite variable, ranging from a few seconds to many hours. It is not usually relieved by nitroglycerin. The heart is often rapid or irregular during episodes of pain, but ST segment elevations or depressions on the ECG are rare.

The dominant clinical feature of this syndrome is the presence of an apical midsystolic click on auscultation. The click generally is late and of low intensity when the patient is supine, moves closer to the first heart sound (S_1) and gets louder when the patient sits, and gets closer yet to S_1 and is of maximal intensity when the patient stands.[50] Echocardiography will frequently demonstrate systolic prolapse of one or both leaflets of the mitral valve.[51] The resting ECG may be abnormal, with T wave changes, ST segment changes, or abnormal Q waves.[50] Exercise ECGs may also be abnormal.[50]

Most patients with mitral click syndrome do not have chest pain, but the syndrome is so common that affected persons with this complaint are frequently encountered. The pain is not due to myocardial ischemia but may be related to traction of the prolapsing valve apparatus on the adjacent myocardium.[50] Since mitral click–murmur syndrome is usually benign, the major problem is that the syndrome is often mistakenly diagnosed as coronary artery disease because of pain, arrhythmias, or abnormal ECGs.[50,53] Careful attention to the pain history and to cardiac auscultation usually reveals the true cause of the symptoms. Patients with coronary disease only rarely have clicks.

Individuals with mitral click–murmur syndrome may have autonomic dysfunction, and symptoms usually respond to beta-adrenergic blocking agents.[54] Although most patients with this syndrome have stable, benign courses, occasionally problems arise from arrhythmias, bacterial endocarditis, or, rarely, from development of substantial mitral regurgitation or emboli.[55]

AORTIC DISSECTION

More than 90% of cases of acute dissection of the aorta present with pain.[56] The pain is usually extremely severe, and although it is generally in the anterior chest, it has a predilection to radiate to the back, where it may be most prominent. It is frequently felt in the abdomen. Prodromata are rare and the pain is generally maximal in intensity from its onset. The pain may change in location, particularly if dissection is progressing. Pleuritic components are often present. Pain may occur in any of the sites typical of cardiac pain. Many cases are mistaken for an acute myocardial infarction, and some dissections involving the ascending aorta result in concomitant infarction by occluding a coronary artery.

Aortic dissection is caused by degeneration of the aortic media that results in blood entering through a tear in the intima and cleaving the media, forming a false channel for a variable distance.[57] Obstruction of vessels in the region of the dissection may occur. Those susceptible to this condition are hypertensives with poor control; pregnant women, especially those with hypertension; persons with certain congenital cardiovascular lesions, particularly coarctation of the aorta; and persons with connective-tissue disorders such as Marfan's syndrome or Ehlers–Danlos syndrome.[56] Patients with connective-tissue disorders differ in that pain tends to be less severe and may even be absent.

Symptoms and signs depend to a large degree on the location of the dissection. If the ascending aorta is involved, aortic regurgitation, pericarditis, and myocardial ischemia or infarction may be prominent features. Neurologic signs will appear if cerebral vessels are obstructed. Renal failure may occur with renal artery involvement. Intestinal ischemia may cause ileus or bloody diarrhea. Differential loss of pulse or decrease in blood pressure in one or more extremities is a common sign in this disorder. Symptoms or signs of obstruction may be confusing, since a lengthy dissection may obstruct some branches of the aorta yet spare others. X-ray films or ultrasonography may give evidence of enlargement of the aorta, and angiography can generally confirm the presence of dissection.

Certain features should lead to a strong suspicion of dissection of the aorta in a patient presenting with chest pain. These include a history of poorly controlled hypertension, pregnancy with toxemia, congenital cardiovascular disorders, or connective tissue disorders. A chest pain that is overwhelmingly severe and radiates to the back or abdomen is characteristic. Loss or diminution of pulses on one side of the body and enlargement of the aorta on x-ray films frequently direct attention to the diagnosis. Arachnodactyly or other stigmata or Marfan's syndrome may be observed.

PULMONARY HYPERTENSION

Conditions with elevation in pulmonary artery pressure may cause acute or chronic chest pain. Mitral stenosis, primary pulmonary hypertension, pulmonary embolus, cor pulmonale due to chronic lung disease, and Eisenmenger's syndrome are common underlying conditions. The pain in many cases is probably due to distention of the pulmonary artery and its branches and resultant stimulation of nerve endings in the adventitia.[25] Since similar pain sometimes occurs with pulmonic valvular stenosis, however, the right ventricle may be the source in some cases.[26] Both mechanical distention of the ventricle and oxygen lack from sudden increase in oxygen demands due to pressure overload are possible factors.

The pain of pulmonary hypertension resembles the chest pain of myocardial ischemia, but, unlike cardiac pain, it rarely radiates to the arms, neck, abdomen, or back. The pain varies widely in intensity, quality, and duration. Typically, mitral stenosis presents as a dull discomfort in the anterior chest that is of mild or moderate intensity and lasts for several hours. Pain with acute pulmonary embolus may be more intense, resembling the pain of myocardial infarction. It is frequently associated with a relatively high general level of physical activity for the person but not necessarily to specific episodes of effort. It does not tend to subside rapidly with rest, and responses to nitroglycerin vary. In those conditions that cause chest pain related to pulmonary hypertension, dyspnea tends to be prominent at the time pain occurs. Physical findings of pulmonary hypertension, particularly a loud pulmonic component of the second heart sound (S_2) and a right ventricular (RV) lift, are usually reliable indicators of these conditions. In mitral stenosis an opening snap and a low-pitched, rumbling apical diastolic murmur are usually present. In primary pulmonary hypertension or pulmonary embolus, pulmonic systolic or, rarely, diastolic, murmurs may be present. Cyanosis and clubbing may be noted with Eisenmenger's syndrome. Signs of RV overload on the ECG and x-ray film or echocardiographic evidence of pulmonary hypertension are often present.

AORTIC OUTFLOW TRACT DISEASE
AND SYSTEMIC HYPERTENSION

Valvular aortic stenosis or insufficiency is frequently associated with chest pain indistinguishable from classical angina. In both aortic stenosis and aortic insufficiency, compression of coronary vessels by the high wall tension in the hypertrophied or dilated myocardium may reduce oxygen delivery, while the pressure and volume overloads increase myocardial oxygen demand.[58] A Venturi effect by a jet stream across the coronaries may be a factor in reducing flow in aortic stenosis. Physical findings of aortic valve disease, LV hypertrophy on the ECG, suggestive x-ray films and distinctive echocardiographic findings generally allow these two valvular diseases to be readily identified.

Obstructive hypertrophic cardiomyopathy (idiopathic hypertrophic subaortic stenosis) occasionally is associated with chronic chest pain. In some cases the pain resembles classical angina. The mechanism of pain production is unknown, but myocardial ischemia due to excessive oxygen demand has been suspected. The frequent presence of large Q waves on the ECG often leads to the disease being confused with coronary artery disease. A systolic apical murmur that increases in intensity during a Valsalva maneuver and a characteristic brisk, bifid arterial pulse may be present. Echocardiography is the most reliable method for confirming the diagnosis. Asymmetric ventricular hypertrophy and systolic anterior motion of the mitral valve are cardinal features.

Occasionally, hypertensive patients with recent, relatively abrupt rises in arterial pressure will have anterior chest pain. Presumably this is due to distention of the root of the aorta and stimulation of nerve endings in the aortic wall. Care must be taken to exclude coronary disease in such cases, since the presence of hypertension is a risk factor for coronary artery disease and the two coexist frequently.

CARDIOMYOPATHY, MYOCARDITIS, AND CARDIAC VASCULITIS

Patients with congestive cardiomyopathy frequently have mild precordial pain poorly related to exertion.[59,60] The origin of this pain is unknown. Although usually free of pain, except myalgias, patients with acute myocarditis sometimes have chest discomfort of varying severity.[61] In rare cases the pain may be a dominant feature and may suggest acute myocardial infarction. Usually, however, with both cardiomyopathy and myocarditis, signs and symptoms of heart failure rather than chest pain are the major presentation.

In conditions with vasculitis, such as periarteritis nodosa or lupus erythematosus, the usual reason for chest pain is pericarditis. Occasionally, however, pain of an ischemic nature occurs due to involvement of the coronary arteries. Myocardial infarction may occur.

GASTROINTESTINAL PAIN

Esophageal Pain

Pain patterns in esophageal diseases resemble those in cardiac diseases, and distinguishing the two can be quite difficult.[32,62] As noted previously, pain from the esophagus can be felt in regions innervated by spinal segments C7–T12. Pain is particularly common in the anterior chest. Reflux esophagitis due to hiatal hernia may have a pain pattern closely resembling angina. Acid reflux into the lower esophagus gives rise to "heartburn," a substernal burning discomfort often associated with regurgitation of sour fluid. Heartburn is relieved by belching, antacids, food, or histamine-2–receptor antagonists such as cimetidine. Heartburn is particularly common at night, when it is aggravated by the supine position, which increases acid reflux. If a stricture develops, dysphagia may occur. The burning quality of the pain, its relation to meals and position, and its relief by belching or antacids are the distinctive features. Since anginal pain is often "burning" and is also sometimes relieved by belching, this esophageal condition may be difficult to recognize. If esophagitis is suspected, x-ray films of the esophagus, esophagoscopy, the Bernstein acid infusion test, and esophageal manometry are useful for confirming the diagnosis.[32]

Esophageal spasm may mimic either angina or acute myocardial infarction.[63] With or without achalasia, in which the esophagus is enlarged due to failure of the esophageal sphincter to relax, strong dyssynergic contractions of the esophagus occur. Dysphagia is usually present. Symptoms are often postprandial and aggravated by drinking cold liquids. Nocturnal pain is also common. The pain resembles cardiac discomfort in location and quality. This condition often responds to nitroglycerin. X-ray films of the esophagus with barium and esophageal manometry will confirm the diagnosis. Methacholine may induce pain.

Cardiaclike chest pain may also be induced by esophageal rupture.[62] This generally occurs with severe retching or after esophagoscopy. Mediastinal or neck emphysema or free air under the diaphragm may be present. Rarely, an esophageal diverticulum following tuberculosis or other mediastinal infections will cause chest pain and dysphagia.[64]

Acute Pancreatitis

Acute pancreatitis most commonly is associated with either alcoholism or biliary tract disease with stones. The pain generally is felt in regions innervated by spinal segments T10–L2 and is usually in the epigastrium and the back. It is often constant but may be paroxysmal. It is frequently position-sensitive and relieved by leaning forward, in which it resembles pericardial pain.[20] ST–T segment changes on the ECG may resemble ischemic cardiac changes or changes found with pericarditis. The patient may be in shock. Abdominal findings, including tenderness, guarding, and ileus, are usual. Serum amylase or lipase is usually elevated, serum calcium is usually decreased.

Peptic Ulcer Disease

Through spinal segments T6–T10, gastric or duodenal ulcer pain or gastritis may cause epigastric pain that can radiate to the lower chest. With perforation the pain may be felt in the back. The relief of pain by antacids, meals, or histamine-2–receptor antagonists; abdominal tenderness; lack of relationship to exertion; and lack of response to nitroglycerin usually distinguish this disorder from cardiac disease. Endoscopy and upper gastrointestinal x-ray films will reveal the pathology.

Biliary Tract Disease

Acute cholecystitis usually presents as abdominal right upper quadrant and epigastric pain with fever, vomiting, or nausea. At times the pain is felt as high as regions innervated by T6, including portions of the left or right anterior chest as well as the back. Pleurisy may occur, the gallbladder may be palpable, and stones may be visible on x-ray film. A history of intolerance to fatty or spicy foods may be obtained. Jaundice may be present. Usually the ECG is normal but, rarely, ST–T changes may occur. Chronic cholecystitis may have some similarity to angina.

Splenic Flexure Syndrome

Gas collections in the splenic flexure of the colon may, through distention, cause precordial or left chest and shoulder pain.[65] Aerophagia and abdominal fullness are frequently present. Pain is often relieved by bowel movements or passage of flatus. Percussion or an abdominal x-ray film can demonstrate the gas.

CHEST PAIN FROM MUSCULOSKELETAL AND NEURAL DISORDERS

Because it shares the same spinal segment innervation, any disorder of the anterior chest wall can mimic cardiac pain. For the same reason, so also can disorders of the cervical or thoracic spine.

Costochondral Junction Pain (Tietze's Syndrome)

This peculiar inflammation of the costochondral or costosternal junction is frequently mistaken for cardiac pain.[66] The second, third, or fourth costochondral junctions on the left are frequently involved. The pain varies in quality and intensity. Palpation of the costochondral junctions reproduces the pain.

Xiphoidalgia (hypersensitive xiphoid syndrome) closely resembles Tietze's syndrome. Direct pressure on the xiphoid produces pain substernally and elsewhere in the precordium, in the epigastrium, and in the shoulders and arms. The pain is often associated with nausea.[29]

It is wise to take care before dismissing a possible cardiac cause for local tenderness in the sternal or costochondral regions. Occasionally, acute myocardial infarction or severe angina will result in such tenderness through activation of the appropriate spinal segment. Similar pain may occur with rib fractures, tumors of the rib cage, or eosinophilic granuloma. In such cases, local rib tenderness and swelling are usually present. X-ray films reveal the lesions. Rheumatoid arthritis and other forms of arthritis may also cause chest pain.

Cervical or Thoracic Spine Disease

Most commonly due to osteoarthritis with or without preceding trauma, damage to the lower cervical vertebrae frequently causes chest pain similar to angina.[29,67] Pain is usually due to compression of the spinal nerves from narrowing of the foramina. Association with certain movements of the head, and sometimes with dizziness, is characteristic. Ankylosing spondylitis in young men may give similar pain by the same mechanism. In ankylosing spondylitis, aortic regurgitation and atrioventricular conduction defects may be present. Other rheumatoid diseases, tuberculosis, fractures, and neoplasms may involve the cervical or thoracic spine with similar effects. X-ray films of the cervical and thoracic spine are valuable for distinguishing these disorders.

Thoracic Outlet Syndrome

Pain in the chest may be due to compression of nerves or vessels by bony elements at the superior aspect of the thoracic cage.[29,68] Typically, subjects are 30 to 50 years old. The syndrome is more common in women. Cervical ribs, abnormalities of the first rib, or abnormalities of the clavicle are the commonest causes. Hypertrophy of the scalenus anticus muscle frequently compresses the brachial plexus and brachial artery. The pectoralis minor tendon may compress vessels at the coracoid process.

Usually, one of the upper extremities is involved in the pain pattern. Deep palpation in the neck or supraclavicular regions may reproduce symptoms. Adson's maneuver (rotation of the head toward the side of symptoms during deep inhalation with the neck extended and hands resting on the knees while sitting) is frequently positive in scalenus anticus syndrome, causing pain or pulse diminution. Compression of the axillary or brachial vessels between the clavicle and first rib or by the pectoralis minor muscle tendon can be detected by loss of pulse when the arm is extended directly overhead (hyperabduction test). Holding the arms stiffly downward and backward with the shoulders braced in an "attention" position (costoclavicular test) may also obliterate the pulse.

Herpes Zoster

Prior to the development of a rash, herpes zoster may cause a sharp, burning pain in the precordium from involvement of posterior root ganglia and peripheral nerves. It is commonest in elderly patients and may appear together with fever, stiff neck, and cutaneous hyperesthesia. Other forms of neuralgia may cause similar chest pain.

PULMONARY CAUSES OF CHEST PAIN

Most pain of pulmonary origin is pleuritic. This is particularly true of pneumonia or pulmonary infarction, where aggravation of chest pain by deep inspiration is pronounced. As noted earlier, large pulmonary emboli may result in nonpleuritic precordial pain with pulmonary hypertension. Pulmonary neoplasm often causes a dull or aching nonpleuritic pain in the area involved by the tumor. Spontaneous pneumothorax may present with very severe chest pain, but usually the pain is pleuritic. The presence of pneumothorax can usually be determined by physical examination and x-ray films. In addition to the pleuritic nature of pain in most pulmonary disease, cough, hemoptysis, chills and rales, rhonchi, or rubs are features often encountered.

OTHER CAUSES OF CHEST PAIN

Mondor's Disease

Mondor's disease is thrombophlebitis of the anterior chest wall and breasts. Trauma or breast surgery may precede its development.[69] Other breast conditions may occasionally cause localized chest pain.

Shoulder–Hand Syndrome

After a myocardial infarction, disuse of the left shoulder may hasten development of a painful osteoarthritis. The pain in the left shoulder, adjacent left chest, and left arm may be mistaken for cardiac pain from ischemia or infarction.

Takayasu's Disease

Also known as "pulseless disease" or "aortic arch syndrome," Takayasu's disease is an inflammation of the aorta and some of its major proximal branches and the pulmonary artery.[70] It affects young women primarily, especially oriental women. Obstruction to flow in the brachiocephalic, subclavian, or carotid arteries may result in loss of the radial or carotid pulses. Pulmonary hypertension may occur.[70] Systemic hypertension is often present despite the low blood pressures in the arms, and this can usually be detected by taking the blood pressure in the legs. Syncope is a frequent occurrence. Chest pain is common. The pain may be due to pulmonary hypertension, active arteritis, pericarditis, aortic valve disease, or, if the coronary arteries are involved, myocardial ischemia or damage.[71]

Precordial Migraine

Rather than an accompaniment to migraine headaches, precordial migraine can be an equivalent that appears instead of a headache in patients with migraine.[29,72] Pain is usually dull and occurs on the left side of the chest but may occur elsewhere in regions generally affected by cardiac pain. Rarely, it is sharp or pleuritic. Palpitations are common. Headache is sometimes present. Pain may last for hours or days but can be of shorter duration.

Neurocirculatory Asthenia

Neurocirculatory asthenia is a vague and dubious entity, described by Da Costa in 1871 and dubbed "soldier's heart" by Lewis and others. It consists of chest pain, dyspnea, sweating, dizziness, palpitations, easy fatigability, and anxiety.[73,74] Hyperventilation is common. Most affected individuals are sedentary or physically deconditioned. If the syndrome exists as a distinct disease process, it is probably psychological in origin. Some of the patients with this diagnosis probably had mitral click–murmur syndrome.

Summary

Cardiac pain, like other deep visceral pain, can be extensively modified by psychological factors and other cerebral functions. A gating mechanism in the substantia gelatinosa of the spinal cord may allow cerebral modulation of pain transmission. Autonomic reflexes may also modify reactions to cardiac pain.

Sensory innervation of the heart is by way of the upper five thoracic segments of the spinal cord, and pain can be referred into cervical or lower thoracic segments as well. Major sites for cardiac pain are the regions of the sternum; the anterior chest, particularly on the left; the medial aspects of the arms, particularly on the left; the ulnar aspects of the forearm, wrist, and hand; and the anterior neck and throat. Less commonly, pain originating in the heart may be felt in the jaws, upper abdomen, and back. Most cardiac pain is due to release of a noxious endogenous biochemical substance as a result of myocardial ischemia or ischemic damage. The agent is unknown but a kinin has been proposed as the mediator.

Classical angina pectoris due to fixed atherosclerotic coronary obstructive lesions is precipitated by exertion and relieved by rest and nitroglycerin. It is related to increased myocardial oxygen requirements, especially with exercise, digestion, and emotional stress. The pain is usually pressurelike, aching, or burning, and lasts between 30 seconds and 30 minutes. In the vast majority of cases, its distribution includes the anterior chest and left arm. Sweating, weakness, dyspnea, and abdominal fullness commonly accompany classical angina.

In variant angina and myocardial infarction, the onset of pain usually is unrelated to increases in myocardial oxygen requirements. More commonly, it is due to severe reduction of regional myocardial flow to levels that cannot sustain basal oxygen need. Variant angina is due to spasm of one or more coronary vessels, with or without the presence of atherosclerosis. Myocardial infarction is most commonly due to thrombosis superimposed at a site of coronary atherosclerosis. In quality and location the pain of myocardial infarction resembles that of classical angina, but it is often more severe and of longer duration.

Pericardial pain resembles pain due to ischemic myocardial disease but can often be distinguished by its pleuritic components, its variation with body position, or its radiation to the region of the trapezius muscle, or by the presence of a pericardial rub and suggestive ECG or echocardiographic signs. Conditions that commonly mimic pain due to myocardial ischemia include mitral click–murmur syndrome, aortic outflow tract disease, esophagitis, and a variety of musculoskeletal disorders, as well as many other disorders.

References

1. Hardy JD, Wolf HG, Goodell H: Pain and Sensations and Reactions. Baltimore, Williams & Wilkins, 1952
2. Mountcastle, VB: Pain and temperature sensibilities. In Mountcastle VB (ed): Medical Physiology, 13th ed. St Louis, CV Mosby, 1974
3. Melzack R, Wall PD: Pain mechanisms: A new theory. Science 150:971, 1965
4. Jenner E: Letter to William Heberden in 1778. In Baron J: The Life of Edward Jenner, Vol. 1, London, Colburn, p 39. 1838
5. Parry CH: An Inquiry into the Symptoms and Causes of the Syncope Anginosa, Commonly Called Angina Pectoris, Illustrated by Dissections. Bath and London, R Crutwell, 1779
6. Warren JC: Remarks on angina pectoris. N Engl J Med Surg 1:1, 1812
7. Herrick JB: Clinical features of sudden obstruction of the coronary arteries. JAMA 59:2015, 1912
8. Keefer CS, Resnik WH: Angina pectoris, a syndrome caused by anoxemia of the myocardium. Arch Intern Med 41:469, 1928
9. Lewis T: Pain in muscular ischemia: Its relation to anginal pain. Arch Intern Med 49:713, 1932
10. Del Bianco PL, Del Bene E, Sicuteri F: Heart pain. Adv Neurol 4:375, 1974
11. Katz LN: Mechanism of pain production in angina pectoris. Am Heart J 10:322, 1935
12. Prinzmetal M, Kennamen R, Merliss R: Angina pectoris. 1. A variant form of angina pectoris. Am J Med 27:375, 1959
13. Maseri A, Mimmo R, Chierchia S: Coronary artery spasm as a cause of acute myocardial ischemia in man. Chest 68:625, 1975
14. Groves B: Variant angina—an electrocardiographic and arteriographic spectrum produced by coronary artery spasm. Curr Probl Cardiol 2:1, 1977
15. Edwards JE: Editorial: The direction of blood flow in coronary arteries arising from the pulmonary trunk. Circulation 29:163, 1964
16. Neufeld HN, Lester RG, Adams P Jr, et al: Congenital communication of a coronary artery with a cardiac chamber or the pulmonary trunk (coronary artery fistula). Circulation 24:171, 1961
17. Chipps HD: Aneurysm of the sinus of Valsalva causing coronary occlusion. Arch Pathol 31:627, 1941
18. Eliot RS, Wollbrink A, Edwards JE: Congenital aneurysm of the left aortic sinus: A rare lesion and a rare cause of coronary insufficiency. Circulation 28:951, 1963
19. Maling HM, Highman B: Exaggerated ventricular arrhythmias and myocardial fatty changes after large doses of norepinephrine and epinephrine in unanesthetized dogs. Am J Physiol 191:590, 1958
20. Rona G, Chappel CI, Balasy T, et al: An infarct-like myocardial lesion and other

toxic manifestations produced by isoproterenol in the rat. Arch Pathol 67:443, 1959

21. Maron BJ, Epstein SE, Roberts WC: Hypertrophic cardiomyopathy and transmural myocardial infarction without significant atherosclerosis of the extramural coronary arteries. Am J Cardiol 43:1086, 1979

22. Rembert JC, Kleinman LH, Fedor JM, et al: Myocardial blood flow distribution in concentric left ventricular hypertrophy. J Clin Invest 62:379, 1978

23. Spodick DH, Littman D: Idiopathic myocardial hypertrophy. Am J Cardiol 1:610, 1958

24. Wenckebach KF: Angina pectoris and the possibility of its surgical relief. Br Med J 1:809, 1924

25. Viar WN, Harrison TR: Chest pain in association with pulmonary hypertension: Its similarity to the pain of coronary disease. Circulation 5:1, 1952

26. Stuckey D: Cardiac pain in association with mitral stenosis and congenital heart disease. Br Heart J 17:397, 1955

27. Rinzler SH: Cardiac Pain. Springfield, Ill, Charles C Thomas, 1951

28. Reich NE, Fremont RE: Chest Pain. New York, Macmillan, 1961

29. Wehrmacher WH: Pain in the Chest. Springfield, Ill, Charles C Thomas, 1964

30. Feinstein R, Langten JNK, Jameson RM, et al: Experiments on pain referred from deep somatic tissues. J Bone Joint Surg (Am) 36(Am):981, 1954

31. Capps JA: An Experimental and Clinical Study of Pain in the Pleura, Pericardium and Peritoneum, p 99. New York, Macmillan, 1932

32. Bernstein L, Fruin RC, Pacina R: Differentiation of esophageal pain from angina pectoris. Medicine 41:143, 1962

33. Wolf HG, Wolf S: Pain, p 54. Springfield, Ill, Charles C Thomas, 1948

34. Heberden W: Some account of a disorder of the breast. Med Trans Roy Coll Physicians 2:59, 1772

35. Robinson BF: Relation of heart rate and systolic blood pressure to the onset of pain in angina pectoris. Circulation 35:1073, 1967

36. Redwood DR, Rosing DR, Epstein SE: Circulatory and symptomatic effects of physical training in patients with coronary-artery disease and angina pectoris. N Engl J Med 286:959, 1972

37. Horwitz LD: The diagnostic significance of anginal symptoms. JAMA 229:1196, 1974

38. Mudge GH Jr, Grossman W, Mills RM Jr, et al: Reflex increase in coronary vascular resistance in patients with ischemic heart disease. N Engl J Med 295:1333, 1976

39. Harrison TR, Reeves TJ: Principles and problems of ischemic heart disease. Chicago, Year Book Medical Publishers, 1968

40. Horwitz LD, Herman MV, Gorlin R: Clinical response to nitroglycerin as a diagnostic test for coronary artery disease. Am J Cardiol 29:149, 1972

41. Ritchie JL, Trobaugh GB, Hamilton GW, et al: Myocardial imaging with thallium-201, at rest and during exercise. Comparison with coronary arteriography and resting and stress electrocardiography. Circulation 56:66, 1977

42. Borer JS, Brensike JF, Redwood DR, et al: Limitations of the electrocardiographic response to exercise in predicting coronary-artery disease. N Engl J Med 293:367, 1975

43. Borer JS, Bacharach SL, Green MV, et al: Real time radionuclide cineangiography in the noninvasive evaluation of global and regional left ventricular function at rest and during exercise in patients with coronary artery disease. N Engl J Med 296:839, 1977

44. Levine SA: Carotid sinus massage: A new diagnostic test for angina pectoris. JAMA 182:1332, 1962

45. Horwitz LD, Groves BM, Walsh RA, et al: Functional significance of coronary collateral vessels in patients with coronary artery disease. Am Heart J 104:221, 1982
46. Linhart JW: Myocardial function in coronary artery disease determined by arterial pacing. Circulation 44:203, 1971
47. Curry RC Jr, Pepine CJ, Salom MB, et al: Effects of ergonovine in patients with and without coronary artery disease. Circulation 56:803, 1977
48. Alonzo AM, Simon AB, Feinleib M: Prodromata of myocardial infarction and sudden death. Circulation 52:1056, 1975
49. Hancock EW, Cohn K: The syndrome associated with midsystolic click and late systolic murmur. Am J Med 41:183, 1966
50. Lobstein HP, Horwitz LD, Curry GC, et al: Electrocardiographic abnormalities and coronary arteriograms in mitral click–murmur syndrome. N Engl J Med 289:127, 1973
51. Procacci PM, Savran SV, Schreiter SL, et al: Prevalence of clinical mitral valve prolapse in 1,169 young women. N Engl J Med 294:1086, 1976
52. Tutassaura H, Gerein AN, Miyagishima RT: Mucoid degeneration of the mitral valve: Clinical review, surgical management and results. Am J Surg 132:276, 1976
53. Mills P, Rose J, Hollingsworth J, et al: Longterm prognosis of mitral valve prolapse. N Engl J Med 297:13, 1977
54. Gaffney FA, Karlsson ES, Campbell W, et al: Autonomic dysfunction in women with mitral valve prolapse syndrome. Circulation 59:894, 1979
55. Kostuk WJ, Boughner DR: Strokes: A complication of mitral leaflet prolapse? Lancet 2:313, 1977
56. Hirst AE Jr, Johns VJ Jr, Kime SW Jr: Dissecting aneurysm of the aorta: Review of 505 cases. Medicine 37:217, 1958
57. Schlatmann TJM, Becker AE: Pathogenesis of dissecting aneurysm of the aorta. Am J Cardiol 39:21, 1977
58. Fallen EI, Elliot WC, Gorlin R: Mechanisms of angina in aortic stenosis. Circulation 36:480, 1967
59. Levene DL, Davies GM, Saibil FG: Chest pain arising from intrathoracic structures. In Levene DL (ed): Chest Pain: An Integrated Diagnostic Approach, p 65. Philadelphia, Lea & Febiger, 1977
60. Harvey WP, Segal JP, Gurel T: The clinical spectrum of primary myocardial disease. Prog Cardiovasc Dis 7:17, 1964
61. Gore I, Saphin O: Myocarditis: A classification of 1402 cases. Am Heart J 34:827, 1947
62. Bennett J, Atkinson M: The differentiation between oesophageal and cardiac pain. Lancet 2:1123, 1966
63. Castell DO: Achalasia and diffuse esophageal spasm. Arch Intern Med 136:571, 1976
64. Reich NE, Fremont RE: Chest Pain, p 151. New York, Macmillan, 1961
65. Machella TE, Dvorken JH, Biel FJ: Observations on the splenic flexure syndrome. Ann Intern Med 37:543, 1952
66. Wolf E, Stern S: Costosternal syndrome: Its frequency and importance in differential diagnosis of coronary heart disease. Arch Intern Med 136:189, 1976
67. Edmeads J: Pain arising from thoracic nerves, nerve roots and spinal cord. In Levene DL (ed): Chest Pain: An Integrated Diagnostic Approach, p 107. Philadelphia, Lea & Febiger, 1977
68. Lord JW Jr, Rosati LM: Thoracic outlet syndromes. Clin Symp 23:3, 1971
69. Lunn CM, Potter JM: Mondor's disease (subcutaneous phlebitis of the breast region). Br Med J 1:1074, 1954

70. Lupi-Herrera E, Sanchez-Torres G, Marcushamer J, et al: Takayasu's arteritis: Clinical study of 107 cases. Am Heart J 93:94, 1977

71. Cipriano PR, Silverman JF, Perlroth MG, et al: Coronary arterial narrowing in Takayasu's aortitis. Am J Cardiol 39:744, 1977

72. Fitz-Hugh T: Precordial migraine: An important form of "angina innocens." Internat Clin 1:141, 1940

73. DaCosta JM: An irritable heart: A clinical form of functional cardiac disorder and its consequences. Am J Med Sci 61:17, 1871

74. Lewis T: The Soldier's Heart and the Effort Syndrome. New York, Paul B Hoeber, 1919

2

DYSPNEA

John V. Weil, M.D.

Definition

Dyspnea, a major cause of distress and disability in cardiac patients, is one of the most important symptoms of heart disease. Yet it is one of the least understood, partly because it is inherently subjective in nature and hence difficult to measure and partly because no single class of receptors, discrete pathway, or mechanism has been found that can account for dyspnea in all the myriad settings in which it occurs. Indeed, despite many decades of investigation summarized in several excellent symposia,[1,2] there is not even universal agreement concerning the definition of dyspnea, although it is commonly regarded as "shortness of breath or an unpleasant intrusion of the normally subconscious sensation of breathing into the conscious domain."[3] It is most commonly seen in patients with disease of the heart or lungs and in patients with mechanical dysfunction of the respiratory apparatus, including the lungs, chest wall, and respiratory muscles. Most would agree that in such patients shortness of breath at rest or during low-level muscular exercise constitutes dyspnea. It is less obvious whether the term dyspnea could also be applied to the respiratory distress experienced by normal individuals during maximal or near-maximal exercise or at the break point of a breath hold. In these cases the term *breathlessness* is often used.[2] Whether the sensation is labeled "dyspnea" or "breathlessness" may depend on whether it is perceived as appropriate or inappropriate to the level of activity. In the case of dyspnea, the respiratory distress seems disproportionate to the degree of activity, and thus is considered pathologic, whereas in breathlessness the sensation is appropriate to the respiratory demands, as in heavy exercise. A few other terms should be defined at the outset. These include *hyperpnea*, the classic response to exercise, in which ventilation increases according to metabolic demands, and, as a result, blood gas tensions, particularly CO_2 tension, remain constant. *Hyperventilation*, in contrast, refers to increases in ventilation that are disproportionate to metabolic demands and thus lead to decreases in arterial CO_2 tension. *Tachypnea* denotes a shift in respiratory pattern to an increased respiratory rate and a decreased tidal volume. All of these objective aspects of ventilation are frequently associated with dyspnea, but, unlike dyspnea, they constitute measurable signs.

Physiology

Dyspnea is in many respects analogous to pain: both are symptoms produced by noxious stimuli, both are subjective warnings that something is wrong, and both may be protective. Pain serves to limit motion in an injured extremity, and dyspnea may serve to limit exertion, thus preserving the balance of gas exchange and metabolic demand. It may also minimize respiratory muscle fatigue. Finally, dyspnea may be a factor in a feedback loop that results in optimal respiratory breathing strategies that, in turn, reduce dyspnea—an analog of the way in which pain in an extremity may lead a person to alter his gait to minimize pain. Unlike pain, however, dyspnea has thus far not been associated with any single class of stimuli or receptors, nor have discrete pathways or central nervous system (CNS) centers analogous to those mediating pain been described for dyspnea.

Indeed, a unifying theory that accounts for stimuli, pathways, and mechanisms of dyspnea and that satisfactorily explains how and why dyspnea arises in so many clinical settings has not been found. Still, a pathogenetic scheme can be formulated that explains many of the characteristics of dyspnea and is helpful in understanding its features (Fig. 2-1).

RESPIRATORY DYSFUNCTION

Ventilatory dysfunction leading to decreased ventilatory capacity is common to a large proportion of patients complaining of dyspnea. Dysfunction can be due to increased airways resistance, as in airways obstruction; to decreased lung compliance, as in restrictive lung disease; to changes in the shape or compliance of the chest wall; to weakness of the respiratory muscles; or to inefficient ventilation caused by alterations in dead space or ventilation–perfusion imbalance.

VENTILATORY CAPACITY–DEMAND IMBALANCE

It is clear that, in addition to dysfunction of the respiratory apparatus, other factors must be considered as, for example, in the case of a patient who breathes easily at rest but in whom profound dyspnea is induced by mild exercise. Hypoxia, hypercapnia, and acidosis, which act to increase ventilation,

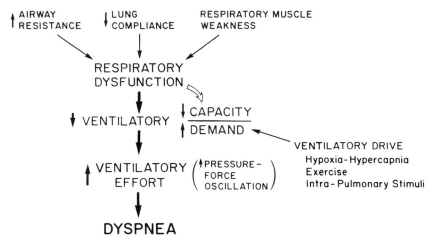

FIG. 2-1. Hypothetical sequence of events involved in the pathogenesis of dyspnea. See text for detailed explanation.

elicit a similar sensation, which suggests that dyspnea is more the result of an unfavorable relationship between ventilatory capacity and ventilatory demand than of decreased capacity alone. Decreased capacity may be well tolerated when ventilatory demands are low but may lead to dyspnea in the face of even modest increases in ventilatory requirements.

Exercise is by far the most common stress leading to increased dyspnea in patients with respiratory dysfunction, and it should be regularly inquired about during history taking. The answers to questions about, for example, how many flights of stairs the patient can climb or the distance he or she can walk on level ground before experiencing disabling dyspnea provide useful semiquantitative information. In addition to exercise, a number of other ventilatory drives may also work to increase ventilatory demand and contribute to the development of dyspnea. These include hypoxemia, which may result from lung disease or from sojourn at high altitude, and acidosis, either respiratory or metabolic, which is a classic stimulus to breathing and may precipitate or augment dyspnea in patients with respiratory dysfunction.

VENTILATORY DRIVES

The extent to which ventilatory drives (ventilatory stimuli) increase ventilation and intensify dyspnea is determined not only by their intensity but also by the individual's sensitivity to them. Sensitivity varies from person to person, and this variation may explain why in some patients mild abnormalities in blood gases are associated with intense dyspnea, whereas in others major blood gas abnormalities produce little dyspnea.[4] Indeed, among patients with chronic obstructive pulmonary disease of similar pathology and functional severity, there is a spectrum of clinical profiles that encompasses, at one end, patients who have nearly normal blood gases and extreme dyspnea (sometimes called "pink puffers") and in whom ventilatory drives appear to be high and, at the other, patients in whom marked hypoxemia and hypercapnia are associated with little dyspnea despite a comparable degree of airways obstruction (the "blue bloaters") and in whom ventilatory drive is decreased.[5-7] The ventilatory drive differences between these two groups appears to have a familial, genetic basis.[8]

Other ventilatory drives of special importance in dyspnea stem from intrapulmonary processes such as vascular congestion, inflammation, abnormal airways stretch, and increased pulmonary arterial pressure. These intrapulmonary stimuli excite a reflex arc leading to hyperventilation, a rapid, shallow, breathing pattern, and the sensation of dyspnea (Fig. 2-2). The receptors involved seem for the most part linked to the afferent vagus nerve. Although some of the relevant receptors have probably not yet been identified, at least three classes, accounting for many of the responses, are known: airway epithelial irritant receptors, small airways stretch receptors, and juxtacapillary "J" receptors.[9,10] Excitation of these receptors leads to an increase in neural transmission to the brain stem by way of the afferent or sensory vagus nerves— which are not to be confused with the efferent parasympathetic vagal fibers. The net effect of this increased neural traffic is to limit the duration and thus

INTRAPULMONARY RECEPTORS

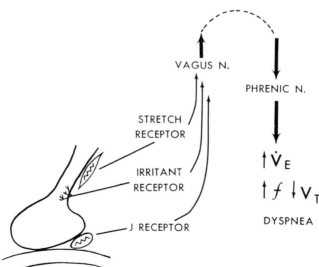

FIG. 2-2. Activation of afferent vagal nerve endings by intrapulmonary processes leads to early termination of inspiratory activity, resulting in a rapid, shallow, breathing pattern (tachypnea), and hyperventilation. These changes are often associated with shortness of breath. Such mechanisms seem to contribute important to the development of dyspnea in a variety of intrapulmonary disease states.

the depth of inspiration and lead to a complementary increase in respiratory frequency. The increased respiratory frequency is usually proportionately greater than the decreased respiratory depth, resulting in hyperventilation. The abnormal, rapid, shallow respiratory pattern seen in various pulmonary diseases and in analogous experimental lung lesions can be normalized by vagal blockade, which in human subjects also decreases dyspnea.[10-12] In dogs with experimental interstitial pneumonitis there is tachypnea and limited capacity for exercise (perhaps an objective counterpart of dyspnea); vagal blockade normalizes this respiratory pattern and increases exercise tolerance.[13] This increase in tolerance may represent a decrease in dyspnea-related limitation of exercise. Thus, in intrapulmonary diseases there exist stimuli to vagal nerve endings that contribute to ventilatory drive and to the development of dyspnea.

DECREASED GAS EXCHANGE EFFICIENCY

Ventilatory demands may also be increased by factors that lead to ventilatory inefficiency because a higher total ventilation is required to achieve a given level of effective alveolar ventilation. This occurs when the ventilation–perfusion (V/Q) pattern is abnormal, especially when there is ventilation of poorly perfused or nonperfused areas of lung (high V/Q). Ventilation of such areas is essentially wasted and must be accompanied by an increase in ventilation to the remainder of the lung if arterial blood gas tensions are to remain normal and classic chemical ventilatory drives satisfied. Another common, but often unappreciated, type of ventilatory inefficiency is a tachypneic breathing pattern in patients with intrapulmonary disease, presumably resulting from stimulation of vagal nerve endings. When the breathing pattern is shallow, a higher proportion of tidal volume, and thus inspiratory effort, is devoted to ventilation of anatomical dead space, which remains relatively constant in volume despite decreased tidal volume. Thus, decreases in tidal volume lead to disproportionate reductions in the alveolar or effective ventilatory components of tidal volume. Consequently, if normal blood gas tensions are to be preserved as the breathing patterns become more shallow, total ventilation must rise by an increase in the respiratory rate.

ABNORMAL BLOOD GASES

If dyspnea is associated with an increase in ventilatory demand relative to capacity, how is this imbalance sensed? One possibility is that blood gas abnormalities arising from respiratory dysfunction, such as hypoxia or hypercapnia, might stimulate dyspnea. Indeed, they may contribute by increasing ventilatory drive and ventilatory demand, but there is ample evidence that abnormal blood gases in themselves are probably not primary causes of the sensation of dyspnea. This is well illustrated by young patients with diabetic ketoacidosis who are free of pulmonary disease. In these patients, acidemia may be severe and associated with an impressive increase in ventilation, with arterial carbon dioxide tensions (P_aCO_2) ranging between 10 mm Hg and 20 mm Hg, yet dyspnea is frequently absent. Paralyzed patients requiring ventilatory support with a tank respirator provide another example of apparent dissociation between abnormality in blood gases and the sensation of dyspnea. These patients experience dyspnea after much smaller increases in P_aCO_2 when ventilation is decreased by lowering the respirator setting, than when P_aCO_2 is raised by adding CO_2 to the inspired air with normal respirator settings.[14] The pattern of breathing, therefore, is somehow important in the genesis of dyspnea.

Another indication of the importance of breathing patterns is the finding that the intense dyspnealike discomfort experienced at the break point of a breath hold is significantly relieved by allowing the subject to take a breath of hypoxic–hypercapnic gas. Following such a breath, the subject experiences relief sufficient to permit resumption of breath holding, even though there is no improvement in blood gases.[15,16] Thus, some factor related to the time elapsed since the previous inspiration and perhaps mediated by the vagal reflexes is involved in the breath hold analog of dyspnea.[17] An experiment carried out by Campbell and coworkers dramatically dissociates blood gas abnormalities from the break point sensation of breath hold.[18] Campbell allowed himself to be paralyzed with curare, which causes muscular paralysis but no sensory deficits. He noted that despite the development of severe hypercapnia, he experienced no sensation of air hunger. Finally, as illustrated by the "pink puffer"–"blue bloater" dichotomy in patients with chronic airways obstruction, nondyspneic patients often have pronounced abnormalities in blood gases, while dyspneic individuals often have near-normal blood gases.[6,19] This may be a consequence of variations in ventilatory drive such that, despite abnormal blood gases, patients with low drives experience little ventilatory stimulation, which reduces the ventilatory demand portion of the capacity–demand balance. In any event, the evidence overall favors the view that abnormalities in arterial blood gases contribute to dyspnea but are not a central cause of it.

RESPIRATORY MUSCLES: WORK AND FORCE DEVELOPMENT

It seems likely that the ventilatory capacity–demand balance is sensed by monitoring respiratory effort rather than blood gases. While abnormal blood gases do not correlate particularly well with dyspnea, increased relative or absolute work of breathing or respiratory effort does.[20] In absolute terms, most dyspneic patients work harder to breathe because of abnormalities in airways resistance or in lung or chest wall compliance. However, the notion that absolute work of breathing is a prominent factor in dyspnea fails to explain the occurrence of dyspnea in partially paralyzed individuals with normal lungs, in whom the work of breathing is, if anything, reduced. This suggests that relative work of breathing, that is, ventilatory work normalized for maximal work, may be a more useful concept. It seems unlikely that respiratory work—the product of the volume of air moved and the pressure difference required to move it—is directly involved in the development of dyspnea. A number of instances can be found in which dyspnea and respiratory work can be dissociated. For example, in the case of paralyzed respirator patients, already alluded to, in whom a reduction of the respirator setting led to increased dyspnea, there was probably little or no increase in respiratory work by the patient compared to the hypercapnic challenge, yet dyspnea increased.[14] Perhaps even more convincing is the common experience that a breath hold, which ultimately leads to an intense dyspnealike sensation at break point, involves no true inspiratory work because no gas is being moved.[9] Some other means of translating the ventilatory capacity–demand imbalance into the subjective sensation of dyspnea must exist.

If increased absolute or relative respiratory work does not offer a satisfactory explanation for dyspnea, perhaps the force or pressure developed in the attempt to breathe provides a better explanation. Indeed, intrapleural or transpulmonary pressures, expressed either in absolute terms or as a proportion of maximum developed pressures, seem to account convincingly for dyspnea thresholds in health and disease, within patients at rest or exercising, and following oxygen administration.[21] Marshall, Stone, and Christie, for example, showed that during increasing muscular exercise, the plateau for ventilation—a presumed objective counterpart of dyspnea—was better correlated with developed intrapleural pressure than with work of breathing.[22] This relationship held true for normal subjects and for patients with mitral stenosis or emphysema. The addition of an external resistance tended to decrease exercise tolerance and was associated with a decrease in respiratory work but with an increase in the intrapleural pressure at which ventilation plateaued. Some investigators have also found a convincing relationship between the development of dyspnea and the tidal change in transpulmonary pressure, the rate of change in pressure, or the relative pressure, that is, absolute pressures expressed as a percentage of maximum voluntary pressures.[23-25]

Just as respiratory force and pressure development may be important in the development of dyspnea, they may also be major determinants of the normal breathing pattern. Otis, Fenn, and Rahn long ago pointed out that normal subjects choose a resting respiratory pattern that requires the least expenditure of effort.[26] Thus, the tidal volume selected is large enough to efficiently ventilate alveoli but small enough to avoid the penalties associated with elastic work, which become marked at high tidal volumes. Concomitantly, breathing frequency is selected to keep airflow low enough to minimize the resistive work penalties associated with high airflows. More detailed studies of breathing patterns in a number of experimental and pathological conditions subsequently confirmed this finding but suggested that the selection of respiratory pattern is linked more closely to the reduction of developed forces or pressures than to the reduction of work.[21,27] It was found that elastic loads, which unduly increase the pressures required to generate normal tidal volumes, result in rapid, shallow breathing, whereas resistive loads, which increase the pressures required to generate airflow, result in slower, deeper breathing with lower flow rates. Thus, equivalent increases in respiratory work lead to different changes in respiratory pattern that have the effect in each case of minimizing the forces or pressures required for ventilation. Respiratory pressures may be used by healthy people as a subconscious error signal to optimize respiratory patterns, and it may be that dyspnea arises when this error signal has become so large as to intrude on consciousness.

Where does the actual sensation of increased pulmonary pressure arise? Much evidence favors respiratory muscles as an important site. There is a growing opinion that, in general, muscles are far more important than joints in sensing motion, position, and force or effort.[28] The diaphragm in particular, seems to be involved: increased activity on the diaphragmatic electromyogram (EMG) is closely correlated with the occurrence of dyspnea, and spinal block, which leaves the diaphragm unaffected, has little effect on the duration of breath hold or the sensation associated with it.[29–33] In chronic obstructive pulmonary disease, dyspnea is increased in the supine position but is promptly relieved with mechanical respiratory assist. Both effects correlate with changes on the diaphragmatic EMG, which is increased in the supine position and suppressed by ventilatory assist.[30] Furthermore, as mentioned above, in paralysis with curare, which, unlike spinal block, does paralyze the diaphragm, the break point sensation during breath hold was virtually abolished.[18] It must be pointed out, however, that these results are at variance with the common complaint of dyspnea in patients with disease-related paralysis or muscle weakness. Perhaps the difference lies in the more uniform effects of curare. If disease-related paralysis leaves some muscle units able to respond and develop force while others cannot, the increased activity of the functional or partly functional units could account for the development of dyspnea.

That dyspnea occurs in patients with paralysis or muscle weakness indicates that absolute force or pressure development, which are reduced in such patients, cannot by themselves account for the sensation. Perhaps, then, the precipitating factor is relative, as opposed to absolute, pressure. Although there is no clear proof that such relative quantities are indeed responsible, nor is the mechanism of their detection certain, such considerations have led Campbell and Howell to propose an intriguing and plausible theory—that appropriateness of change in respiratory muscle length and tension is critical in the pathogenesis of dyspnea.[34] The notion here is that individuals are able to appreciate the relationship between an applied effort and the resulting response. A person quickly becomes aware that a well-defined effort will be sufficient to lift a familiar object such as a baseball; but if the baseball contained a concealed lead core, greatly increasing its weight, the person would be startled by the unexpected effort required to lift it. Similarly, at high altitude, individuals unaccustomed to such altitudes are surprised by the increased shortness of breath (dyspnea?) associated with commonplace activities. In both cases, the sensation arises from the apparent inappropriateness of the increased effort required to carry out familiar tasks. Specifically, in the case of respiratory and other muscles this sensation might arise through monitoring of developed muscle tension and the resulting change in muscle length, that is, length–tension inappropriateness.[35] There are two types of sensors that could provide information about such a relationship. The Golgi tendon organ is capable of providing a measure of muscle tension, and the muscle spindle can monitor muscle length. The spindle is a complex sensor containing at least two muscle systems, intra- and extrafusal, and at least two motor innervations, gamma and alpha, as well as intrafusal stretch receptors. It is capable of sensing changes in relative tension because its intrinsic muscles respond to intensity of alpha motoneuron transmission to the parent muscle, which adjusts the length of the spindle. This, in turn, alters the tension sensed by the spindle. Thus, the spindle can serve as a comparator capable of determining whether a change in muscle length corresponds to that called for by the CNS. These concepts are appealing in that they unify several diverse causes of dyspnea. In cases of lung dysfunction, where disproportionately high muscle tension is required to develop the high pressures needed to maintain normal ventilation, spindles may produce a signal proportional to the inappropriateness of the length–tension relationship. Similarly, in diseases with muscle weakness or paralysis, the muscle spindle may sense a disparity between the intensity of the command it receives and the reduced extent of muscle shortening that results.

Clearly, many of the conditions that precipitate dyspnea may also lead to respiratory muscle fatigue, and it is possible that the two are interrelated in some fashion.[36] Fatigue could contribute to the sensation of dyspnea. Alternatively, dyspnea might lead either to changes in respiratory pattern or to limitations in physical activity that would prevent or postpone the development of muscle fatigue. Indeed, recent studies suggest that, in exercise, patients with chronic obstructive pulmonary disease select respiratory patterns that produce relatively high transdiaphragmatic pressures of short duration that lead to dyspnea but little or no fatigue. In contrast, imposed changes in breathing pattern designed to prolong inspiratory time with lower pressures but greater pressure–time products lead to diaphragmatic fatigue but less dyspnea.[37]

VAGAL AFFERENT PATHWAYS

Dyspnea can arise from a variety of chemical and mechanical disturbances within the lung as well as from mechanical events in respiratory muscles, especially the diaphragm. It is less clear, however, which nervous conduits are involved in the transmission of this information to the CNS, and no critical or essential pathway has been identified. Attention has largely focused on the vagus nerve, as outlined above, because vagal blockade prolongs breath hold, decreases dyspnea in a number of disease states in patients, and abolishes the hyperventilation and tachypnea that are so closely associated with dyspnea in experiments in both animals and humans.[12,13,17] Although the vagus seems to be of considerable importance, it is unclear whether vagal traffic constitutes merely another form of ventilatory drive that aggravates dyspnea, or is specifically involved in sensing dyspnea. In any event, it is not likely to be the sole pathway for such stimuli, and other nerves, such as dorsal thoracic afferents and afferent fibers in the phrenic nerve, may also be important. It is unclear how stimuli are integrated when they reach the CNS in such a fashion that they act to feed back control of the respiratory pattern, as discussed earlier, and how they lead to the conscious sensation of respiratory distress. There are two current theories: one proposes that nerves activated by peripheral receptors may project directly to the cortex, and the other that these receptors may be linked to brain stem or midbrain respiratory integration systems in such a way that only when activity in these lower centers reaches some critical level do they lead to spill-over activation of the cortex to produce the conscious sensation of respiratory distress. In either case, it is clear, from the impressive effects of exogenous opiates in reducing the sensation of dyspnea without influencing any of the stimuli leading to it, that the relevant pathways, like others concerned with responses to noxious stimuli, may be modulated by opiate receptors. This will be discussed in the context of therapeutic approaches to cardiac dyspnea.

Clinical Presentation

PATHOGENESIS OF DYSPNEA IN THE CARDIAC PATIENT

Two major pathophysiologic factors are responsible for dyspnea in the cardiac patient: pulmonary congestion and increased pulmonary arterial pressure. Of the two, pulmonary congestion is by far the more common. Indeed, this relationship is so close that the occurrence of dyspnea at rest or on exertion in a patient with known heart disease should cause the physician to suspect that pulmonary congestion is present. This relationship also underlies differences in the chronologic development of dyspnea in relation to various cardiac defects. It occurs early and is quite prominent in mitral stenosis, a condition in which pulmonary congestion is an early manifestation. In contrast, dyspnea is a late and ominous development in patients with aortic stenosis, in whom, during most of the course, left ventricular (LV) end-diastolic pressures are low and in whom there is no pulmonary congestion. Only later, when LV failure develops, leading to pulmonary congestion, does dyspnea become evident. Pulmonic stenosis typically does not lead to pulmonary congestion, and there is little or no dyspnea. Thus, there appears to be overall a clear association, across various kinds of cardiac disorders, between pulmonary congestion and the occurrence of dyspnea.[38] This relationship is also evident both in comparisons between different patients and within individual patients. For example, in patients with heart disease in whom exercise is limited by dyspnea, striking exercise-induced increases in pulmonary arterial wedge pressure are a consistent finding, whereas in those patients in whom exercise is limited by muscle weakness, such elevations are not seen.[39] Similarly, within individual patients, factors that increase dyspnea, such as exercise, volume overload, or recumbency, are all associated with increased pulmonary arterial wedge pressure, whereas decreased wedge pressures accompany the relief of dyspnea by diuretics.[40,41]

Although reduced cardiac output may play a role in the pathogenesis of dyspnea, it is probably of minor importance. Cardiac lesions such as severe pulmonic stenosis may decrease cardiac output but leave the pulmonary circulation relatively unaffected, and in such circumstances dyspnea is uncommon.[38] In patients with mitral stenosis, the occurrence of dyspnea is closely correlated with increased pulmonary arterial wedge pressure, an index of pulmonary congestion, but is poorly related to cardiac output.[40] Similarly, the administration of diuretic agents commonly leads to reductions in cardiac output but a decrease in dyspnea, apparently related to decreases in pulmonary capillary wedge pressures.[41]

It seems likely that this relationship between wedge pressure and dyspnea is mediated by several pulmonary consequences of circulatory congestion (Figure 2-3). First, and most commonly documented, is increased lung stiffness, that is, a decrease in compliance of the congested lung that may reflect in varying degrees the combined effects of increased circulatory filling *per se* together with varying degrees of interstitial and gross alveolar edema.[42-48] There is also evidence of closure of small airways in pulmonary congestion, which lowers the volume of lung available for ventilation.[45,47] A less consistent finding, especially in milder cases of pulmonary congestion, is increased airways resistance and decreased dynamic compliance, which may reflect narrowing of the airway lumen by mucosal edema and possibly by active bronchoconstriction.[44-46] The contribution of bronchoconstriction is difficult to determine because virtually all bronchodilators also have positive inotropic, vasodilator, diuretic, or other effects that lead to hemodynamic improvement; it is uncertain whether resolution of dyspnea following their use is due to bronchomotor effects or to improved hemodynamic function. Other consequences of pulmonary congestion that may contribute to dyspnea include disturbed gas exchange, (*i.e.*, decreased diffusing capacity or impaired ventilation–perfusion relationships) which may act by increasing ventilatory demands.[49]

In simple pulmonary congestion, deranged blood gases probably make only a minor contribution to development of dyspnea, since the associated hyperventilation typically minimizes blood gas abnormalities. In fact, P_aCO_2 is usually below normal and P_aO_2 is only slightly depressed. In cases of frank pulmonary

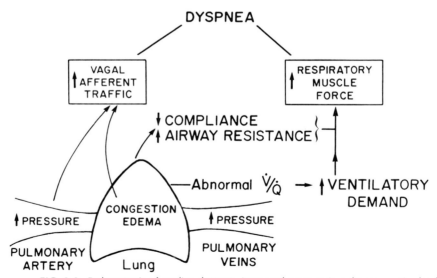

FIG. 2-3. Pathogenesis of cardiac dyspnea. Increased pressure in pulmonary veins leads to pulmonary congestion or edema, which increases vagal afferent traffic directly and also indirectly through effects on lung compliance and airway resistance. Associated adverse effects on ventilation perfusion balance may also lead to increased ventilatory demand, which further increases dyspnea.

edema, however, there may be hypoventilation with hypercapnia and severe hypoxemia, which may contribute substantially to respiratory demand and hence to the severity of dyspnea.

Several lines of evidence suggest that dyspnea arising from intrapulmonary effects of congestion is probably mediated largely by vagal pathways. First, cardiac dyspnea is typically associated with tachypnea and hyperventilation, which are common features of a number of other syndromes involving increased afferent vagal activity.[46] This respiratory pattern, when produced by pulmonary congestion, can be blocked by vagal section or blockade in animals and humans, where it also reduces the sensation of dyspnea.[12,50,51] Hyperventilation, a characteristic accompaniment of dyspnea, is useful because it is objectively measurable. The phenomenon is most impressively demonstrated during exercise, where it is seen as an alteration in the ventilation–oxygen consumption relationship with a marked increase in the ventilation per unit oxygen consumption—that is, an increased ventilatory equivalent for oxygen, representing a disproportionate ventilatory response to a metabolic load. This response is correlated with increased pulmonary arterial wedge pressure but not with changes in cardiac output.[40]

Although the vagus nerve represents a major afferent pathway in the production of cardiac dyspnea, it is far less clear which receptors may be involved. As mentioned, changes in compliance and airways resistance could contribute to the generation of afferent traffic by stimulating stretch receptors, but there is disagreement about whether stretch receptor traffic is, in fact, increased.[12,52,53] Airway mucosal changes could activate irritant receptors, or interstitial edema could activate juxtacapillary (J) receptors, but there is no direct evidence to indicate whether these play important roles.

Just as pulmonary congestion leads to dyspnea, dyspnea may also lead to increased pulmonary congestion, producing a vicious cycle in which the sympathetic nervous system may be of critical importance. Heart failure augments sympathetic activity in exercise, and increased respiratory effort may also contribute to sympathetic activation.[54-56] Sympathetic activation, through its arterial vasoconstrictor effects, may increase LV afterload and increase central blood volume and LV preload. Both could contribute to increases in LV end-diastolic, left atrial, and pulmonary venous pressures and in pulmonary congestion.

While pulmonary congestion as a cause of dyspnea deserves special attention because of its frequency, it is also clear that increased pulmonary arterial pressure, independent of pulmonary congestion, is a cause of dyspnea. This is impressively illustrated by patients with primary pulmonary hypertension in whom there is increased pulmonary arterial pressure and resistance but normal pulmonary wedge and left atrial pressures. In such cases, dyspnea is typically a major feature of the syndrome and is commonly the earliest and ultimately the most disabling symptom.[57] Respiratory distress is usually initially evident on exertion but may progress to being marked at rest. Other than raised pulmonary arterial pressure, there are few obvious contributors to dyspnea. Arterial blood gas chemistry is often normal or nearly normal and pulmonary function test abnormalities are inconsistent. Although the pathogenesis of dyspnea in such cases is poorly understood, vagal factors again appear to be important. These patients exhibit the hyperventilation and tachypnea that accompany vagal stimulation in other settings. In animals, distention of the main pulmonary artery produces a similar tachypneic ventilatory pattern that can be blocked by vagal section, suggesting the existence of vagal receptors located in the walls of large pulmonary vessels.[58] The receptors seem to be located in the pulmonary artery beyond the pulmonic valve, since isolated increased right ventricular (RV) pressure in patients with pulmonic stenosis seems not to share the propensity of pulmonary hypertension to produce dyspnea. It must also be remembered that the pathogenesis of primary pulmonary hypertension is unknown. To the extent that a chronic injury process is involved, other classes of intrapulmonary vagal receptors might be activated by inflammatory or other aspects of the process, contributing to hyperventilation, tachypnea, and dyspnea.

Primary pulmonary hypertension is a fairly pure, albeit rare, example of the link between increased precapillary pulmonary arterial pressure and dyspnea, but such a relationship may also contribute significantly to the development of dyspnea in a number of more complex disorders. These include pulmonary hypertension with congenital heart disease, as in Eisenmenger's complex, where high pulmonary blood flows and left-to-right intra- or extracardiac shunts lead to pulmonary hypertension and shunt reversal. Pulmonary arterial pressures are also increased in patients with left-sided cardiac defects, such as mitral stenosis, partly as a passive consequence of increased downstream (left atrial) pressures, but also because increased left atrial or pulmonary venous pressure is often associated with a disproportionate increase in pressure at the arterial level in the pulmonary circulation.[59] This is common in patients with mitral stenosis, where pulmonary arterial pressures are often increased to a greater extent than can be directly accounted for by the increase in left atrial pressure and where there is an increase in the pressure gradient and vascular resistance across the lung. Although the mechanism of increased pulmonary vascular resistance in a setting of increased pulmonary venous pressure remains unknown, the resulting pulmonary hypertension may contribute significantly to dyspnea, since increased pulmonary vascular resistance seems to correlate with the severity of dyspnea in patients with mitral stenosis. Increased pulmonary vascular resistance may also explain the delayed resolution of dyspnea that follows the initial dramatic improvement after surgical correction of mitral stenosis. The later improvement coincides with a gradual fall in pulmonary vascular resistance related, perhaps, to regression of anatomical changes.

Precapillary pulmonary hypertension is probably also an important factor in the prominent dyspnea of patients with an acute pulmonary embolus. In major embolic episodes, pulmonary hypertension is common, but dyspnea, hyperventilation, and tachypnea also occur even in localized, small, peripheral, embolic events in which pulmonary arterial pressure is probably not increased. Tachypnea and hyperventilation can be readily demonstrated in animals that have emboli confined to small segments of lung and that show no increase in pulmonary arterial pressure.[60] Tachypnea and hyperventilation can be abolished by vagal blockade, and it seems likely that emboli are in some way able to excite intrapulmonary vagal nerve endings, stimulated in part by increased pulmonary arterial pressure but also by other factors. Finally, pulmonary hypertension may contribute to dyspnea in patients with lung disease. Pulmonary dysfunction is commonly associated with pulmonary hypertension, and at least two fundamental pathogenic mechanisms are thought to be involved. First, and perhaps most common, is active pulmonary arterial vasoconstriction in response to alveolar hypoxia or hypoventilation.[61] When alveolar hypoxia and hypercapnia are localized, as in regional hypoventilation, local vasoconstriction serves the useful purpose of diverting blood flow to better-ventilated areas of lung. In patients with diffuse lung dysfunction and general hypoventilation, however, global vasoconstriction leads to pulmonary hypertension. This is common in the patient with the "blue-bloater" variety of chronic airways obstruction. Another recognized mechanism of pulmonary hypertension in lung disease is disease-induced loss of pulmonary vascular bed, which leads to anatomically determined increases in pulmonary vascular resistance and pulmonary arterial pressure. This is common in the normally ventilated "pink puffer" obstructive patient and in patients with a restrictive lung disease, such as interstitial fibrosis. It is, of course, difficult to determine how much of the dyspnea is due to the lung disease itself and how much is contributed by pulmonary hypertension, but as new therapeutic approaches aimed at pulmonary vasodilatation are employed in such patients, it will be intriguing to determine the extent to which dyspnea can be improved independent of changes in lung function.

CARDIAC DYSPNEA SYNDROMES

Dyspnea on Exertion

Exercise is the common setting for dyspnea in general and for cardiac dyspnea in particular.[35] As previously mentioned, dyspnea in cardiac patients largely reflects the presence of pulmonary congestion or increased pulmonary arterial pressure, or both, and exercise typically aggravates these problems. Dyspnea is most common in patients with left-sided cardiac dysfunction arising either from anatomical obstruction, as in mitral stenosis, or from decreased ventricular function stemming from cardiomyopathies of rheumatic, ischemic, or other causes. In the case of myocardial ischemia, the ventricular dysfunction may be episodic, occurring as a feature of an anginal syndrome. In patients who do not experience ischemic pain, ventricular dysfunction may be the sole manifestation of episodic ischemia, that is, it may be an angina equivalent. In all these patients, exercise leads to increased pulmonary arterial wedge pressure, either because exercise-induced increases in cardiac output across a fixed obstruction lead to increased upstream pressure; because heart failure leads to a depressed preload–cardiac output relationship so that an increased preload is required to generate an elevated cardiac output; or because exercise-induced ischemia leads to an acute depression in myocardial function with increased preload.[62] Exertional dyspnea related to pulmonary hypertension occurs in patients whose pulmonary hypertension is due to congenital heart disease, to mitral stenosis, or to pulmonary emboli or lung disease. Exercise-induced pulmonary congestion leads, in turn, to lung dysfunction and increased respiratory effort. Because of its adverse effects on ventilation–perfusion balance, congestion also impairs gas exchange efficiency and increases ventilatory demands, thereby further contributing to the intensity of dyspnea in exercise. Again, the most common primary factor is an exercise-induced increase in pulmonary venous pressure, resulting either from the increased left atrial pressure required to generate increased cardiac output across an elevated or fixed mitral value resistance, as in mitral stenosis, or from exercise-induced increases in LV end-diastolic pressure due to defects in myocardial function. Accordingly, dyspnea on exertion should lead to a search for pulmonary congestion due to left-sided valvular obstruction or LV dysfunction, or to pulmonary hypertension due to a variety of causes.

Orthopnea

Orthopnea refers to postural dyspnea that is induced when a person lies flat, typically supine, and that is usually relieved by elevating the head and upper torso above the horizontal or by sitting. It is generally said to be most common in individuals with left-sided cardiac defects that are either obstructive, as in mitral stenosis, or due to left ventricular dysfunction, as in congestive heart failure. In either case, several factors seem to contribute to its development. Greater effort is required to breathe when lying flat than when upright, due, perhaps, to increases in central blood volume and to the fact that respiratory muscles are working at a positional disadvantage.[49] In individuals with LV dysfunction, gravity helps to distribute blood to dependent venous reservoirs in the abdomen and legs (Fig. 2-4). In the supine position, however, blood is redistributed from dependent toward central, intrapulmonary reservoirs, increasing pulmonary venous volume and pressure and thereby promoting pulmonary congestion with decreased compliance, increased airways resistance, and dyspnea.[63] It should be remembered, however, that orthopnea is a fairly nonspecific finding because it is generally more difficult, even for normal individuals, to breathe when supine, and that patients with a variety of respiratory problems find breathing more difficult when lying down. Patients with severe exacerbations of asthma, for example, typically sleep sitting up because they find it easier to breathe in that position, and the same is true of patients with chronic obstructive pulmonary disease.[30] Many normal people use two pillows to prop their head up at night, because if they fail to do so, they feel sensations of choking or suffocation. These sensations should not be confused with true orthopnea, which depends upon a shift in blood volume for its relief and thus requires the whole upper torso, and not just the head, to be propped up.

Paroxysmal Nocturnal Dyspnea

Paroxysmal nocturnal dyspnea consists of the sudden onset of dyspnea a few hours after the patient has gone to sleep. It typically awakens the patient and is usually relieved by sitting, standing, or walking about. It is closely related to orthopnea, occurring in the same types of patient, having its onset with recumbency, and being relieved by the assumption of a more upright

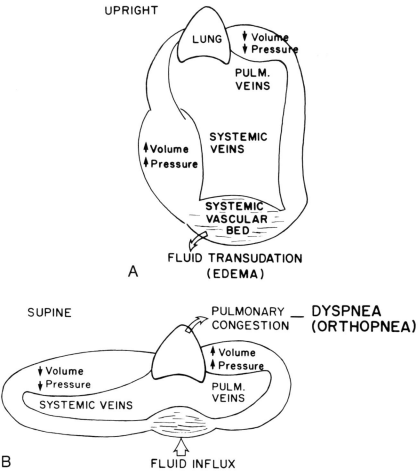

UPRIGHT

LUNG ↓ Volume
      ↓ Pressure

PULM.
VEINS

SYSTEMIC
VEINS

↑Volume
↑Pressure

SYSTEMIC
VASCULAR
BED

FLUID TRANSUDATION
(EDEMA)

A

SUPINE

PULMONARY — DYSPNEA
CONGESTION   (ORTHOPNEA)

↑ Volume
↑ Pressure

↓ Volume
↓ Pressure

PULM.
VEINS

SYSTEMIC VEINS

B   FLUID INFLUX

FIG. 2-4. Postural influences on the circulation and the pathogenesis of orthopnea and paroxysmal dyspnea. (*A*) In the upright posture, intravascular volume is shifted toward dependent systemic venous reservoirs and is decreased by fluid transudation and edema formation. Both effects tend to reduce pulmonary venous volume, pulmonary venous pressure, and congestion of the lungs. (*B*) In the supine position, decreased pressure in dependent systemic veins leads to resorption of interstitial fluid and expansion of blood volume. There is a redistribution of intravascular volume toward the pulmonary veins, leading to increased pulmonary venous pressure and pulmonary congestion.

position. The major difference is that whereas orthopnea typically designates dyspnea that occurs within a few minutes of lying down, paroxysmal nocturnal dyspnea occurs after a delay of several hours. Like orthopnea, paroxysmal nocturnal dyspnea is probably a consequence of the redistribution of blood volume toward the pulmonary circulation, with increased pulmonary venous and capillary pressures with recumbency. The temporal delay is probably explained by an increase in total blood volume resulting from the resorption of dependent peripheral edema fluid into the intravascular compartment when the patient is in the horizontal position. Indeed, impressive hemodilution and blood volume expansion over several hours of recumbency are described in patients with heart failure and other edematous states.[64,65] Thus, paroxysmal nocturnal dyspnea can be viewed as having the pathogenetic features of orthopnea with the added stress of hypervolemia due to resorption of dependent edema fluid.

Cardiac Asthma

Cardiac asthma is closely related to, if not identical with, paroxysmal nocturnal dyspnea. Whereas the latter diagnosis is based on historical recounting of symptoms by the patient, the diagnosis of cardiac asthma is based on the results of physical examination at the time of the event, and the two diagnoses probably often represent different interpretations of the same event. In other words, a physician witnessing an episode of paroxysmal nocturnal dyspnea would commonly observe a patient who fulfills the basic criteria of asthma—paroxysmal wheezing dyspnea—with widespread wheezes evident on physical examination. In fact, in a cardiac patient any episode of asthma that begins abruptly a few hours after going to sleep could be considered as a potential episode of paroxysmal nocturnal dyspnea. The origin of the wheezes is unclear, but they may reflect edema of airway mucosa and bronchoconstriction.

Acute Pulmonary Edema

Acute pulmonary edema is an extreme life-threatening circumstance in which pulmonary congestion, present in the syndromes discussed previously, has progressed to frank alveolar flooding. The underlying cardiac conditions are essentially the same as those already described for the milder syndromes. The major difference is that the patient is usually in great distress and has derived little relief from sitting or standing. Dyspnea is extreme. Physical examination shows a patient in obvious respiratory distress with cyanosis who is insisting on sitting upright. Heart rate is commonly high, as is the systemic blood pressure, even in patients who may ordinarily be normotensive. Auscultation of the chest may show widespread wheezes but, in contrast to the syndromes discussed earlier, diffuse rales are prominent. The pathogenesis of pulmonary edema is, in most respects, similar to that of the syndromes described earlier. In pulmonary edema, however, measurements of blood catecholamine levels provide evidence of marked sympathetic activation, which may contribute to systemic arterial vasoconstriction and hypertension and to systemic venoconstriction with increased central blood volume.[66] This increased sympathetic activity may add elements of a vicious cycle to the pathogenesis of this disorder. Often the precipitating event is unclear. In some patients the episode can be attributed to a new myocardial infarct, but in others no clear reason is found. Perhaps in some cases a transient arrhythmia resulting in a sudden increase in ventricular dysfunction may be responsible, but this is commonly not susceptible to direct proof.

DIFFERENTIAL DIAGNOSIS OF CARDIAC
VERSUS NONCARDIAC DYSPNEA

Differentiation between cardiac and noncardiac causes of dyspnea is usually relatively straightforward when a careful history and physical examination have been performed and the results of chest x-ray and pulmonary function tests are available. In patients with cardiac dyspnea, the physical examination usually shows corroborating evidence manifested as murmurs, gallop rhythms, cardiomegaly, neck vein distention, hepatic congestion, or peripheral edema. The chest x-ray films commonly reveal an enlarged heart, pulmonary blood flow redistribution suggestive of pulmonary congestion, and, in long-standing cases, prominent septal lymphatics—so-called Kerley "B" lines. Pulmonary function tests usually reveal mild abnormalities. In contrast, the patient with predominantly noncardiac, usually pulmonary, dyspnea will have features on history, physical examination, and chest x-ray films suggestive of pulmonary dysfunction. In borderline cases, especially in interstitial fibrosis, it may be necessary to add the measurement of diffusing capacity to the usual battery of pulmonary function tests to demonstrate the abnormality. In most cases differentiation between cardiac and pulmonary dyspnea follows easily from available information, but in some patients differentiation may be exceedingly difficult, and occasionally impossible. In some instances it may be very difficult to determine whether interstitial changes on chest x-ray films are attributable to interstitial fibrosis or represent interstitial edema due to pulmonary congestion. Past history and prior chest x-ray films can be useful because chronicity of many years' duration favors the diagnosis of interstitial lung disease. Careful reexamination of the patient for "silent" or subtle mitral stenosis with physical examination and ultrasound studies of mitral valve motion and left atrial diameter can also be useful. On some occasions a therapeutic trial of diuretic administration may be necessary to resolve the issue convincingly.

In some patients dyspnea is prominent in the face of apparently normal physical examinations, chest x-ray films, electrocardiograms (ECGs), and pulmonary function studies. Some of these patients may have dyspnea of no discernible cause. In others dyspnea may be the manifestation of chronic salicylate ingestion. In some, dyspnea may represent the initial clinical manifestation of pulmonary hypertension, which can easily be missed, since in such a setting physical findings, chest x-ray films, ECGs, and pulmonary function tests are often normal or only nonspecifically or mildly abnormal. To make this diagnosis, a high index of suspicion is essential, especially in young women with Raynaud's phenomenon, who represent the largest class of patients in whom primary pulmonary hypertension is seen. In such patients a careful review of the physical examination and ECG is necessary. New noninvasive ultrasound techniques are being developed that may provide useful screening data to indicate the magnitude of pulmonary arterial pressure. (See Chap. 15, Pulmonary Hypertension.) Ultimately, the definitive diagnosis in such cases rests on cardiac catheterization.

Finally, dyspnea of uncertain cause may also be a prominent feature of multiple, recurrent pulmonary emboli. In this disorder, episodic dyspnea may occur during embolic events, and the resulting pulmonary hypertension may lead to chronic dyspnea on exertion or even at rest, as occurs in other patients with pulmonary arterial hypertension. Careful review of the history, physical examination, and other available data for risk factors, as well as episodic hemoptysis or pleuritic pain suggestive of embolic events, may be very helpful in establishing a diagnosis. Most commonly, cardiac catheterization with pulmonary angiography is required to make a definitive diagnosis. In a few cases, a therapeutic trial of anticoagulants may be useful.

THERAPEUTIC CONSIDERATIONS

With few exceptions, therapeutic measures aimed at ameliorating cardiac dyspnea seem to work largely through their ability to reduce pulmonary congestion (Fig. 2-5). Probably the oldest, and most dramatic, treatment for cardiac dyspnea was phlebotomy, which is quite effective in the pulmonary congestive syndromes leading to dyspnea, including acute pulmonary edema. In modern times phlebotomy has been replaced by less invasive methods of reducing total or pulmonary blood volume, such as rotating tourniquets, which act to sequester blood volume in the peripheral systemic bed, with complementary reductions in pulmonary blood volume and pressure. This remains an effective and acceptable technique for treatment of acute pulmonary edema. Another effective approach has been the use of positive-pressure breathing, which probably acts, as do rotating tourniquets, to redistribute blood volume from central to peripheral venous reservoirs. In this case the increase in intrathoracic pressure probably acts to preferentially retard venous return to the central circulation and cause a redistribution of blood toward the periphery.

While detailed discussion of pharmacologic mechanisms is beyond the scope

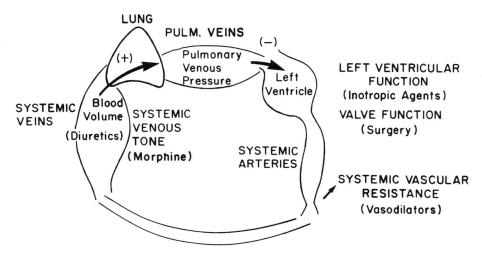

FIG. 2-5. Mechanism and locus of action of principal therapeutic approaches to cardiac dyspnea.

of this chapter, the following few essential aspects of drug action on dyspnea will be described. Diuretics are very useful for the management of cardiac dyspnea. Their major action appears to be to reduce both total and pulmonary blood volumes, with resultant decreases in pulmonary congestion as measured by decreased pulmonary wedge pressure.[41] Most diuretic agents are also vasodilators and may also act as unloading agents to decrease cardiac work requirements, leading to further decreases in pulmonary congestion. A variety of other vasodilators have also proven effective in reducing left ventricular work loads, with resulting improvements in pulmonary congestion and dyspnea. Morphine has long been known to be especially effective in the acute management of dyspnea, although its mechanisms of action are not entirely clear. The drug may work in part by improving pulmonary congestion by reducing adrenergically mediated constriction of systemic veins, with consequent decreases in central blood volume and pulmonary congestion.[67] The drug may also work through its modulating effects on pathways concerned with responses to noxious stimuli, and its effects on dyspnea may be analogous to its well-known analgesic effects. Finally, a number of inotropic agents have been effective in the management of pulmonary congestion and dyspnea. The best known of these are the digitalis glycosides. Other agents with positive inotropic properties have been useful, including the xanthines, and even beta-adrenergic agonists have been effective, although usually only transiently. More recently, inotropic agents with longer periods of effectiveness have been described.[68]

Surgical intervention may be highly effective in amenable cases. Probably the most dramatic relief of dyspnea afforded by surgery is seen following surgical correction of mitral valve disease.

Summary

Dyspnea, the intrusion of the normally unconscious act of breathing into the conscious domain, is appreciated as a sense of difficulty in breathing or as respiratory distress. It is a symptom of great importance in the cardiac patient because of its frequency and because of the extent to which the discomfort it engenders and the limitation that it imposes on capacity for physical activity interfere with the lifestyle of the cardiac patient. It has been suggested that dyspnea arises from an imbalance between ventilatory demands and capacity to breathe. This imbalance is translated into increased respiratory muscle effort that may be gauged in terms of the appropriateness of the resulting ventilatory response. These forces and other stimuli appear to be sensed by a variety of nerve endings, many of them associated with afferent fibers running in the vagus nerve, and this increased vagal sensory traffic appears to be important in the production of symptoms of dyspnea. In cardiac patients, congestion of the lungs and increased pulmonary arterial pressure seem to be the most common abnormalities that trigger dyspnea. Reversal of these abnormalities through a variety of therapeutic approaches constitutes the most effective management of shortness of breath in the cardiac patient.

References

1. Howell JBL, Campbell EJM (eds): Breathlessness. Proceedings of an International Symposium, University of Manchester, p 243. Oxford, Blackwell Scientific Publications, 1966
2. Porter R (ed): Breathing: Hering-Breuer Centenary Symposium. London, J & A Churchill, 1970
3. Lukas DS: Dyspnea. In MacBryde CM, Blacklow RS (eds): Signs and Symptoms: Applied Pathologic Physiology and Clinical Interpretation, p 341. Philadelphia, JB Lippincott, 1970
4. Hirshman CA, McCullough RE, Cohen PJ, et al: Effect of pentobarbitone on hypoxic ventilatory drive in man: Preliminary study. Br J Anaesth 47:963, 1975
5. Dornhorst AC: Respiratory insufficiency. Lancet 1:1185, 1955
6. Lane DJ, Howell JBL: Relationship between sensitivity to carbon dioxide and clinical features in patients with chronic airways obstruction. Thorax 25:150, 1970
7. Matthews AW, Howell JBL: Assessment of responsiveness to carbon dioxide in patients with chronic airways obstruction by rate of isometric inspiratory pressure development. Clin Sci Molec Med 50:199, 1976
8. Collins DD, Scoggin CH, Zwillich CE, et al: Hereditary aspects of decreased hypoxic response. J Clin Invest 21:105, 1978
9. Comroe JH: Physiology of Respiration: An Introductory Text. Chicago, Year Book Medical Publishers, 1974
10. Widdicombe JG: Respiratory reflexes. In Fenn WO, Rahn, H (eds): Handbook of Physiology, Section 3, Respiration, p 585. Washington, DC, American Physiological Society, 1964
11. Guz A: Regulation of respiration in man. Ann Rev Physiol 37:303, 1975
12. Guz A, Noble MIM, Eisele JH, et al: Experimental results of vagal block in cardiopulmonary disease. In Porter R (ed): Breathing: Hering-Breuer Centenary Symposium, p 315. London, J & A Churchill, 1970
13. Phillipson EA, Murphy E, Kozar LF, et al: Role of vagal stimuli in exercise ventilation in dogs with experimental pneumonitis. J Appl Physiol 39:76, 1975
14. Opie LH, Smith AC, Spalding JMK: Conscious appreciation of the effects produced by independent changes of ventilation volume and of end-tidal pCO_2 in paralysed patients. J Physiol 149:494, 1959
15. Hill L, Flack M: The effect of excess carbon dioxide and of want of oxygen upon the respiration and the circulation. J Physiol 37:77, 1908
16. Fowler WS: Breaking point of breath holding. J Appl Physiol 6:539, 1954
17. Noble MIM, Eisele JH, Trenchard D, et al: Effect of selective peripheral nerve blocks on respiratory sensations. In Porter R (ed): Breathing: Hering-Breuer Centenary Symposium, p 233. London, J & A Churchill, 1970
18. Campbell EJM, Freedman S, Clark TJH, et al: The effect of muscular paralysis induced by tubocurarine on the duration and sensation of breath-holding. Clin Sci 32:425, 1967
19. Editorial: The fighter versus the nonfighter: Control of ventilation in chronic obstructive pulmonary disease. Arch Environ Health 7:125, 1963
20. McIlroy MB: Dyspnea and the work of breathing in diseases of the heart and lungs. Prog Cardiovasc Dis 1:284, 1959
21. Christie RV: Dyspnoea in relation to the visco-elastic properties of the lung. Proc R Soc Med 46:381, 1953
22. Marshall R, Stone RW, Christie RV: The relationship of dyspnoea to respiratory effort in normal subjects, mitral stenosis and emphysema. Clin Sci 13:625, 1954
23. Suero JT, Woolf CR: Alterations in the mechanical properties of the lung during dyspnea in chronic obstructive pulmonary disease. J Clin Invest 49:747, 1970

24. Nisell O: The respiratory work and pressure during exercise, and their relation to dyspnea. Acta Med Scand 166:113, 1960
25. O'Connell JM, Campbell AH: Respiratory mechanics in airways obstruction associated with inspiratory dyspnea. Thorax 1:669, 1976
26. Otis AB, Fenn WO, Rahn H: Mechanics of breathing in man. J Appl Physiol 2:592, 1950
27. Mead J: Control of respiratory frequency. J Appl Physiol 15:325, 1960
28. McCloskey DI: Kinesthetic sensibility. Physiol Rev 58:763, 1978
29. Guz A: Sensory aspects of the diaphram: Review of the problem. Am Rev Respir Dis 119:65, 1979
30. Rochester DF, Braun NMT: Diaphragm and dyspnea: Evidence from inhibiting diaphragmatic activity with respirators. Am Rev Respir Dis 119:77, 1979
31. Agostoni E: Diaphragm activity during breath holding: Factors related to its onset. J Appl Physiol 18:30, 1963
32. Noble MIM, Eisele JH, Frankel HL, et al: The role of the diaphragm in the sensation of holding the breath. Clin Sci 41:275, 1971
33. Eisele J, Trenchard D, Burki N, et al: The effect of chest wall block on respiratory sensation and control in man. Clin Sci 35:23, 1968
34. Campbell EJM, Howell JBL: The sensation of breathlessness. Br Med Bull 19:36, 1963
35. Killian KJ, Campbell EJM: Dyspnea and exercise. Ann Rev Physiol 45:465, 1983
36. Derrenne JP, Macklem PT, Roussos CH: The respiratory muscles: Mechanics, control and pathophysiology. Am Rev Respir Dis 118:581, 1978
37. Grassino A, Bellemare F, Laporta D: Diaphragm fatigue and the strategy of breathing in COPD. Chest (in press)
38. McIlroy MB: Breathlessness in cardiovascular disease. In Howell JBL, Campbell EJM (eds): Breathlessness. Proceedings of an International Symposium, University of Manchester, p 187. Oxford, Blackwell Scientific Publications, 1966
39. Mauck HP, Shapiro W, Patterson JL: Pulmonary venous (wedge) pressure: Correlation with onset and disappearance of dyspnea in acute left ventricular heart failure. Am J Cardiol Vol 13, p 301, March 1964
40. Ebnother CL, Selzer A, Stone AO, et al: The ventilatory response to exercise in patients with mitral stenosis and its relationship to circulatory dynamics. Am J Med Sci Vol 233, p 46, January 1957
41. Stampfer M, Epstein SE, Beiser GD, et al: Hemodynamic effects of diuresis at rest and during intense upright exercise in patients with impaired cardiac function. Circulation 37:900, 1968
42. Bondurant S, Hickam JB, Isley JK: Pulmonary and circulatory effects of acute pulmonary vascular engorgement in normal subjects. J Clin Invest 36:59, 1957
43. Cook CD, Mead J, Schreiner GL, et al: Pulmonary mechanics during induced pulmonary edema in anesthetized dogs. J Appl Physiol 14:177, 1959
44. Wilhemsen L, Varnauskas E: Effects of acute plasma expansion on the mechanics of breathing. Clin Sci 33:29, 1967
45. Sharp JT, Griffith GT, Bunnell IL, et al: Ventilatory mechanics in pulmonary edema in man. J Clin Invest 37:111, 1958
46. Turino GM, Fishman AP: The congested lung. J Chron Dis 9:510, 1959
47. Collins JV, Clark TJH, Brown DJ: Airway function in healthy subjects and in patients with left heart disease. Clin Sci Molec Med 49:217, 1975
48. Marshall R, McIlroy MB, Christie RV: The work of breathing in mitral stenosis. Clin Sci 13:137, 1954
49. Bates DV, Christie RV: Pulmonary function in heart disease and in pulmonary hypertension. In Bates DV, Macklem PT, Christie RV (eds): Respiratory Function in Disease, p 301. Philadelphia, WB Saunders, 1971

50. Heyer HE, Holman J, Shires GT: The diminished efficiency and altered dynamics of respiration in experimental pulmonary congestion. Am Heart J 35:463, 1948
51. Churchill ED, Cope O: The rapid shallow breathing resulting from pulmonary congestion and edema. J Exp Med 49:531, 1929
52. Marshall R, Widdicombe JG: The activity of pulmonary stretch receptors during congestion of the lungs. Q J Exp Physiol 43:320, 1958
53. Bulbring E, Whitteridge D: The activity of vagal stretch endings during congestion in perfused lungs. J Physiol 103:477, 1945
54. Chidsey CA, Braunwald E, Morrow AG: Catecholamine excretion and cardiac stores of norepinephrine in congestive heart failure. Am J Med 39:442, 1965
55. Bolton B, Carmichael EA, Sturup G: Vaso-constriction following deep inspiration. J Physiol 86:83, 1936
56. Duggan JJ, Love VL, Lyons RH: A study of reflex venomotor reactions in man. Circulation 7:869, 1953
57. Voelkel N, Reeves JT: Primary pulmonary hypertension. In Moser KM (ed): Pulmonary Vascular Diseases, p 573. New York, Marcell Dekker, 1979
58. Kan WO, Ledsome JR, Bolter CP: Pulmonary arterial distention and activity in phrenic nerve of anesthetized dogs. J Appl Physiol 46:625, 1979
59. Dexter L: Pulmonary vascular disease in acquired heart disease. In Moser KM (ed): Pulmonary Vascular Diseases, p 427. New York, Marcell Dekker, 1979
60. Horres AD, Bernthal T: Localized multiple minute pulmonary embolism and breathing. J Appl Physiol 16:842, 1961
61. Grover RF, Wagner WW, McMurtry IF, et al: The pulmonary circulation. In Abboud F (ed): The Handbook of Physiology. Bethesda, Md., American Physiological Society, 1979
62. Braunwald E, Ross J Jr, Sonnenblick EH: Mechanisms of Contraction of the Normal and Failing Heart. Boston, Little, Brown & Co, 1968
63. Cherniack RM, Cuddy TE, Armstrong JB: Significance of pulmonary elastic and viscous resistance in orthopnea. Circulation 15:859, 1957
64. Perera GA, Berliner RW: The relation of postural hemodilution to paroxysmal dyspnea. J Clin Invest 22:5, 1943
65. Berson SA, Yalow RS, Azulay A, et al: The biological decay curve of P^{32} tagged erythrocytes: Application to the study of acute changes in blood volume. J Clin Invest 31:581, 1952
66. Hayashi KD, Moss AJ, Yu PM: Urinary catecholamine excretion in myocardial infarction. Circulation 60:473, 1969
67. Ward JM, McGrath RF, Weil JV: Effects of morphine on the peripheral vascular response to sympathetic stimulation. Am J Cardiol 29:659, 1972
68. Baim DS, McDowell AV, Cherniles J, et al: Evaluation of a new bipyridine inotropic agent—milrinone—in patients with severe congestive heart failure. N Engl J Med 309:748, 1983

3

SYNCOPE

JoAnn Lindenfeld, M.D.

Definition

The term *syncope* (Greek *synkope*, "a cutting short") is generally used to refer to a relatively abrupt loss of consciousness that is transient and rapidly reversible. *Presyncope* and *near-syncope* describe episodes of "near-loss of consciousness" that are usually caused by lesser degrees of the same problems that lead to syncope. Although many terms in everyday usage, such as "faint", "spell," "swoon," "blackout," and so on, may be used synonymously with syncope, it is critical that the physician probe behind these words to determine their exact meaning to the patient. For example, "spells" may actually represent "drop attacks," typical transient ischemic attacks, (TIAs), vertigo, or merely severe muscular weakness. Each of these diverse meanings can lead the physician on a very different diagnostic course.

Syncope is a symptom, not a primary disease, and has many possible causes. Current usage defines syncope as a transient loss of consciousness caused by a reduction in cerebral oxygen or glucose delivery that is due either to decreased amounts of these constituents in blood or, more commonly, to decreased cerebral blood flow. Other causes of transient loss of consciousness that might be termed neuropsychologic are discussed here as well because they are frequently part of the differential diagnosis (Table 3-1).

Table 3–1.   Etiology of Transient Loss of Consciousness

I. Syncope: cerebral hypoxia (hypoglycemia)
  A. Quantitative decrease in cerebral blood flow
    1. Decreased cerebral perfusion pressure
      a. Decreased arterial pressure
        1. Faulty arterial pressure homeostasis
        2. Decreased cardiac output due to a primary cardiac abnormality
        3. Obstruction to venous return
      b. Increased venous or intracranial pressure
    2. Increased cerebral vascular resistance
  B. Qualitative decrease in cerebral blood flow
II. Neuropsychologic causes
  A. Epilepsy
  B. Hysterical syncope

Physiology

REGULATION OF CEREBRAL BLOOD FLOW

Because the brain has no appreciable store of high-energy phosphate compounds, a sudden decrease in cerebral oxygen delivery will lead almost immediately to a shortage of these high-energy compounds, resulting in cerebral cellular dysfunction and unconsciousness.[1] In fact, if the cerebral circulation is cut off completely, loss of consciousness occurs in a few seconds.[2] If cerebral oxygen delivery is restored quickly, cellular dysfunction is rapidly reversed, and consciousness returns as rapidly as it was lost.

Although the brain makes up only 2% of total body mass, it receives 13% of the cardiac output and is responsible for 19% of total body oxygen consumption.[3] The importance of cerebral oxygen delivery and the necessity for understanding its overall control and component parts are thus apparent. Cerebral oxygen delivery is the product of cerebral blood flow and the oxygen content of blood. The brain requires approximately 3.5 cc O_2 per 100 g of brain tissue per minute for normal functioning.[1,4] Below this level of oxygen delivery, consciousness is affected. Fortunately, there is a wide margin of safety in cerebral oxygen delivery. Cerebral blood flow in a supine, healthy, normal person is approximately 50 cc to 55 cc per 100 g brain tissue per minute, and the normal oxygen content of blood is 17 cc to 19 cc O_2 per 100 ml of blood.[1,4] This results in a cerebral oxygen delivery of 9.0 cc to 10.5 cc O_2 per 100 g brain tissue per minute and an arteriovenous oxygen difference of 6 cc to 7 cc O_2 per 100 g brain tissue per minute.[5] Although the brain generally receives much more oxygen than is necessary to maintain normal functioning and consciousness, it is capable of extracting most of the oxygen delivered to it.[5] However, the oxygen safety margin may be narrowed in many common situations in which cerebral oxygen delivery is decreased due to a fall either in the effective oxygen content of blood or in the cerebral blood flow. The effective oxygen content of blood may be reduced by variations in red blood cell oxygen affinity, red blood cell concentration, or the partial pressure of oxygen in the blood. However, even when the oxygen content of blood is lowered by such disorders as anemia or hypoxemia, there remains an additional margin of safety for cerebral oxygen delivery that is provided by the careful regulation of both systemic arterial pressure and cerebral blood flow.[3,4,6] Maintenance of arterial pressure is a very high priority of the regulatory systems of the intact organism, but, in spite of this high priority, variations of blood pressure in both directions do occur. Cerebral blood flow, however, remains remarkably constant over a wide range of arterial pressures.[3,4,6]

Cerebral blood flow has two major determinants: cerebral perfusion pressure and cerebral vascular resistance.[3,4,6] Cerebral perfusion pressure is the difference between the arterial and venous pressures. In humans, venous pressure is low (5 mm Hg or less) under normal circumstances, making arterial pressure the major determinant of cerebral perfusion pressure.[3] The critical mean arterial pressure for maintenance of normal cerebral blood flow in a normal person is approximately 60 mm Hg to 70 mm Hg; below this pressure, cerebral blood flow falls off rapidly (Fig. 3-1).[3,4,6-8] In normal supine subjects, symptoms of cerebral hypoxia begin at a mean arterial pressure of about 40 mm Hg.

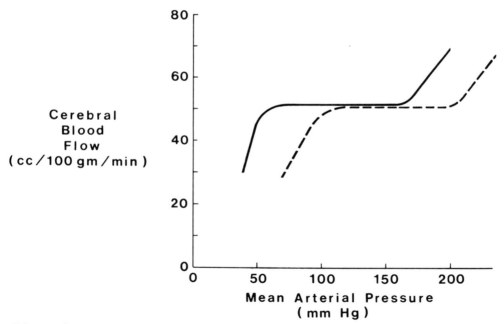

FIG. 3-1. The relationship between cerebral blood flow and mean arterial pressure in normotensive man (*solid line*) and hypertensive man (*dotted line*). (Data from Lassen NA: Cerebral blood flow and oxygen consumption in man. Physiol Rev 39:183, 1959; Strandgaard S, Oleson J, Skinhoj E, et al: Autoregulation of brain circulation in severe arterial hypertension. Br Med J 1:507, 1973; Zijlstra WG: Physiology of the cerebral circulation. In Minderhoud JM (ed): Cerebral Blood Flow: Basic Knowledge and Clinical Implications, pp 79–85. Amsterdam, Exerpta Medica, 1981)

Effective mean arterial pressure for the brain may be different in the supine and upright positions. In a person in the upright position, the base of the brain is about 240 mm above the heart. Thus, the brain "sees" a mean arterial pressure that is effectively 18 mm Hg less than the actual mean arterial pressure.[6] Cerebral perfusion pressure does not decrease by this amount, since standing also leads to a fall of several mm Hg in venous pressure. Cerebral blood flow in the standing position is only about 80% of that measured in the supine position.[9,10] The drop could be due to the change in cerebral perfusion pressure or to the fall in arterial carbon dioxide pressure (P_aCO_2) that accompanies the upright posture. As we shall see, P_aCO_2 is an extremely important variable in the regulation of cerebral vascular resistance.[6] If falls in cerebral perfusion pressure were the sole cause of falls in cerebral blood flow, however, standing upright would reduce cerebral blood flow to the point where autoregulation is lost. Since consciousness is well preserved in the upright position, it seems most likely that the fall in cerebral blood flow with standing is due to changes in P_aCO_2.

High venous pressures (240 mm H_2O, or 18 mm Hg) decrease cerebral perfusion pressure, but usually not enough to affect cerebral blood flow.[11] It is conceivable, however, that when combined with low arterial pressures, high venous pressures might lower cerebral perfusion pressures enough to decrease cerebral blood flow. Very high venous pressures alone may lead to diminished cerebral blood flow, but mechanisms other than just reduced cerebral perfusion pressure may be involved.[3,12] As intracranial pressure increases above venous pressure, cerebral perfusion pressure becomes arterial pressure minus intracranial pressure.[13,14] The effects of high intracranial pressure on cerebral blood flow have been studied in several situations. In an experimental model, raising intracranial pressure to very high levels (500 mm H_2O, or 37 mm Hg) led to a significant decrease in cerebral blood flow that was reversed when the high intracranial pressure was relieved.[6] In studies of patients with high intracranial pressures due to tumors and other such conditions, cerebral blood flow was also decreased, but relieving the high intracranial pressure with intraventricular puncture did not restore cerebral blood flow.[15] Thus, it is unclear whether increases in intracranial pressure affect cerebral blood flow only by reducing cerebral perfusion pressure or whether other mechanisms are involved. However, it seems likely that intracranial pressure, like venous pressure, may demonstrably affect cerebral perfusion pressure and thus cerebral blood flow when it is very high or when arterial pressure is low. That cerebral perfusion pressure, and not just arterial pressure, is important is highlighted when positive gravitational forces are considered. With forces of 4 G to 5 G, the effective arterial pressure at the base of the brain is nearly zero. However, the venous pressure is −50 mm Hg to −60 mm Hg, leading to a cerebral perfusion pressure adequate to maintain cerebral blood flow and consciousness.[16]

The second major determinant of cerebral blood flow is cerebral vascular resistance. Over a wide range of mean arterial pressures (which usually are nearly the same as cerebral perfusion pressure, since venous pressure is normally very low) cerebral blood flow remains remarkably constant. This process, called *autoregulation*, occurs in many vascular beds in the body, but it is particularly refined in the brain. As Figure 3-1 demonstrates, cerebral blood flow (and thus cerebral oxygen delivery) is remarkably constant for mean arterial pressures of between 60 mm Hg and 160 mm Hg. Autoregulation is managed by changes in cerebral vascular resistance.

Cerebral vascular resistance is determined by the length and diameter of the cerebral vessels themselves, the chronic arterial pressure, the neural and metabolic effects on the cerebral resistance vessels, the viscosity of blood, and the temperature. Obstructive disease that leads to either generalized or localized changes in cerebral vascular resistance can change the diameter of cerebral blood vessels. As can be seen in Figure 3-1, arterial pressure plays a determining role in cerebral blood flow only when it is very high or very low. As arterial pressure falls below normal, cerebral vessels dilate, and thus constant cerebral blood flow is maintained. However, below a mean arterial pressure of 60 mm Hg to 70 mm Hg, cerebral blood vessels are maximally vasodilated and can no longer maintain normal cerebral blood flow.[4] Likewise, above a mean pressure of approximately 160 mm Hg, cerebral vascular resistance can no longer increase, and increments in mean arterial pressure lead to similar increments in cerebral vascular flow which often results in disruption of the delicate endothelial lining of the blood–brain barrier.[3] With longstanding increases in arterial pressure, the autoregulation curve shifts to the right.[17] (See Fig. 3-1.) Although this shift affords additional protection at high blood pressure levels, it has the consequence that arterial pressure cannot fall as low before autoregulation is lost. Thus, in a group of patients with hypertension, symptoms of cerebral hypoxia were noted when mean arterial pressure was acutely decreased below 68 mm Hg—a much higher level than the 40 mm Hg at which symptoms of cerebral hypoxia are first noted in normotensive subjects.[17] There is minute-to-minute regulation of cerebral vascular resistance, but controversy remains about the actual controlling mechanisms. Some claim autoregulation occurs by means of a myogenic reflex (the Bayliss effect), but most argue that control is exerted through either neural or metabolic factors,[4,6,18–21] with local metabolic factors being the most likely candidates.[19]

Perhaps the most powerful known regulator of cerebral vascular resistance is carbon dioxide (CO_2). Inhalation of 5% to 7% CO_2 (P_aCO_2 of 50 mm Hg and 59 mm Hg, respectively) leads to increases of 50% to 100% in cerebral blood flow without changes in arterial pressure or cerebral oxygen utilization.[6,22] Likewise, hyperventilation to a P_aCO_2 of 26 mm Hg leads to marked rise in cerebral vascular resistance and a 40% fall in cerebral blood flow. Cerebral blood flow changes by about 0.9 ml to 1.7 ml per 100 g brain tissue per minute for each 1 mm Hg change in P_aCO_2, with responsiveness being greatest when P_aCO_2 is near normal.[6] Chronic adaptation of cerebral blood flow to hypocapnia does occur.[23,24] Cerebral vascular resistance also responds to changes in P_aO_2. For increases in P_aO_2 above 50 mm Hg, arterial oxygen content increases by only a small amount, but as P_aO_2 falls below 50 mm Hg, oxygen content falls markedly. Thus, hyperoxia (100% O_2 in inspired air) leads to only small decreases in cerebral blood flow (11% to 14%), while mild hypoxia (P_aO_2 of 50 mm Hg) leads to about a 30% rise in cerebral blood flow.[4,6] More severe degrees of hypoxia lead to even greater increments in cerebral blood flow.[3,4,6,21] Cerebral metabolic activity is also an important determinant of cerebral vascular resistance. Although it was once thought that cerebral oxygen utilization changed very little over a wide range of activities, it is now known that *regional* cerebral oxygen uptake varies with cerebral activity.[19] However, with the exception of coma states, where metabolic activity and oxygen uptake are very low, or seizure states, where oxygen uptake is very high, these changes in regional oxygen uptake are reflected in local cerebral resistance changes that do not often have a very large effect on overall cerebral vascular resistance or blood flow. Thus with exercise, anxiety, or arithmetic calculations we see little change in overall cerebral blood flow or oxygen consumption. Viscosity is said to affect resistance, and, indeed, cerebral blood flow does decrease with polycythemia and increase with anemia. However, it seems likely that these changes may not occur because of changes in viscosity alone but that they may also be affected by changes in oxygen delivery and, possibly, in P_aCO_2.[6,20,25] Cerebral blood flow falls with hypothermia; although many factors may contribute to this fall, the most important is probably the fall in cerebral oxygen consumption.[6] Thus, it appears that, with the exception of, P_aCO_2 effects, changes in cerebral vascular resistance are ultimately linked to oxygen uptake and the metabolic by-products. The actual local regulator that leads to changes in cerebral vascular resistance remains uncertain. Adenosine, potassium ion concentration, and local hydrogen concentration are the most likely possibilities.[19] Although autoregulation in the cerebral vascular bed is highly refined, there are several situations in which autoregulation may be lost. These include extreme changes in arterial pressure, hypercapnia, severe hypoxia, head trauma, cerebral ischemia, and cerebral tumors.[26,27]

Cerebral blood flow is carefully regulated to maintain cerebral oxygen delivery. There are, however, many factors that may reduce cerebral oxygen delivery by leading to a reduction in either arterial oxygen content or cerebral blood flow. While syncope is often caused by a sudden change in only one variable—for instance, a marked fall in arterial pressure—it is easy to see how a combination of less severe changes might decrease the safety margin for cerebral oxygen delivery. Thus, moderate falls in arterial pressure or P_aO_2, which would rarely cause any problems alone, may lead to syncope when combined.

The brain utilizes glucose as its major fuel supply. Because glycogen stores are very limited in the brain, metabolism and thus consciousness are dependent on a nearly continuous supply of glucose.[1] Loss of consciousness occurs somewhat more slowly with acute hypoglycemia than with cerebral hypoxia.

We have seen that cerebral blood flow is carefully maintained over a wide range of arterial pressures. However, if there are large falls in arterial pressure, cerebral perfusion may be compromised. Fortunately, a complex neurohumoral regulatory system prevents large falls in blood pressure in most situations.

ARTERIAL PRESSURE HOMEOSTASIS

Arterial pressure is the product of cardiac output and systemic vascular resistance. Cardiac output is the product of stroke volume and heart rate. Systemic vascular resistance is a function of the length, diameter, and thickness of the systemic vessels; the muscular tone in these vessels; and the extrinsic compression of these vessels by soft tissue. Changes in blood volume influence both cardiac output and systemic vascular resistance. Heart rate, stroke volume, vascular tone, some aspects of soft tissue compression, and blood volume may all be affected by neurohumoral regulation. The widespread effects and importance of this regulation in humans can be demonstrated by a description of the changes that occur with assumption of the upright position—a constant, daily test of arterial pressure homeostasis.

Man's initial attempts to attain an upright position were very likely stymied by inadequate mechanisms for arterial pressure homeostasis. Indeed, most four-legged mammals, if placed in an upright position, are unable to maintain an adequate arterial pressure for any length of time.[28,29] In humans, standing results in gravitational forces that lead to pooling of 500 ml to 750 ml of blood in the veins of the buttocks and legs.[30] In addition to venous pooling with quiet standing, extravasation of fluid from the intravascular to the interstitial space results in hemoconcentration and decreased blood volume. Blood volume may be decreased by 10% after 10 minutes of quiet standing and may decrease up to as much as 15% with more prolonged standing.[30,31] The blood that pools in the legs with standing has been displaced from the intrathoracic ("central") blood compartment.[32] This displacement results in decreased cardiac filling, leading to a fall in stroke volume and cardiac output. Without effective compensatory mechanisms, this decline in cardiac output would lead to a severe fall in arterial pressure, just as it does in four-legged mammals placed in the upright position.[28] Fortunately, powerful compensatory mechanisms, operating primarily through the autonomic nervous system, do exist in humans, and standing actually results in little change in mean arterial pressure.[33] These compensatory mechanisms include baroreceptor activation, increased respiration, increased muscle and interstitial pressure in the legs, activation of the renin–angiotensin system, and, probably, release of vasopressin. With venous pooling and decreased cardiac output, there is less stretch of the carotid and aortic baroreceptors, which results in parasympathetic withdrawal and increased sympathetic activity.[30,34,35] Vasoconstriction of resistance vessels in muscle, skin, renal, and splanchnic beds increases systemic resistance, thus mobilizing blood to restore filling of the heart. Increases in heart rate and contractility further improve cardiac output. Increased sympathetic activity may also stimulate renin release. Decreased cardiac filling simultaneously affects the cardiopulmonary baroreceptors.[30,34–36] One set of cardiopulmonary receptors is in the atria, at the junctions of the superior vena cava and inferior vena cava with the right atrium and at the junctions of the pulmonary veins and the left atrium. Two additional networks of receptors are present throughout all the chambers of the heart. The input from these receptors is carried by both the vagus nerve and the sympathetic nerves. Decreased stretch of the cardiopulmonary receptors leads to changes similar to those produced by decreased stretch of the carotid and aortic baroreceptors as well as to an antidiuretic effect.[35,37]

Although the responses of arterial and low-pressure baroreceptors to standing are similar, in other situations they can generate opposing responses, and the ultimate result of their action is often not predictable.[35,38] Some of these situations will be discussed later. The increased sympathetic activity elicited by these reflexes is reflected by an increase in circulating catecholamines. In normal resting subjects, standing results in a 50% increase in norepinephrine levels in 2 minutes and a doubling in 10 minutes.[39,40] Increased respiration and increased tone in the abdominal and lower limb musculature augment venous return.[41-43] Activation of the renin–angiotensin system further augments blood volume but is somewhat more delayed.[44-46] It remains unclear whether active venoconstriction is an important part of the baroreceptor responses to standing.[30,47-49] With walking or just tensing of the leg muscles, the "muscular venous pump" in the legs (the combination of venous valves preventing back-flow and increased venous pressure) leads to rapid lowering of pressure at the ankles, preventing venous pooling and aiding venous return.[43,50]

The transfer of blood from the intrathoracic intravascular space to dependent veins that occurs with standing and the resulting compensatory changes lead to a characteristic pattern of hemodynamic changes.[33,51-55] Stroke volume falls by about 30% to 50%. Heart rate increases by 10 to 20 beats per minute but not enough to maintain cardiac output, which falls by about 20%. Peripheral vascular resistance increases. Since there is little change in oxygen consumption, the arteriovenous oxygen difference widens from about 4 to 6 vol %. Systolic pressure usually does not change or falls slightly while diastolic pressure rises slightly or shows no change. Thus, mean arterial pressure remains constant or rises slightly with a narrowing in pulse pressure. These changes are characteristic after at least 2 minutes of quiet standing. It should be noted that, in normal subjects, within the first 30 seconds after standing there may be a transient 5 mm Hg to 40 mm Hg fall in systolic blood pressure and a rise in heart rate of 20 to 30 beats per minute.[51,56]

With higher ambient temperatures, venous pooling increases.[30,41] Prolonged quiet standing may also lead to additional venous pooling because of the loss of the effects of the muscle pump. In both of these situations, an additional burden is placed on compensatory mechanisms.[51] The importance of venous pooling is emphasized by studies demonstrating that if venous pooling is prevented by water immersion or G-suit inflation, the usual hemodynamic changes of orthostasis are largely prevented.[30] Thus, it is not surprising that patients with an increased blood volume, such as occurs with congestive heart failure, tolerate orthostatic stress much better than normal people.[57]

It is evident that the compensatory mechanisms regulating arterial pressure involve many parts of the nervous system. Afferent nerves must carry impulses from the carotid sinuses, aorta, atria, ventricles, and muscles to the spinal cord and the vasomotor center in the medulla. Synapses connect the vasomotor center to the hypothalamus and cerebral cortex. Efferent impulses are carried through the autonomic ganglia and sympathetic and parasympathetic nerves to local organ beds, which must be responsive if changes are to occur. Complex hormonal systems regulate blood volume. An abnormality in any part of this system, from sensory organ to end organ, may lead to defective compensatory changes, resulting in defective arterial pressure control.

Clinical Presentation

Syncope is a result of cerebral hypoxia or hypoglycemia. Either quantitative or qualitative decreases in cerebral blood flow may be responsible (see Table 3-1). Quantitative decreases in cerebral blood flow may occur with decreased cerebral perfusion pressure or increased cerebral vascular resistance. Problems that lead to syncope by decreasing cerebral perfusion pressure are considered first.

QUANTITATIVE DECREASE IN CEREBRAL BLOOD FLOW

Decreased Cerebral Perfusion Pressure: Decreased Arterial Pressure

Significant decreases in cerebral perfusion pressure leading to syncope may result from decreased arterial pressure, from increased venous or intracranial pressure, or from combinations of these. The most common cause, however, is a decrease in arterial pressure to a level at which cerebral autoregulation cannot maintain cerebral blood flow. Falls in arterial pressure occur when there is faulty arterial pressure homeostasis, when there is an intrinsic abnormality in cardiac function, or when there is an obstruction to venous return.

FAULTY ARTERIAL PRESSURE HOMEOSTASIS. Table 3-2 lists the causes of faulty arterial pressure homeostasis. Many of the diseases listed lead to chronic orthostatic hypotension. When severe, the orthostatic hypotension may result in syncope. Chronic orthostatic hypotension will not usually be found with problems such as vasodepressor syncope, carotid sinus syndrome, and afferent nerve stimulation, which have a more paroxysmal presentation.

ORTHOSTATIC HYPOTENSION. Orthostatic hypotension is an abnormal fall in both systolic and diastolic blood pressure that occurs with standing and leads to symptoms of dizziness, presyncope, or actual syncope. Although there are no specific criteria for abnormal orthostatic changes in blood pressure, it is generally agreed that if there is a *persistent* decrease of 30 mm Hg or more in systolic blood pressure and of 15 mm Hg or more in diastolic blood pressure after 2 minutes of standing, the clinical diagnosis of orthostatic hypotension may be made, provided the changes are accompanied by symptoms.[45] The blood pressure and heart rate should be taken with the patient supine, immediately on standing, and after 2 minutes and 5 minutes of standing. Orthostatic hypotension may be classified as *hypoadrenergic* (asympathicotonic) or *hyperadrenergic* (sympathicotonic).[30,58]

Hypoadrenergic orthostatic hypotension may be primary (idiopathic) or secondary. Since hypoadrenergic orthostatic hypotension is caused by defects in or interference with the autonomic nervous sytem, it might more correctly be termed primary and secondary autonomic insufficiency.

Patients with primary or idiopathic orthostatic hypotension can be divided into two groups. Those who present with symptoms of dysautonomia—that is, orthostatic hypotension, anhidrosis, impotence, nocturnal polyuria, and heat intolerance—but with no evidence of central nervous system (CNS) disease are classified as having idiopathic orthostatic hypotension (Bradbury–Eggleston syndrome).[59] Patients who present with the same dysautonomia plus CNS disease (usually corticospinal, corticobulbar, cerebellar, or extrapyramidal) fit a

Table 3–2.   Causes of Faulty Arterial Pressure Homeostasis

I. Orthostatic Hypotension
   A. Hypoadrenergic orthostatic hypotension
      1. Primary orthostatic hypotension (autonomic insufficiency)
         a. Idiopathic orthostatic hypotension (Bradbury–Eggleston syndrome)
         b. Shy–Drager syndrome
      2. Secondary orthostatic hypotension (autonomic insufficiency)
         a. Due to underlying diseases
             Diabetes mellitus
             End-Stage renal disease
             Polyneuropathy
             Guillain–Barré
             Parkinson's disease
             Intracranial tumors
             Spinal cord tumors
             Cerebral infarction
             Syringomyelia
             Amyloid
             Porphyria
             Traumatic and inflammatory myelopathies
             Tabes dorsalis
             Familial dysautonomia (Riley–Day syndrome)
             Multiple sclerosis
             Alcoholism
             Holmes–Adie syndrome
             Neoplasm
             Vacor
             Vincristine
             ? Primary aldosteronism with hypokalemia
             ? Aging
         b. Surgical sympathectomy
   B. Hyperadrenergic orthostatic hypotension
      Decreased venous return due to
      a. Hypovolemia
      b. Decreased venous tone or function
      c. Defective volume regulation
   C. Drug-induced orthostatic hypotension
  II. Vasovagal syncope
 III. Carotid sinus syncope
 IV. Afferent nerve stimulation

category entitled Shy–Drager syndrome.[45,60–62] In the Shy-Drager syndrome, autonomic insufficiency may antedate the appearance of CNS disease by 2 years to 5 years.[45] Both are diseases of the autonomic nervous system, but the site of the lesion differs. Patients with the Shy–Drager syndrome have a normal supine level of norepinephrine but the level fails to rise with standing or exercise.[39] Response to tyramine and sensitivity to infused norepinephrine are normal. Although agreement is not universal, these data suggest that there is a normal peripheral sympathetic system but a central defect in activation of the sympathetic nervous system.[39,63,64] Patients with idiopathic orthostatic hypotension have low supine levels of circulating norepinephrine that fail to rise significantly with standing or exercise.[39] There is no response to infused tyramine (indicating an abnormality in release or storage of norepinephrine at the nerve terminal), and catecholamine fluorescent studies demonstrate decreased norepinephrine in the nerve terminals.[62,65] Although these patients also have a marked increase in sensitivity to infused norepinephrine, suggesting "denervation supersensitivity," it has been pointed out that the increase may reflect the underlying baroreceptor malfunction.[64] All of these results suggest that idiopathic orthostatic hypotension is caused by a defect in the peripheral sympathetic nervous system. These results are summarized in Figure 3-2 and Table 3-3. Both idiopathic orthostatic hypotension and Shy–Drager syndrome are diseases of middle age and occur more commonly in men than in women.[45] In both forms, the symptoms of dysautonomia may appear gradually over a period of years.[45,66] The CNS signs in patients with Shy–Drager syndrome usually become evident within 2 years to 5 years of the onset of orthostatic hypotension and may be indistinguishable from idiopathic Parkinson's disease.[66] The cause of the lesions in these diseases is unknown and there is no known cure. However, the prognosis is much worse for patients with Shy–Drager syndrome than for those with idiopathic orthostatic hypotension.[45,62] Death often results from general debility and its complications: pulmonary embolism, malnutrition, and pneumonia.[67]

Secondary autonomic insufficiency has many underlying causes (see Table 3-2). These diseases involve the CNS or the peripheral autonomic nervous system, or both. CNS disease that involves the autonomic nervous system usually also involves other systems. Thus, movement disorders, parkinsonism, weakness, and bulbar disorders may accompany disorders of the vasomotor center. Spinal cord diseases are most often associated with paralysis and spasticity.[61,62] Orthostatic hypotension due to spinal cord disease usually results when the lesion is above T_6.[66] Neoplasms outside the CNS may be associated with a polyneuropathy leading to orthostatic hypotension.[66] Disorders of the peripheral autonomic nervous system generally show low resting norepinephrine levels with subnormal or absent rises in norepinephrine levels with standing and exercise.[45,62] There is hypersensitivity to infused norepinephrine and a lack of norepinephrine release with tyramine. This is the same pattern described for idiopathic orthostatic hypotension, which is also felt to be a disorder of the peripheral autonomic nervous system (see Table 3-3). The quantitative defect in norepinephrine response will depend on the severity of the autonomic involvement. CNS lesions are associated with changes similar to those previously described for the Shy–Drager syndrome (see Table 3-3). Patients with autonomic insufficiency generally have involvement of both the sympathetic and parasympathetic systems. Thus, as well as postural hypotension symptoms can include anhidrosis, sphincter dysfunction (bladder and bowel), various degrees of impotence, fixed heart rate, constipation or nocturnal diarrhea, and heat intolerance.[45,62] Supine arterial pressure may be high, since venous pooling of blood is reversed and fluid returns to the intravascular space. The same mechanisms that fail to maintain arterial pressure with standing, fail to lower pressure with recumbency. This is emphasized by the absence of a

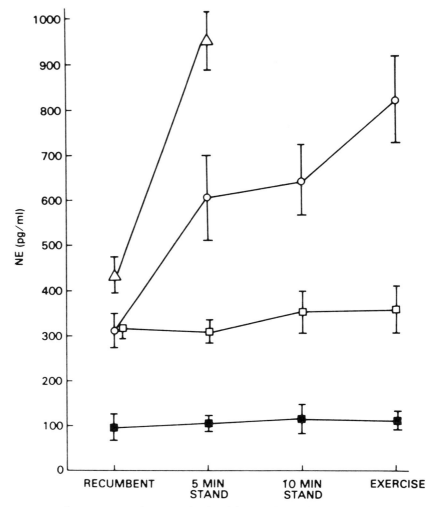

FIG. 3-2. Plasma norepinephrine (NE) levels while recumbent, after standing for 5 and 10 minutes, and after 5 minutes of isometric exercise while standing. Solid squares represent idiopathic orthostatic hypotension; open squares, Shy–Drager syndrome; open circles, normal subjects; and open triangles, normal subjects after furosemide diuresis. Values show one standard error of the mean. (Zeigler MG: Postural Hypotension Annu Rev Med 31:239 1980. Reproduced with permission)

heart rate response when hypertension is induced by pressor agents.[68] Patients with orthostatic hypotension are often most symptomatic early in the morning, perhaps because the activity of the renin–angiotensin system is lowest in the morning and gradually increases throughout the day in response to the decrease in effective blood volume.[45,69] In patients with hypoadrenergic orthostatic hypotension, compensatory mechanisms are often inadequate or com-

Table 3–3. Comparison of Idiopathic Orthostatic Hypotension and
Shy–Drager Syndrome

	IOH*	SDS†
Supine norepinephrine	Decreased	Normal
Standing and exercise norepinephrine	No increase	No increase
Tyramine response	Absent	Normal
Sensitivity to infused norepinephrine	Increased	Normal
Proposed site of autonomic nervous system defect	Peripheral	Central

*IOH = idiopathic orthostatic hypotension
†SDS = Shy–Drager syndrome

pletely absent. Consequently, these patients may not report the tachycardia, pallor, nausea, or sweating preceding a syncopal event that would be expected if compensatory mechanisms were intact.[61]

Several forms of secondary orthostatic hypotension deserve special comment. Diabetes mellitus is one of the most common causes of autonomic neuropathy. Parasympathetic function is generally affected earlier than sympathetic function.[70] As a result, postural abnormalities in heart rate appear before orthostatic hypotension does, making these heart rate changes sensitive indicators of autonomic dysfunction in diabetics.[71] Diabetics with autonomic neuropathy have a worse prognosis than those without neuropathy, and it has been suggested that the neuropathy itself may be partly responsible for the difference.[70,72] Cerebral infarction or cerebral vascular disease is often included among the causes of autonomic insufficiency.[45] Although there is some evidence for this association, it is likely that age, general debility, and drugs play a more important role.[39,66,73–75] Amyloidosis may present as an idiopathic autonomic neuropathy but may also manifest a sensory neuropathy.[76–78] Infiltration of vessel walls by amyloid may decrease the response to sympathetic stimulation.[79] Low voltage on the electrocardiogram (ECG) may serve as a clue to the presence of amyloid.[80] Vincristine, a cancer chemotherapeutic agent, may lead to orthostatic hypotension because of a widespread peripheral neuropathy.[81] A rodenticide, "Vacor Rat Killer," which was sold for only a short time, causes severe autonomic insufficiency when ingested.[82] Patients with primary aldosteronism and hypokalemia may have orthostatic hypotension.[83] It is not yet clear whether this is a manifestation of hypokalemia alone, which may alter vascular reactivity, or whether there is additional autonomic dysfunction.[84] The orthostatic hypotension resolves with repletion of potassium or removal of the tumor. Rarely, carcinomas may lead to orthostatic hypotension. This may be a nonmetastatic complication, as illustrated by a patient with bronchial carcinoma whose orthostatic hypotension disappeared following irradiation of the primary tumor.[85] Orthostatic hypotension has been reported in other thoracic neoplasms, in pancreatic carcinoma, and in posterior fossa tumors.[86–88] Familial dysautonomia (the Riley–Day syndrome) is an autosomal recessive disorder seen in Ashkenazic Jews.[89] It is characterized by autonomic insufficiency, which appears shortly after birth and progresses to death in early adult life. Postural hypotension occurs, as do paroxysms of hypertension caused by defective blood pressure regulation, denervation hypersensitivity, and release of catecholamines from the adrenal medulla in response to hypoglycemia.[90] Tissue and resting levels of catecholamines are normal but circulating levels fail to rise with standing.[31]

Orthostatic hypotension is relatively common in the elderly. A drop of 20 mm Hg or more in systolic pressure occurs in 10% to 20% of both hospitalized and healthy people over the age of 65.[91-94] The causes of this high incidence of orthostatic hypotension have not been carefully investigated. Signs of autonomic insufficiency have been found in some, but not all, of these patients.[92] A study by MacLennan and associates showed a strong correlation between orthostatic hypotension and high supine systolic arterial pressure.[94] These authors suggested that the orthostatic hypotension might be related to an abnormally stiff vascular bed. A stiff vascular bed might be poorly responsive to vasoconstrictor stimuli but could also lead to decreased baroreceptor deformation, resulting in an abnormality in the afferent arc of this reflex. Indeed, high supine arterial pressures are quite compatible with autonomic insufficiency. The normal increase in heart rate with standing is delayed in some elderly patients with orthostatic hypotension.[95] This delayed heart rate response is likely to exacerbate orthostatic hypotension and may be a reflection of abnormal autonomic reflexes. In another study of 494 patients over the age of 65 living at home, factors such as heart disease, organic brain disease, absent ankle jerks, varicose veins, potentially hypotensive drugs, anemia, bacteriuria, and hyponatremia were correlated with the presence of postural falls in systolic blood pressure of greater than 20 mm Hg to 30 mm Hg. Patients with orthostatic hypotension had two or more of these factors more commonly than patients without orthostatic hypotension. Thus, it seems likely that the high incidence of orthostatic hypotension in the elderly is the result of a combination of many factors. Secondary orthostatic hypotension may also be caused by surgical sympathectomy or by drugs. (Drug-induced orthostatic hypotension is considered later in this chapter.)

The integrity of the autonomic nervous system can be assessed with tests that analyze circulatory function, pupillary responses, or urogenital function.[45,71,84,96] In general, the heart rate and blood pressure responses to standing, tilting, lower-body negative pressure, or to a Valsalva maneuver provide information about the entire sympathetic and parasympathetic autonomic reflex arcs. The afferent limb of both the sympathetic and parasympathetic arcs is the baroreceptor sensory system, whose function cannot be independently tested, although recent work suggests that vasopressin responses may reflect afferent function.[97] At present, dysfunction of the afferent limb is assumed when the total reflex response is abnormal but the efferent limb of the arc is normal. The central and efferent limbs of the circulatory system are tested by noting the heart rate and blood pressure response to stimuli transmitted by afferents other than the baroreceptors. In the case of the sympathetic system, one could assess the blood pressure response to stress, mental concentration, or the application of ice packs. The absence of sweating in response to an increased central temperature or abnormal sensitivity to infused norepinephrine or tyramine are indications of abnormalities in the sympathetic system.

Sympathetic preganglionic and postganglionic lesions could be assessed by measuring resting norepinephrine levels. The central and efferent limbs of the vagus nerve might be tested either by measuring the heart rate response to atropine or by measuring respiratory variations in heart rate.[84,96]

Hyperadrenergic orthostatic hypotension is a term used to describe a type of orthostatic hypotension in which, in contrast to autonomic insufficiency, patients show signs of exaggerated sympathetic activity. Tachycardia and signs of increased vasoconstriction such as pallor and cold extremities are present. This type of orthostatic hypotension has also been termed *sympathicotonic orthostatic hypotension.*[30,58,98] Norepinephrine levels are often high at rest and increase even more with standing.[62] Patients do not usually have signs of autonomic insufficiency unless a combined problem is present. Table 3-4 summarizes the differences between the presenting features of hypoadrenergic and hyperadrenergic orthostatic hypotension. The cause of hyperadrenergic orthostatic hypotension is a decrease in venous return, particularly prominent with standing, that leads to exaggerated compensatory mechanisms. The fall in venous return may be due to hypovolemia, to decreased venous tone or function, or to defective blood volume regulation (see Table 3-2). Causes of hypovolemia include:

> Blood loss
> Gastrointestinal loss (vomiting, diarrhea)
> Diuretics
> Skin loss (sweating)
> Addison's disease
> Third space sequestration
> Renal loss

Decreased venous tone can lead to accentuated venous pooling and orthostatic hypotension. Causes of decreased venous tone or function include:

> Varicose veins
> Absent venous valves
> Drugs (sympatholytics, nitrates)
> Hyperbradykinism
> Heat

Drugs such as prazocin or nitroglycerin, which dilate veins, are common causes. Excessive venous pooling resulting from venous insufficiency due to varicose veins or absent venous valves does occur but is uncommon as an actual cause of symptoms.[99-101] Heat may lead to increased venous pooling and orthostatic hypotension, especially if combined with prolonged standing.[30] A syndrome of hyperbradykinism has been described in five members of a family.[102] This syndrome is associated with excessive arterial and venous vasodilation and is believed to be due to a deficiency in the enzyme that accelerates bradykinin breakdown.

In a number of situations, the regulation of blood pressure is faulty because

Table 3–4. Differences in the Presenting Features of Hypoadrenergic and Hyperadrenergic Orthostatic Hypotension

Presenting Feature	Hypoadrenergic	Hyperadrenergic
Presyncope, syncope	Yes	Yes
Other symptoms (nausea, palpitations)	Sometimes	Yes
Signs (pallor, sweating)	No	Yes
Increased heart rate	No	Exaggerated increase
Other (anhidrosis, impotence incontinence, etc.)	Yes	No
Supine blood pressure	Normal or increased	Normal or decreased
Supine norepinephrine	Normal or decreased	Normal or increased
Standing norepinephrine	No change	Increases

there is defective volume regulation. Causes of defective volume regulation include:

> Pheochromocytoma
> ? Orthostatic dysregulation
> ? Mitral valve prolapse
> ? End-stage renal disease
> Malignant hypertension
> Deconditioning
> Weightlessness

With pheochromocytoma, high levels of circulating catecholamines cause chronic arterial and venous constriction, leading to a decreased blood volume. With standing, little further constriction can occur. Thus, venous pooling results in orthostatic hypotension.[79,103] A similar situation may exist in some patients with malignant hypertension where there is vasoconstriction and extreme volume contraction.[104,105] These patients are likely to be very sensitive to antihypertensive drugs. Recent work suggests that there are several other situations in which blood volume regulation is faulty. Pheochromocytomas that secrete epinephrine may also result in hypotension because of the vasodilating properties of epinephrine.

Patients with end-stage renal disease who are being treated with chronic dialysis often have problems with dialysis-induced hypotension and syncope. Although it is known that these patients may have diffuse autonomic dysfunction, there is no agreement that this is the cause of dialysis-induced hypotension.[106–109] However, it does appear that these patients have more vasoconstriction than similar patients who do not develop hypotension on dialysis. Such patients may have a hyperadrenergic form of hypotension.[110] Indeed, preventing volume loss in these patients during dialysis apparently prevents hypotension.[111]

Patients with mitral valve prolapse may have symptoms of dyspnea, chest pain, palpitations, poor exercise capacity, easy fatigability, and orthostatic hypotension.[112,113] Several studies have demonstrated an apparent autonomic imbalance in these patients.[40,55,113–116] Although some studies suggest that beta-adrenergic hypersensitivity is the underlying problem, other studies have shown that these patients are abnormally vasoconstricted both at rest and with orthostatic stress.[55,116] This is supported by data demonstrating higher-than-normal plasma catecholamines both at rest and with standing and a plasma volume that is lower than normal.[40,55] The cause of the increased sympathetic tone is not known, but the relative hypovolemia may predispose to orthostatic hypotension. This syndrome is remarkably similar to what has been variably termed "soldier's heart" or "neuroregulatory asthenia" in the past.[117]

Prolonged bed rest leads to decreased exercise capacity ("deconditioning") as well as to orthostatic hypotension.[118-122] The causes of the orthostatic hypotension are not entirely understood, but a major factor is probably a decrease in blood volume that reflects decreases in both plasma and red blood cell volume.[121] This conclusion is supported by studies showing that gravitational stresses such as lower-body negative pressure in patients subjected to prolonged bed rest prevent both decreases in blood volume and orthostatic hypotension.[120,123] Such factors as decreases in venous tone or reduced efficiency of the muscular venous pump with prolonged bed rest may also be important in reducing venous return.

A number of illnesses may exhibit both hyperadrenergic and hypoadrenergic orthostatic hypotension. Chronic renal failure has already been discussed. Patients with diabetes mellitus may have orthostatic hypotension due to autonomic neuropathy. However, diabetic patients may also have orthostatic hypotension with exaggerated supine and upright norepinephrine levels, that is, hyperadrenergic orthostatic hypotension.[58] Possible causes of this hyperadrenergic form in diabetes include an increased resistance of blood vessels to norepinephrine and intravascular volume depletion caused by "leaky" capillaries. Some patients with diabetes may have a combination of these two forms of orthostatic hypotension. Furthermore, there is now evidence that insulin itself may alter blood pressure regulation. The administration of insulin, especially in the upright position, may lead to a marked fall in blood pressure and a rise to heart rate that is especially dramatic in diabetics with autonomic neuropathy.[124-126] The possibility of insulin-induced orthostatic hypotension should be considered when diabetics experience hypoglycemic symptoms but have no hypoglycemia. The actual mechanism of insulin-induced hypotension is unknown, but several possibilities have been suggested, including alterations in baroreceptor sensitivity, decreases in plasma volume, and changes in the responsiveness of peripheral blood vessels to norepinephrine.[127-129]

Drug-induced orthostatic hypotension is quite common. Drugs may lead to orthostatic hypotension by decreasing total blood volume (diuretics), by increasing venous pooling (nitrates), or by interfering with the compensatory reflexes that maintain blood pressure with standing (guanethidine, hydralazine, beta-adrenergic blocking agents) (Table 3-5). Many underlying conditions make patients more likely to develop orthostatic hypotension with drugs. These include autonomic insufficiency, volume depletion or decreased venous tone, and abnormal chronotropic responses. The elderly patient is also more sensitive, perhaps because the elderly often have many of these predisposing problems. Diuretics make a patient more sensitive to many of the other drugs listed in Table 3-5. Hot weather, exercise, and alcohol consumption all cause periperal

Table 3–5. Drugs Implicated in Orthostatic Hypotension

Antihypertensives	Antidepressants
Centrally acting	Tricyclic antidepressants
Clonidine	Monoamine oxidase inhibitors
Alpha-methyldopa	Antipsychotics
Guanabenz	Phenothiazines
Ganglionic blockers	Butyrophenones
Trimethaphan	Antiparkinsonian
Postganglionic adrenergic blockers	L-dopa
Guanethidine	L-dopa and carbidopa
Reserpine	Bromocriptine
Alpha adrenergic receptor blockers	Beta adrenergic blockers
Phenoxybenzamine	CNS Depressants
Phentolamine	Morphine
Prazocin	Benzodiazepines
Pargyline	Phenobarbital
Converting enzyme inhibitors	Alcohol
Captopril	Diuretics
Direct vasodilators	Thiazides
Hydralazine	Loop diuretics
Minoxidil	
Diazoxide	
Sodium nitroprusside	
Other vasodilators	
Nitrates	
Calcium channel blockers	

asodilation and may predispose to orthostatic hypotension. Other factors that lead to decreased venous return, such as prolonged quiet standing or a Valsalva manueuver during micturition or defecation, may increase susceptibility to postural hypotension.[130]

Several drugs are particularly likely to cause orthostatic hypotension. These include guanethidine, pargyline, prazosin, antiparkinsonian drugs, antipsychotic and antidepressant drugs, and loop diuretics. Guanethidine may lead to hypotension with standing or with exercise.[131] Prazosin is most likely to cause orthostatic hypotension after the first dose, particularly in patients with a diminished intravascular volume.[131] The antipsychotic and antidepressant drugs commonly lead to orthostatic hypotension due to a combination of CNS effects and alpha-adrenergic blockade.[132,133] The antiparkinsonian drugs L-dopa, bromocriptine, and, particularly, L-dopa plus carbidopa may all reduce standing blood pressure, but the mechanism is not well understood.[132] In patients with congestive heart failure, captopril may lead to postural hypotension.[134]

VASOVAGAL SYNCOPE. Vasovagal syncope (vasodepressor syncope, the common faint) most often occurs in normal people but may also occur in subjects with heart disease.[46,135] It is usually precipitated by emotionally stressful or painful situations, such as venipuncture, surgical manipulation, phlebotomy, or the sight of blood. These stimuli seem to provoke vasovagal reactions more readily in association with fatigue, hunger, or sleep-deprivation, and in hot, crowded environments. Vasovagal syncope usually occurs when the subject is standing, though, rarely, it may occur in a supine patient.[136] Premonitory signs and symptoms are almost always present and begin with pallor and sweating. Nausea, epigastric discomfort, yawning, sighing, hyperventilation, and mydriasis follow shortly thereafter. Blurred vision, impaired hearing, and a feeling of decreased awareness appear just before the loss of postural tone and unconsciousness.[79,135] It is interesting that subjects do not describe these premonitory feelings as unpleasant, nor do they report feelings of fear or apprehension.[137] The presyncopal period may last from a few seconds to several minutes. Syncope can be prevented if the subject lies down. Once syncope occurs, consciousness is regained almost immediately if the subject is laid flat with the legs elevated. The pallor, nausea, and weakness persist for several minutes, however, and presyncope or syncope may recur if the subject is allowed to stand too soon after the initial vasovagal episode.

Partial understanding of the vasovagal reaction came to John Hunter in 1793 while he was performing a therapeutic phlebotomy. When the patient fainted, he noted that "the colour of the blood that came from the vein was a fine scarlet."[138] This description of the arterialization of venous blood made it clear that vasodilation was an important part of vasovagal syncope. Despite many subsequent studies, we still do not fully understand the actual triggering mechanisms, though the sequence of hemodynamic events is fairly clear.[139–145]

Much of the research on vasovagal syncope has been done in subjects undergoing head-up tilt or lower-body negative pressure, both of which simulate the venous pooling seen with standing. Nitrates, venesection, and occlusion thigh cuffs have also been used. A decreased effective circulating blood volume is the common factor in all these maneuvers. However, many episodes of vasovagal syncope are precipitated by fear, pain, or emotional trauma. While the circulatory changes may not be identical to those precipitated by decreased effective blood volume, the vasovagal reactions appear so similar that it is assumed that a similar hemodynamic pattern occurs regardless of the precipitant.

The vasovagal reaction has been separated into two phases.[139–141] The early phase is characterized by a gradual fall in arterial pressure, with little change in cardiac output or forearm venous tone. Changes in heart rate are variable. In the second phase, there is a sudden decrease in heart rate and a profound decrease in blood pressure. Central venous pressure and cardiac output drop abruptly. The cause of the decreasing arterial pressure in the early phase is unknown. Mild peripheral vasodilation could explain this fall in blood pressure, though early vasodilation is not seen in all studies.[139] Later events result from a sudden decrease in skeletal muscle vascular resistance. Muscle blood flow increases, but muscle oxygen utilization is unchanged. Thus, venous blood turns "scarlet." While relative bradycardia occurs simultaneously with the fall in blood pressure, it is not the major factor: preventing the bradycardia with atropine does not restore either the fall in arterial pressure or consciousness.[141,144] As a result of the severe fall in arterial pressure, renal, mesenteric, and cerebral blood flows decrease. It is not known why the fall in arterial pressure does not provoke a reflex increase in heart rate and cardiac output.

During this later phase of a vasovagal episode, the normal rise in plasma renin is blunted, presumably decreasing angiotensin-mediated vasoconstriction.[46] The sudden fall in resistance in the muscle beds may be mediated by intracardiac receptors, particularly those in the left ventricle.[79,146] Thus, hypotension might lead to increased sympathetic stimulation of the heart, increased myocardial wall tension, and stimulation of the left ventricular (LV) receptors, triggering reflex vasodilation.[35,79] Another possible cause of skeletal muscle vasodilation is stimulation of efferent cholinergic vasodilator fibers to skeletal muscle arterioles.[79] Although this type of vasodilation can be triggered by emotion, its physiologic significance in humans is unknown.[35,147] The oliguria that lasts for up to 90 minutes after a vasovagal reaction appears to be mediated by release of arginine vasopressin.[148] An intriguing study suggests that the vasopressin might also have a role in the pallor and nausea of vasovagal syncope.[149]

Episodes like vagovagal syncope may be seen in patients with aortic stenosis, primary pulmonary hypertension, and other forms of cardiovascular disease. Thus, it should not be assumed that the patient presenting with a vasovagal reaction does not have serious underlying disease.

CAROTID SINUS HYPERSENSITIVITY. Since 1799, pressure over the carotid artery has been known to induce cardiac slowing.[150] The reflex was thought to be due to pressure on the vagus nerve until Hering demonstrated, in 1920, that it was due to pressure on the carotid sinus.[150] Each carotid sinus is a fusiform dilation of the terminal common carotid and the root of the internal carotid artery. Stretch receptors (mechanoreceptors) located in the adventitia of the carotid sinus are stimulated by stretching or distention.[35] A nerve (the carotid sinus nerve) from these receptors joins the glossopharyngeal nerve and conducts impulses to the medullary vasomotor and cardioinhibitory centers. The efferent arc of the carotid sinus reflex is made up of the vagal and cervical sympathetic nerves. The carotid sinus receptors, together with similar receptors in the aortic arch, make up the arterial baroreceptors. An increase in arterial pressure leads to stretching of the baroreceptors and causes an increase in afferent nerve activity, triggering a reflex decrease in heart rate, peripheral vascular resistance, and myocardial contractility. The effects result from decreased sympathetic vasoconstrictor activity and increased parasympathetic activity to the heart. Activation of sympathetic vasodilator pathways plays a much smaller role.[35] Pressure over either carotid sinus simulates increased baroreceptor stretch and may result in bradycardia or decreased blood pressure. When the resultant hypotension leads to symptoms of dizziness, presyncope, or syncope, it is termed the *hypersensitive carotid sinus syndrome* or *carotid sinus syncope*. Three forms of this syndrome are described: cardioinhibitory, vasodepressor, and cerebral.[151] The cardioinhibitory (vagal) type is the most common and is manifested by symptoms of hypotension due to sinus bradycardia, sinus arrest, or atrioventricular (AV) block. Atrial conduction defects with alterations in amplitude or morphology of the P wave may also be seen on the ECG.[150] The cardioinhibitory form of the carotid sinus syndrome can be prevented by atropine. The vasodepressor form of the carotid sinus syndrome consists of a fall in systemic vascular resistance leading to hypotension without bradyarrhythmias. It can be prevented by epinephrine but not by atropine.[151] Patients may have a combination of the cardioinhibitory and vasodepressor forms. The cerebral form of the carotid sinus syndrome is manifested by a sudden loss of consciousness unassociated with changes in heart rate or blood pressure when pressure is applied to the carotid sinus. The pathophysiology of the cerebral form is unclear and its actual existence has been questioned, with the suggestion that it may represent obstruction of carotid blood flow by carotid sinus pressure.[150,152]

Carotid sinus syncope is uncommon in patients under 30 years of age and increases in frequency with age. Patients may report symptoms of presyncope or syncope with activities that cause pressure over the carotid sinus, such as shaving or wearing a tight collar or extreme movements of the neck, such as those entailed in driving a car in reverse.[151,153] Clear precipitating factors are not always present.[152] Manual pressure over the carotid sinus may confirm or suggest the diagnosis of carotid sinus syncope. The patient should be supine, with the head in a neutral position. If auscultation over the carotids demonstrates a bruit or bruits, manual carotid sinus stimulation should not be performed.[150] The carotid sinus is found 2 cm to 3 cm below the angle of the jaw posterior to the anterior belly of the sternocleidomastoid muscle. To avoid a sudden decrease in cerebral blood flow, pressure should never be applied over both carotid arteries simultaneously. Pressure should be gentle initially and should last for only a few seconds, since the decrease in blood flow is related to the intensity of the pressure.[151] Pressure may then be increased but should not last for more than 20 seconds. To be sure that the carotid blood flow is not occluded, one may palpate the ipsilateral superficial temporal artery.[150] Heart rate and blood pressure should be monitored carefully. The largest falls in heart rate and blood pressure occur immediately after carotid sinus pressure is applied.[151] There is a wide range of responses to carotid sinus pressure. Both cardioinhibitory and vasodepressor responses are increased in frequency and magnitude in men; with increasing age; in patients with hypertension, atherosclerosis, or diabetes; and in patients with scars, enlarged lymph nodes, or tumors close to or involving the carotid sinus.[150–152,154–156] In healthy young people, carotid sinus pressure often leads to a fall in blood pressure of less than 10 mm Hg, with heart rate decreasing only a few beats.[150,151,156] In healthy elderly subjects, carotid sinus pressure may lead to a fall in systolic arterial pressure of 20 mm Hg to 40 mm Hg. Right and left carotid sinuses should be tested separately, since the responses may be very different.[150,155,156] Vasodilation tends to persist longer than the decreased heart rate.[151] When the cardioinhibitory form of carotid sinus hypersensitivity is present, carotid sinus stimulation should be repeated after atropine is given. If hypotension results from carotid sinus stimulation following atropine, a vasodepressor component is present. Both ventricular asystole for 3 seconds or more and a fall in systolic arterial pressure of greater than 50 mm Hg are considered definitely abnormal responses to carotid sinus pressure.[152] However, many patients with this degree of carotid sinus hypersensitivity may not have carotid sinus syncope.[152,157] Furthermore, carotid sinus hypersensitivity is so common in the elderly that its presence in an elderly patient with syncope should not prevent a careful search for other causes of syncope. Indeed, it has been estimated that in elderly patients with carotid sinus hypersensitivity and syncope, syncope is caused by the hypersensitive carotid sinus in only about one-third of the patients.[158] Ambulatory ECG monitoring may often help in determining if carotid sinus hypersensitivity is actually causing symptoms.

Complications with carotid sinus pressure are very rare, but cardiac standstill and strokes do occur. They are much more common in elderly hypertensive patients with cerebral vascular disease.[150] Atropine, epinephrine, and norepinephrine should be readily available. Digoxin, beta-adrenergic blockers, and alpha-methyldopa plus digoxin have all been reported to accentuate the carotid sinus response and lead to carotid sinus syncope.[157]

If a tumor or enlarged lymph node is causing carotid sinus syncope, surgical removal may be curative. If no anatomical cause is found and symptoms persist after the patient has been instructed to avoid stimulation of the carotid sinus, several forms of therapy are available. With the cardioinhibitory form, permanent ventricular pacing often prevents symptoms. When there is a major vasodepressor component, treatment is more difficult and is usually directed toward blood volume expansion, pharmacologic vasoconstriction or denervation, or surgical resection of the carotid sinus.[79]

AFFERENT NERVE STIMULATION.   Conditions in which afferent nerve stimulation may cause syncope include:

> Glossopharyngeal neuralgia
> Deglutition (swallow) syncope
> Vertiginous syncope
> Micturition syncope
> Defecation syncope
> Diver's syncope

Stimulation, particularly painful stimulation, of endobronchial, pharyngeal, laryngeal, or esophageal mucosal linings may occasionally precipitate hypotension and syncope. Hypotension and syncope may also occur when the peritoneum or pleura are stimulated by paracentesis or thoracentesis. Afferent impulses from these areas trigger a vagal response with resultant sinus bradycardia, sinus arrest, or heart block. This reflex response has been described in patients with *glossopharyngeal neuralgia*.[159,160] A similar reaction has been described during swallowing in some patients with esophageal tumors, diverticulae, spasm, or stenosis, and is called *deglutition* or *swallow syncope*.[161-164] In one patient, attacks could be reproduced by inflating a balloon at the level of an esophageal diverticulum. Esophageal endoscopy and bronchosocopy may cause similar reactions. Atropine or local anesthesia may prevent some of them. Phenytoin may improve glossopharyngeal neuralgia and prevent syncopal spells. Correction of the esophageal problem may also prevent attacks. In one patient, dilation of an esophageal stenosis eliminated the episodes. The same reflex response is very likely the cause of the syncope that occasionally follows severe vertigo.

Micturition syncope probably results, at least in part, from a similar reflex.[165-167] The syndrome typically occurs in adult men with nocturia, often after alcohol consumption. Syncope occurs during or immediately after voiding. Several factors are probably involved in micturition syncope, including vasodilation brought on by both a warm bed and alcohol. Straining to start the urinary stream may simulate the Valsalva maneuver. All of these factors, which decrease venous return, plus sudden emptying of a distended bladder may lead to reflex bradycardia and hypotension. *Defecation syncope* probably results from similar mechanisms in elderly subjects.[168]

Syncope that occurs among divers is poorly understood. When afferent nerves in the trigeminal nerve distribution or nasal mucosa are stimulated by cold water or smelling salts, reflex vasoconstriction and marked bradycardia may occur.[35] It has been speculated that this "diving reflex" as well as hypoxia and other unknown factors may be involved.[135]

PRIMARY CARDIAC ABNORMALITY

ARRHYTHMIA-INDUCED SYNCOPE AND STOKES–ADAMS DISEASE.   Syncope commonly results from a sudden decrease in cardiac output due to a rapid change in heart rate or rhythm. These attacks have been termed *Stokes–Adams attacks* after the researchers who correctly described their etiology.[169] Although the term was originally applied to patients with AV block, it is sometimes used to refer to episodes of cerebral ischemia resulting from any arrhythmia. However, the term Stokes–Adams syndrome (or Stokes–Adams disease) can most appropriately be applied to cases of syncope due to high-grade AV block and the term *arrhythmia-induced syncope* should be used for cases of syncope caused by arrhythmias.[170]

A fall in cardiac output sufficient to cause syncope may be the result of bradycardia, tachycardia, or a combination of the two. Following is a list of arrhythmias often implicated in syncope:

TACHYARRHYTHMIAS
   Ventricular fibrillation or flutter
   Ventricular tachycardia
   Supraventricular tachycardia
      Paroxysmal atrial or junctional tachycardia
      Atrial fibrillation with rapid ventricular response
      Atrial flutter with rapid ventricular response

BRADYARRHYTHMIAS
   Sinus arrest
   Sinus exit block
   Sinus bradycardia
   AV block
      Proximal (AV node)
      Distal (His–Purkinje system)

PACEMAKER FAILURE

In normal, healthy people, only extreme changes in heart rate will lead to syncope. However, less severe changes in heart rate may lead to syncope in patients already compromised by underlying heart disease, cerebrovascular disease, or volume depletion. Syncope due to either bradyarrhythmias or tachy-arrhythmias is much more likely in an upright patient but may occur in a supine patient. Several ways in which cardiac arrhythmias affect cardiac output are listed below:

> Heart rate
> > Ventricular filling
> > Contractility effects (Bowditch)
> > Myocardial oxygen consumption
>
> Loss of AV synchrony
> > Atrial booster pumps
> > Closure of AV valves
> > AV valve regurgitation
> > Cannon A waves
>
> Loss of ventricular synchrony
> > Myocardial performance
> > Mitral regurgitation
>
> Effects on circulatory reflexes
> > Arterial baroreceptors
> > Atrial and ventricular "low pressure" baroreceptors
>
> Effects on regional organ flow
> > Coronary
> > Cerebral
> > Renal
> > Mesenteric

Changes in heart rate are the most obvious result of arrhythmias or conduction disease. Normally, there is a reciprocal relationship between stroke volume and heart rate so that cardiac output is maintained over a wide range of heart rates. As heart rate falls, ventricular filling increases and stroke volume is increased by the Frank–Starling mechanism.[171] Eventually, even in the normal heart, there is a point at which stroke volume can no longer increase. Once this point is reached, continued slowing of the heart rate will result in a falling cardiac output. Patients with intrinsic heart disease may have less ability to increase stroke volume and thus may have less tolerance for slow heart rates. As heart rate increases, diastole is shortened more than systole. In normal subjects, fortunately, most ventricular filling occurs early in diastole, and the rapid filling phase is not affected until the heart rate exceeds about 160 beats per minute.[172] Above this rate, stroke volume declines more than heart rate increases, and cardiac output falls. In patients in whom filling of the ventricles is more prolonged during diastole (*e.g.*, in patients with mitral stenosis), ven-tricular filling, and thus cardiac output, will be compromised at much lower heart rates.[173] Two other independent effects of heart rate must be considered. The first, the *treppe* phenomenon of Bowditch, describes the positive inotropic effect of increasing heart rate, an effect which is probably due to sustained mobilization of calcium during the tachycardia.[174] The second effect is that of tachycardia on myocardial oxygen consumption. For the same cardiac output per minute, the rapidly beating heart requires more oxygen than a heart beating more slowly. This generally does not present any difficulties unless coronary flow is restricted by such factors as coronary atherosclerosis. If ischemia results, myocardial function and cardiac output may be further compromised.

AV synchrony provides several hemodynamic benefits, including the atrial contribution to ventricular filling ("the booster pump"), a contribution to normal AV valve closure, and the prevention of mitral or tricuspid regurgitation in early systole. Atrial systole benefits cardiac output most when the P–R interval is between 0.1 and 0.2 seconds.[175] In the normal resting heart, atrial contraction adds 5% to 15% to cardiac output, and in diseased hearts atrial contraction may increase cardiac output even more.[176-178] Atrial contraction is particularly important in poorly compliant ventricles, such as may occur with aortic stenosis, cardiac hypertrophy, or acute myocardial infarction. In patients with mitral stenosis and atrial fibrillation, the loss of atrial contraction is particularly deleterious with abbreviation of ventricular filling brought on by a rapid heart rate. Atrial contraction can add significantly to ventricular filling without large increases in mean left atrial pressure. Since dyspnea and left atrial pressure are closely related, the potential benefit on symptomatology is obvious.[179] A properly timed atrial contraction contributes to the normal closure of the AV valves and helps prevent mild mitral and tricuspid regurgitation.[172] These contributions are minor in comparison to the atrial "booster pump" function. When AV synchrony is lost but atrial activity remains, the atria contract against closed AV valves. This results in *cannon A waves* in the left atria and pulmonary veins as well as in the right atria and great veins. If atrial activity is frequent, as in ventricular tachycardia with retrograde atrial activation, ventricular filling may be decreased because of a reverse flow of blood in the great veins limiting ventricular filling.[180] Further, it is conceivable that these cannon A waves significantly increase mean left atrial pressure, resulting in dyspnea.

Ventricular asynchrony occurs whenever conduction through the ventricles is altered. This may result from a primary ventricular arrhythmia, aberrant conduction, abnormal His–Purkinje system conduction, or artificial pacing. Normally, ventricular contraction moves from the apex of the heart and inflow tract and papillary muscles to the outflow tract.[180] With ventricular asynchrony there is a slower rate of rise of LV pressure and a less effective cardiac performance.[181-183] Ventricular ejection becomes more efficient as conduction becomes more normal, and less efficient as conduction becomes more abnormal.[181] The diminished ventricular performance is probably primarily due to uncoordinated ventricular contraction with some AV valve regurgitation. If the papillary muscles are activated late rather than early, their normal anchoring function for the AV valves is lost, and regurgitation may occur.[184] Thus, ventricular tachycardias of similar rates but different origins may have different hemodynamic effects. Cardiac performance, however, is affected much less by the loss of ventricular synchrony than by the loss of AV synchrony.[185]

It seems likely that arrhythmias affect peripheral circulatory reflexes both by changes in atrial and ventricular volumes and pressures and by the associated changes in arterial pressure. Activation of low-pressure baroreceptors in the atria may be influenced by high atrial pressures. Indeed, it has been postulated that the low-pressure baroreceptors are responsible for the polyuria described during paroxysmal tachycardia.[186-188]

Blood flow in the regional organs is affected by many factors, including arterial pressure, reflex mechanisms, circulating hormones, local disease, and the degree of autoregulation in each local vascular bed. In normal subjects, cerebral blood flow is autoregulated over a wide range of arterial pressure. The effects of arrhythmia will be primarily due to the resultant arterial pressure.[189] Coronary blood flow is also autoregulated, but the majority of LV flow occurs during diastole. Since tachyarrhythmias limit diastole, coronary blood flow may be compromised, particularly as myocardial oxygen requirements are increased by the tachycardia.[190] This is particularly important in patients with coronary obstruction. Flow in renal and mesenteric beds is diminished during tachyarrhythmias as a result of both the actual fall in cardiac output and the degree of compensatory response to this fall.[191] Obviously, local disease, such as atherosclerosis, is likely to exaggerate the effects of arrhythmias on blood flow to regional organs.

Arrhythmias that frequently result in syncope were listed earlier in this chapter. Ventricular fibrillation and flutter always result in severe hemodynamic compromise. However, these arrhythmias are very uncommon causes of syncope, since spontaneous reversion is rare in humans. Ventricular tachycardia leads to syncope much more commonly than does supraventricular tachycardia for the reasons already discussed and because patients with ventricular tachycardia often have more serious underlying heart disease. Supraventricular tachycardias lead to syncope only if the rate is very fast or if the patient has a compromised cardiovascular system. Patients with accessory conduction pathways (Wolff–Parkinson–White or Lown–Ganong–Levine syndrome) are particularly likely to have very rapid supraventricular tachycardias.[192,193] Some patients with paroxysms of tachycardia will have a period of sinus arrest following reversion of the arrhythmia. In some patients, this period of bradycardia may actually cause the syncope. Ventricular tachycardia and fibrillation are usually associated with significant underlying heart disease. An unusual form of ventricular tachycardia, *torsades de pointes,* may be associated with underlying heart disease or other precipitating factors.[194] This arrhythmia is often the cause of quinidine-induced syncope.[195] It is important to recognize that antiarrhythmic drugs may precipitate both *torsades de pointes* and the more common form of ventricular tachycardia. A detailed discussion of the etiology of ventricular tachycardia is provided elsewhere.[196,197]

Bradyarrhythmias resulting in syncope are a result of either the sick sinus syndrome or AV block. The sick sinus syndrome refers to a disease of the sinus node (and often the AV node) that may present in one of several ways: persistent, severe, sinus bradycardia; sinus arrest; sinoatrial block; atrial fibrillation with a slow ventricular response; and the brady–tachy syndrome, in which tachycardias are followed by sinoatrial bradycardias.[198,199] Drugs that may exacerbate the sick sinus syndrome include:

Digitalis glycosides
Antiarrhythmic drugs (quinidine, procainamide, disopyramide)
Beta-adrenergic blocking drugs
Calcium channel blocking drugs (verapamil, diltiazem)
Antihypertensive drugs (alpha-methyldopa, clonidine, reserpine, guaneth-
    idine)
Miscellaneous (lithium, phenytoin)[198,200,201]

AV block can be divided into proximal (AV nodal) or distal (His–Purkinje) system disease. Presyncope and syncope are caused less often by proximal AV block than by distal complete block because the junctional escape rhythm is usually faster and more reliable than the corresponding ventricular escape rhythm seen with distal conduction disease. Drugs may also effect both proximal and distal AV conduction.

If a syncopal spell due to a paroxysmal arrhythmia or conduction defect was not witnessed, a proper diagnosis may not be easy to make. Ambulatory ECG monitoring is often helpful in detecting paroxysmal arrhythmias or conduction defects, but a careful correlation of symptoms to arrhythmia is essential. Particularly in older people, episodes of asymptomatic sinus bradycardia and supraventricular and ventricular arrhythmias are very common.[202] The importance of correlating symptoms with arrhythmias is also clear in patients with conduction disease. When bifascicular or trifascicular block is discovered in a patient with syncope, it might be assumed that transient AV block is the cause of the syncope. However, in studies of patients with heart block and syncope, heart block was actually responsible for the syncope in only 20% of cases.[203,204] Finally, when chest pain precedes syncopal events, coronary artery spasm should be considered. In this syndrome, unlike typical angina, syncope frequently results from both brady- and tachyarrhythmias.[205]

CARDIAC OBSTRUCTION OR DYSFUNCTION. When cardiac obstruction or myocardial dysfunction is severe, cardiac output is relatively fixed and cannot adequately increase with stress. During exercise, metabolic products accumulate in muscle and cause vasodilation. If cardiac output cannot increase, arterial pressure will fall. Thus, exertional hypotension and syncope are often characteristic of cardiac obstruction. However, obstruction to flow is not the only pathophysiologic mechanism of syncope. Stimulation of cardiovascular reflexes as well as arrhythmias often play an important role. Exertional syncope is characteristic of these diseases, but it is not always present. Causes of cardiac obstruction or myocardial dysfunction leading to syncope include:

Aortic stenosis
Prosthetic valve dysfunction
Idiopathic hypertrophic cardiomyopathy
Myocardial infarction
Atrial myxoma
Cardiac tamponade
Aortic dissection
Acute pulmonary embolism

Primary pulmonary hypertension
Pulmonary stenosis
Tetrology of Fallot
Eisenmenger's syndrome

Syncope is a grave symptom in aortic stenosis and usually indicates severe obstruction. Once patients with aortic stenosis present with syncope, the average duration of survival is only 3 years.[206] Syncope in aortic stenosis often follows exertion.[207-209] With exercise, LV intracavitary pressure rises to very high levels, activating mechanoreceptors in nonexercising muscle, which results in a withdrawal of sympathetic tone, vasodilation, and a fall in arterial pressure.[208,210] Following corrective surgery in these patients, forearm vascular resistance increases with exercise as it does in normal people.[208] Arrhythmias may follow vasodilation and prolong the episode of unconsciousness.[209] Several other potential mechanisms for syncope exist in aortic stenosis. Severe elevation of LV end-diastolic pressure could lead to subendocardial ischemia, resulting in diminished LV function or arrhythmia. Arrhythmias may occur spontaneously in aortic stenosis. Less commonly, calcium may be deposited in the conduction system, resulting in heart block. When syncope is due to aortic stenosis, aortic valve replacement is usually indicated.

Syncope may result from prosthetic valve dysfunction. Chronic obstruction of an aortic valve by a thrombus or fibrous ingrowth may cause syncope similar to that seen in aortic stenosis. More acute dysfunction of a mitral or aortic valve may lead to a sudden severe fall in cardiac output.

Syncope occurs in 15% to 30% of patients with *idiopathic hypertrophic cardiomyopathy.*[211,212] Syncope may not be as ominous a sign in this disease as in aortic stenosis, and some patients with this disease have a history of syncope over many years.[212,213] Other studies suggest that syncope may still indicate a poor prognosis.[214] Idiopathic hypertrophic cardiomyopathy is a disease of unknown etiology characterized by a nondilated hypertrophied left ventricle. Obstruction to outflow often occurs in the subaortic area and is worsened by a decrease in cardiac volume or an increase in cardiac contractility. Thus, diuretics, vasodilators, and positive inotropic agents may worsen the LV obstruction.[215] While outflow tract obstruction has long been considered the important pathophysiologic property of this disease, others would argue that the obstruction to LV inflow caused by the effects of hypertrophy on LV compliance is of critical importance.[216] The actual cause of syncope in most patients is not known. Since exertional syncope is often seen in this disease, it is conceivable that exercise leads to gradually increasing obstruction to LV outflow because of the increased contractility caused by high levels of sympathetic stimulation. Syncope might result from reflex vasodilation, as already described for aortic stenosis, or just from progressive decreases in cardiac output. Impaired ventricular filling due to catecholamine-induced decreases in ventricular compliance might have the same effect. That syncope can be caused by either of these mechanisms, rather than by arrhythmia, is supported by a report of sinus tachycardia occurring during an episode of syncope in a patient with hypertrophic cardiomyopathy.[217] However, the potential importance of arrhythmias in this disease cannot be ignored, since it is associated with a high incidence of supraventricular and ventricular arrhythmias.[218,219] In addition, asystole, heart block, and an accessory pathway resulting in rapid AV conduction and eventual ventricular fibrillation have all been reported in hypertrophic cardiomyopathy.[220-222]

Syncope is not a common presenting feature of myocardial infarction in general but must be considered as part of the differential diagnosis in the elderly.[203] Transient arrhythmias, heart block, or sudden decreases in myocardial function may all be causes. Mechanoreceptors in a dyskinetic inferior wall might be stimulated, with resultant vasodilation and hypotension.[223]

Left atrial myxomas are often suspended from a stalk attached to the interatrial septum. Sudden changes in posture may cause the myxoma to move into the mitral valve orifice and obstruct left ventricular filling.[224] A similar situation may occur with a large thrombus. A careful history of initiation of syncope by specific postures and careful auscultation for a "tumor plop" may aid in the diagnosis, which can be confirmed by echocardiography.

In cardiac tamponade, the main cause of syncope is probably the severely limited filling of the left ventricle. It is conceivable that the high venous pressures combined with low arterial pressure may also lead to a diminished cerebral perfusion pressure. Syncope in acute aortic dissection seems to be most often caused by tamponade.[225]

Syncope may be a presenting feature of acute pulmonary embolus.[226,227] Among patients with pulmonary embolus, hypotension, hypoxemia, greater than 50% obstruction of the pulmonary circulation, and right heart failure are much more common in those who experience syncope.[226,227] Thus, along with hypoxemia, sudden obstruction to RV outflow appears to be a major cause. However, sudden distention of the pulmonary artery or right ventricle may also lead to a reflex vagal activation and resultant bradycardia.[228]

Effort-related syncope in a young woman should suggest primary pulmonary hypertension. In fact, effort syncope may be the presenting symptom of this disease.[229] Several mechanisms are possible. Inability to increase cardiac output in the face of the increased peripheral metabolic activity and consequent vasodilation in muscle is a possible cause. Because some patients have been observed to have an absent pulse during these episodes, it has been postulated that high pressures in the right ventricle or pulmonary artery lead to reflex vagal activation and sympathetic withdrawal.[152] Hypoxemia may also be a contributing factor. Syncope occurs in pulmonary stenosis, though less commonly than in primary pulmonary hypertension.[230] The mechanisms are likely to be similar to those described for primary pulmonary hypertension.

Syncope may occur in congenital heart defects with right-to-left shunts and either pulmonic stenosis or pulmonary hypertension. The most common of these defects is tetralogy of Fallot.[231] The spells are called *cyanotic hypoxic spells*. In tetralogy, extended episodes of crying, feeding, or exercise may lead to these spells. In the past, increased infundibular spasm with resultant increased right-to-left shunt was felt to be responsible.[232] More recent data suggests that sudden increases in cardiac output brought on by crying or exercise lead to increases in the right-to-left shunt, resulting in increased hypoxemia and hypercarbia. A particularly sensitive respiratory center further provokes hyperpnea in response to these metabolic stimuli by increasing cardiac output and venous return and further increasing the right-to-left shunt and the hypoxemia.[233] In addition, in all of these defects, exercise may lead to peripheral vasodilation, which increases the right-to-left shunt, resulting in more severe hypoxemia.

OBSTRUCTION TO VENOUS RETURN. Sudden decreases in venous return cause syncope by a reduction in cardiac output. Three situations deserve comment. *Cough syncope* (tussive syncope) usually occurs in stocky, middle-aged men with chronic bronchitis. A paroxysm of coughing results in a marked increase in intrathoracic pressure and a decrease in venous return.[234] However, several other factors play at least as important a role. Large increases in cerebrospinal fluid pressure decrease cerebral perfusion pressure, compromising cerebral blood flow.[235] Stimulation of pulmonary receptors may lead to reflex vasodilation and bradycardia and, in rare cases, to heart block.[236] Increased cerebrovascular resistance due to hypocapnia may also play a role. Rarely, Valsalva maneuvers can cause syncope in competitive weight lifting, strenuous stretching, or straining at stool. School children may voluntarily cause syncope by use of the Valsalva maneuver. The child squats and hyperventilates then suddenly stands and performs a Valsalva maneuver. Pregnant women may occasionally have a peculiar form of syncope that occurs while lying supine and is relieved by rolling to one side. The *supine hypotensive syndrome of pregnancy* results when the large uterus compresses the inferior vena cava, obstructing venous return.[237] Rolling to one side relieves the obstruction.

Decreased Cerebral Perfusion Pressure: Increased Venous or Intracranial Pressure

Although there is experimental evidence that increases in venous or intracranial pressure may lead to a decrease in cerebral perfusion pressure, only rare clinical correlates are well described. Cough syncope, as already discussed, is caused in large part by the high intracranial pressures generated with coughing. Cerebral perfusion pressure and thus cerebral blood flow are compromised.[234] Very rarely, colloid cysts of the third ventricle intermittently obstruct that cavity, with an increase in intracranial pressure, a decrease in cerebral perfusion pressure, and syncope. One might keep this potential mechanism for syncope in mind for other diseases in which there are marked increases in intracranial pressure (tumors, hematomas, and other such conditions) or for diseases where central venous pressure is very high and arterial pressure is low (cardiac tamponade, congestive heart failure). It is possible that cerebral perfusion pressure is barely adequate in these diseases, and any transient minor change in cardiac output might lead to syncope.

Increased Cerebral Vascular Resistance

When cerebral vascular resistance is increased, there is a fall in cerebral blood flow. Increased cerebral vascular resistance may result from a fixed obstruction or from compression of intracranial or extracranial vessels. Causes of syncope due to increased cerebral vascular resistance include:

Vascular disease
  Intracranial
    Atherosclerosis
    Vasospasm
  Extracranial
    Takayasu's arteritis
    Subclavian steal
    Klippel–Feil syndrome
Cerebral emboli
Hyperventilation
Migraine

Typical intracranial atherosclerosis may lead to transient ischemic attacks (TIAs) of either the cerebral or vertebral basilar circulation. Syncope is rare in TIAs involving the carotid circulation but common when atherosclerotic disease involves the vertebrobasilar system. It is postulated that the medullary arousal center may be affected. Vertebrobasilar TIAs are accompanied by other vertebrobasilar signs such as vertigo, diplopia, dysarthria, and ataxia.

Cerebral vasospasm may lead to a marked increase in cerebral vascular resistance and a fall in cerebral blood flow. Severe cerebral vasospasm occurs in malignant hypertension but usually results in a generalized disorder of cerebral function rather than in syncope.

Obstruction of extracranial vessels may also lead to a syncope. Syncope is common in Takayasu's arteritis, in which large intrathoracic arteries are obstructed.[238] Cerebral blood flow may fall precipitously when peripheral vascular resistance in other areas falls, as occurs with exercise. A similar problem is the *subclavian steal syndrome.* The subclavian artery is severely involved by atherosclerosis distal to the takeoff of the carotid artery but proximal to the origin of the vertebral artery. With arm exercise, peripheral resistance in the arm falls, causing blood to flow through the circle of Willis and retrograde through the vertebral artery into the subclavian artery.[234,239] Along with a history of syncope induced by upper-extremity exercise, subclavian bruits and unequal arm blood pressures are the key to this diagnosis.[240]

Rarely, cervical spondylosis, or the Klippel–Feil syndrome, may be severe enough to lead to compression of the vertebral arteries. Usually syncope occurs with severe rotation or hyperextension of the neck and may mimic carotid sinus hypersensitivity. Syncope is often preceded by vertigo, nausea and vomiting, and scotomas.[61]

Cerebral emboli lead to TIAs and strokes but rarely to syncope. Causes of cerebral emboli are listed below:

Atherosclerotic plaques
Intracardiac thrombus
Thrombi from prosthetic valves
Endocarditis
Mitral valve prolapse
Calcified valves
Paradoxical emboli

Hyperventilation often causes a feeling of faintness but only very rarely leads to syncope. Hyperventilation, however, may precipitate syncope when cerebral oxygenation is already compromised. Hyperventilation usually is initiated by anxiety.[241] It often begins insidiously with a gradual, almost imperceptible, increase in the rate and depth of respiration. Hypocapnia and respiratory alkalosis ensue. Cerebral blood flow may fall by as much as 40% due to the hypocapnia-induced increase in cerebral vascular resistance. Respiratory alkalosis results in a leftward shift of the oxyhemoglobin dissociation curve, and less oxygen is released to the tissues at any given oxygen tension.[242] The respiratory alkalosis reduces ionized calcium, leading to paresthesias and carpopedal spasm. Initially, patients complain of circumoral and extremity paresthesias, a feeling of suffocation, and chest tightness. These symptoms may last for as long as 30 minutes. Relief may be obtained by relieving anxiety or by having the patient breathe into a paper bag, thus increasing P_aCO_2 and lowering cerebral vascular resistance. Symptoms of the hyperventilation syndrome may be reproduced by having the patient voluntarily hyperventilate.

Syncope associated with migraine headaches is rare and has been described primarily in adolescent girls. It is suggested that vasospasm in the basal arterial system leads to decreased cerebral blood flow and syncope.[243] No hemodynamic changes are evident, but subjects usually awake with a severe occipital headache.

QUALITATIVE DECREASE IN CEREBRAL BLOOD FLOW

Hypoxemia and Hypoglycemia

Sudden transient hypoxemia severe enough to produce syncope is an unusual event. The exceptions are patients with congenital heart disease who have right-to-left shunts with either severe pulmonary hypertension or pulmonary stenosis. Any cause of increased cardiac output may lead to exaggerated right-to-left shunting, increased hypoxemia, and syncope. Exercise is a particular problem because the decreased systemic vascular resistance increases right-to-left shunting to an even greater degree. Although chronic hypoxemia alone does not often cause syncope, it is probably a predisposing factor in many cases. Hypoxemia stimulates cerebral vessels to dilate, increasing cerebral oxygen delivery. With a second challenge to cerebral vasodilatory reserve, such as a decrease in arterial pressure, cerebral vasodilatory reserve may be inadequate to maintain cerebral oxygen delivery. In the absence of hypoxemia, the same decrease in arterial pressure could be tolerated without difficulty.

The symptoms of hypoglycemia usually unfold over a matter of minutes rather than seconds. Initially there is diaphoresis, hunger, tachycardia, fine tremor, headache, irritability, and epigastric discomfort. Many of these symptoms are due to epinephrine release. If hypoglycemia progresses, impairment of consciousness followed by loss of consciousness results. Myoclonic twitches and seizures may occur. Syncope resulting from hypoglycemia is unrelated to posture and is not usually associated with hypotension. Loss of consciousness often lasts several minutes. The diagnosis is made by testing the blood sugar level during the event. Further evaluation of hypoglycemia is discussed elsewhere.[244]

NEUROPSYCHOLOGIC CAUSES OF TRANSIENT LOSS OF CONSCIOUSNESS

The differentiation of syncope from a convulsive disorder may be particularly difficult if there are no witnesses to the event or if the seizures are akinetic seizures. Fortunately, akinetic seizures occur primarily in children. While tonic–clonic movements, urinary and fecal incontinence, tongue-biting, absence of prodromal and postictal confusion, and headache may all occur with syncope, the presence of this constellation of symptoms strongly favors a seizure disorder. The electroencephalogram (EEG) may be helpful. Unfortunately, however, as many as 40% of subjects with grand mal epilepsy show a normal EEG pattern between attacks.[61] The sensitivity of the test may be increased by using special activating procedures and additional recording electrodes.[245]

Several features suggest a diagnosis of hysterical syncope. The patient is usually involved in a dramatic situation when syncope occurs. Heart rate and blood pressure are unaffected, and the patient is rarely injured. Syncope may last for many minutes, even after the patient is supine, and upon awakening the patient demonstrates little anxiety or concern about the episode.

Clinical Evaluation

The cause of syncope is often evident after a careful history, physical examination, and ECG.[246] A description of the syncopal event or events by witnesses is particularly valuable. A complete history and physical examination is always important, but certain areas are particularly so in patients with syncope. These are listed in Table 3-6. The type of onset is often helpful. A prolonged onset lasting minutes suggests hyperventilation or hypoglycemia. When premonitory symptoms last only a few seconds, a sudden fall in arterial pressure is often the cause. These few seconds, however, may allow the patient to avoid severe injury when syncope does occur. Patients with orthostatic hypotension due to severe autonomic insufficiency may have no premonitory symptoms because appropriate sympathetic response to hypotension is lacking. The events immediately preceding syncope often help in detecting the cause. Has the patient recently used insulin or antihypertensive drugs? Severe emotional stress or pain preceding the event would be common with hyperventilation or vasovagal syncope. Exertional syncope would suggest any of the causes of cardiac obstruction or Takayasu's arteritis. Syncope after upper-extremity exertion should lead to a careful evaluation for the subclavian steal syndrome. Syncope precipitated by extreme movement of the head and neck suggests either carotid sinus hypersensitivity or cervical spine abnormalities. If angina precedes syncope, think of coronary artery spasm. A primary intra-

Table 3–6. Clinical Evaluation of the Patient with Syncope

I. History	
Type of onset:	Sudden, gradual
Preceding events:	Food and drug intake, angina, emotional stress, exercise (what type), coughing, movements of head, micturition, alcohol, environment, trauma
Position at onset:	Supine, upright, prolonged standing, change in position
Associated symptoms:	Palpitations, diaphoresis, epigastric discomfort, neurologic symptoms, aura, headache, tonic–clonic movements, chest pain
Duration:	Seconds to minutes; minutes to an hour
Clearing of sensorium:	Rapid, slow
Postevent signs and symptoms:	Incontinence, tongue biting, injury, headache, neurologic deficit, immediate recurrence
II. Physical Examination	
Heart and respiratory rate	
Blood pressure	
Supine and standing	
Both arms and legs	
Palpation and auscultation of major vessels	
Cardiac and chest examination	
Skin and mucous membranes	
Extremities	
Neurologic examination	
Carotid sinus massage	
Voluntary coughing	
Voluntary hyperventilation	
Tests of autonomic nervous system function	
III. ECG and Chest X-Ray Film	
IV. Additional Tests That May Be Indicated	
EEG	
Ambulatory ECG monitoring	
Echocardiogram	
Exercise testing	
Electrophysiologic Testing	

cranial process might be associated with a severe headache. Orthostatic hypotension is likely if syncope occurs shortly after rising from a supine position. Prolonged standing with little muscular activity may lead to vasovagal syncope. Although syncope most often occurs in a standing patient, hypoglycemia, hyperventilation, seizures, and Stokes–Adams attacks may cause syncope in a supine subject. Syncope usually last for only a few seconds or a minute if the patient is placed in a supine position. More prolonged episodes suggest hyperventilation, hypoglycemia, or hysteria. Following a syncopal episode, the patient's mental status usually returns to normal very rapidly. Following a seizure the patient is often confused for 20 to 30 minutes. While incontinence, tongue-biting, tonic–clonic movements, and postevent confusion may occur with other causes of syncope, this constellation of symptoms suggests a seizure disorder.

Clues to the etiology of syncope are often available from the physical examination. If the patient is seen immediately, heart rate, respiratory rate, blood pressure, and a careful neurologic examination may provide a diagnosis that is obscured once the patient recovers. Blood pressure should be taken in both arms and both legs. Differences in blood pressure may suggest the subclavian steal syndrome or Takayasu's arteritis. Blood pressure should be taken after the patient has been supine for 2 or 3 minutes. It should then be recorded again, along with heart rate, immediately on standing, and at 2 and 5 minutes after standing. The patient should be asked about symptoms with standing. Occasionally, elderly patients will have a marked but transient fall in blood pressure immediately on standing.[98] Careful auscultation over the carotid and subclavian arteries may reveal bruits. Cardiac examination may show murmurs, clicks, or tumor plops suggestive of an intracardiac obstruction. The skin and mucous membranes should be evaluated for dehydration and the extremities for clubbing or cyanosis suggesting congenital heart disease. A careful neurologic examination is mandatory. The technique of carotid sinus massage has been described: both sides should be tested individually, with the patient supine and with careful monitoring of heart rate and blood pressure. If suggested by the history, having the patient cough or hyperventilate may reproduce the patient's symptoms and lead to a diagnosis. If orthostatic hypotension is present, several tests, such as the Valsalva maneuver and cold pressor tests, can be used to further evaluate autonomic nervous system function. An ECG may give a clue to the possibility of tachyarrhythmias or bradyarrhythmias or pacemaker malfunction.

If the etiology of syncope has not been determined after this evaluation, it becomes more difficult to establish. Electroencephalography should be performed if seizures are suspected, but in between episodes EEGs are positive in only 60% of patients with grand mal seizures.[245] Echocardiography can detect many of the intracardiac obstructive lesions. Ambulatory ECG monitoring can be quite helpful in detecting conduction disease and arrhythmias, particularly when a patient's symptoms coincide with rhythm abnormalities. Exercise testing may be useful for precipitating arrhythmias but is not as helpful as ambulatory monitoring. In patients for whom no etiology can be inferred from these procedures, the EEG may need to be repeated with more aggressive stimulation techniques.[245] Repeated ambulatory ECG monitoring may be necessary. Electrophysiologic testing may be of value for detecting occult arrhythmias or sinus node or conduction system disease when other studies are negative, but its sensitivity and specificity are not firmly established.[247-249]

Summary

Syncope is caused by a sudden transient decrease in cerebral oxygen or glucose delivery. Although the margin of safety for cerebral oxygen delivery is wide, it can be narrowed in two ways. A sudden severe drop in cerebral oxygen or glucose delivery may by itself lead to syncope. In addition, a less severe fall in cerebral oxygen or glucose delivery may cause syncope if delivery of these substances is already compromised by other abnormalities. Indeed, especially in the elderly, it is very often a combination of factors that actually leads to syncope.

The cause of syncope is usually evident after the initial history, physical examination, and ECG. If the cause remains unclear after this evaluation, establishing a diagnosis may be much more difficult. The vigor with which additional diagnostic tests are pursued will depend on the degree to which the physician suspects that an underlying life-threatening disorder has led to syncope.

Finally, it is obvious that a precise diagnosis is required if therapeutic interventions are to succeed. Many abnormalities, such as arrhythmias, conduction abnormalities, or carotid sinus hypersensitivity, occur commonly but may not necessarily be the cause of syncope. The association of these abnormalities with the patient's symptoms is especially valuable. Unfortunately, this association cannot always be made, and the physician may need to try various therapeutic measures in a blind fashion, particularly if the syncope has been recurrent. In some of these patients, electrophysiologic testing may prove helpful in reaching the correct diagnosis.

References

1. Zijlstra WG: Cerebral metabolism. In Minderhoud JM (ed): Cerebral Blood Flow: Basic Knowledge and Clinical Implications, pp 56–78. Amsterdam, Exerpta Medica, 1981
2. Rossen R, Kabat H, Anderson JP: Acute arrest of cerebral circulation in man. Arch Neurol Psychiatr 51:510, 1943
3. Zijlstra WG: Physiology of the cerebral circulation. In Minderhoud JM (ed): Cerebral Blood Flow: Basic Knowledge and Clinical Implications, pp 34–55. Amsterdam, Exerpta Medica, 1981
4. Lassen NA: Cerebral blood flow and oxygen consumption in man. Physiol Rev 39:183, 1959
5. McHenry LC Jr, Fazekas JF, Sullivan JF: Cerebral hemodynamics of syncope. Am J Med Sci 241:173, 1961
6. Reivich M: Physiology of the cerebral circulation. In Goldensohn EJ, Appel SH (eds): Scientific Approaches to Clinical Neurology, pp 728–748. Philadelphia, Lea & Febiger, 1977
7. Lassen NA: Autoregulation of cerebral blood flow. Circ Res (Suppl 1) 15:201, 1964
8. Rapela CE, Green HD: Autoregulation of canine cerebral blood flow. Circ Res (Suppl 1) 15:205, 1964
9. Scheinberg P, Stead EA Jr: The cerebral blood flow in male subjects as measured by the nitrous oxide technique: Normal values for blood flow, oxygen utilization, glucose utilization and peripheral resistance with observations on the effect of tilting and anxiety. J Clin Invest 28:1163, 1949
10. Tindall GT, Craddock A, Greenfield J Jr: Effect of the sitting position on blood flow in the internal carotid artery of man during general anesthesia. J Neurosurg 26:383, 1967
11. Moyer J, Miller S, Snyder H: Effects of increased jugular pressure on cerebral hemodynamics. J Appl Physiol 7:245, 1954

12. Raisis JE, Kindt GW, McGillicuddy JE, et al: The effects of primary elevation of cerebral venous pressure on cerebral hemodynamics and intracranial pressure. J Surg Res 26:101, 1979

13. Kjallquist A, Siesjo BK, Zwetnow N: Effects of increased intracranial pressure on cerebral blood flow and on cerebral venous pO_2, pCO_2, pH, lactate and pyruvate in dogs. Acta Physiol Scand 75:267, 1969

14. Nakagawa Y, Tsuru M, Kenzoh Y: Site and mechanism for compression of the venous system during experimental intracranial hypertension. J Neurosurg 41:427, 1974

15. Shenkin HA, Spitz EB, Grant FC, et al: The acute effects on the cerebral circulation of the reduction of increased intracranial pressure by means of intravenous glucose or ventricular drainage. J Neurosurg 5:466, 1948

16. Henry JP, Gauer OH, Kety SS, et al: Factors maintaining cerebral circulation during gravitational stress. J Clin Invest 30:292, 1951

17. Strandgaard S, Oleson J, Skinhoj E, et al: Autoregulation of brain circulation in severe arterial hypertension. Br Med J 1:507, 1973

18. Mchedlishvili G: Physiological mechanisms controlling cerebral blood flow. Stroke 11:240, 1980

19. Berne RM, Winn HR, Rubio R: The local regulation of cerebral blood flow. Prog Cardiovasc Dis 24:243, 1981

20. Kety SS: The physiology of the cerebral circulation. In Vinken PJ, Bruyn GW (eds): Handbook of Clinical Neurology, Vol 11, Vascular Diseases of the Nervous System, pp 118–127. New York, American Elsevier, 1972

21. Betz E: Cerebral blood flow: Its measurement and regulation. Physiol Rev 52:595, 1972

22. Kety SS, Schmidt CF: The effects of active and passive hyperventilation on cerebral blood flow, cerebral oxygen consumption, cardiac output, and blood pressure of normal young men. J Clin Invest 25:107, 1946

23. Severinghaus JW, Chiodi H, Eger I, et al: Cerebral blood flow in man at high altitudes. Circ Res 19:274, 1966

24. Skinhøj E: Cerebral blood flow adaptation in man to chronic hypo- and hypercapnia and its relation to CSF pH. Scand J Clin Lab Invest Vol 22(Suppl 102), p viiiA, 1968

25. Haggendal E, Nilsson NJ, Norback B: Effect of viscosity on cerebral blood flow. Acta Chir Scand (Suppl 364) 1966

26. Scheinberg P: The cerebral circulation. In Zelis R (ed): The Peripheral Circulations, pp 151–162. New York, Grune & Stratton, 1975

27. Zwetnow NN: Pathophysiology of autoregulation. In Minderhoud JM (ed): Cerebral Blood Flow: Basic Knowledge and Clinical Implications, pp 79–85. Amsterdam, Exerpta Medica, 1981

28. Hill L: The influence of the force of gravity on the circulation of the blood. J Physiol 18:15, 1895

29. Hill L, Barnard H: The influence of the force of gravity on the circulation. J Physiol 21:323, 1897

30. Gauer OH, Thron HL: Postural changes in the circulation. In Visscher MB (ed): Handbook of Physiology, pp 2409–2440. Baltimore, Williams & Wilkins, 1965

31. Ziegler MG, Lake CR, Kopin IJ: Deficient sympathetic nervous response in familial dysautonomia. N Engl J Med 294:630, 1976

32. Sjostrand T: Regulation of the blood distribution in man. Acta Physiol Scand 26:312, 1952

33. Currens JH: A comparison of the blood pressure in the lying and standing positions: A study of five hundred men and five hundred women. Am Heart J 35:646, 1947

34. Shepherd JT, Vanhoutte PM: *The human cardiovascular system: Facts and concepts.* New York, Raven Press, 1979
35. Abboud FM, Heistad DD, Mark AL, et al: Reflex control of the peripheral circulation. Prog Cardiovasc Dis 28:371, 1976
36. Donald DE, Shepherd JT: Cardiac receptors: Normal and disturbed function. Am J Cardiol 44:873, 1979
37. Linden RJ: Atrial reflexes and renal function. Am J Cardiol 44:879, 1979
38. Abboud FM: Integration of reflex responses in the control of blood pressure and vascular resistance. Am J Cardiol 44:903, 1979
39. Ziegler MG, Lake CR, Kopin IJ: The sympathetic nervous system defect in primary orthostatic hypotension. N Engl J Med 296:293, 1977
40. Pasternac A, Tubua JF, Puddu PE, et al: Increased plasma catecholamine levels in patients with symptomatic mitral valve prolapse. Am J Med 73:783, 1982
41. Hamilton JE, Lichty JS, Pitts WR: Cardiovascular response of healthy young men to postural variations at varied temperatures. Am J Physiol 100:383, 1932
42. Franseen EB, Hellebrandt FA: Postural changes in respiration. Am J Physiol 138:364, 1943
43. Pollack A, Wood EH: Venous pressure in the saphenous vein at the ankle in man during exercise and changes in posture. J Appl Physiol 1:649, 1948
44. Guyton AC: Arterial Pressure and Hypertension, pp 1–9. Philadelphia, WB Saunders, 1980
45. Thomas JE, Schirger A, Fealy RD, et al: Orthostatic hypotension. Mayo Clin Proc 56:117, 1981
46. Oparil S, Vassaux C, Sanders CA, et al: Role of renin in acute postural homeostasis. Circulation 41:89, 1970
47. Epstein SE, Beiser GD, Stampfer M, et al: Role of the venous system in baroreceptor-mediated reflexes in man. J Clin Invest 47:139, 1968
48. Boreus LO, Hollenberg NK: Venous constriction in response to head-up tilt in man. Can J Physiol Pharmacol 50:317, 1972
49. Samueloff SL, Browse NL, Shepherd JT: Response of capacity vessels in human limbs to head-up tilt and suction on lower body. J Appl Physiol 21:47, 1966
50. Stegall HF: Muscle pumping in the dependent leg. Circ Res 19:180, 1966
51. Wald H, Guernsey M, Scott FH: Some effects of alteration of posture on arterial blood pressure. Am Heart J 14:319, 1937
52. Hellebrandt FA, Franseen EB: Physiology study of vertical stance in man. Physiol Rev 23:220, 1943
53. Bevegard SA, Holmgren A, Jonssan B: The effect of body position on the circulation at rest and during exercise with special reference to the influence on the stroke volume. Acta Physiol Scand 49:279, 1960
54. Reeves JT, Grover RF, Blount SG Jr, et al: Cardiac output response to standing and treadmill walking. J Appl Physiol 16:283, 1961
55. Gaffney FA, Bastian BC, Lane LB, et al: Abnormal cardiovascular regulation in the mitral valve prolapse syndrome. Am J Cardiol 52:316, 1983
56. Ewing DJ, Hume L, Campbell IW, et al: Autonomic mechanisms in the initial heart rate response to standing. J Appl Physiol 49:809, 1980
57. Abelmann WH: Alterations in orthostatic tolerance after myocardial infarction and in congestive heart failure. Cardiology (Suppl 1) 61:236, 1976
58. Cryer PE, Silverberg AB, Santiago JV, et al: Plasma catecholamines in diabetes. The syndromes of hypoadrenergic and hyperadrenergic postural hypotension. Am J Med 64:407, 1978
59. Bradbury S, Eggleston C: Postural hypotension: A report of three cases. Am Heart J 1:73, 1925

60. Shy GM, Drager GA: A neurologic syndrome associated with orthostatic hypotension: A clinical pathologic study. Arch Neurol 2:511, 1960
61. Adams RD, Victor M: Faintness and syncope. In Principles of Neurology, pp 248–257. New York, McGraw-Hill, 1981
62. Ziegler MG: Postural hypotension. Ann Rev Med 31:239, 1980
63. Diamond MA, Murray RH, Schmid PG: Idiopathic postural hypotension: Physiologic observations and report of a new mode of therapy. J Clin Invest 49:1341, 1970
64. Bannister R, Sever P, Gross M: Cardiovascular reflexes and biochemical responses in progressive autonomic failure. Brain 100:327, 1977
65. Kontos HA, Richardson DW, Norvell JE: Norepinephrine depletion in idiopathic orthostatic hypotension. Ann Intern Med 82:336, 1975
66. Johnson RH, Spalding JMK: Arterial hypotension. In Disorders of the Autonomic Nervous System, pp 79–113. London, Blackwell Scientific Publications, 1974
67. Schirger A, Thomas JE: Idiopathic orthostatic hypotension: Clinical spectrum and prognosis. Cardiology (Suppl 1) 61:144, 1976
68. Demanet JC: Usefulness of noradrenaline and tyramine infusion tests in the diagnosis of orthostatic hypotension. Cardiology (Suppl 1) 61:213, 1976
69. Johnson RH: Orthostatic hypotension in neurological disease. Cardiology (Suppl 1) 61:150, 1976
70. Ewing DJ, Campbell IW, Clarke BF: Assessment of cardiovascular effects in diabetic autonomic neuropathy and prognostic implications. Ann Intern Med 92:308, 1980
71. Ewing DJ, Campbell IW, Murray A, et al: Immediate heart-rate response to standing: Simple test for autonomic neuropathy in diabetics. Br Med J 1:145, 1978
72. Watkins PJ, Mackay JD: Cardiac denervation in diabetic neuropathy. Ann Intern Med 92:304, 1980
73. Johnson RH, Smith AC, Spalding JMK, et al: Effect of posture on blood pressure in elderly patients. Lancet 1:731, 1965
74. Hammarstrom S, Lindgren AGH: Postural hypotension in a patient with multiple encephalomalacias. Acta Med Scand 111:537, 1942
75. Gross M, Marshall J: Blood pressure lability in ischemic cerebrovascular disease. Clin Sci 38:563, 1970
76. Brown JW, Monroe LS, Palmer L: Intractible vomiting, diarrhea and orthostatic hypotension in amyloidosis of the peripheral nervous system. Am J Dig Dis 13:836, 1968
77. Gaan D, Mahoney MP, Rowlands DJ, et al: Postural hypotension in amyloid disease. Am Heart J 84:395, 1972
78. Kyle RA, Kottke BA, Schirger A: Orthostatic hypotension as a clue to primary systemic amyloidosis. Circulation 34:883, 1966
79. Sobel BE, Roberts R: Hypotension and syncope. In Braunwald E (ed): Heart Disease: A Textbook of Cardiovascular Medicine, pp 952–963. Philadelphia, WB Saunders, 1980
80. Buja LM, Khoi NB, Roberts WC: Clinically significant cardiac amyloidosis. Am J Cardiol 26:394, 1970
81. Aisner J, Weiss HD, Chang P, et al: Orthostatic hypotension during combination chemotherapy with vincristine. Cancer Chemother Rep 58:927, 1974
82. LeWitt PA: The neurotoxicity of the rat poison Vacor: A clinical study of 12 cases. N Engl J Med 302:73, 1980
83. Biglieri EG, McElroy MB: Abnormalities of circulatory reflexes in primary aldosteronism. Circulation 33:78, 1966
84. Heinrich WL: Autonomic insufficiency. Ann Intern Med 142:339, 1982

85. Park DM, Johnson RH, Crean GP, et al: Orthostatic hypotension in bronchial carcinoma. Br Med J 3:510, 1972
86. Boasberg PD, Henry JP, Rosenbloom AA, et al: Case reports and studies of paraneoplastic hypotension: Abnormal low pressure baroreceptor responses. Med Pediatr Oncol 3:59, 1977
87. Riedel G, Frewin DB, Gladstone L, et al: Orthostatic hypotension following surgery on brain stem neoplasms: Report of two cases. Arch Phys Med Rehabil 55:471, 1974
88. Thomas JP, Shields R: Associated autonomic dysfunction and carcinoma of the pancreas. Br Med J 4:32, 1970
89. Riley CM, Day RL, Greeley DM, et al: Central autonomic dysfunction with defective lacrimation. I. Report of 5 cases. Pediatrics 3:468, 1949
90. Dancis J, Smith AA: Familial dysautonomia. N Engl J Med 274:207, 1966
91. Rodstein M, Zeman FD: Postural blood pressure changes in the elderly. J Chronic Dis 6:581, 1957
92. Johnson RH, Smith AC, Spalding JMK, et al: Effect of posture on blood pressure in elderly patients. Lancet 1:731, 1965
93. Caird FI, Andrews GR, Kennedy RD: Effect of posture on blood pressure in the elderly. Br Heart J 35:527, 1973
94. MacLennan WJ, Hall MRP, Timothy JI: Postural hypotension in old age: Is it a disorder of the nervous system or of blood vessels? Age Aging 9:25, 1980
95. White NJ: Heart-rate changes on standing in elderly patients with orthostatic hypotension. Clin Sci 58:411, 1980
96. Johnson RH, Spalding JMK: The nervous control of the circulation and its investigation. In Disorders of the Autonomic Nervous System, pp 33–58. London, Blackwell Scientific Publications, 1974
97. Zerbe RL, Henry DP, Robertson GL: Vasopressin response to orthostatic hypotension: Etiologic and clinical implications. Am J Cardiol 74:265, 1983
98. Thulesius O: Pathophysiological classification and diagnosis of orthostatic hypotension. Circulation (Suppl 1) 61:180, 1976
99. Bevegard S, Lodin A: Postural circulatory changes at rest and during exercise in five patients with congenital absence of valves in the deep veins of the legs. Acta Med Scand 172:21, 1962
100. Grimby G, Nilsson NJ, Sanne H: Cardiac output during exercise in patients with varicose veins. Scand J Clin Lab Invest 1:21, 1964
101. Zsoster T, Cronin RFP: Venous distensibility in patients with varicose veins. JAMA 94:1293, 1966
102. Streeten DH, Kerr CB, Kerr LP, et al: Hyerbradykinism: A new orthostatic syndrome. Lancet 2:1048, 1972
103. Brunjes S, Johns VJ, Crane MG: Pheochromocytoma. N Engl J Med 262:393, 1960
104. Cohn JN: Paroxysmal hypertension and hypovolemia. N Engl J Med 275:643, 1966
105. Laragh JH: Personal views on the mechanisms of hypertension. In Genest J, Kuchel O, Hamet P, et al (eds): Hypertension, pp 620–621. New York, McGraw-Hill, 1983
106. Ewing DJ, Winney R: Autonomic function in patients with chronic renal failure on intermittent hemodialysis. Nephron 15:424, 1975
107. Kersh ES, Kronfield SJ, Unger A, et al: Autonomic insufficiency in uremia as a cause of hemodialysis induced hypotension. N Engl J Med 290:650, 1974
108. Pickering TG, Gribben B, Oliver DO: Baroreflex sensitivity in patients on long term haemodialysis. Clin Sci 43:645, 1972
109. Nies AS, Robertson D, Stone WJ: Hemodialysis hypotension is not the result of uremic peripheral autonomic neuropathy. J Lab Clin Med 94:395, 1979

110. Lilley JJ, Golden J, Stone RA: Adrenergic regulation of blood pressure in chronic renal failure. J Clin Invest 57:1190, 1976
111. Heinrich WL, Woodard TD, Blachley JD, et al: Role of osmolality in blood pressure stability after dialysis and ultrafiltration. Kidney Int 18:480, 1980
112. Devereux RB, Perloff JK, Reichek N, et al: Mitral valve prolapse. Circulation 54:3, 1976
113. Santos AD, Mathew PK, Hilal A, et al: Orthostatic hypotension: A commonly unrecognized cause of symptoms in mitral valve prolapse. Am J Med 71:746, 1981
114. Coughlan HC, Phares P, Cowley M, et al: Dysautonomia in mitral valve prolapse. Am J Med 67:236, 1979
115. De Carvallo JA, Messerli FA, Frohlich ED: Mitral valve prolapse and borderline hypertension. Hypertension 1:518, 1979
116. Boudoulas H, Reynolds JC, Mazzaferri E, et al: Metabolic studies in mitral valve prolapse syndrome: A neuroendocrine-cardiovascular process. Circulation 61:1200, 1980
117. Wooley CF: Where are the diseases of yesteryear? DaCosta's syndrome, soldiers heart, the effort syndrome, neurocirculatory asthenia and the mitral valve prolapse syndrome. Circulation 53:749, 1976
118. Taylor HL, Henschel A, Brozek J, et al: Effects of bed rest on cardiovascular function and work performance. J Appl Physiol 2:223, 1949
119. Miller PB, Johnson RL, Lamb LE: Effects of four weeks of absolute bed rest on circulatory functions in man. Aerospace Med 35:1194, 1964
120. Stevens PM, Miller PB, Lynch TN, et al: Effects of lower body negative pressure on physiologic changes due to four weeks of hypoxic bed rest. Aerospace Med 37:466, 1966
121. Vogt FB, Mack PB, Johnson PC, et al: Tilt table response and blood volume changes associated with fourteen days of recumbency. Aerospace Med 38:43, 1967
122. Saltin B, Blomquist B, Mitchell JH, et al: Response to submaximal and maximal exercise after bed rest and training. Circulation (Suppl 7) 38:1, 1968
123. Convertino VA, Sandler H, Webb P, et al: Induced venous pooling and cardiorespiratory response to exercise after bedrest. J Appl Physiol 52:1343, 1982
124. Page MM, Smith RBW, Watkins PJ: Cardiovascular effects of insulin. Br Med J 1:430, 1976
125. Miles DW, Hayter CJ: The effect of intravenous insulin on the circulatory responses to tilting in normal and diabetic subjects with special reference to baroreceptor reflex block and atypical hypoglycemic reactions. Clin Sci Molec Med 34:419, 1968
126. Page MM, Watkins PJ: Provocation of postural hypotension by insulin in diabetic autonomic neuropathy. Diabetes 25:90, 1976
127. Appenzeller O, Goss JE: Glucose and baroreceptor function. Arch Neurol 23:137, 1970
128. Mackay JD, Hayakawa H, Watkins PJ: Cardiovascular effects of insulin: Plasma volume changes in diabetics. Diabetologia 15:453, 1978
129. Alexander WD, Oake RJ: The effect of insulin on vascular reactivity to norepinephrine. Diabetes 26:611, 1977
130. Talbot S, Smith AJ: Factors predisposing to postural hypotensive symptoms in the treatment of high blood pressure. Br Heart J 37:1059, 1975
131. Prichard BNC and Owens CWI: Drug treatment of hypertension. In Genest J, Kuchel O, Heimet P, et al (eds): Hypertension, pp 1171–1209. New York, McGraw-Hill, 1983
132. Drugs causing postural hypotension. Med Lett Drugs Ther 16:15, 1978

133. Drugs for psychiatric disorders. Med Lett Drugs Ther 25:45, 1983
134. Captopril Multicenter Research Group: A placebo-controlled trial of captopril in refractory chronic congestive heart failure. J Am Coll Cardiol 2:755, 1983
135. Weissler AM, Lewis RF, Boudoulas H, et al: Syncope. In Hurst JW (ed): The Heart, pp 576–588. New York, McGraw-Hill, 1982
136. Verill PJ, Aellig WH: Vasovagal faint in the supine position. Br Med J 4:348, 1970
137. Karp HR, Weissler AM, Heyman A: Vasodepressor syncope: ECG and circulatory changes. Arch Neurol 5:94, 1961
138. Hunter J: Works of John Hunter, Vol 3. London, JF Palmer, 1937
139. Epstein SE, Stampfer M, Beiser GD: Role of capacitance and resistance vessels in vasovagal syncope. Circulation 37:524, 1968
140. Glick G, Yu PN: Hemodynamic changes during spontaneous vasovagal reactions. Am J Med 34:42, 1963
141. Weissler AM, Warren JV, Estes EH Jr, et al: Vasodepressor syncope: Factors influencing cardiac output. Circulation 15:875, 1957
142. Barcroft H, Edholm OG, McMichael J, et al: Post-hemorrhagic fainting: Study by cardiac output and forearm flow. Lancet 1:489, 1944
143. Barcroft H, Edholm OG: On the vasodilation in human skeletal muscle during post-hemorrhagic fainting. J Physiol 104:161, 1945
144. Lewis T: Vasovagal syncope and the carotid sinus mechanism. Br Med J 1:893, 1972
145. Murray RH, Thompson LJ, Bowers JA, et al: Hemodynamic effects of graded hypovolemia and vasodepressor syncope induced by lower body negative pressure. Am Heart J 76:799, 1968
146. Aviado DM Jr, Schmidt CF: Cardiovascular and respiratory reflexes from the left side of the heart. Am J Physiol 196:726, 1959
147. Blair DA, Glover WE, Greenfield ADH, et al: Excitation of cholinergic vasodilator nerves to human skeletal muscles during emotional stress.
148. Brun C, Knudsen EOE, Raashar F: Kidney function and circulatory collapse, postsyncopal oliguria. J Clin Invest 25:568, 1946
149. Stead EA Jr, Kunkel P, Weiss S: Effect of pitressin in circulatory collapse induced by sodium nitrate. J Clin Invest 18:673, 1939
150. Lown B, Levine SA: The carotid sinus: Clinical value of its stimulation. Circulation 23:766, 1961
151. Weiss S, Baker JP: The carotid sinus reflex in health and disease: Its role in the causation of fainting and consciousness. Medicine 12:297, 1933
152. Lesser LM, Wenger NK: Carotid sinus syncope. Heart Lung 5:453, 1976
153. Wright KE Jr, McIntosh HD: Syncope: A review of pathophysiological mechanisms. Prog Cardiovasc Dis 13:580, 1971
154. Sigler LH: Hyperactive vasodepressor carotid sinus reflex. Arch Intern Med 70:983, 1942
155. Heidorn GH, McNamara AP: Effect of carotid sinus stimulation on the electrocardiograms of clinically normal individuals. Circulation 14:1104, 1956
156. Purks WK: Electrocardiographic findings following carotid sinus stimulation. Ann Intern Med 13:270, 1939
157. Lipsitz LA: Syncope in the elderly. Ann Intern Med 99:92, 1983
158. Johnson RH: Blood pressure and its regulation. In Caird FI, Dall JLC, Kennedy RD (eds): Cardiology in Old Age, pp 101–126. New York, Plenum Press, 1976
159. Khero BA, Mullins CB: Cardiac syncope due to glossopharangeal neuralgia. Arch Intern Med 128:806, 1971
160. Kong Y, Heyman A, Entman ML, et al: Glossopharyngeal neuralgia associated with bradycardia, syncope and seizures. Circulation 30:109, 1964
161. Wik B, Hillestead L: Deglutition syncope. Br Med J 3:747, 1975

162. Tolman KG, Ashworth W: Syncope induced by dysphagia corrected by esophageal dilation. Am J Dig Dis 16:1026, 1971
163. Levin B, Posner JB: Swallow syncope. Neurology 22:1086, 1972
164. Waddington JKB, Matthews HR, Evans CC, et al: Carcinoma of the esophagus with swallow syncope. Br Med J 3:232, 1975
165. Haldane JH: Micturition syncope. Can Med Assoc J 101:712, 1969
166. Lyle CB Jr, Monroe JT Jr, Flinn DE, et al: Micturition syncope: Report of 24 cases. N Engl J Med 265:982, 1961
167. Godec CJ, Cass AS: Micturition syncope. J Urol 126:551, 1981
168. Pathy MS: Defecation syncope. Age Aging 7:233, 1978
169. MacMurray FG: Stokes–Adams disease: A historical review. N Engl J Med 256:643, 1957
170. Pomerantz B, O'Rourke RA: The Stokes–Adams syndrome. Am J Med 46:941, 1969
171. Stein E, Damato AN, Kosowsky BD, et al: The relation of heart rate to cardiovascular dynamics: Pacing by atrial electrodes. Circulation 33:925, 1966
172. Silber EB, Katz LN: Pathophysiologic basis and effects of arrhythmias. In *Heart Disease*, pp 135–170. New York, Macmillan, 1975
173. Benchimol A, Liggett MS: Cardiac haemodymanics during stimulation of the right atrium, right ventricle and left ventricle in normal and abnormal hearts. Circulation 33:933, 1966
174. Covell JW, Ross J Jr, Taylor R, et al: Effects of increasing frequency of contraction on the force velocity relation of the left ventricle. Cardiovasc Res 1:2, 1967
175. Brockman SK: Cardiodynamics of complete heart block. Am J Cardiol 16:72, 1965
176. Mitchell JH, Gupta DN, Payne RN: Influence of atrial systole on effective ventricular stroke volume. Circ Res 17:11, 1965
177. Samet P, Bernstein W, Levine S: Significance of atrial contribution to ventricular filling. Am J Cardiol 15:195, 1965
178. Samet P, Castillo C, Bernstein WH: Hemodynamic sequelae of atrial, ventricular, and sequential atrioventricular pacing in cardiac patients. Am Heart J 72:725, 1966
179. Braunwald E: Symposium on cardiac arrhythmias: Introduction with comments on the hemodynamic significance of atrial systole. Am J Med 37:665, 1964
180. DeMaria AW, Tabuie H, Kamiyama T, et al: The deleterious hemodynamic consequences of retrograde ventriculoatrial conduction in ventricular tachycardia. Circulation 46:145, 1972
181. Wiggers CJ, Katz LN: The contour of the ventricular volume curves under different conditions. Am J Physiol 58:439, 1922
182. Lister JW, Klotz DH, Jomain SL, et al: Effect of pacemaker site on cardiac output and ventricular activation in dogs with complete heart block. Am J Cardiol 14:494, 1964
183. Bourassa G, Boiteau GH, Allenstein BJ: Hemodynamic studies during intermittent left bundle branch block. Am J Cardiol 10:792, 1962
184. McIntosh HD, Morris JJ Jr: Hemodynamic consequences of arrhythmias. Prog Cardiovasc Dis 8:330, 1966
185. Sinno MZ, Gunnar RM: Hemodynamic consequences of cardiac dysrhythmias. Med Clin North Am 60:69, 1976
186. Wood P: Polyuria in paroxysmal tachycardia and paroxysmal atrial flutter and fibrillation. Br Heart J 25:273, 1963
187. Kinney MJ, Stein RM, DiScala VA:The polyuria of paroxysmal atrial tachycardia. Circulation 50:429, 1974
188. Boykin J, Cadnapaphornchai P, McDonald KM, et al: Mechanism of diuretic response associated with atrial tachycardia. Am J Physiol 229:1486, 1975

189. Corday E, Irving DW: Effect of cardiac arrhythmias on the cerebral circulation. Am J Cardiol 6:803, 1960
190. Corday E, Gold H, DeVera LB, et al: Effect of cardiac arrhythmias on the coronary circulation. Ann Intern Med 50:535, 1959
191. Irving DW, Corday E: Effect of cardiac arrhythmias on the renal and mesenteric circulations. Am J Cardiol 8:32, 1961
192. Wolff L, Parkinson J, White PD: Bundle-branch block with short P–R interval in healthy young people prone to paroxysmal tachycardia. Am Heart J 5:685, 1930
193. Lown B, Ganong WF, Levine SA: The syndrome of short P–R interval, normal QRS complex and paroxysmal rapid heart action. Circulation 5:693, 1952
194. Smith WM, Gallagher JJ: "Les Torsades de Pointes": An unusual ventricular arrhythmia. Ann Intern Med 93:578, 1980
195. Reynolds EW, VanderArk CR: Quinidine syncope and delayed repolarization syndromes. Med Concepts Cardiovasc Dis 55:117, 1976
196. Bigger JT: Mechanisms and diagnosis of arrhythmias. In Braunwald E (ed): Heart Disease: A Textbook of Cardiovascular Medicine, pp 630–690. Philadelphia, WB Saunders, 1980
197. Lown B: Cardiovascular collapse and sudden cardiac death. In Braunwald E (ed): *Heart Disease: A Textbook of Cardiovascular Medicine*, pp 778–817. Philadelphia, WB Saunders, 1980
198. Bigger JT, Reiffel JA: Sick sinus syndrome. Annu Rev Med 30:91, 1979
199. Moss AJ, Davis RJ: Brady-tachy syndrome. Prog Cardiovasc Dis 16:439, 1974
200. Scheinman MM, Strauss HC, Evans GT, et al: Adverse effects of sympatholytic agents in patients with hypertension and sinus node dysfunction. Am J Med 64:1013, 1978
201. Strauss HC, Gilbert M, Svenson RH, et al: Electrophysiologic effects of propranolol on sinus node function in patients with sinus node dysfunction. Circulation 54:452, 1976
202. Lindenfeld J, Groves BM: Cardiovascular function and disease in the aged. In Schrier RW (ed): Clinical Internal Medicine in the Aged, pp 87–123. Philadelphia, WB Saunders, 1982
203. McAnulty JH, Rahimtoola SH, Murphy E, et al: Natural history of "high risk" bundle-branch block: Final report of a prospective study. N Engl J Med 307:137, 1982
204. Dhingra RC, Denes P, Wu D, et al: Syncope in patients with bifascicular block: Significance, causative mechanisms and clinical implications. Ann Intern Med 81:302, 1974
205. Heupler FA: Syndrome of symptomatic coronary arterial spasm with nearly normal coronary arteriograms. Am J Cardiol 45:873, 1980
206. Ross J Jr, Braunwald E: The influence of corrective operations on the natural history of aortic stenosis. Circulation (Suppl V) 38:61, 1968
207. Flamm MD, Braiff BA, Kimball R, et al: Mechanism of effort syncope in aortic stenosis. Circulation (Suppl II) 36:109, 1967
208. Mark AL, Kioschos JM, Abboud FM, et al: Abnormal vascular responses to exercise in patients with aortic stenosis. J Clin Invest 52:1138, 1973
209. Schwartz LS, Goldfisher J, Sprague GJ, et al: Syncope and sudden death in aortic stenosis. Am J Cardiol 23:647, 1969
210. Mark AL, Abboud FM, Schmid PG, et al: Reflex vascular responses to left ventricular outflow obstruction and activation of baroreceptors in dogs. J Clin Invest 52:1147, 1973
211. Adelman AG, Wigle ED, Ranganathan N, et al: The clinical course in muscular

subaortic stenosis: A retrospective and prospective study of 60 hemodynamically proved cases. Ann Intern Med 77:515, 1972

212. Shah PM, Adelman AG, Wigle ED, et al: The natural and unnatural history of hypertrophic obstructive cardiomyopathy. Circ Res (Suppl II) 34–35:179, 1974

213. Braunwald E, Lambrew CT, Rockoff S, et al: Idiopathic hypertrophic subaortic stenosis. Circulation (Suppl IV) 29–30:1, 1964

214. McKenna WJ, Deanfield J, Faruqui A, et al: Prognosis in hypertrophic cardiomyopathy. Am J Cardiol 47:532, 1981

215. Braunwald E, Brockenbrough ED, Frye RL: Studies on digitalis. V. Comparison of the effects of ouabain on left ventricular dynamics in valvular aortic stenosis and hypertrophic subaortic stenosis. Circulation 26:166, 1962

216. Murgo JP: Does outflow obstruction exist in hypertrophic cardiomyopathy? N Engl J Med 307:1008, 1982

217. McKenna W, Harris L, Deanfield JE: Syncope in hypertrophic cardiomyopathy. Br Heart J 47:177, 1982

218. Savage DD, Seides BF, Maron BJ, et al: Prevalence of arrhythmias during 24-hour electrocardiographic monitoring and exercise testing in patients with obstructive and nonobstructive hypertrophic cardiomyopathy. Circulation 59:866, 1979

219. McKenna WJ, Chetty S, Oakley CM, et al: Arrhythmia in hypertrophic cardiomyopathy: Exercise and 48 hour ambulatory electrocardiographic assessment with and without beta blocking therapy. Am J Cardiol 45:1, 1980

220. Joseph S, Balcon R, McDonald L: Syncope in hypertrophic obstructive cardiomyopathy due to asystole. Br Heart J 34:974, 1972

221. Chmielewzki CA, Riley RS, Mahendran A, et al: Complete heart block as a cause of syncope in asymmetric septal hypertrophy. Am Heart J 93:91, 1977

222. Krikler DM, Davies MJ, Rowland E, et al: Sudden death in hypertrophic cardiomyopathy: Associated accessory atrioventricular pathways. Br Heart J 43:245, 1980

223. Thames MD, Klopfenstein HS, Abboud FM, et al: Preferential distribution of inhibitory cardiac receptors with vagal afferents in the inferoposterior wall of the left ventricle activated during coronary occlusion in the dog. Circ Res 43:512, 1978

224. Selzer A, Sakai FD, Popper RW: Protean clinical manifestations of primary tumors of the heart. Am J Med 52:9, 1972

225. Slater EE, DeSanctis RW: The clinical recognition of dissecting aortic aneurysm. Am J Med 60:625, 1976

226. Thames MD, Alpert JS, Dalen JE: Syncope in patients with pulmonary embolism. JAMA 238:2509, 1977

227. Bell WR, Siman TL, DeMets DL: The clinical features of submassive and massive pulmonary emboli. Am J Med 62:355, 1977

228. Simpson RJ Jr, Podolak R, Mangano CA Jr, et al: Vagal syncope during recurrent pulmonary embolism. JAMA 249:390, 1983

229. Dressler W: Effort syncope as an early manifestation of primary pulmonary hypertension. Am J Med Sci 223:131, 1952

230. Johnson LW, Grossman W, Dalen JE, et al: Pulmonic stenosis in the adult: Long-term follow up results. N Engl J Med 287:1159, 1959

231. Perloff JK: The Clinical Recognition of Congenital Heart Disease, 2nd ed, p 457. Philadelphia, WB Saunders, 1978

232. Friedberg CK: Syncope: Pathologic physiology: Differential diagnosis and treatment. Mod Concepts Cardiovasc Dis 40:55, 1971

233. Guntheroth WG, Morgan BC, Mullins GL: Physiologic studies of paroxysmal hy-

pernea in cyanotic congenital heart disease. Circulation 31:70, 1965

234. Sharpey-Schafer EP: The mechanism of syncope after coughing. Br Med J 2:860, 1953

235. McIntosh HD, Estes EH, Warren JV: The mechanism of cough syncope. Am Heart J 52:70, 1956

236. Hart G, Oldershaw PJ, Cull RE, et al: Syncope caused by cough-induced complete atrioventricular block. PACE 5:564, 1982

237. Perloff JK: Pregnancy and cardiovascular disease. In Braunwald E (ed): Heart Disease: A Textbook of Cardiovascular Medicine, p 1872. Philadelphia, WB Saunders, 1980

238. Currier RD, DeJong RN, Bole GG: Pulseless disease, central nervous system manifestations. Neurology 4:818, 1954

239. Reivich N, Holling HE, Roberts B, et al: Reversal of blood flow through the vertebral artery and its effect on cerebral circulation. N Engl J Med 265:878, 1961

240. Mannick JA, Sutter CG, Hume DG: The "subclavian steal" syndrome: A further documentation. JAMA 182:254, 1962

241. Engel GL, Ferris EB, Logan M: Hyperventilation: Analysis of clinical symptomatology. Ann Intern Med 27:683, 1947

242. Missri JR, Alexander S: Hyperventilation syndrome: A brief review. JAMA 240:2093, 1974

243. Bickerstaff ER: Impairment of consciousness in migraine. Lancet 2:1057, 1961

244. Foster DW, Rubenstein AH: Hypoglycemia, insulinoma and other hormone-secreting tumors of the pancreas. In Harrison TR (ed): Principles of Internal Medicine, pp 1758–1763. New York, McGraw-Hill, 1980

245. Adams RD, Victor M. Special techniques for neurologic diagnosis. In Adams RD, Victor M (eds): Principles of Neurology, pp 10–28. New York, McGraw-Hill, 1981

246. Silverstein MD, Singer DE, Mulley AG, et al: Patients with syncope admitted to medical intensive care units. JAMA 248:1185, 1982

247. DiMarco JP, Garan H, Harthorne JW, et al: Intracardiac electrophysiologic techniques in recurrent syncope of unknown cause. Ann Intern Med 95:542, 1981

248. Gulamhusein S, Nacarelli GV, Ko PT, et al: Value and limitations of clinical electrophysiologic study in assessment of patients with unexpected syncope. Am J Med 73:700, 1982

249. Hess DS, Morady F, Scheinman MM: Electrophysiologic testing in the evaluation of patients with syncope of undetermined origin. Am J Cardiol 50:1309, 1982

4

MUSCULOSKELETAL ABNORMALITIES AND HEART DISEASE

Antonio C. de Leon, Jr., M.D.

Musculoskeletal abnormalities are fairly common findings in a physical examination. In most cases, they are isolated findings. In some instances, they can serve as a clue to the presence of disease by virtue of frequently observed association. In other instances, the musculoskeletal abnormality is in itself a typical manifestation of the disease process. Thus, in the clinical recognition of heart disease, an awareness of the relationships that may exist between particular types of cardiac and musculoskeletal abnormalities can be very useful.

Habitus and General Appearance

MARFAN'S SYNDROME typically presents with a tall individual who has inappropriately long limbs and other associated musculoskeletal findings, such as arachnodactyly, pectus excavatum, joint laxity, and ectopia lentis (Fig. 4-1). Recognition of this entity from its physical manifestation should immediately alert one to the possible presence of associated cardiovascular disease. It is estimated that 60% of patients with Marfan's syndrome have mitral or aortic regurgitation, aneurysm of the ascending aorta, or a dilated aortic root.[1,2] Mitral valve prolapse has been noted echocardiographically in as many as 80% of patients.[3]

Other cardiovascular lesions noted in Marfan's syndrome include coarctation of the aorta, aneurysm of the pulmonary artery, dilatation of the sinuses of Valsalva, and patent ductus arteriosus. Aortic aneurysm dissection is the cause of death in 29% to 43% of patients.[4]

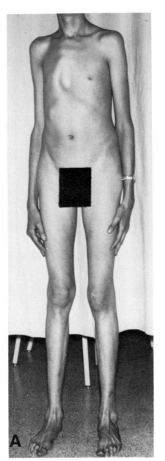
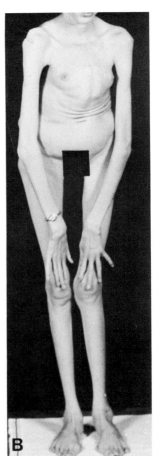

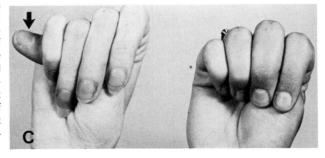

FIG. 4-1. Marfan's syndrome. (*A*) Male and (*B*) Female adults with typical body habitus demonstrating disproportionately long arms and legs, arachnodactyly, and pectus deformities. (*C*) Clenched hand of woman with Marfan's syndrome and normal hand. Note the marked protrusion of the thumb due to arachnodactyly and excessive joint laxity (*arrow*). (*A* and *B* courtesy of Ray Pryor, M.D., and S. Gilbert Blount, Jr., M.D. *C* courtesy of Bertron M. Groves, M.D.)

PSEUDOXANTHOMA ELASTICUM like Marfan's syndrome, is a form of connective tissue disorder. The typical physical appearance is that of unusual skin laxity, resulting in a "plucked chicken" appearance (Fig. 4-2). It is a multisystem disease involving, among other things, the cardiovascular system. Premature peripheral vascular atherosclerosis is noted in 28% to 60% of cases, hypertension in 25%, angina pectoris in 50%, and congestive heart failure in 70%.[5] Less commonly, mitral stenosis and insufficiency and tricuspid insufficiency have been noted in this entity.[6] A case of restrictive cardiomyopathy from diffuse endocardial fibroelastosis has been reported.[7]

EHLERS–DANLOS SYNDROME is an autosomal dominant disorder of connective tissue that presents with hyperextensible skin, hypermobile joints, skin nodules, susceptibility to bruising, and musculoskeletal abnormalities (Fig. 4-3). In hospitalized patients, the prevalence of cardiovascular abnormalities was noted to be high (47%). The most frequent abnormality noted was mitral valve prolapse, followed by aortic root dilation, sinus of Valsalva dilation, or both. Bicuspid aortic valve and aortic stenosis, pulmonic stenosis, dilated pulmonary artery and annulus with regurgitation, atrial septal defect, and ventricular septal defects have also been noted.[8]

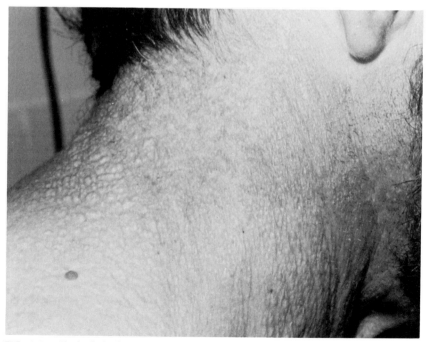

FIG. 4-2. "Plucked chicken" appearance of the nuchal skin in a patient with pseudoxanthoma elasticum. (Courtesy of J. Clark Huff, M.D.)

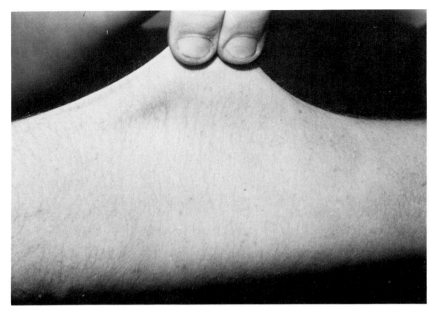

FIG. 4-3. Hyperextensible skin in a patient with Ehlers–Danlos syndrome. (Courtesy of J. Clark Huff, M.D.)

HUTCHINSON–GILFORD PROGERIA SYNDROME is an uncommon autosomal recessive heritable disorder that presents as premature aging. The skin is thin, warm, and dry, with sparse hair. Prominent spots of brownish pigmentation may be present in areas exposed to sunlight. Alopecia is present and the cranium appears large in relation to the face and body. The limbs are of proportionate length, but marked coxa valga is present after the age of 2 to 3 years. The most striking associated abnormality is that of varying degrees of generalized atherosclerosis, with death occurring between the ages of 7 and 27 years.[9]

HURLER'S SYNDROME (GARGOYLISM) is a heritable disorder characterized by dwarfism and characteristic facial appearance. Coronary artery disease is an important and frequently noted cardiovascular lesion.[10] The abnormal intracellular accumulation of mucopolysaccharide has resulted in damage to mitral and aortic valves, resulting in valvular regurgitation. Mitral stenosis has also been reported.[11]

OSTEOGENESIS IMPERFECTA is an inherited disorder of connective tissue characterized by deformity resulting from recurrent fractures, especially of the long bones. It is additionally characterized by deafness and bluish coloration of sclerae, tympanic membranes, and nail lacunae. Although cardiovascular abnormalities appear to be much less common than in Marfan's syndrome, such pathologic findings as dilation of the aortic root and aortic valve cusps, mitral ring dilation, and redundant mitral valve cusps have been described. The most commonly noted cardiac lesions are aortic insufficiency and, much less commonly, mitral insufficiency.[12,13]

ANKYLOSING SPONDYLITIS is a form of rheumatic disorder associated with arthritic changes, especially of the sacroiliac joints, zygapophyseal and costovertebral articulations, interspinous ligaments, and paravertebral tissues. This sort of involvement results in the characteristic "poker back." Dilation of the ascending aorta and sinuses of Valsalva is present with thickening of the adventitia and intimal proliferation of the aortic wall behind and immediately above the sinuses. The fibrous thickening behind the commissures causes the cusps to sag toward the left ventricle, resulting in aortic regurgitation.[14] Aortic regurgitation, which is by far the most common associated cardiac phenomenon, tends to be more frequently encountered in the older patient with spondylitis of longer duration. The prevalence of aortic regurgitation in patients with spondylitis of 15 years' duration is 3.5%, rising to 10.1% after 30 years of spondylitis.[15]

TURNER'S SYNDROME presents as a female patient with XO chromosomal anomaly, typically with a short stature, webbing of the neck, cubitus valgus, and a typical facies brought about by a small mandible, prominent ears, low posterior hair line, ptosis, and epicanthic fold. The most common cardiovascular anomaly noted in this entity is coarctation of the aorta. In one study, the incidence was 68%.[16]

ULLRICH–NOONAN SYNDROME represents a group of patients who have the physical characteristics of Turner's syndrome in conjunction with XX or XY (male Turner) chromosomes (Fig. 4-4). In Ullrich–Noonan syndrome, coarctation of the aorta is rare. Thirty-five percent of patients have cardiovascular anomalies, most frequently pulmonic stenosis with a dysplastic valve. Asymmetric septal hypertrophy and pulmonary artery branch stenosis are also frequent. In some patients, atrial septal defects occur in association with the pulmonic stenosis. It is noteworthy the the XO/XX Turner mosaic also tends to be associated with pulmonic stenosis rather than coarctation of the aorta.[17]

MULTIPLE LENTIGINES OR LEOPARD SYNDROME (the explanation for the acronym LEOPARD is: *L*entigenes, *E*lectrocardiographic abnormities, *O*cular hypertelorism, *P*ulmonary valve stenosis, *A*bnormalities of genitalia, *R*etardation of growth, and *D*eafness) is characterized by the presence of numerous small focal areas of hyperpigmentation that can occur throughout the body, sparing only the mucosal surfaces. It is associated with growth retardation, sensorineural deafness, genital abnormalities (especially gonadal hypoplasia), ocular hypertelorism, and cardiac abnormalities. Electrocardiographic abnormalities described have included left axis deviation, prolonged P–R interval and bundle branch block. Valvular and subvalvular pulmonic stenosis are the most commonly noted cardiac lesions.[18]

ELLIS–VAN CREVELD SYNDROME is characterized by symmetric dwarfism, polydactyly, and dysplastic nails and teeth. Congenital cardiac lesions are

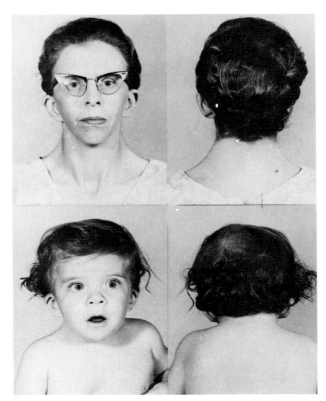

FIG. 4-4. Mother and daughter with Ullrich–Noonan syndrome (XX Turner's syndrome). Both had short stature, webbing of the neck, cubitus valgus, low posterior hairline, small mandible, prominent ears, inner epicanthic fold, short fifth finger, and valvular pulmonary stenosis. (From Nora JJ, Sinha AK: Direct familial transmission of the Turner phenotype. Am J Dis Child 116:346, 1968. By permission of American Medical Association)

noted in 50% to 60% of cases, the majority of which involve patients with a single atrium or a large atrial septal defect.[19,20]

The Head and Face

SUPRAVALVULAR AORTIC STENOSIS SYNDROME is characterized by the "elfin facies," which consist of protruding lips, low-set eyes, epicanthic folds, and strabismus. A history of infantile hypercalcemia may be present. A consistent cardiac lesion is localized narrowing of the aorta immediately above the sinus of Valsalva. In some, the aorta is hypoplastic throughout its course. Associated peripheral pulmonary artery stenosis is also common (Fig. 4-5).[21-23]

The characteristics of a group of patients with facial features similar to those of supravalvular stenosis, and with associated short stature and mental retardation, have been named *cardiofacial syndrome*. Pulmonary valvular dysplasia is the associated cardiac lesion.[24] The term cardiofacial syndrome has also been used for a group of patients with unilateral partial lower facial weakness thought to be due to subclinical viral infection during the 5th or 6th week of

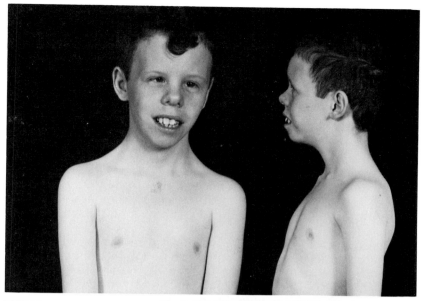

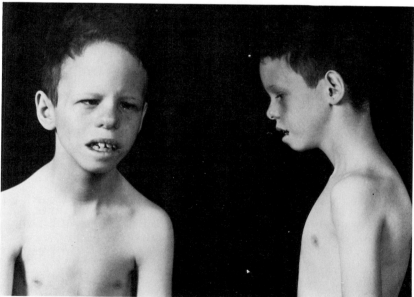

FIG. 4-5. Physical appearance characteristic of supravalvular aortic stenosis in ten-year-old mentally retarded twins with associated peripheral pulmonary artery branch stenosis. (Top) In this twin, cardiac catheterization revealed severe supravalvular aortic stenosis, mild right ventricular infundibular stenosis, and mild proximal right pulmonary artery stenosis. (Bottom) In this twin, catheterization demonstrated supravalvular aortic stenosis, severe right pulmonary artery branch stenosis, and a ventricular septal defect. (From Páge HL, Vogel JHK, Pryor R, Blount, SG: Supravalvular aortic stenosis: Unusual observations in three patients. Am J Cardiol 23:270, 1969)

gestation. In this group, as many as 50% have associated cardiac abnormalities, most frequently ventricular septal defect, patent ductus arteriosus, and tetralogy of Fallot.[25]

DOWN'S SYNDROME (trisomy 21) is well known for its characteristic "mongoloid" appearance, which is produced by the widely set eyes, upward-slanting palpebral fissure, epicanthal folds, and large tongue. Various congenital cardiac malfunctions have been noted, the most common being persistent common atrioventricular (AV) canal (60%), isolated ventricular septal defect (29%), and tetralogy of Fallot (14.5%).[26] In another study, the overall incidence of cardiac anomaly in Down's syndrome was 52% and in those patients, atrial septal defect, ostium primum and atrioventricularis communis combined, was the most common lesion, followed by ventricular septal defect.[27]

TRISOMY 13–15 is associated with cardiac malfunction in 84% of cases, the most common defects being ventricular septal defect, patent ductus arteriosus, and atrial septal defect. In trisomy 18 the incidence of associated cardiac defects is 98%, the most common being ventricular septal defect, patent ductus arteriosus, pulmonic stenosis, and bicuspid aortic valve. Atrial septal defect is comparatively rare.[27]
Severe congenital anomalies of the eyes, including microphthalmia, anophthalmia, colobomata, and cataracts, characterize trisomy 13–15. Facial clefts are more common in trisomy 13–15 than in trisomy 18.

CARCINOID SYNDROME results from metastatic gastrointestinal carcinoid tumor, usually with hepatic involvement. A striking feature is the occurrence of flushing, mostly involving the face, neck, and other sun-exposed areas of the body and extremities. The flush may range from a bright red to a violaceous hue. Serotonin is believed to be responsible for the resulting associated cardiac lesions which are, most frequently, tricuspid insufficiency and pulmonic stenosis. Tricuspid stenosis and pulmonary valve insufficiency are less common.[28,29]

FABRY'S DISEASE (angiokeratoma corporis diffusum universale) is an inborn error of glycosphingolipid metabolism and presents with telangiectatic lesions, keratosis, and corneal opacities (Fig. 4-6). Because glycolipid deposits occur in all cardiac structures, cardiac complications are frequently noted. Conduction abnormalities, abnormal left ventricular (LV) function, and mitral regurgitation have been described.[30]

ACROMEGALY is the result of increased secretion of growth hormone from acidophilic or mixed acidophilic and chromophobe adenoma of the pituitary gland. It results in enlargement of the cartilaginous and bony structures of the head, face, hands, and feet. The most common cardiovascular complication is systemic hypertension. Cardiomegaly, arrhythmias, intraventricular conduction abnormalities, and cardiomyopathy have been described. In some patients, asymmetric septal hypertrophy has been noted.[31-34] Concentric LV hypertrophy, in some series, is a far more frequent finding.[35]

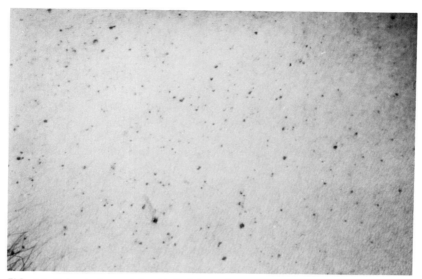

FIG. 4-6. Telangiectases of the skin in Fabry's disease. (Courtesy of J. Clark Huff, M.D.)

GOLDENHAR'S SYNDROME consists of a complex of deformities consisting of ocular, auricular, and vertebral dysplasia. The incidence of associated congenital heart disease is about 47%. Although no specific cardiac anomaly is noted, the most common lesion is ventricular septal defect.[36,37]

SMITH–LEMLI–OPITZ SYNDROME consists of a typical facies brought about by anteverted nares, micrognathia, a broad maxillary ridge, and low-set ears. It is associated with mental retardation, hypospadias, and cryptorchidism in the male, and cutaneous syndactyly of the second and third toes. Twenty percent have associated cardiovascular anomalies consisting of endocardial cushion defects, ventricular septal defect, patent ductus arteriosus, and atrial septal defect.[38]

DE LANGE SYNDROME consists of a characteristic facies with a wide upper lip, upturned nose, horizontal cleft in the chin, hairy eyebrows, and low-set ears. It is associated with mental retardation, widely spaced nipples, bilateral hemimelia, and rocker-bottom feet. Between 15% and 17% percent have associated congenital cardiac malformations. The most common lesions reported have been ventricular septal defect, patent ductus arteriosus, and pulmonic stenosis.[39]

RUBINSTEIN–TAYBI SYNDROME presents with a facies characterized by a small mouth, abnormally shaped and positioned ears, bushy eyebrows, epicanthal folds, and a squint. Associated findings include angulation of the thumbs and toes, overlapping of the toes, and broad terminal phalanges of the digits.

Patent ductus arteriosus, double aortic arch, and pulmonic stenosis have been noted.[40]

The Thorax

Various forms of thoracic cage abnormalities are common physical findings and do not necessarily imply the presence of heart disease. In some instances, the thoracic cage deformity may result in physical findings that can mimic and suggest pathology.[41,42] In patients with heart disease, however, thoracic skeletal abnormalities are frequently found. Sixty-one percent of patients with mitral valve prolapse can have associated pectus excavatum, straight thoracic spine, or scoliosis.[43]

Scoliosis has been noted in 66% of patients with cyanotic congenital heart disease and in 24% of patients with acyanotic congenital heart disease. Interestingly, the major convexity of the scoliosis tends to be opposite the side in which the aortic arch is present.[44]

Unilateral, high left parasternal bulge has been noted to be frequently a clue to atrial septal defect. Bilateral anterior chest bulge invading the midsternal region, or a low left parasternal bulge in the 4th and 5th chondrosternal junction, on the other hand, have been more frequently associated with a ventricular septal defect.[45]

The Extremities

Many of the previously discussed disease entities are associated with abnormalities of the limbs, hands, and feet. Among them are Marfan's syndrome, the mucopolysaccharidoses such as Hurler's syndrome, osteogenesis imperfecta, Turner's syndrome, trisomy 21, trisomy 13–15, and trisomy 18, Ellis–van Creveld syndrome, acromegaly, and de Lange syndrome. Cardiovascular abnormalities also occur in association with abnormalities that involve the limbs, joints, and hands.

HOLT–ORAM SYNDROME commonly presents with the physical finding of hypoplasia of the greater multangular carpal bone on the radial side, resulting in a small thumb on the same plane as the fingers (Fig. 4-7A). The most common associated cardiac anomaly is a secundum atrial septal defect.[46] In cases with radial hypoplasia or aplasia, usually associated with absent or residual thumbs, ventricular septal defects may be the most common associated cardiac lesion.[47] There appears to be a spectrum of upper-limb abnormalities in which any one of the upper limb bones may be absent, hypoplastic, or deformed (Fig. 4-7B). The term *upper limb–cardiovascular syndrome* has been used to encompass the reported cases. Viewed from this standpoint, ostium secundum atrial septal defect, (present in 32 out of 99 cases), and ventricular septal defect

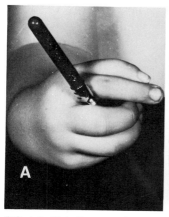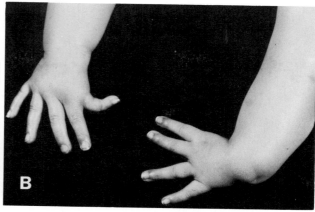

FIG. 4-7. Holt–Oram syndrome (*A*) Right hand of child with a fingerlike hypoplastic thumb which cannot be opposed. (*B*) Six-week-old infant with left radial club hand with absent thumb and hypoplastic fingerlike thumb on right hand. Several of the child's relatives also had Holt–Oram syndrome. (Courtesy of Bertron M. Groves, M.D.)

(present in 30 out of 99 cases), lead the list of congenital cardiac lesions clinically diagnosed.[48]

POLYDACTYLY is associated most frequently with ventricular septal defect.[49] When associated with atrial septal defect, the ostium primum variety predominates.[50] Polydactyly is also a feature of the Ellis-van Creveld syndrome in which the most common cardiac lesion is single atrium or large atrial septal defect, and of the Laurence–Moon–Biedl syndrome, in which no one congenital cardiac anomaly predominates, although it has been associated with patent ductus arteriosus, great vessel transposition, pulmonic stenosis, dextrocardia, and hypoplastic aorta.[51]

SCLERODERMA is a disease involving blood vessels and connective tissue. Its cutaneous manifestation is taut, thickened, or edematous skin, especially evident in the hands and fingers, less often in the feet and toes. Normal skin folds at the knuckles disappear, and chronic, recurrent ulcerations at the tip of the digits develop (Fig. 4-8). Although there is proliferation of connective tissue and degeneration of myocardial fibers, the cardiomegaly associated with the disease is thought to be the result of pulmonary or systemic hypertension. The most common cardiovascular lesion (present in 36% of cases) is chronic adhesive pericarditis.[52] Echocardiography commonly reveals thickening of the LV wall, left atrial enlargement, pericardial effusion, and decreased closing velocity of the anterior mitral valve leaflet.[53]

RHEUMATOID ARTHRITIS presents with characteristic joint abnormalities. The characteristic hand deformity results from subluxation of metacarpophalangeal joints, with ulnar deviation of the digits and hyperextension deformity of proximal interphalangeal joints. As many as 60% of patients may have cardiac involvement. By echocardiography, 46% have pericardial in-

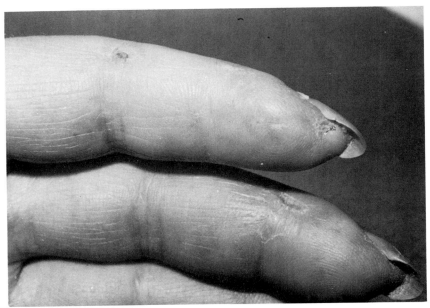

FIG. 4-8. Subcutaneous calcinosis and recurrent ulcerations of fingertips in patient with scleroderma. (Courtesy of J. Clark Huff, M.D.)

volvement (effusion, thickening, or both). Thirty percent have valve abnormality (reduced diastolic descent rate of 40 mm–60 mm per second), presumably due to fibrosis of the valve structures. Granulomatous infiltration of the valve or myocardium have also been proposed as mechanisms.[54]

JACCOUD'S ARTHRITIS (chronic post–rheumatic fever arthritis) presents with ulnar deviation and flexion of the metacarpophalangeal joints, with extension of the interphalangeal joints. Although it may mimic rheumatoid arthritis in initial appearance, the associated ulnar deviation is correctable (Fig. 4-9).[55]

CYANOSIS AND CLUBBING of the nail beds are useful clinical clues to the presence of right-to-left shunting. When symmetrical, right-to-left shunting is commonly at atrial or ventricular level. Reversal of shunt across a patent ductus arteriosus with pulmonary hypertension results in differential cyanosis (*i.e.*, cyanosis that is evident in the feet but is less evident or absent in the hands). Reversed differential cyanosis (*i.e.*, greater cyanosis of the hands than the feet) should suggest the possibility of complete great vessel transposition with severe pulmonary hypertension and reversal of flow through a patent ductus arteriosus. A similar presentation can occur with complete transposition of the great vessels combined with complete interruption of the aortic arch.[56]

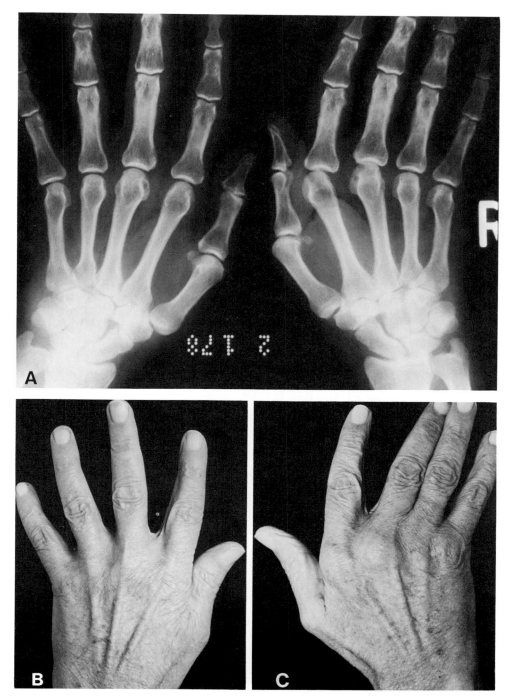

FIG. 4-9. Man with rheumatic mitral valve stenosis and Jaccoud's arthritis. (*A*) Hand x-rays. The left hand has been straightened and the right hand is relaxed with ulnar deviation evident. Note preservation of joint architecture. (*B*) Left hand with ulnar deviation corrected. (*C*) Right hand demonstrating ulnar deviation mimicking rheumatoid arthritis deformity. (Courtesy of Bertron M. Groves, M.D.)

The Neuromuscular Disorders

DUCHENNE'S MUSCULAR DYSTROPHY is a heredo-familial myopathic disorder that is clinically manifest in males and presents with calf pseudohypertrophy (Fig. 4-10). Tall right precordial R waves and deep limb lead and left precordial Q waves characterize the electrocardiogram of most of these patients. These ECG changes are caused by selective scarring of the posterobasal portion of the left ventricle.[57]

By echocardiography, there is a lower than normal LV ejection fraction and percent shortening of LV diameter.[58] Mitral valve prolapse has been noted in 25% to 35% of patients.[59–61]

Pathologic studies on three patients with Duchenne's muscular dystrophy and features of mitral valve prolapse suggest that degenerative changes including the posterior papillary muscle and posterobasal segment of the left ventricle may be the underlying mechanism for prolapse in these patients.[62]

LIMB-GIRDLE DYSTROPHY is an autosomal recessive myopathic disorder that usually has its onset during adolescence. Muscular weakness begins in the pelvic or shoulder girdle and subsequently invades both areas. Cardiac involvement is uncommon, but ECG abnormalities such as a prolonged P–R interval, abnormal Q waves, and an abnormal R wave in lead V_1 have been noted.[63]

FACIOSCAPULOHUMERAL DYSTROPHY is an autosomal dominant myopathic disorder that has its onset in adolescence. Cardiac involvement in this entity is considered rare.

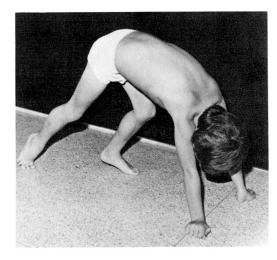

FIG. 4-10. Duchenne's muscular dystrophy with pseudohypertrophy of the calves in a young boy overcoming hip weakness by supporting his weight on both feet and hands as he initiates the effort to arise from the floor. (Ringel SP: Clinical presentations in neuromuscular disease. In Vinken PJ, Bruyn GW (eds): Handbook of Clinical Neurology, Vol 40, Diseases of Muscle, p 315. Amsterdam, Elsevier/North-Holland, 1979)

MYOTONIC DYSTROPHY   is an autosomal dominant myopathic disorder. Cranial muscles are often affected, resulting in ptosis, facial weakness, and dysarthria (Fig. 4-11). Limb weakness is initially distal, that is, hand weakness precedes shoulder weakness, and foot drop precedes pelvic weakness. There is difficulty in muscular relaxation (myotonia). Conduction abnormalities (AV block, right bundle branch block, left axis deviation [LAD] have been observed. Abnormalities noted in ventricular function parameters suggest that this disorder has a cardiomyopathic component.[64] A 17% incidence of mitral valve prolapse has also been reported.[59] Papillary muscle dysfunction may also play a role in the genesis of this disease, as it does in Duchenne muscular dystrophy.[65]

FRIEDREICH'S ATAXIA   is an autosomal recessive or dominant disorder resulting in spinocerebellar degeneration. Gait impairment and poor coordination are present. Progressive skeletal deformities including kyphoscoliosis and pes cavus occur (Fig. 4-12). Approximately 50% of patients manifest cardiac abnormalities, including cardiomegaly and conduction disturbances such as AV and bundle branch block.

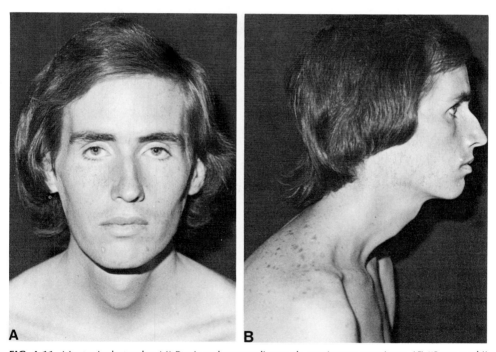

A   **B**

FIG. 4-11. Myotonic dystrophy. (*A*) Ptosis and temporalis muscle wasting are prominent. (*B*) "Swan neck" appearance caused by weakness and wasting of neck muscles. (From Ringel SP: Clinical presentations in neuromuscular disease. In Vinken PJ, Bruyn GW (eds): Handbook of Clinical Neurology, Vol 40, Diseases of Muscle, p 305. Amsterdam, Elsevier/North Holland, 1979)

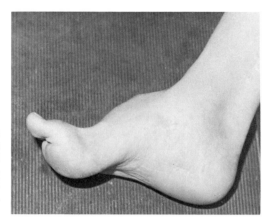

FIG. 4-12. Pes cavus deformity of the foot seen in patients with long-standing weakness of the muscles of the feet. (From Ringel SP: Clinical presentations in neuromuscular disease. In Vinken PJ, Bruyn GW (eds): Handbook of Clinical Neurology, Vol 40, Diseases of Muscle, p 321. Amsterdam, Elsevier/North-Holland, 1979)

Summary

An in-depth knowledge of the numerous relationships between musculoskeletal abnormalities and underlying cardiovascular disease allows a clinician to suspect heart disease from careful inspection of his patient. To minimize the possibility of oversight, observations should be made in the following categories:

1. Habitus and general appearance
2. Head and face
3. Thorax
4. Extremities
5. Neuromuscular abnormalities

Once an underlying cardiac abnormality is suspected, the physical examination and noninvasive studies can then be focused to confirm or reject its presence.

References

1. Pyeritz RE, McKusick VA: The Marfan's syndrome: Diagnosis and management. N Engl J Med 300:772, 1979
2. Brown OR, De Mots KPE, Roberts A, et al: Aortic root dilation and mitral valve prolapse in Marfan's syndrome: An echocardiographic study. Circulation 52:652, 1975
3. Spangler RD, Nora JJ, Lortscher RH, et al: Echocardiography in Marfan's syndrome. Chest 69:72, 1976
4. Hirst AE, Gore I: Marfan's syndrome: A review. Prog Cardiovasc Dis 16:187, 1973
5. Przybojewski JZ, Maritz F, Tiedt FAC, et al: Pseudoxanthoma elasticum with cardiac involvement: A case report and review of the literature. S Afr Med J p 268, 21 Feb. 1981

6. Coffman JD, Sommers SC: Familial pseudoxanthoma elasticum and valvular heart disease. Circulation 59:600, 1959
7. Navarro–Lopez F, Llorian A, Ferrer–Roca O, et al: Restrictive cardiomyopathy in pseudoxanthoma elasticum. Chest 78:113, 1980
8. Leier CV, Call TD, Fulkerson PK, et al: The spectrum of cardiac defects in the Ehlers–Danlos syndrome, types I and III. Ann Intern Med 92:171, 1980
9. De Busk FL: The Hutchinson–Gilford progeria syndrome. J Pediatr 80:697, 1972
10. Brosius FC, Roberts WC: Coronary artery disease in the Hurler syndrome. Am J Cardiol 47:649, 1981
11. Schieken RM, Kerber RE, Ionasescu VV, et al: Cardiac manifestations of the mucopolysaccharidoses. Circulation 52:700, 1975
12. Stein D, Kloster FE: Valvular heart disease in osteogenesis imperfecta. Am Heart J 94:637, 1977
13. Heppner RL, Babitt HJ, Bianchine JW, et al: Aortic regurgitation and aneurysm of sinus of Valsalva associated with osteogenesis imperfecta. Am J Cardiol 31:654, 1973
14. Bulkley BH, Roberts WC: Ankylosing spondylitis and aortic regurgitation. Circulation 48:1014, 1973
15. Graham DC, Smythe HA: The carditis and aortitis of ankylosing spondylitis. Bull Rheum Dis 9:171, 1958
16. Nora JJ, Torres FG, Sinha AK, et al: Characteristic cardiovascular anomalies of XO Turner syndrome, XX and XY phenotype and XO/SS Turner mosaic. Am J Cardiol 25:639, 1970
17. Nora JJ, Nora AA, Sinha AK, et al: The Ullrich–Noonan syndrome (Turner phenotype). Am J Dis Child 127:48, 1974
18. Gorlin RJ, Anderson RC, Blaw M: Multiple lentigenes syndrome. Am J Dis Child 117:652, 1969
19. McKusick VA, Egeland JA, Eldridge R, et al: Dwarfism in the Amish: I. The Ellis–Van Creveld syndrome. Bull Johns Hopkins Hosp 115:306, 1964
20. Blackburn MG, Belliveau RE: Ellis–Van Creveld syndrome. Am J Dis Child 122:267, 1971
21. Williams JCP, Barratt–Boyes BG, Lowe JB: Supravalvular aortic stenosis. Circulation 24:1311, 1961
22. Beuren AJ, Schulze C, Eberle P, et al: The syndrome of supravalvular aortic stenosis, peripheral pulmonary stenosis, mental retardation and similar facial appearance. Am J Cardiol 13:471, 1964
23. Martin EC, Moseley IF: Supravalvular aortic stenosis. Br Heart J 35:758, 1973
24. Line LM, Turner SW, Sparkes RS: Pulmonary valvular dysplasia, a cardiofacial syndrome. Br Heart J 35:301, 1973
25. Cayler GG, Blumenfield CM, Anderson RL: Further studies of patients with cardiofacial syndrome. Chest 60:161, 1971
26. Tandon R, Edwards JE: Cardiac malformations associated with Down's syndrome. Circulation 47:1349, 1973
27. Warkany J, Passarge E, Smith LB: Congenital malformations in autosomal trisomy syndromes. Am J Dis Child 112:502, 1966
28. Trell E, Rausing A, Ripe J, et al: Carcinoid heart disease. Clinicopathologic findings and follow-up in 11 cases. Am J Med 54:433, 1973
29. Roberts WC, Sjoerdsma A: The cardiac disease associated with the carcinoid syndrome. Am J Med 35:5, 1964
30. Becker AE, Schoorl R, Balk AG, et al: Cardiac manifestations of Fabry's disease. Am J Cardiol 36:829, 1975
31. McGuffin WL Jr, Sherman BM, Roth J, et al: Acromegaly and cardiovascular disorders: A prospective study. Ann Intern Med 81:11, 1974

32. Hejtmanick MR, Beadfield JU, Herman GR: Acromegaly and the heart: A clinical and pathologic study. Ann Intern Med 34:1445, 1951

33. Hearne M, Sherber H, de Leon AC: Asymmetric septal hypertrophy in acromegaly. Circulation (Suppl II)52:35, 1975

34. Luboshirtzki R, Hammerman H, Barzilia D, et al: The heart in acromegaly: Correlation of echocardiographic and clinical findings. Isr J Med Sci 16:378, 1980

35. Savage DD, Henry WL, Eastman RC, et al: Echocardiographic assessment of cardiac anatomy and function in acromegalic patients. Am J Med 67:823, 1979

36. Friedman S, Saraclar M: The high frequency of congenital heart disease in oculo-auriculo-vertebral dysplasia (Goldenhar's syndrome). J Pediatr 85:873, 1974

37. Mellor DH, Richardson JE, Douglas DM: Goldenhar's syndrome. Arch Dis Child 48:537, 1973

38. Robinson CD, Perry LW, Barlee A, et al: Smith–Lemli–Opitz syndrome with cardiovascular abnormality. Pediatrics 47:844, 1971

39. Rao PS, Sissman NJ: Congenital heart disease in the de Lange syndrome. J Pedriatr 79:674, 1971

40. Kushnick T: Brachydactyly, facial abnormalities, and mental retardation. Am J Dis Child 111:96, 1966

41. de Leon AC, Perloff JK, Twigg H, et al: The straight back syndrome: Clinical cardiovascular manifestations. Circulation 32:193, 1965

42. Guller B: Cardiac findings in pectus excavatum in children: Review and differential diagnosis. Chest 66:165, 1974

43. Bon Tempo CP, Ronan JA, de Leon AC, et al: Radiographic appearance of the thorax in systolic click–late systolic murmur syndrome. Am J Cardiol 36:27, 1975

44. Jordan CE, White RI Jr, Fischer KC, et al: The scoliosis of congenital heart disease. Am Heart J 84:463, 1972

45. Arosemena E, Elliott LP, Eliot RS: Chest deformity in adults with congenital heart disease. Am J Cardiol 20:309, 1967

46. Silverman ME, Copeland AJ Jr, Hurst JW: The Holt–Oram syndrome; the long and short of it. Am J Cardiol 25:11, 1970

47. Harris LC, Osborne WP: Congenital absence or hypoplasia of the radius with ventricular septal defect: Ventriculoradial dysplasia. J Pediatr 68:265, 1966

48. Braus UW, Lintermans JPL: The upper limb-cardiovascular syndrome. Am J Dis Child 124:779, 1972

49. Silverman ME, Hurst JW: The hand and the heart. Am J Cardiol 22:718, 1968

50. Sanches Casos A: Genetics of atrial septal defect. Arch Dis Child 47:581, 1972

51. McLaughlin TE, Krovetz LJ, Schiebler GL: Heart disease in the Laurence–Moon–Biedl–Bardet syndrome. J Pediatr 65:388, 1964

52. Sackner MA, Heinz ER, Steinberg AJ: The heart in scleroderma. Am J Cardiol 17:542, 1966

53. Gottdiener JS, Moutsopoulos HM, Decker JL: Echocardiographic identification of cardiac abnormality in scleroderma related disorders. Am J Med 66:391, 1979

54. Nomeir AM, Turner R, Watts E, et al: Cardiac involvement in rheumatoid arthritis. Ann Intern Med 79:800, 1973

55. Zwaifler NJ: Chronic postrheumatic fever (Jaccoud's) arthritis. N Engl J Med 267:10, 1962

56. Buckley MJ, Mason DT, Ross J Jr, et al: Reversed differential cyanosis with equal desaturation of the upper limbs: Syndrome of complete transposition of the great vessels with complete interruption of the aortic arch. Am J Cardiol 15:111, 1965

57. Perloff JK, Roberts WC, de Leon AC, et al: The distinctive electrocardiogram of Duchenne's progressive muscular dystrophy. Am J Med 42:179, 1967

58. Farah MG, Evans EB, Vignos PJ Jr: Echocardiographic evaluation of left ventricular function in Duchenne's muscular dystrophy. Am J Med 69:248, 1980
59. Reeves WC, Griggs R, Nanda NC, et al: Echocardiographic evaluation of cardiac abnormalities in Duchenne's dystrophy. Arch Neurol 37:272, 1980
60. Sanyal SK, Leung RKF, Tierney RC, et al: Mitral valve prolapse syndrome in children with Duchenne's progressive muscular dystrophy. Pediatrics 63:116, 1979
61. Biddison JH, Dembo DH, Spalt H, et al: Familial occurrence of mitral valve prolapse in X-linked muscular dystrophy. Circulation 59:1299, 1979
62. Sanyal SK, Johnson WW, Dische MR, et al: Dystrophic degeneration of papillary muscle and ventricular myocardium: A basis for mitral valve prolapse in Duchenne's muscular dystrophy. Circulation 62:430, 1980
63. Perloff JK, de Leon AC Jr, O'Doherty E: The cardiomyopathy of progressive muscular dystrophy. Circulation 33:625, 1966
64. Beulcke G, Casazza F, Columbo B, et al: On some cardiological aspects of Steinert's disease (myotonic dystrophy). Z Kardiol 68:848, 1979
65. Strasburg B, Shinger RC, Rosen K: Myotonia dystrophica and mitral valve prolapse. Chest 78:845, 1980

5

CYANOSIS

Roy V. Ditchey, M.D.

Definition

Cyanosis is a bluish discoloration that results from an increased amount of deoxygenated hemoglobin or hemoglobin derivatives in the small blood vessels of the skin and mucous membranes, as well as in other organs that are not usually visible.[1] The appearance and degree of cyanosis depend on the amount of deoxygenated hemoglobin present, the color of the blood plasma, and the thickness and pigmentation of the skin. It usually is most marked in the lips, earlobes, nail beds, and malar eminences but may be more apparent in the retina or mucous membranes of the mouth in patients with dark complexions. Since the vascular contents are responsible for the abnormal color, cyanotic skin blanches with pressure. Other disorders that cause bluish skin color do so through an accumulation of extravascular skin pigments (see Causes of Blue or Gray Skin Color, below). As a result, the discoloration persists despite application of pressure sufficient to empty the cutaneous vessels of blood.

CAUSES OF BLUE OR GRAY SKIN COLOR*

Genetic causes
   Hyperpigmentation of the eyelids, axillae, and nailbeds of some normal individuals

    *Excluding disorders causing well-circumscribed lesions with clearly identifiable borders.

Metabolic causes
  Hemochromatosis
  Ochronosis

Nutritional causes
  Chronic nutritional insufficiency

Chemical causes
  Heavy metal intoxication
    Silver (argyria)
    Gold
    Bismuth
    Lead
  Topical mercury (contained in face creams)
  Fixed drug eruptions (*e.g.,* due to phenothiazines)

Neoplastic causes
  Metastatic melanoma with melanuria and generalized dermal pigmentation

Circulatory causes
  Cyanosis

The causes of cyanosis fall into two general categories (see Causes of Cyanosis, below). Cyanosis is said to be *central* in origin when it results from increased amounts of unsaturated hemoglobin or abnormal hemoglobin derivatives in arterial blood. The skin and mucous membranes generally are both affected (since all tissues receive arterial blood), and the cyanosis does not depend on decreased tissue perfusion. Clubbing of the fingers and toes often accompanies arterial unsaturation of long standing, and its presence usually means that cyanosis is central in origin. In *peripheral* cyanosis, arterial oxygen saturation is normal, but slow blood flow through peripheral tissues leads to increased oxygen extraction and abnormally high concentrations of deoxygenated hemoglobin in capillary and venous blood. Although clinical differentiation between central and peripheral cyanosis is not always possible, decreased blood flow is often accompanied by a redistribution of flow away from the extremities. As a result, the mucous membranes of the mouth sometimes are spared when cyanosis is peripheral in origin.

CAUSES OF CYANOSIS

Central cyanosis
  Decreased arterial hemoglobin saturation
    Decreased inspired oxygen tension (high altitude). (See Table 5-2)
    Impaired respiratory function
      Hypoventilation
      Perfusion of underventilated lung areas
      Impaired oxygen diffusion
    Anatomical right-to-left shunts
      Cyanotic congenital heart disease (See Cyanotic Congenital Heart Diseases, below)
      Pulmonary arteriovenous fistulae

Hemoglobin variants with low affinity for oxygen
  Stable
  Unstable
Abnormal hemoglobin derivatives
  Methemoglobinemia
    Hereditary
      M hemoglobins
      Methemoglobin reductase deficiency
    Acquired
  Sulfhemoglobinemia

Peripheral cyanosis
  Cold exposure
  Low cardiac output
  Arterial obstruction or spasm
  Venous obstruction

Physiology

NORMAL SKIN COLOR AND THE THRESHOLD FOR CYANOSIS

Light impinging on human skin is partly reflected and partly transmitted inward to successive cell layers in the epidermis, dermis, and subcutaneous tissues.[2,3] Each layer of tissue contains pigments that act as color screens or biologic optical filters, absorbing specific wavelengths of light in the visible spectrum. As a result, light striking each layer is absorbed, or scattered, or transmitted to the layer below until the energy of the incident beam is dissipated. A small fraction of absorbed radiation then is re-emitted at longer wavelengths, a phenomenon known as fluorescence. The color perceived at the skin's surface is determined by the wavelengths ultimately *remitted*, or passed back, from various depths by backward scattering of optical radiation. For example, if all wavelengths within the visible spectrum were absorbed, the skin would appear pure black; if all visible wavelengths were remitted, it would appear pure white; intermediate colors result from the optical mix of remitted wavelengths, that is, the wavelengths not absorbed by cutaneous and subcutaneous pigments.

Light reflected at the outer surface of the skin does not contribute significantly to skin color, since surface reflectance is relatively constant for all wavelengths.[3] Rather, normal skin color is determined by the absorption patterns, density, and distribution of four major pigments in the inner layers of the skin and subcutaneous tissues.[2,3] Melanin, a brown pigment with broad absorption characteristics in the visible and ultraviolet range, is the dominant pigment in the epidermis and is responsible for the various degrees of dark skin color present in normal individuals. It acts largely as a neutral filter, diminishing remittance of light from underlying tissue layers. Carotene (a term used to describe a group of related substances known as carotenoids) is present in the cornified layer of the epidermis, and in sebaceous glands and subcutaneous fat. It is responsible for the yellow tint often present in highly keratinized and relatively amelanotic skin areas. The remaining two pigments are in the blood perfusing the skin, rather than in the skin and subcutaneous tissues themselves. Oxygenated and deoxygenated hemoglobin are the major pigments of the dermis and contribute substantially to both normal and abnormal skin color. Oxygenated hemoglobin has two characteristic peak absorption bands and is bright red in appearance; deoxygenated hemoglobin has a single absorption band and is darker and less red (or more blue) in appearance; other pigments in blood plasma normally are pale yellow and contribute relatively little to the color perceived at the skin's surface.

In general, the contribution of blood pigments to skin color depends on the density and distribution of blood vessels in the skin, the total concentration and saturation of hemoglobin in the blood, and the extent to which the effects of these pigments are masked by melanin. In dark races, the effects of melanin on skin color are sufficiently dominant that contributions from other skin pigments, including hemoglobin, often can be appreciated only in areas where the melanin content is reduced, such as the mucous membranes of the mouth. Even under these conditions, however, *rapid* changes in skin color invariably are due to changes in either the caliber of cutaneous blood vessels or the concentration or saturation of hemoglobin in cutaneous blood.

It generally is stated that clinical recognition of cyanosis requires a deoxygenated hemoglobin concentration of more than 5g/100 ml in the capillaries of the skin.[1,4,5] This axiom is based on early work by Lundsgaard, who estimated capillary hemoglobin saturation from arterial and brachial venous oxygen contents and capacities in normal and cyanotic subjects.[1,4] He found that cyanosis usually was detectable when a simple average of arterial and venous oxygen unsaturations exceeded 6 to 7 vol%. This corresponds to a deoxygenated hemoglobin concentration of approximately 5g/100 ml and is valid as an empiric observation. However, it is unlikely that this actually represents the critical concentration of deoxygenated hemoglobin responsible for cyanosis, for several reasons. First, Lungsgaard recognized that the degree of unsaturation of capillary blood cannot be determined precisely by averaging arterial and venous unsaturations.[1,4] Reasoning that the hemoglobin saturation of capillary blood must be intermediate between arterial and venous values, he intended an average of the two only as an approximation. In fact, the oxygen content of capillary blood may resemble either arterial or venous content more closely, depending on the local balance between blood flow and tissue oxygen consumption. Furthermore, the brachial veins drain a nonhomogeneous group of tissues with widely varying metabolic rates and local venous oxygen contents. As a result, the degree of unsaturation of brachial venous blood may not indicate accurately the amount of deoxygenated hemoglobin present in veins draining the skin. This is particularly true since cutaneous blood flow not only serves the metabolic requirements of the skin, but also plays an important role in heat exchange and body temperature regulation. When external temperature rises, cutaneous blood flow increases out of proportion to increases in local metabolic rate. As a result, cutaneous venous oxygen contents are high relative to other organ systems. Finally, in most areas of the body, skin color probably is influenced less by the hemoglobin concentration and saturation of blood in the cutaneous capillaries than by that in other cutaneous and subcutaneous vessels. For the most part, superficial capillaries follow a course that is perpendicular to the surface of the skin, so that only the small apical segments of the capillary loops within each dermal papilla are visible from the skin surface.[6,7] Except in the nail folds, where capillary loops lie parallel to the surface of the skin, and in the nail beds, where they are especially dense, the pigments contained in these vessels contribute relatively little to skin color. In contrast, the subpapillary venous plexuses into which cutaneous capillaries drain are both extensive and oriented parallel to the skin surface.[8] It is likely that the pigments coursing through these vessels make the major vascular contribution to skin color.

HEMOGLOBIN CONCENTRATION AND SATURATION

Although the precise concentration required is uncertain, cyanosis clearly results from an increased amount of deoxygenated hemoglobin in the small vessels of the skin. Furthermore, it appears that cyanosis is related more closely to the *absolute* concentration of deoxygenated hemoglobin than to the ratio of deoxygenated to oxygenated hemoglobin concentrations. Confirmation by direct measurement of cutaneous capillary and venous hemoglobin concentrations and saturations is lacking. However, the presence of cyanosis correlates closely with the average of arterial and brachial venous unsaturated hemoglobin concentrations, regardless of the amount of saturated hemoglobin present.[1,4] This suggests that, although total and saturated hemoglobin concentrations may influence the hue or color of cyanotic skin, it is the concentration of deoxygenated hemoglobin that determines whether or not cyanosis is present.

The concentration of deoxygenated hemoglobin in cutaneous blood is determined by the total hemoglobin concentration and the percent saturation of hemoglobin with oxygen; hemoglobin saturation is determined in turn by the partial pressure of oxygen in blood (PO_2) and the shape of the oxygen–hemoglobin dissociation curve. These interrelationships are important in the pathogenesis of cyanosis, since abnormalities at any step potentially can cause or prevent cyanosis independently of other variables. For example, in patients with severe anemia, the absolute concentration of deoxygenated hemoglobin may not be sufficient to cause cyanosis despite complete unsaturation of cutaneous blood. Conversely, polycythemic patients may have abnormally high deoxygenated hemoglobin concentrations (and therefore cyanosis), despite normal or increased oxygen content and hemoglobin saturation. If one accepts that a deoxygenated hemoglobin concentration of approximately 5g/100 ml is necessary for the clinical detection of cyanosis, hemoglobin unsaturation cannot cause cyanosis in patients with total hemoglobin concentrations below this level. As the total hemoglobin concentration increases above 5g/100 ml the degree of unsaturation required for cyanosis progressively declines (Table 5-1). Theoretically, a polycythemic patient with a total hemoglobin concentration of 25 g/100 ml could be cyanotic despite an oxygen saturation of 80%.

Table 5–1.   Influence of Total Hemoglobin Concentration on the Oxygen Saturation Threshold for Cyanosis*

Total Hemoglobin Concentration (g/100 ml)	Oxygen saturation (%)
< 5	not possible
5	0
6	17
7	29
8	37
9	44
10	50
11	55
12	58
13	62
14	64
15	67
16	69
17	71
18	72
19	74
20	75
21	76
22	77
23	78
24	79
25	80

*Assuming detection of cyanosis requires a concentration of deoxygenated hemoglobin of 5 g/100 ml.

Under normal conditions, hemoglobin is more than 90% saturated whenever PO_2 is greater than approximately 70 mm Hg. However, the shape of the normal oxygen–hemoglobin dissociation curve is sigmoid, so that hemoglobin saturation falls abruptly with only modest further reductions in PO_2. The shape and position of this curve (and, therefore, the precise relationship between PO_2 and hemoglobin saturation) depend on body temperature and intracellular concentrations of hydrogen ion, carbon dioxide, and 2,3 diphosphoglycerate (2,3-DPG), an organic mediator of hemoglobin function. Specifically, an increase in the concentration of one or more of these variables will shift the oxygen–hemoglobin dissociation curve to the right, decreasing hemoglobin saturation at any given oxygen tension. These factors make the concentration of deoxygenated hemoglobin in cutaneous blood (and, therefore, cyanosis) a complex function of total hemoglobin concentration, oxygen tension, and a potentially dynamic or changing relationship between PO_2 and oxygen saturation. The shape and position of the oxygen–hemoglobin dissociation curve also can differ significantly from normal as a result of either primary or drug-induced abnormalities in hemoglobin structure. These abnormalities are discussed in detail in the following section.

Clinical Presentation

CENTRAL CYANOSIS

By definition, central cyanosis is due to increased amounts of unsaturated hemoglobin or abnormal hemoglobin derivatives in arterial blood. Arterial unsaturation results in abnormally high capillary and venous concentrations of deoxygenated hemoglobin despite normal blood flow and oxygen extraction by peripheral tissues. It results from either decreased arterial oxygen tension (hypoxemia) or abnormalities of hemoglobin that reduce its affinity for oxygen.

At high altitudes, the oxygen tension in arterial blood (P_aO_2) may be low enough to cause significant hemoglobin unsaturation even in the absence of disease. This is because barometric pressure is an important determinant of the partial pressures and relative concentrations of respiratory gases in ambient and alveolar air. For example, oxygen and nitrogen, the major gases in the earth's atmosphere, are present in relatively constant proportions in dry air at all altitudes. As a result, ambient PO_2 and PN_2, which account for approximately 20.94% and 78.09% of total barometric pressure, respectively, are lower at high altitudes because of decreased atmospheric pressure.[9] *Alveolar* PO_2 (P_AO_2) is even more sensitive to changes in altitude because of higher (and relatively fixed) local concentrations of carbon dioxide and water vapor. Specifically, P_AH_2O is determined entirely by body temperature (equalling 47 mm Hg at 37°C), and is independent of barometric pressure. P_ACO_2 is determined by the balance between carbon dioxide production in the body and its removal through alveolar ventilation. Although it tends to fall at higher altitudes due to hypoxemia-induced hyperventilation, it decreases less than either ambient PO_2 or P_AO_2. As a result, both P_ACO_2 and P_AH_2O occupy progressively larger fractions of total alveolar pressure as altitude increases (Table 5-2).

P_aO_2 is slightly lower than P_AO_2 at all altitudes because of small amounts of venous admixture, but still is sufficient to maintain hemoglobin saturation above 90% at elevations of up to 8,000 to 10,000 feet above sea level (depending on the extent of compensatory hyperventilation). This is because normal oxygen–hemoglobin dissociation characteristics prevent significant arterial unsaturation despite moderate hypoxemia. However, further ascent eventually results in significant (and precipitous) unsaturation of arterial blood. For example, at an elevation of 15,000 feet above sea level, the effects of decreased barometric pressure and proportionately greater concentrations of carbon dioxide and water vapor in alveolar air decrease P_AO_2 to approximately 45 mm Hg, a level of hypoxemia sufficient to cause cyanosis in the absence of anemia. Oxygen breathing decreases the P_AN_2, but has no effect on P_ACO_2 or P_AH_2O. As a result, hypoxemia and hemoglobin unsaturation develop at very high altitudes even when pure oxygen is being breathed. For example, inhalation of (unpressurized) 100% oxygen at an altitude of approximately 43,000 feet results in levels of arterial hypoxemia and hemoglobin unsaturation comparable to those present when breathing ambient air at 15,000 feet.[9] At an altitude of approximately 50,000 feet, the sum of P_ACO_2 and P_AH_2O nearly equals bar-

Table 5–2. Barometric and Respiratory Gas Pressures as a Function of Altitude

Altitude (Feet)	Barometric Pressure	Dry Ambient Air				Alveolar Air*			
		PO_2 (mm Hg)	PCO_2 (mm Hg)	PH_2O (mm Hg)	PN_2 (mm Hg)	P_AO_2 (mm Hg)	P_ACO_2 (mm Hg)	P_AH_2O† (mm Hg)	P_AN_2 (mm Hg)
0	760	159	<1	0	593	103	40	47	570
5,000	632	132	<1	0	494	81	38	47	466
10,000	523	110	<1	0	408	61	36	47	379
15,000	429	90	<1	0	335	45	33	47	304
20,000	349	73	<1	0	273	35	30	47	237

*Approximations based on several sources (10).

†At 37°C. P_AO_2 and P_AN_2 are lower than ambient levels because P_ACO_2 and P_AH_2O are higher; in addition, oxygen and nitrogen tensions vary relative to each other, depending on the balance between respiratory delivery of oxygen to alveoli and its removal by circulating blood.

123

ometric pressure, and, unless pressure is restored artificially, the lungs contain little or no oxygen, regardless of the composition of inspired air.

Arterial hypoxemia and hemoglobin unsaturation frequently result from respiratory or cardiovascular disorders that interfere with lung function or shunt systemic venous blood into the arterial circuit. Serious abnormalities in lung function (particularly alveolar hypoventilation or perfusion of poorly ventilated lung areas) are common causes of central cyanosis. These may be acute and reversible, as in drug-induced respiratory depression, pulmonary edema, or severe pneumonia; or chronic and irreversible (without supplemental oxygen), as in emphysema. Theoretically, impaired oxygen diffusion across alveolar membranes also can cause arterial hypoxemia, although the clinical importance of this effect is disputed. Lung diseases such as diffuse interstitial fibrosis cause thickening of alveolar membranes and decreases in diffusing capacity but also interfere with normal ventilation and blood flow patterns. Arterial hypoxemia in these conditions results primarily from ventilation–perfusion inequalities, rather than "alveolar–capillary block." Although a variety of disorders cause obliteration or loss of pulmonary capillary beds, this effect does not contribute to arterial hypoxemia or cyanosis, since it does not itself result in perfusion of underventilated lung areas.

Certain types of congenital heart disease cause cyanosis by shunting systemic venous blood directly into left-sided cardiac chambers or great vessels. Since blood flows from high to low pressure areas, right-to-left shunting between cardiac chambers or from the pulmonary artery to the aorta requires not only a direct communication between right- and left-sided structures, but also an increase in right heart or pulmonary arterial pressure. For this reason, such shunts are usually associated with either increased pulmonary vascular resistance or an anatomical obstruction within the right heart or pulmonary artery distal to the shunt site. The most common form of cyanotic congenital heart disease is the tetralogy of Fallot, the essential components of which are a ventricular septal defect and either valvular or muscular (subvalvular) pulmonary outflow tract obstruction. The presence and degree of cyanosis depend on the severity of the obstruction, which determines right ventricular (RV) pressure and the amount of right-to-left shunting. Other forms of cyanotic congenital heart disease are listed under Cyanotic Congenital Heart Diseases, below. Ventricular septal defects and other disorders that initially produce large left-to-right shunts often lead to structural changes that substantially (and irreversibly) increase pulmonary vascular resistance (the so-called Eisenmenger's syndrome). Compensatory increases in RV pressure eventually lead to shunt reversal (*i.e.,* right-to-left shunting) and cyanosis.When pulmonary hypertension complicates a large left-to-right shunt through a patent ductus arteriosus, shunt reversal causes differential cyanosis; that is, the distribution of cyanosis depends on the location of the ductus in relation to the major branches of the aortic arch. In the usual circumstance, when the ductus arises distal to the origin of the left subclavian artery, right-to-left shunting through the ductus typically causes cyanosis of the trunk and lower extremities, while arterial blood flowing to the upper extremities, head and neck remains normally saturated.[10,11] Cyanosis may extend to the left arm if either the ductus inserts more proximally or unsaturated blood streams into the left subclavian artery.

When pulmonary hypertension and right heart failure develop in this setting, diffuse cyanosis often results from right-to-left shunting through a patent foramen ovale.

CYANOTIC CONGENITAL HEART DISEASES

Disorders not requiring increased pulmonary vascular resistance
  Relatively common
    Tetralogy of Fallot
    Pulmonic atresia with ventricular septal defect
    Pulmonary stenosis with atrial right-to-left shunting
  Uncommon
    Single ventricle with pulmonic stenosis or atresia
    Tricuspid atresia
    Transposition of the great vessels
    Ebstein's anomaly with atrial right-to-left shunting
  Rare
    Double outlet right ventricle
    Vena caval to left atrial communication
    Mitral atresia
    Double outlet left ventricle
    Total anomalous pulmonary venous return

Disorders requiring increased pulmonary vascular resistance (Eisenmenger's syndrome)
  Relatively common
    Ventricular septal defect
    Patent ductus arteriosus
    Atrial septal defect
  Uncommon
    Single ventricle
    Truncus arteriosus

Pulmonary arteriovenous fistulae also shunt deoxygenated blood directly into the systemic circulation. Such communications may be either congenital or acquired and occur either as isolated anomalies or in association with systemic diseases such as hereditary telangiectasia.[12] The physiologic significance of these fistulae depends on their size and number. Multiple pulmonary arteriovenous fistulae as well as direct portal vein–pulmonary vein anastamoses may be responsible for significant right-to-left shunting in some patients with cirrhosis.[13–15]

The degree of arterial hemoglobin unsaturation and cyanosis caused by a right-to-left shunt depends on the size of the shunt relative to systemic blood flow and the saturation of systemic venous blood. Except in the case of pulmonary arteriovenous fistulae, shunt flow depends at least in part on the relative resistances to flow through the pulmonary and systemic circulations. As a result, drugs or physiologic stresses (such as physical exercise) that decrease systemic vascular resistance increase the magnitude of right-to-left shunts. This presents a specific risk and limitation to the use of vasodilating agents in an attempt to decrease pulmonary vascular resistance in patients with congenital heart disease and Eisenmenger physiology. Both physiologic and pathologic increases in body metabolism and oxygen extraction by peripheral tissues (*e.g.*, due to exercise or fever), worsen arterial desaturation in patients with central cyanosis by decreasing the hemoglobin saturation of systemic venous blood. This is true whether the cause of cyanosis is a right-to-left shunt or ventilation–perfusion inequality in the lung. Patients with right-to-left shunts tolerate exercise poorly because of the combined effects of a fall in systemic vascular resistance (which increases shunt flow) and an increase in oxygen extraction by the exercising muscles (which decreases systemic venous hemoglobin saturation). Cyanosis in such patients is worsened, both during exercise and at rest, by the secondary polycythemia that develops as a result of long-standing arterial hemoglobin unsaturation.

Several types of abnormal hemoglobin produce central cyanosis by causing arterial unsaturation despite normal P_aO_2. These consist of both stable and unstable hemoglobin variants with decreased affinity for oxygen, and represent rare, familial causes of cyanosis. In the past 20 years, more than 40 stable hemoglobin tetramers with altered oxygen-binding characteristics have been identified.[16] Most bind oxygen more avidly than normal, but several types (*e.g.*, hemoglobins Kansas and Beth Israel) have markedly decreased oxygen affinity and cause significant arterial unsaturation. Both stable and unstable hemoglobin variants are inherited in an autosomal dominant pattern, and result from structural changes at alpha- or beta-chain sites important in hemoglobin function. Unstable hemoglobins are variants in which the molecular changes involved cause structural instablility, leading to intracellular precipitation, Heinz body formation, and variable degrees of hemolysis. They are important primarily as rare causes of congenital, nonspherocytic, hemolytic anemia. However, the amino acid substitutions responsible for structural instability often involve sites important for normal hemoglobin function. As a result, unstable hemoglobins commonly have abnormal oxygen-binding characteristics (either increased or decreased oxygen affinity). Changes in oxygen affinity usually are mild, although unstable variants with decreased affinity for oxygen occasionally have been associated with significant arterial unsaturation and cyanosis. The onset of cyanosis with both stable and unstable hemoglobin variants depends on the globin chain involved in the structural defect. Cyanosis is present at birth with alpha-chain variants, but may be delayed with beta-chain variants until 3 to 6 months of age, when fetal hemoglobin (HbF), which contains gamma-chains rather than beta-chains, is replaced by adult hemoglobin (HbA).

Rarely, central cyanosis results from the presence of an abnormal hemoglobin derivative (specifically, methemoglobin or sulfhemoglobin) in arterial blood, rather than an increased concentration of deoxygenated hemoglobin. Reversible oxygen binding by hemoglobin depends on the maintenance of heme iron in the reduced or ferrous (Fe^{2+}) state. Methemoglobin is hemoglobin containing ferric (Fe^{3+}) iron and is formed continuously in erythrocytes through processes of auto-oxidation. Since this change in heme iron prevents oxygen binding, normal hemoglobin function depends on enzymatic reduction of methemoglobin according to the reaction

$$Hb^{3+} + NADH \xrightarrow[\text{(diaphorase I)}]{\text{methemoglobin reductase}} Hb^{2+} + NAD$$

This process normally keeps methemoglobin levels at less than 1% of total hemoglobin concentration. Although increased concentrations of methemoglobin decrease arterial saturation, cyanosis is related more to the absorption characteristics of methemoglobin as a pigment than to an increased concentration of deoxygenated hemoglobin. This is illustrated by the fact that methemoglobin concentrations above 1.5 g/100 ml (approximately 10% of total hemoglobin) usually result in cyanosis, compared to the approximately 5 g/100 ml of deoxygenated hemoglobin required for cyanosis under other circumstances.[17] Methemoglobin also differs from the other hemoglobin variants that cause cyanosis in that the oxygen affinity of the functional (ferrous) heme subunits present is actually *increased*. This is because the structural conformation of methemoglobin is similar to that of oxyhemoglobin; as a result, oxidation of one of the four heme irons (from ferrous to ferric) in a hemoglobin tetramer increases the affinity of the remaining heme subunits for oxygen.[18] This effect interferes with oxygen unloading in peripheral tissues and adds to the functional consequences of a loss of oxygen-binding sites in patients with significantly increased methemoglobin concentrations.

Congenital methemoglobinemia results either from an inherited, structural abnormality of hemoglobin or from a deficiency of the enzyme methemoglobin reductase. The so-called M hemoglobins are inherited in an autosomal dominant pattern and result from alpha-chain or beta-chain amino acid substitutions that lead to irreversible oxidation of heme iron. The affinity of these hemoglobins for oxygen is either normal or decreased. Although there is no effective treatment, heterozygous patients generally have only mild methemoglobinemia and asymptomatic cyanosis. As with other abnormal hemoglobins, the onset of cyanosis is determined by the globin chain involved, occurring at birth with alpha-chain variants and at 3 to 6 months of age with beta-chain variants. Methemoglobin reductase deficiency follows an autosomal recessive pattern of inheritance and usually results in mild to moderate methemoglobinemia.[19,20] Most patients are asymptomatic except for cyanosis, which can be decreased or eliminated by administering agents (such as methylene blue or ascorbic acid) that directly oxidize heme iron.

Acquired methemoglobinemia results from exposure to drugs or toxins that oxidize heme iron either directly (*e.g.*, nitrites, nitrates, and quinones) or after biochemical transformation in the intestine or liver (*e.g.*, phenacetin, sulfonamides, and aniline dyes).[19,21] Drugs currently used in medical practice rarely, if ever, cause clinically significant methemoglobinemia except in unusually susceptible persons (such as patients heterozygous for methemoglobin reductase deficiency). Oxidant drugs and toxins also may cause accumulation of a poorly characterized hemoglobin derivative known as sulfhemoglobin. This substance derives its name from the fact that it can be formed *in vitro* by mixing hemoglobin with hydrogen sulfide. The absorption characteristics of sulfhemoglobin lead to cyanosis at concentrations even less than those required with methemoglobin.[17]

PERIPHERAL CYANOSIS

Peripheral cyanosis is due to increased extraction of oxygen from normally saturated arterial hemoglobin and usually results from decreased tissue blood flow. When blood flow is slow relative to local oxygen needs, a greater than normal amount of oxygen is removed from each unit of blood as it passes through tissue capillaries. As a result, the concentration of deoxygenated hemoglobin in capillary and venous blood is increased. Factors that cause peripheral cyanosis also commonly result in a redistribution of blood flow from peripheral to central organs, making cyanosis more apparent in the extremities. However, the term *peripheral* refers to the local mechanisms responsible for decreased capillary and venous hemoglobin saturation, not to the distribution of cyanosis.

Cold exposure causes cutaneous vasoconstriction and decreases blood flow to the skin. These responses, aimed at reducing heat loss, override the usual effects of oxygen demand on local blood flow. As a result, exposure to cold often causes peripheral cyanosis in normal people by increasing oxygen extraction and decreasing cutaneous capillary and venous hemoglobin saturation. However, at very low temperatures, the effects of decreased blood flow may be offset by inhibition of skin metabolism and an increase in the affinity of hemoglobin for oxygen. These latter effects limit tissue oxygen extraction, and may prevent cyanosis despite near-cessation of cutaneous blood flow.

Low output states such as congestive heart failure and shock are associated with changes in vascular resistance that redistribute blood flow from peripheral to central organs. Even when arterial blood is normally saturated, cutaneous vasoconstriction results in decreased local blood flow and increased oxygen extraction. Systemic venous hypertension which is present in this setting, probably intensifies cyanosis by dilating subpapillary venous plexuses.

Obstructive arterial disease can produce cyanosis by decreasing local blood flow, although pallor is a more consistent feature of major artery occlusion. In contrast, venous obstruction typically results in marked localized cyanosis of the involved extremity, due to both decreased blood flow and dilation of cutaneous veins.

Theoretically, peripheral cyanosis could also result from an increase in tissue oxygen consumption rather than a primary decrease in blood flow. However, because of the skin's role in body temperature regulation, cutaneous blood flow normally is much greater than would be necessary simply to meet local oxygen needs. This allows skin metabolism to increase substantially without causing significant unsaturation of cutaneous capillary and venous blood. Furthermore, disorders and physiologic stresses that increase tissue oxygen requirements, such as fever and exercise, typically cause a disproportionate rise in cutaneous blood flow because of an increased need to dissipate heat. As a result, oxygen extraction per unit of blood actually decreases, as do cutaneous capillary and venous deoxygenated hemoglobin concentrations. These effects tend to *lessen* peripheral forms of cyanosis except when cutaneous blood flow is limited by vascular disease.

COMBINED CENTRAL AND PERIPHERAL CYANOSIS

A variety of disorders cause cyanosis through a combination of central and peripheral mechanisms. For example, severe left ventricular (LV) failure often results in both pulmonary edema (which causes arterial hemoglobin unsaturation) and low cardiac output (which increases peripheral oxygen extraction). Likewise, cardiac output frequently is low in patients with cyanotic congenital heart disease and an anatomical right-to-left shunt. In these and other conditions in which hypoxemia results from venous admixture, increased peripheral oxygen extraction intensifies cyanosis both directly and by worsening arterial hemoglobin unsaturation. The latter effect results from a decrease in the oxygen content of venous blood effectively shunted into the arterial circulation.

Summary

Cyanosis results from an increased amount of deoxygenated hemoglobin or hemoglobin derivatives in blood. Correct identification of the cause of cyanosis depends on thoughtful integration of the patient's history and physical findings with the results of selected laboratory tests.

Key features of the history include the duration of cyanosis, possible exposure to drugs or toxins that produce abnormal hemoglobin derivatives, and symptoms indicative of cardiovascular or respiratory disease. The duration of cyanosis is particularly important, since cyanosis present since birth is usually due to an anatomical right-to-left shunt. Other, rare possibilities include hereditary methemoglobinemia and alpha-chain hemoglobin variants with decreased affinity for oxygen. Patients with beta-chain hemoglobin variants typically become cyanotic at 3 to 6 months of age, when HbF is replaced by HbA.

Physical examination may help differentiate between central and peripheral forms of cyanosis, and, when combined with a chest x-ray film, often establishes the presence of cardiovascular or respiratory disease. Cyanosis that spares the lips and mucous membranes of the mouth usually is peripheral in origin. Cyanosis confined to an extremity indicates peripheral arterial or, more commonly, venous obstructive disease, while differential cyanosis (sparing the upper extremities) suggests right-to-left shunting through a patent ductus arteriosus. Clubbing of the fingers and toes is an important, but nonspecific, clinical finding, which may be present both with and without cyanosis in a variety of medical disorders. In cyanotic subjects, it suggests long-standing arterial unsaturation, and is present most often in patients with cyanotic congenital heart disease. Clubbing does not occur as a result of either peripheral or recently developed central cyanosis. Finally, massage or warming of an extremity increases cutaneous blood flow and often eliminates peripheral, but not central cyanosis.

The most important laboratory tests in the differential diagnosis of cyanosis are the measurement of P_aO_2 and hemoglobin saturation. The presence of arterial unsaturation indicates that cyanosis is, at least partly, central in origin, whereas a normal value excludes all forms of central cyanosis except methemoglobinemia and sulfhemoglobinemia. When necessary (*i.e.*, when central cyanosis is suspected despite normal arterial hemoglobin saturation), specific tests can be used to screen for these derivatives. Arterial unsaturation in the presence of normal P_aO_2 suggests an abnormal hemoglobin with decreased affinity for oxygen, a diagnosis that can be confirmed by hemoglobin electrophoresis. The presence of polycythemia, which may either cause or intensify cyanosis, is readily confirmed or excluded with a simple hematocrit.

References

1. Lundsgaard C, Van Slyke DD: Cyanosis. Medicine 2:1, 1923
2. Edwards EA, Dunthy SQ: The pigments and color of living human skin. Am J Anat 65:1, 1939
3. Parrish JA, White HAD, Pathak MA: Photomedicine. In Fitzpatrick TB, Eisen AZ, Wolff K, et al: Dermatology in General Medicine, 2nd ed, p 949. New York, McGraw-Hill, 1979
4. Lundsgaard C: Studies on cyanosis I and II. J Exper Med 30:259, 1919
5. Braunwald E: Cyanosis, hypoxia, and polycythemia. In Isselbacher KJ, Adams RD, Braunwald E, et al: Harrison's Principles of Internal Medicine, 9th ed, p 166. New York, McGraw-Hill, 1980
6. Montagna W, Parakkal PF: The Structure and Function of Skin, 3rd ed, p 142–156. New York, Academic Press, 1974
7. Braverman IM, Yen A: Ultrastructure of the human dermal microcirculation II. The capillary loops of the dermal papilla. J Invest Dermatol 68:44, 1977
8. Yen A, Braverman IM: Ultrastructure of the human dermal microcirculation: The horizontal plexus of the papillary dermis. J Invest Dermatol 65:131, 1976
9. Lambertson CJ: Hypoxia, altitude, and acclimatization. In Mountcastle VB (ed): Medical Physiology, 14th ed, p 1843. St Louis, CV Mosby, 1980
10. Lukas DS, Araujo J, Steinberg I: The syndrome of patent ductus arteriosus with reversal of flow. Am J Med 17:298, 1954
11. Whitaker W, Heath D, Brown JW: Patent ductus arteriosus with pulmonary hypertension. Br Heart J 17:121, 1955
12. Dines DE, Arms RA, Bernatz PE, et al: Pulmonary arteriovenous fistulas. Mayo Clin Proc 49:460, 1974
13. Berthelot P, Walker JG, Sherlock S, et al: Arterial changes in the lungs in cirrhosis of the liver–lung spider nevi. N Engl J Med 274:291, 1966
14. Kravath RE, Scarpelli EM, Bernstein J: Hepatogenic cyanosis: Arteriovenous shunts in chronic active hepatitis. J Pediatr 78:238, 1971
15. Calafresi P, Abelman WH: Portacaval and portopulmonary anastomosis in Laennec's cirrhosis and heart failure. J Clin Invest 36:1257, 1957
16. Wintrobe MM, Lee GR, Boggs DR, et al: Clinical Hematology, 8th ed, p 803. Philadelphia, Lea & Febiger, 1981
17. Finch CA: Methemoglobinemia and sulfhemoglobinemia. N Engl J Med 239:470, 1948
18. Darling RC, Roughton FJW: The effect of methemoglobin on the equilibrium between oxygen and hemoglobin. Am J Physiol 137:56, 1942

19. Winthrobe MM, Lee Gr, Boggs DR, et al: Clinical Hematology, 8th ed, p 1011. Philadelphia, Lea & Febiger, 1981
20. Jaffe E, Hsieh HS: DPNH—methemoglobin reductase deficiency and hereditary methemoglobinemia. Semin Hematol 8:417, 1971
21. Smith RP, Olson MV: Drug-induced methemoglobinemia. Semin Hematol 10:253, 1973

6

VENOUS AND ARTERIAL PULSATIONS

Gordon A. Ewy, M.D.

The evaluation of the jugular venous and arterial pulsations is an integral part of the cardiovascular examination. The correct interpretation of these impulses can provide important clues to the hemodynamics of the patient. Their evaluation can be accomplished with ease and an economy of time, but, like all skills, optimal development requires practice and, at times, tutelage.

Physiology of the Venous Pulse

IDENTIFICATION OF THE JUGULAR VENOUS PULSE

The jugular venous pulse is recognized by its location in the neck and by its characteristic pulsations.[1] The internal jugular vein is a relatively deep structure lying lateral to the carotid artery. In the mid- and lower neck, this large vein runs beneath the sternocleidomastoid muscle. The lower end of the sternocleidomastoid muscle splits into two heads that originate from the clavicle. The triangle formed by the two heads of the sternocleidomastoid muscle and the clavicle, the *internal jugular triangle,* marks the location of the internal jugular bulb. Normally, the pulsations from the internal jugular vein are reflected in the lower portion of the neck by the motion of the skin over the internal jugular triangle and the sternocleidomastoid muscle. The external jugular vein, which is smaller and has more discrete pulsations, is superficial and located more laterally. Because of its superficial location, the external jugular vein is prominent in patients who have chronic elevation of venous pressure. Characteristically, the venous pulse is a series of weak, wavy, nonpalpable impulses, contrasting with the stronger, easily palpable carotid arterial pulse. An important exception to this generalization is the venous pulse of patients with severe tricuspid regurgitation. With severe incompetence of the tricuspid valve, the high right ventricular (RV) systolic pressure is transmitted to the right atrium and hence to the veins, resulting in a pulse that is large and sometimes palpable. These prominent systolic venous impulses could be mistaken for prominent arterial pulsations. However, the discrepancy between the forceful pulsation in the neck and a relatively weak radial arterial pulse should arrest one's attention and suggest that the prominent neck pulsations are venous.

Pressure at the base of the neck will obliterate venous pulsations but has little effect on arterial pulsations. Another differential diagnostic feature is that venous pulsations are likely to be altered by changes in position. Arterial pulsations are little changed with varying positions. Venous pulsations are subject to a much greater respiratory variation than arterial pulsations. Finally, abdominal compression may result in changes in the height of venous pulsation but has no effect on arterial pulsations. With attention to these details, venous pulsations can be reliably recognized.

EVALUATING THE JUGULAR VENOUS PULSE

Evaluation of the jugular venous excursions requires the patient to be in an optimal position. This position varies depending upon the venous pressure. The patient's head and thorax are gradually raised or lowered until the venous pulsations are optimally visible.

The evaluation of the jugular venous pulses should be divided into three general categories: estimating the jugular venous pressure, assessing the response of the venous pressure to abdominal compression, and interpreting the jugular venous waveform.

Estimating Central Venous Pressure

When estimating the venous pressure, one is estimating the hydrostatic filling pressure of the right heart.[2] Because hydrostatic fluid pressure is measured vertically, regardless of the shape of the fluid container, venous pressure is measured as the vertical distance between the mid right atrium and the mean venous pulsations at the top of the column of venous blood. The reference point for estimating the height of venous pressure is the sternal angle or the angle of Lewis.[1] Sir Thomas Lewis called attention to the fact that the angle between the manubrium and the body of the sternum bears a near-constant relationship to the right atrium irrespective of whether the patient is in the supine, the sitting, or any intermediate position (Fig. 6-1). The sternal angle, then, is the benchmark for the noninvasive determination of venous pressure. This angle can be felt as a transverse ridge formed by the angulation between the manubrium and the body of the sternum at the ar-

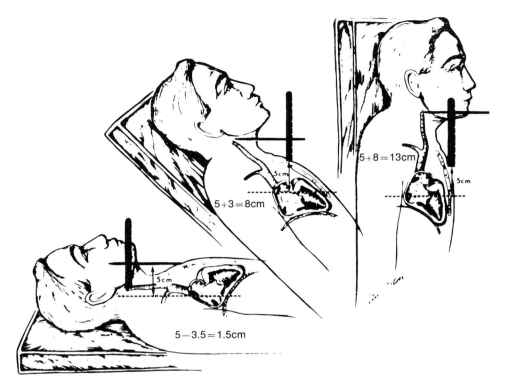

FIG. 6-1. Technique for estimating venous pressure. As shown, the sternal angle, or angle of Lewis, is approximately 5 cm above the mid-right atrium with the patient in any position from supine to upright. The patient is positioned so that the jugular venous pulsations are best seen. A centimeter ruler is placed vertically on the sternal angle if the venous pressure is above the angle of Lewis. The distance above the sternal angle is then determined by forming a right angle to the ruler with a pencil or other straight edge, as shown. The supine patient has a normal venous pressure. Since the pulsations are below the sternal angle, the vertical distance is subtracted from the reference point. The second patient is in an intermediate position, as this is where his venous pulsations are best seen. The venous pressure is 3 cm above the sternal angle, or about 8 cm H_2O. The third patient has a marked elevation of venous pressure. The venous pulsations at the top of the venous blood column are visible only in the upright position. Again measured vertically, the venous pulsations are 8 cm above the sternal angle, equivalent to a venous pressure of approximately 13 cm H_2O.

ticulation of the second ribs. For practical purposes, if the venous pulsations are equal to or lower than the sternal angle, the venous pressure is normal. Pressure is said to be elevated when the top of the venous column in the neck is 2 cm to 3 cm above the sternal angle, that is, indicating a mean right atrial pressure of 7 cm to 8 cm H_2O. It is a common misconception that patients must be examined with the trunk at an angle of 45 degrees from the horizontal. This is incorrect: the patient should be placed in the position where the venous pulsations are best seen. The patient with normal venous pressure must be nearly horizontal if the venous pulsations are to be seen. On the other hand, in a patient with markedly elevated venous pressure, the summit of the venous column may not be appreciated unless the patient is sitting bolt upright (see Fig. 6-1).

The patient's head should be resting comfortably on the bed or on a small pillow. A large pillow may need to be removed before one can accurately evaluate the venous pulse because large pillows tend to bend the neck, placing the patient's chin near the chest and thus interfering with the evaluation. Since the internal jugular pulse is often reflected by motion of the skin over the sternocleidomastoid, this muscle must be relaxed. The pulses of the veins of the neck are best seen when the lighting is tangential, so that shadows are cast, causing the pulses to stand out in relief. Directing the beam of a pocket flashlight tangentially across the veins often helps. The shadow of the pulsations on the bed tends to magnify the venous pulsation and may help in their interpretation.

The technique of estimating venous pressure has distinct limitations, and these deserve emphasis. Obstruction of the superior vena cava will result in bilateral venous engorgement, in which the veins fill from above and not from below. Absence of the venous pulsation suggests a block between the right atrium and the jugular veins. Unilateral venous obstruction also occurs. Estimation of the venous pressure is usually not possible in patients in shock because of the marked venous constriction that accompanies the increased sympathetic tone. In pulmonary disease, there is often such marked fluctuation of intrathoracic pressures that accurate assessment is difficult. Finally, in the morbidly obese patient, estimation of the venous pressure is often impossible.

The patient with extreme elevation of venous pressure may have such venous distention that the pulsations may not be appreciated even when the patient is sitting upright. In these cases, the neck often appears full (a bullneck appearance), and the fact that the venous pressure is elevated may be overlooked. If this question arises, palpation of the neck may be helpful. Distended veins have a characteristic soft feeling, in contrast to the relatively noncompliant nature of the neck in the very muscular person with a so-called bullneck. In some patients with markedly elevated venous pressure, the pulsations can be visualized only after the venous pressure decreases with therapy. A marked increase of venous pressure may be indicated by engorgement of the veins under the tongue when the patient is in the sitting or upright position.

The point of the venous pulsation used to estimate the height of the venous pressure is usually not the peak of the waves. One wants to estimate the RV end-diastolic pressure, and thus the height of the pulse just preceding the C wave is used. This point is difficult to see but is usually located near the midpoint of the venous excursion. The jugular venous pressure is then estimated by measuring the height of mean venous pulsation above the angle of Lewis. The two exceptions to this rule are patients with tricuspid regurgitation and patients with constrictive pericarditis. In tricuspid regurgitation the RV filling pressure correlates with the trough of the venous pulse, since the peak of the wave occurs during systole. The height of the regurgitant wave reflects the degree of regurgitation rather than the filling pressure of the right ventricle. In constrictive pericarditis, the RV filling pressure correlates with the peak of the venous pulse.

Abdominal Compression

Patients with heart failure may have an elevated jugular venous pressure. However, if the patient is taking diuretics the venous pressure may be normal in spite of impaired ventricular function. In these patients, sustained pressure applied to the abdomen while the patient is breathing normally may unmask occult abnormalities of circulatory function. In the normal person, there will be little or no increase in the jugular venous pressure. If the venous pressure increases by 2 cm or 3 cm and remains elevated until the pressure is released from the abdomen, compromised ventricular function should be suspected. This test is useful when the jugular venous pressure is normal or questionably elevated. It has no value if the venous pressure is already elevated.

Contour of the Jugular Venous Pulse

Jugular venous pulsations are normally the result of repeated interference with the relatively steady flow of venous return by the contractions and relaxations of the right atrium and ventricle.[1,3] The normal venous pulse, therefore, consists of intermittent increases in the volume of blood in the veins caused by intermittent slowing or halting of blood flow in the right atrium.[2] Because they are low-pressure impulses, venous pulsations are interpreted by inspection rather than by palpation.

The normal venous pulsation is classically taught to consist of two major waves and two major troughs (Fig. 6-2). The A wave results from atrial contraction and is presystolic in timing, peaking near the time of the first heart sound (S_1). The second major wave, the V wave, is caused by continuous venous return to the right atrium during systole, a time when the tricuspid valve is closed. The X descent follows the A wave, and the Y descent follows the V wave (see Fig. 6-2). The relaxation of the atrium is the major factor contributing to the normal X descent. The V wave is terminated and the Y descent initiated by the fall in right atrial pressure coincident with the opening of the tricuspid valve. Thus, the V wave peaks just after the second heart sound (S_2). The A wave is larger than the V wave and the X descent is more prominent than the Y descent.

On occasion, the X descent is interrupted by another wave, the C wave (Fig. 6-3). The C wave in the neck is partly due to transmitted carotid artery pul-

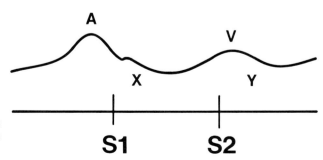

FIG. 6-2. A normal jugular venous pulse, illustrating the A and V waves and the X and the Y descents.

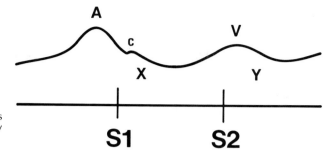

FIG. 6-3. A normal jugular venous pulse, showing the A, C, and V waves with the X and Y descents.

sations and partly due to the upward bulging of the closing tricuspid valve early in ventricular systole. The normal C wave is difficult to recognize as a separate wave.

This idealized description of the venous pulsation has confused many physicians. In many normal people, the A and V waves may not be at all prominent. The most clearly discernible venous motion is a rhythmic collapse, or inward motion, of the jugular venous pulse during systole. Instead of two distinct peaks and two distinct troughs, one sees low-amplitude, undulant venous motion and one dominant collapsing motion. Timing of this inward or collapsing motion shows it to be systolic, and recordings, reveal it to be the X descent. The reason for these findings is the presence of a third positive wave, the H wave (Fig. 6-4). The H wave follows the Y descent and is the result of passive filling of the right atrium and ventricle during diastole.[4] The H wave is present only at normal or slow heart rates, since at faster heart rates diastole is shortened. In the normal person, the subtle changes in venous amplitude from the H to the A wave and the low-amplitude motion of the V wave make these waves difficult to appreciate (see Fig. 6-4). Large changes in amplitude are easier to recognize than small undulations, and, therefore, the most obvious event of the jugular venous pulse is the X descent. Fortunately, recognition of these subtle changes in the H, A, C, and V waves is usually unnecessary, since one can conclude that no significant abnormality of the venous pulsation is present when there is regular systolic collapse of the venous pulsation.[5] The X descent can be timed by observing the jugular venous pulse on the right side of the neck while palpating the opposite carotid (Fig. 6-5). The X descent occurs during systole, at the same time as the carotid pulse. The X descent can also

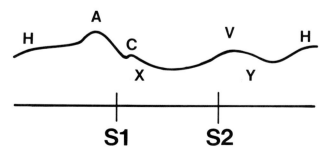

FIG. 6-4. Normal venous pulse, showing the H wave.

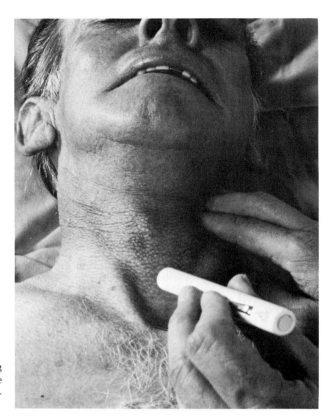

FIG. 6-5. Technique of examining venous pulsations while timing the venous waves by palpating the opposite carotid artery.

be timed by observing the jugular venous pulsations while auscultating over the precordium. As illustrated in Figures 6-2 to 6-4, the X descent occurs during systole.

The need for more detailed analysis is indicated by the absence of the X descent; by the presence of prominent systolic waves, or of easily appreciated A or V waves; or by prominent diastolic collapse of the venous pulse.

Clinical Presentation of the Venous Pulse

ABNORMALITIES OF THE VENOUS WAVE FORM

The A Wave

Abnormal increases in the A wave occur when the force of atrial contraction increases in response to an increased resistance to atrial emptying. Causes of increased resistance to atrial emptying include tricuspid stenosis, decreased compliance of the right ventricle, and, rarely, clots or tumors of the right ventricle. Most causes of RV hypertrophy, the most common of which is pulmonary hypertension, result in an increase in the A wave of the venous pulse. Tetralogy of Fallot is said to be the exception to this rule.[6] RV outflow obstruction and hypertrophic cardiomyopathy must be considered in patients with prominent A waves. As A waves increase in height they become more conspicuous and easier to recognize. When very large, these waves are termed *giant A waves* (Fig. 6-6).

Small A waves may occur because of a poorly contracting right atrium. In atrial flutter, small, rapid F waves may appear as shimmerings on the surface of the venous pulsations. The A wave completely disappears with atrial fibrillation or with atrial standstill.

Cannon A Waves

When the right atrium contracts against the closed tricuspid valve, the full force of atrial contraction is transmitted into the venous system. The resultant impulses are called *cannon A waves* or *cannon waves*. These waves differ from the giant A wave in two respects. First, the cannon A wave is systolic in timing, whereas the giant A wave is presystolic. Second, the cannon A wave tends to have a more rapid rate of rise and therefore appears to have a more flicking motion.

Intermittent cannon A waves may occur with premature ventricular or nodal contractions. They are classically seen in patients with complete heart block. Intermittent cannon A waves may also occur in patients with ventricular pacemakers and dissociation between the independent atrial and the paced ventricular contractions. Regular cannon A waves may accompany paroxysmal supraventricular or junctional tachycardias (Fig. 6-7) or may occur in patients with ventricular pacemakers and normal AV nodal retrograde conduction.

The X Descent

The explanation for the X descent has been the subject of some controversy. Since the X descent is often decreased in patients who do not have atrial contraction, such as those with atrial fibrillation, the X descent has

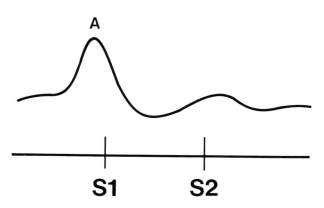

FIG. 6-6. Giant A wave.

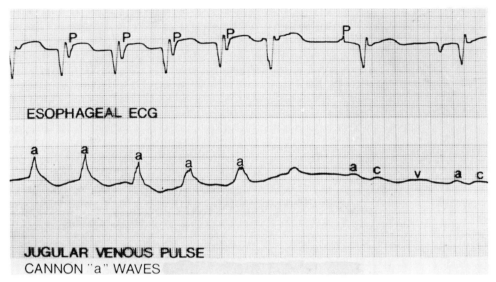

FIG. 6-7. Cannon A waves in patient with junctional tachycardia.

been thought to be related to atrial relaxation. The trough of the X descent is usually the lowest point by the jugular venous pulsation, dropping well below the onset of the A wave. This observation does not preclude the explanation that the X descent is due to atrial relaxation, since some atrial filling (inscribing the H wave) occurs before the onset of active atrial contraction. Atrial fibrillation could decrease the X descent by interfering with atrial relaxation. Another factor contributing to the genesis of the X descent is the descent of the tricuspid valve toward the RV cavity during systole. Some authors divide the X descent in two components, referring to the initial descending limb of the A wave as the X descent and the continued descent following the C wave as the X prime (X') descent (Fig. 6-8). These authors ascribe the X descent to atrial relaxation and the X' descent to tricuspid valve motion towards the right ventricle during systole.[7]

In cardiac tamponade, the venous pressures may be so elevated that the specific wave form is difficult to determine; if recorded, the X descent may be prominent. In experimentally produced tamponade, the dominant right atrial pressure wave is the X descent.[5]

The C Wave

The C wave of the jugular venous pulse was originally thought to be secondary to transmitted carotid pulsations. Wood agreed with this opinion, since he could not find a wave of similar magnitude in right atrial tracings.[1] Rich and Tavell demonstrated that the C wave of the jugular venous pulse occurred at a similar distance from the QRS complex in controls and in patients with left bundle branch block but that, in the latter group, the onset of the

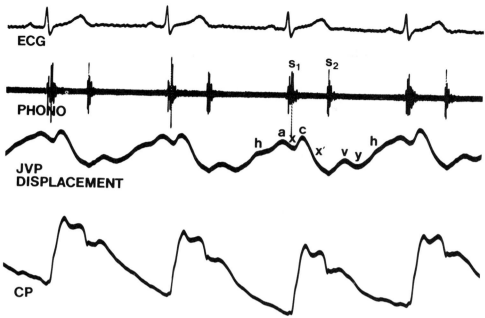

FIG. 6-8. Electrocardiogram (*ECG*), phonocardiogram (*phono*), jugular venous pulse (*JVP* displacement) tracing, and carotid pulse (*CP*) tracing illustrating a normal jugular venous pulse. Note the H wave and C wave. Note that the dominant motion is the systolic collapse of the venous pulse.

carotid pulse was significantly delayed.[8] They concluded that the C wave was not transmitted from the carotid. Tavell recorded jugular venous pulsations by placing a funnel-shaped sensor, held with some pressure, between the two heads of the sternocleidomastoid muscle over the internal jugular bulb and directed posteriorly and caudally. This method produces tracings that can resemble right atrial pressure tracings more than jugular venous tracings that are recorded over the sternocleidomastoid by displacement techniques.

As Coleman emphasized, there are, in all probability, two mechanisms producing the C wave in the jugular venous pulse: one transmitted from the right atrium due to bulging of the tricuspid valve in early systole and one due to transmission from carotid pulsations.[9]

The V Wave

Normally, the A wave is the dominant venous wave. In patients with an atrial septal defect, the V wave is increased in height so that in amplitude it equals or is slightly greater than the A wave (Fig. 6-9).[10] In contrast, the normal left atrial V wave is larger than the left atrial A wave. In patients with large atrial septal defects, the venous pulse may be influenced by the left atrial pressure tracing.

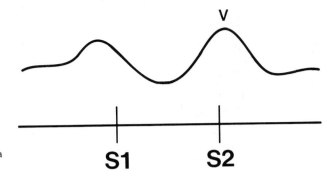

FIG. 6-9. Prominent V wave in a patient with atrial septal defect.

The most common cause of an increase in the magnitude of V waves is incompetence of the tricuspid valve. The waves associated with incompetence of the tricuspid valve are more than just augmented V waves, however, since when severe they begin with the C wave. Therefore, they are often referred to as *CV waves, regurgitant CV waves,* or systolic *S waves* (Fig. 6-10). The appearance of the CV wave will depend not only upon the amount of blood that is regurgitated into the atrium during RV systole, but also upon the compliance or stiffness of the right atrium. Mild degrees of tricuspid regurgitation may be manifest only be a slight obliteration of the X descent. With increasing degrees of tricuspid insufficiency, the height of the V wave will usually increase. Patients with severe tricuspid regurgitation can have very prominent systolic venous pulsations. At times these waves are so forceful that they can be palpated and, thus, are an exception to the generalization that venous pulsations are visible but not palpable. Patients with chronic tricuspid regurgitation usually have associated atrial fibrillation. In this rhythm, the CV wave is not preceded by an A wave.

In patients with severe aortic regurgitation, the forceful arterial pulse may produce a dominant transmitted C wave. In these patients, the examining physician should apply pressure to the base of the neck. Venous pulsations will be abolished.

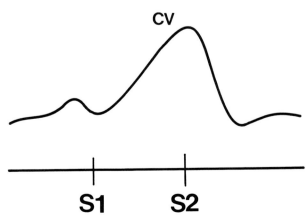

FIG. 6-10. Regurgitant CV wave of tricuspid regurgitation. Note the small A wave prior to the onset of the CV wave.

The Y Descent

The most obvious abnormality of the venous wave form in patients with constrictive pericarditis or restrictive myocardial disease is the striking diastolic collapse of the venous pulse. The distended veins not only collapse suddenly, but often redistend just as suddenly (Fig. 6-11). In pericardial constriction or myocardial restriction disease, the veins are distended because of resistance to filling of the right ventricle. When the tricuspid valve opens, the column of blood falls into the right ventricle. Since the right ventricle has decreased compliance, it quickly fills and the Y ascent is nearly as rapid as the Y descent. The rapid drop and rise in venous pulse pressure of several mm Hg with each arterial pulse is readily apparent on inspection. It should be emphasized that it is not possible to differentiate between restrictive cardiomyopathy and constrictive pericardial disease by inspection of or recordings of the venous pulsations, since both conditions result in similar venous pulsations.

A rapid Y descent is not diagnostic of constrictive pericarditis or restrictive heart disease. Since the Y descent is caused by a fall in venous pressure with the opening of the tricuspid valve, whenever the venous pressure is elevated, the Y descent will be prominent and rapid, provided there is no obstruction in the atrium or the tricuspid valve. Thus, the Y descent is prominent in patients with large CV waves due to tricuspid regurgitation and in patients with right heart failure. When tricuspid stenosis is present, the Y descent is slowed and the Y trough may be absent.[1]

Respiratory Variation and Kussmaul's Sign

The mean jugular venous pressure normally falls with inspiration, passively following the intrathoracic pressure. In some patients with decreased RV compliance, the relative height of the A wave will increase with inspiration even though the mean venous pressure falls. This is thought to be related to an increase in the force of atrial contraction with atrial distention caused by the ventilatory increase in the venous return.

In patients with a marked decrease in RV compliance, such as those with constrictive pericarditis, there is a rise in the mean height of the jugular venous pulse during inspiration. This is known as Kussmaul's sign, and it is present in about 40% of the patients with constrictive pericarditis.[11-13] Kussmaul's sign is generally not seen in patients with pericardial tamponade (Table 6-1).

Right Ventricular Infarction

RV myocardial infarction is virtually always associated with transmural infarction of the inferior or posterior wall of the left ventricle.[14,15] This diagnosis should be suspected in any patient with inferior or posterior myocardial infarction who develops an elevated venous pressure without evidence of significant pulmonary congestion. RV infarction is usually well tolerated but, when extensive, can lead to cardiogenic shock and serious cardiac dysrhythmia.[16-20] It may mimic cardiac tamponade or pulmonary embolism. Hemodynamic alterations gradually appear within the first two days. An early hemo-

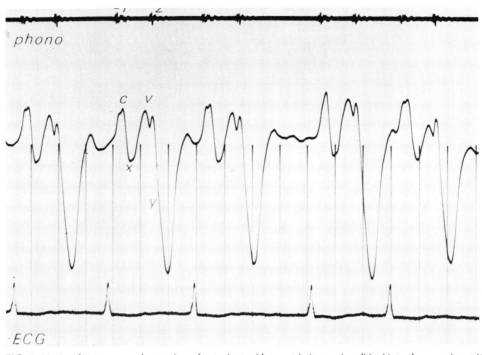

FIG. 6-11. Jugular venous pulse tracing of a patient with constrictive pericarditis. Note the prominent Y descent followed by a rapid ascent.

dynamic sign is an otherwise unexplained elevation of the jugular venous or central venous pressure. In patients with RV infarction, jugular venous pressures in the range of 12 cm to 15 cm H_2O are common. The venous pressure may not fall or may even rise with inspiration (Kussmaul's sign). Associated pericarditis is frequent, and pulsus paradoxus in excess of 10 mm Hg has been reported in 40% of patients in some series.[16–20] Thus, the clinical triad of pericardial rub, pulsus paradoxus, and hypotension is present, strongly suggesting cardiac tamponade. However, closer analysis reveals that the hemodynamics are those of cardiac constriction and not cardiac tamponade. An inspiratory increase in venous pressure is distinctly uncommon in tamponade. Balloon-tipped catheter recordings will show that the morphology of the right heart pressure tracings more closely resembles that of constrictive pericarditis than tamponade. This morphology includes a prominent X and Y descent in the right atrial pressure recording, an early diastolic "dip and plateau" configuration in the RV pressure tracing, and loss of the normal inspiratory decrease of right atrial and RV pressures. In cardiac tamponade, Y descents are not ordinarily seen, the dip and plateau phenomenon in the right ventricle is usually absent, and an inspiratory increase in right atrial pressure is distinctly uncommon.

Table 6–1.   Clinical Profiles of Pericardial Diseases

	Pericardial Effusion	Cardiac Tamponade	Subacute Constriction	Chronic Constriction
Typical etiologies	Numerous	Neoplasm Hemorrhage Uremia	Idiopathic Radiation Rheumatoid	Idiopathic Open heart surgery Tuberculosis
Duration of symptoms	None or variable	Hours to days	Weeks to months	Years
Paradoxical pulse	Absent	Virtually always*	Usually prominent	Usually absent
Kussmaul's Sign	Absent	Absent	Rare	Moderately frequent

*See text for exceptions.

(From Hancock EW: Pericardial disease: Differential diagnosis and management. Hosp Pract 18:101, 1983)

It has been postulated that the constrictive hemodynamics of acute RV infarction are due to the abrupt limitation of diastolic filling of the dilated, infarcted right ventricle by the relatively nondistensible pericardium. Because of this, intravascular volume depletion may mask the hemodynamic signs of RV infarction. It is therefore important to ensure that the patient's volume is adequately expanded before this diagnosis is excluded. Occasionally, regurgitant CV or systolic waves can be seen in the right atrial tracing or the jugular venous pulse as a result of tricuspid insufficiency secondary to dysfunction of an infarcted RV papillary muscle.

Physiology and Clinical Manifestations of Arterial Pulsations

Interest in arterial pulsations dates to antiquity. The common disorders of rate and rhythm were well described in the early part of this century by Sir James MacKenzie and Sir Thomas Lewis, who used recordings of the venous pulse to reflect atrial activity and simultaneous recordings of the apex beat or arterial pulse to reflect ventricular activity. Although a trained observer can on occasion diagnosis a dysrhythmia by simultaneously observing the venous pulse and palpating an artery, few would initiate therapy based on these observations without first confirming and documenting the abnormality with an electrocardiogram. Nevertheless, the routine examination of the arterial pulse for rate and rhythm and observation of the jugular venous pulse frequently suggest when an electrocardiogram is necessary.

Careful evaluation of the character or contour of the carotid pulse and an evaluation of the peripheral pulse for volume alterations (*pulsus alternans*) and abnormal respiratory variations (*pulsus paradoxus*) as well as for rate and rhythm, will reward the examiner with invaluable diagnostic information.

ARTERIAL PULSE CONTOUR

The arterial rate and rhythm can be assessed from any palpable pulse. However, since the arterial pulse contour is altered as it travels to the peripheral arterial vessels, the arterial pulse closest to the heart, that is, the carotid pulse, is evaluated when pulse contour is being assessed.[5] During peripheral transmission of the arterial pulse, however, the pulse pressure increases and the rate of rise of the arterial pulse is accentuated, so that pulsus alternans and pulsus paradoxus can more readily be appreciated in the peripheral pulses.

When the carotid pulse is being assessed, the examining finger is placed lightly over the artery, high in the neck but below the carotid sinus. Increasing pressure is applied until the pulse is readily appreciated. One should assess selectively the upstroke, the peak, and the collapse of the carotid pulse.

ASCENDING LIMB OR UPSTROKE

The rate of rise of the carotid pulse upstroke is altered by various disease states. The rate of rise is increased in patients with hyperdynamic contractions, which occur in anxiety and hypertrophic cardiomyopathy, and in patients with increased aortic run-off, which occurs with aortic regurgitation. The pulse of mitral regurgitation associated with good ventricular function is sometimes referred to as a "small water-hammer" pulse. Even though the pulse pressure is small, the rate of rise can be quite brisk and nonsustained. The rate of rise is decreased in patients with fixed obstruction to the LV outflow tract or with severe heart failure from any cause.

Slow-rising carotid pulsations may be found in patients with significant fixed obstruction of LV outflow caused by discrete subvalvular, valvular, or supravalvular aortic stenosis. Figure 6-12 illustrates the normal pulse and Figure 6-13 the slow-rising pulse of aortic stenosis. The presence or absence of a palpable thrill does not correlate with the severity of stenosis. Patients with significant aortic regurgitation may have a palpable carotid thrill in the absence

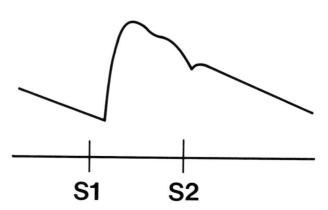

FIG. 6-12. Normal carotid pulse tracing.

of aortic stenosis. Since the carotid pulse contour changes with age, hypertension, and atherosclerosis, the rate of rise of the carotid pulse loses some of its diagnostic value in elderly patients. Elderly patients with significant aortic stenosis can have a normal rate of rise of the arterial pulse.[21]

The aortic and carotid pulses of some patients with aortic valve stenosis have an anacrotic notch in addition to the slow rate of rise. This anacrotic notch is appreciated as a shoulder on the ascending limb of the carotid pulse (see Fig. 6-13). The anacrotic notch is thought to relate to the decreased velocity of flow.

A slow-rising carotid pulse is not necessarily an indication of LV outflow obstruction. A poorly functioning ventricle develops pressure more slowly, and the rate of rise of the carotid pulse may also be slow. However, a slow-rising carotid pulse associated with an anacrotic notch should suggest the presence of aortic stenosis.

PEAK OF THE CAROTID PULSE

The peak of the carotid pulse can be nonsustained, sustained, or bisferiens. Freis and associates have shown that the externally recorded carotid pulse has an early and a late systolic component.[22] In youth, the first component is dominant. With age the second component increases relative to the first, producing a more sustained carotid impulse.[22] Disease states such as systemic hypertension or atherosclerosis also increase the relative height of the second peak. Thus, in these patients the peak of the carotid pulse is more sustained.

On occasion there are two distinctly palpable pulsations in systole. This type of pulse (Fig. 6-14) is said to be *bisferiens* ("twice beating"). The presence of a bisferiens arterial pulse should immediately bring to the clinician's mind three diagnoses: aortic regurgitation, combined aortic stenosis and regurgitation, and obstructive hypertrophic cardiomyopathy. Figure 6-15 illustrates a bisferiens carotid pulse of a patient with hypertrophic cardiomyopathy. In its most florid form, the contour of the carotid pulse of hypotrophic cardiomyopathy has a "spike–dome" configuration. It should be emphasized, however, that in the majority of patients with obstructive or nonobstructive hypertrophic cardiomyopathy, a bisferiens pulse is not present. A bisferiens pulse suggests

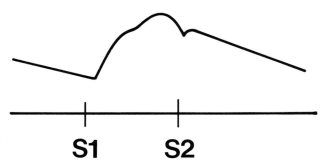

FIG. 6-13. Slow-rising carotid pulse with anacrotic shoulder in patient with aortic stenosis.

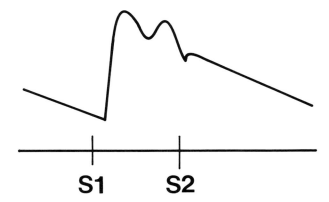

FIG. 6-14. Bisferiens carotid pulse.

that the obstruction is severe. Most patients with hypertrophic cardiomyopathy have only a rapidly rising carotid pulse.

DESCENDING LIMB OF THE CAROTID PULSE

Normally, the carotid pulse collapses rather briskly. In a small subset of patients the dicrotic pulse is very prominent and is palpable. The *dicrotic pulse* is a twice-beating pulse in which the first peak is in systole and the second is in early diastole (Fig. 6-16).[23] The second peak is an exaggeration of the normal dicrotic wave that occurs following the closure of the aortic valve. The characteristics of the dicrotic pulse are a slow rate of rise, small pulse pressure, low dicrotic notch, and a large dicrotic wave.[23] Measurement of systolic time intervals of the dicrotic pulse revealed a prolonged pre-ejection period and a shortened LV ejection time.

Although the exact cause of the dicrotic pulse is unknown, the hemodynamic correlates are clear: low stroke volume, low cardiac output, and high peripheral vascular resistance in a relatively young adult.[23] This constellation is found most often in the young patient with congestive cardiomyopathy. Many elderly patients have a low stroke volume and a high peripheral vascular resistance but, presumably because of less compliant or less resilient arterial vascular systems, do not have a dicrotic arterial pulse. Dicrotic pulses have been recorded in young patients with advanced states of cardiac decompensation due to ischemic heart disease.[5] A striking dicrotic pulse was recorded in a 42-year-old man with a Starr-Edwards aortic valve prosthesis. The presence of clots resulted in malfunction of the valve, with severe compromise of his cardiac stroke volume.[5] Following valve replacement, the striking dicrotic pulse was no longer present.

The importance of low stroke volume in the genesis of the dicrotic pulse has been confirmed by two other observations. First, in patients with a dicrotic arterial pulse, the postpremature beat, a beat with a larger stroke volume, is

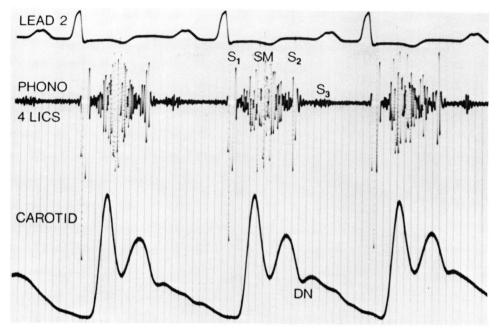

FIG. 6-15. Lead II electrocardiogram, phonocardiogram from the fourth left intercostal space, and carotid pulse tracing from a patient with hypertrophic subaortic stenosis. Note the two systolic impulses. The dicrotic notch (DN) is marked. (Courtesy of Bertron M. Groves, M.D.)

frequently normal.[23] Second, a dicrotic arterial pulse has been observed in young patients with cardiac tamponade only during inspiration—that is, when LV filling is compromised and stroke volume is low.[23]

A dicrotic pulse may also be seen in patients previously operated on for aortic or mitral regurgitation. When observed, it reflects poor ventricular function and, when persistent, indicates a poor prognosis.[24]

PERIPHERAL ARTERIAL PULSES

Peripheral arterial pulses should be routinely checked in all four extremities and in both carotid arteries in patients being evaluated for hypertension, possible aortic dissection, cerebral ischemia, subclavian steal syndrome, claudication, or suspected cardiac decompensation or cardiac tamponade. Figure 6-17 shows the arterial pressure tracings from the central aorta and lower aorta in a patient with severe coarctation of the aorta. Note that the onset of the rise in femoral artery pressure is only slightly delayed but that the rate of rise is much slower, imparting a distinct impression to the palpating fingers that there is a radial or carotid–femoral delay. Simultaneous

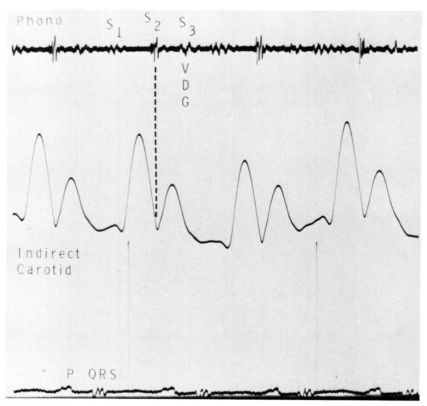

FIG. 6-16. Dicrotic pulse. Note that the dicrotic notch occurs near S_2 and that the second wave is in early diastole. Ventricular diastolic gallop (*VDG*), or S_3, is prominent.

palpation of the radial and femoral pulses should be carried out in all patients with hypertension to rule out the presence of coarction of the aorta.

Atherosclerotic lesions in the subclavian artery can result in a significant discrepancy between the blood pressures in the two upper extremities.

PULSUS ALTERNANS

Pulsus alternans (Fig. 6-18) is a peripheral manifestation of LV decompensation. Simultaneous recordings of arterial pressure changes and of their first derivative show that there is alteration in the height of the pressure pulse and also in the rate of rise.[5] Some have suggested that it is the latter phenomenon that is appreciated during palpation rather than small alterations in peak systolic pressure.

Although a more central arterial pulse is used to evaluate pulse contour, pulsus alternans is best detected by palpation of the more distal radial or

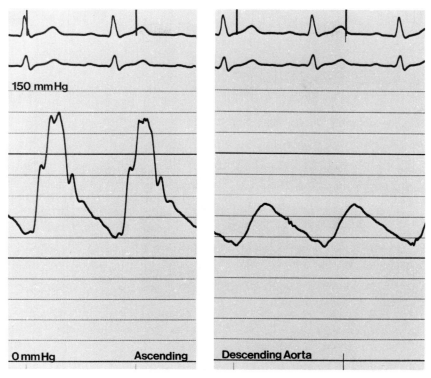

FIG. 6-17. Pressure recordings from a patient with coarctation of the aorta.

femoral artery pulsations. The rate of rise and the peak pressure developed are accentuated during peripheral transmission of the arterial pulse pressure, accentuating the degree of alteration and making pulsus alternans more easily appreciable in the distal arteries. Light pressure, resembling that generated by blowing on your fingertips, is applied over the pulse. Mild degrees of pulsus alternans can be detected by using the blood pressure cuff and deflating it very slowly around systole. Rarely, the weak pulse is too small to feel, in which case *total alternans* is said to be present.

PULSUS PARADOXUS

Pulsus paradoxus was described by Kussmaul over a century ago when he found an inspiratory increase in venous pressure but a decrease in arterial pulse volume in patients with chronic constrictive pericarditis. It is now known that arterial pulsus paradoxus is distinctly rare in constrictive pericarditis but is almost invariably present in pericardial tamponade (see Table

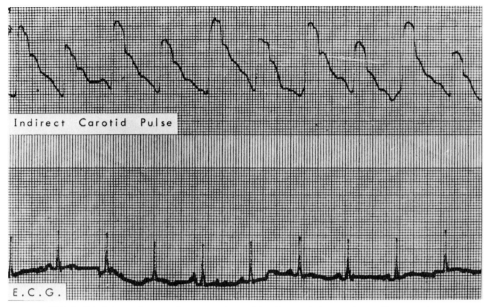

FIG. 6-18. Pulsus alternans from a patient with advanced rheumatic cardiomyopathy.

6-1). Tamponade can occur without pulsus paradoxus as will be discussed below. Pericardial effusion without tamponade does not produce pulsus paradoxus, for only when the pericardium is filled and tensed does hemodynamic embarrassment of the heart ensue. Recognition of pericardial tamponade and appropriate therapy are often life-saving.

Pulsus paradoxus (Fig. 6-19) is generally ascribed to a fall in systolic blood pressure of at least 10 mm Hg to 12 mm Hg during normal inspiration. The technique for the bedside measurement of pulsus paradoxus is illustrated in Figure 6-20. Pulsus paradoxus is most commonly found in patients with obstructive lung disease. In this condition, the marked decrease in intrathoracic pressure with forceful inspiration is transmitted to the intrathoracic arterial structures, resulting in a fall in systolic pressure. The presence of pulsus paradoxus in patients with chronic obstructive lung disease correlates with the degree of pulmonary obstruction.[25]

Shabetai, Fowler, and their coworkers have shown that, in patients with cardiac tamponade, pulsus paradoxus is related to the inspiratory increase in RV filling that causes a decrease in LV filling.[26,27] Because the fluid-filled pericardial sac has reached its limits of distensibility, right heart volume can further increase only if there is a compensating decrease in the volume of the other intrapericardial structures. Echocardiograms have demonstrated a decrease in LV diameter and a decrease in excursion of the mitral value opening during inspiration in patients with pericardial tamponade.[28,29]

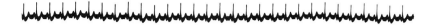

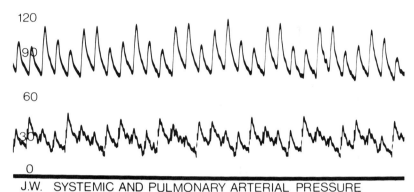

120

90

60

30

0

J.W. SYSTEMIC AND PULMONARY ARTERIAL PRESSURE

FIG. 6-19. Systemic and pulmonary artery pressures in a patient with pulsus paradoxus.

Decreased LV filling on inspiration results in a smaller stroke volume and a lower arterial pressure. Tamponade can occur without pulsus paradoxus in patients with aortic regurgitation or atrial septal defects. These cardiac lesions compensate for inadequate LV filling during inspiration in spite of tamponade. Tamponade can also occur without pulsus paradoxus in patients with marked elevation of LV filling pressure prior to the onset of tamponade.[30]

Cardiac dysrhythmias can cause "pseudo" pulsus paradoxus. Some patients with atrioventricular dissociation can have phasic swings in systolic blood pressure that mimic pulsus paradoxus.

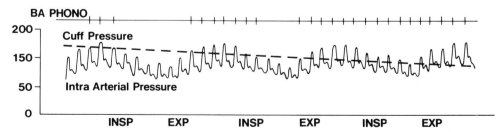

BA PHONO

200

Cuff Pressure

150

50

Intra Arterial Pressure

0

INSP   EXP   INSP   EXP   INSP   EXP

FIG. 6-20. Technique for measuring the degree of pulsus paradoxus is illustrated. A brachial artery phonocardiogram reveals the onset of intermittent Korotkoff sounds on the left and continuous sounds on the right. The pressure difference between the onset of Korotkoff sounds and continuous Korotkoff sounds indicates the degree of pulsus paradoxus. The measurement should be taken while the patient is breathing normally.

References

1. Wood P: Disease of the Heart and Circulation, 2nd ed, pp 42–57. Philadelphia, JB Lippincott, 1956
2. Ewy GA, Marcus FI: Bedside estimation of venous pressure. Heart Bull 17:41, 1968
3. Coleman AL: Clinical Examination of the Jugular Venous Pulse, pp 11–68. Springfield, Ill, Charles C Thomas, 1966
4. Hirschfelder AD: Some variations in the form of the venous pulse. Johns Hopkins Med J 18:265, 1907
5. Ewy, GA, Groves BM: Venous and Arterial Pulsations. New York, Medcom, 1973
6. Perloff JK: The Clinical Recognition of Congenital Heart Disease, p 363. Philadelphia, WB Saunders, 1970
7. Constant, J: Bedside Cardiology, pp 60–64. Boston, Little, Brown & Co, 1969
8. Rich LL, Tavel ME: The origin of the jugular C wave. N Engl J Med 284:1309, 1971
9. Colman AL: Jugular C wave. N Engl J Med 285:462, 1971
10. Tavell ME, Bard RA, Franks LC, et al: The jugular venous pulse in atrial septal defect. Arch Intern Med 121:524, 1968
11. Lange RL, Botticelli JT, Tsagaris TJ, et al: Diagnostic signs in compressive cardiac disorder: Constrictive pericarditis, pericardial effusion and tamponade. Circulation 33:763, 1966
12. Hancock EW: On the elastic and rigid forms of constrictive pericarditis. Am Heart J 100:917, 1980
13. Hancock, EW: Pericardial disease: Differential diagnosis and management. Hosp Pract 18:101, 1983
14. Wade WG: The pathogenesis of infarction of the right ventricle. Br Heart J 21:545, 1959
15. Isner JM, Roberts WC: Right ventricular infarction complicating left ventricular infarction secondary to coronary heart disease. Am J Cardiol 42:885, 1978
16. Cohn J, Tristani FE, Khatri IM: Studies in clinical shock and hypotension: Relationship between left and right ventricular function. J Clin Invest 48:2008, 1969
17. Lorell B, Leinbach RC, Pohost GM, et al: Right ventricular infarction: Clinical diagnosis and differentiation from cardiac tamponade and pericardial constriction. Am J Cardiol 43:465, 1979
18. Coma-Cannella I, Lopez-Sandon J, Gamallo C: Low output syndrome in right ventricular infarction. Am Heart J 98:613, 1979
19. Shah PK, Shellock F, Berman D, et al: Predominant right ventricular dysfunction in acute myocardial infarction: Frequency, clinical, hemodynamic, and scintigraphic findings. Circulation 62:III–313, 1980
20. Sharpe DN, Botvinick EH, Shames DM, et al: The non-invasive diagnosis of right ventricular infarction. Circulation 57:983, 1978
21. Roberts WC, Perloff JK, Costantino T: Severe valvular aortic stenosis in patients over 65 years of age: A clinicopathologic study. Am J Cardiology 27:497, 1971
22. Freis ED, Heath WC, Luchsinger PC, et al: Changes in carotid pulse which occur with age and hypertension. Am Heart J 71:757, 1966
23. Ewy GA, Rios JC, Marcus FI: The dicrotic arterial pulse. Circulation 39:655, 1969
24. Orchard RC, Craige E: Dicrotic pulse after open heart surgery. Circulation 62:1107, 1980
25. Rebuck AS, Pengelly LD: Development of pulsus paradoxus in the presence of airway obstruction. N Engl J Med 288:66–69, 1973

26. Shabetai R, Fowler NO, Fenton JC, et al: Pulsus paradoxus. J Clin Invest 44:1882, 1965
27. Fowler NO: Physiology of cardiac tamponade and pulsus paradoxus II. Mod Concepts Cardiovasc Dis 47:115, 1978
28. Feigenbaum H: Echocardiography, 2nd ed, pp 255–262. Philadelphia, Lea & Febiger, 1976
29. Felner JM, Schlant RC: Echocardiography: A Teaching Atlas, p 523. New York, Grune & Stratton, 1976
30. Reddy PS, Curtiss EJ, O'Toole JD, et al: Cardiac tamponade: Hemodynamic observations in man. Circulation 58:265, 1978

7

PRECORDIAL PALPATION

Jonathan Abrams, M.D.

Definition

Precordial palpation is that aspect of the cardiac physical examination that detects cardiac activity on the chest wall. In the normal individual, cardiac motion is reflected by the *apical beat* or *apical impulse* formed by left ventricular (LV) muscle; right ventricular (RV) activity is not usually palpable. When cardiac hypertrophy or dilatation is present, abnormal systolic and diastolic events emanating from the left or right ventricle may be detected on palpation, and, on unusual occasions, left and right atrial impulses may be felt.

A review of the history of medicine shows that for over 3,500 years physicians have been aware that cardiac activity can be detected with the examining hand.[1] Such eminent scientists as William Harvey, Rene Laennec, and Sir James MacKenzie have made important and remarkably accurate observations about palpable cardiac movements. Modern-day medicine has increased the precision of this field, particularly with respect to the effects of specific chamber hypertrophy and dilatation on the characteristics of the cardiac impulse.

Experienced clinicians can derive a great deal of information about intracardiac size and function from a careful analysis of precordial motion and may often obtain the first clue to ventricular enlargement in this manner. This chapter outlines for the physician a practical approach to precordial palpation that should permit optimal use of this important physical diagnostic technique.

Physiology of the Precordial Impulse

NORMAL PRECORDIAL ACTIVITY

The palpable apical impulse in a normal subject is produced by an anterior movement of the left ventricle during early systole.[2] As isovolumic intraventricular pressure rises, the left ventricle rotates in a counterclockwise direction on its long axis as the cardiac apex lifts and makes contact with the left anterior chest wall.[3] Following aortic valve opening and the first half of ejection, the LV chamber moves away from the chest wall and continues to diminish in size until systole is completed. Thus, the impulse felt or recorded on the precordium is made up of an early outward thrust followed by retraction during the last part of systole; normal palpable cardiac activity occurs only during the first half of systole (Fig. 7-1, Fig. 7-2A). The retraction wave can be seen but is not felt. Diastolic events, such as the LV rapid filling phase or left atrial contraction, are normally not palpable.

In angiographic studies, the intraventricular septum (composed mostly of LV muscle) and the anteroseptal aspect of the left ventricle make contact with

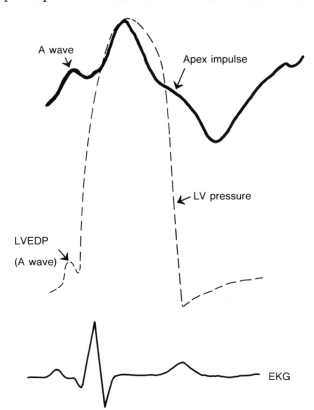

FIG. 7-1. Relationship of the normal LV apex impulse to intraventricular pressure. *LVEDP*=Left ventricular end-diastolic pressure.

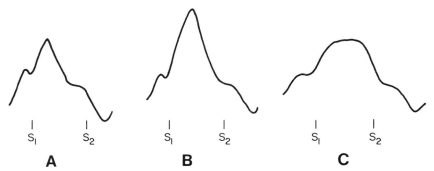

FIG. 7-2. Major types of precordial motion. (*A*) Normal. (*B*) Hyperdynamic. (*C*) Sustained (See text for discussion)

the inner thoracic cage to form the palpable apical impulse.[3] The true anatomical LV apex is actually slightly lower and more lateral than the palpable apical impulse.

Right Ventricular Activity

Although the right ventricle, located just beneath the sternum and left third to fifth ribs, is closer than the left ventricle to the chest wall, RV activity is not normally felt. This is probably because the right ventricle is thin-walled (2 mm–3 mm wall thickness), because peak pressure is low (20 mm Hg–25 mm Hg peak systolic pressure), and because the right ventricle pulls *away* from the anterior chest as the heart rotates in a counterclockwise fashion in early systole. In children and young adults, or thin subjects who have a narrow anteroposterior thoracic diameter, gentle RV activity may occasionally be felt. Careful subxiphoid palpation during held inspiration may also bring out RV motion that is not pathologic.

Diastolic Events

The low pressure and volume transients of mid- and late diastole are normally undetectable by precordial palpation. With alterations in ventricular diastolic volume, pressure, or compliance, these events (palpable third and fourth heart sounds [S_3 and S_4]) can be transmitted to the chest wall by the left or right ventricle and may be felt by the examining fingers.

ABNORMALITIES OF PRECORDIAL MOTION

When there are alterations in ventricular size, shape, or function, precordial activity is more easily detected. The systolic LV and RV precordial impulse may be changed in *location, amplitude, size,* and *contour.*[4,5] (See Clinical Presentation below.)

Systolic Events

HYPERDYNAMIC STATES.   Anxiety, tachycardia, exertion, or catechol excess from any cause will increase cardiac contractility and often systolic blood pressure, resulting in an increase in the force and amplitude of the apical impulse (see Fig. 7-2B). In such situations, the location and contour of the precordial impulse are unchanged.

LEFT VENTRICLE.   Characteristic changes may occur in the apical impulse with LV enlargement, depending on whether there is dominant hypertrophy or dilatation. Such abnormalities may provide the clinician with the first clue to organic heart disease. LV wall-motion abnormalities, whether focal or global, are often manifested by an abnormal apical motion pattern.

VOLUME OVERLOAD.   Early or mild degrees of mitral or aortic regurgitation do not usually alter the contour of the LV impulse. The classic response to such lesions is an increase in the amplitude (hyperdynamic impulse) of the LV impulse without a change in contour: early systolic outward and late systolic inward motion is preserved (see Fig. 7-2B).[4] In severe volume overload states, particularly with depression of LV contractility and a decreased ejection fraction, the LV impulse may become prolonged or sustained into the second half of systole (see Fig. 7-2C). This may be due both to a longer ejection time and to a chamber configuration that is more globular or spherical than the normal elliptical LV shape. LV dilatation with a major increase in LV end-diastolic volume results in leftward and downward displacement of the apical impulse, as well as an increase in the size of the actual contact area of the apical beat.

PRESSURE OVERLOAD.   The initial response of the left ventricle to increased outflow resistance (aortic stenosis, hypertension) is concentric hypertrophy without an increase in cavity size. Systolic function is well maintained. The LV impulse becomes prolonged in duration, reflecting an increased LV ejection time (see Fig. 7-2C). This produces a sustained LV heave or thrust. The force of contraction is increased, but there is relatively little chamber dilatation. Thus, the apical impulse is not usually displaced but has an increased force. With long-standing disease and depression of cardiac function, the left ventricle dilates and the impulse is located more laterally. The area of the chest wall over which the apical beat is felt in pressure-loaded hearts is not usually as large as that in chronic severe volume-overload states.

ABNORMALITIES OF LEFT VENTRICULAR SYSTOLIC FUNCTION.   When LV contractile performance is deranged, the apical impulse can be altered in several ways: (1) the normal brief outward contour may become sustained into the last half of systole (see Fig. 7-2C). This may result either from ischemic dysfunction due to fibrosis or to depressed myocardial contractile performance, or from LV dilatation and a globally depressed ejection fraction; (2) a mid- or late systolic impulse (bulge) may be present, reflecting a disordered contraction pattern (coronary heart disease or cardiomyopathy); (3) an ectopic impulse may be present, that is, an impulse at a site away from the normal apical impulse, usually superior and medial to it.[6,7] This is most likely to occur with LV aneurysm, but may be seen with anterior wall dyskinesis in the absence of an aneurysm; (4) inferolateral displacement and enlargement of the area of the apical beat will be present whenever the LV chamber is substantially dilated, particularly if there is a depressed ejection fraction.

RIGHT VENTRICLE. The RV response is similar to the LV response in volume and pressure overload states. Because the right ventricle is not usually involved in ischemic dysfunction, there are fewer variations to the abnormal RV impulse.

PRESSURE OVERLOAD. Pulmonary hypertension from any cause results in sustained RV activity, manifest as a palpable or visible anterior motion in the lower left sternal area. The RV inflow area is generally located at the left fourth to fifth intercostal space adjacent to the sternum, while the infundibular area is located more superiorly at the third to fourth left intercostal space.[8]

VOLUME OVERLOAD. The volume-loaded right ventricle (atrial septal defect, tricuspid regurgitation without RV dysfunction) produces a hyperdynamic, high-amplitude impulse that retains the pattern of mid- or late systolic retraction. Thus, the motion is a brief anterior thrust. With a very large RV end-diastolic volume or depressed RV contractile function, this anterior parasternal motion becomes sustained.

MITRAL REGURGITATION. In severe mitral regurgitation, there may be an apparent RV impulse reflecting systolic expansion of an enlarged left atrium with subsequent anterior displacement of the right ventricle (Fig. 7-3).[9] This phenomenon requires a dilated left atrium and large mitral leak. The actual palpable parasternal motion is out of synchrony with the earlier LV apical impulse and can be identified with careful examination.

Diastolic Events

LEFT VENTRICLE. LV diastolic filling comprises two phases: initial rapid filling following mitral valve opening and late diastolic augmentation resulting from left atrial contraction. In the normal heart, LV pressure throughout diastole is low; these filling events (and their resultant heart sounds) are neither palpable nor audible.

When ischemia, fibrosis, hypertrophy, or dilatation are present, the compliance, diastolic volume, and filling pressure of the left ventricle are altered, and the two peaks of blood flow from the left atrium to the left ventricle may result in large pressure transients and increased distending forces. In such situations, the rapid filling phase and left atrial systole may result in audible and palpable events (S_3 and S_4).

PALPABLE S_3. An abnormal increase in transmitral flow, a large LV end-diastolic volume, and significant depression of LV function are all asso-

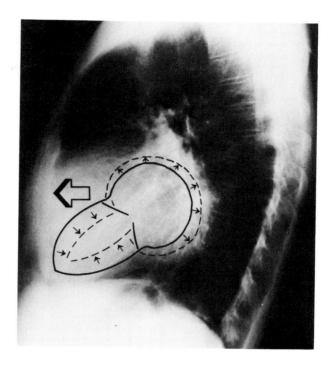

FIG. 7-3. Mechanism of parasternal impulse in severe mitral regurgitation. Systolic expansion of an enlarged left atrium thrusts the right ventricle anteriorly, producing a late systolic impulse at the lower left sternal border.

ciated with the presence of an audible S_3, which may be palpable as well. It is not clear why the S_3 can be detected by palpation in some people and not in others, nor do we know if the presence of a palpable S_3 carries any prognostic or physiologic implications. It is likely that audibility and palpability are more related to factors associated with the coupling of the heart to the chest wall.[10]

A palpable S_3 is found in patients with an enlarged left ventricle and a major elevation in LV filling pressure and end-diastolic volume. In such patients, early and mid-diastolic LV pressure is often elevated; left atrial contraction may not result in any additional pressure augmentation at end-diastole. Typically, these hearts have a decreased ejection fraction. Patients with aortic valve disease, hypertensive heart disease, and coronary heart disease may develop a loud or palpable S_3 when LV function deteriorates, with or without overt congestive heart failure. Congestive cardiomyopathy patients typically have a palpable LV filling sound. The pericardial knock of constrictive pericarditis is actually an early, exaggerated filling event, comparable to a loud S_3, and is usually palpable.

In subjects with an increased volume and rate of blood flow across the mitral valve, an S_3 may be audible and palpable in the presence of good LV function. Classically, severe mitral regurgitation results in such filling events; a large volume of blood returns to the left ventricle from the left atrium during the rapid filling phase. LV end-diastolic volume is usually elevated in such cases, but systolic function and ejection fraction are well preserved.

PALPABLE S_4. A palpable S_4 is related to decreased LV compliance, usually a result of hypertrophy without dilatation or ischemia with increased diastolic stiffness (Fig. 7-4).[11] A palpable S_4 is always associated with an LV end-diastolic pressure that is elevated, sometimes strikingly so, although early and mid-diastolic pressure is often normal. Thus, a palpable S_4 is typical of aortic valve disease, hypertrophic cardiomyopathy, hypertensive heart disease, coronary artery disease, and, occasionally, of congestive cardiomyopathy. The implications of a palpable S_4 are quite different from those of a palpable S_3; in the former case, LV systolic function is usually well preserved and the ejection fraction is normal. A palpable S_3 (in the absence of significant mitral regurgitation) is associated with high LV filling pressures, a dilated ventricle, and decreased systolic function.[12]

RIGHT VENTRICLE. The pathophysiology of a palpable S_3 and S_4 generated in the right ventricle is similar to that in the left heart. Compliance changes (RV hypertrophy secondary to pulmonary hypertension) may result in a palpable RV S_4. Increased blood flow across the tricuspid valve may produce a prominent S_3. Tricuspid regurgitation is a good example of this, and a large left-to-right shunt and atrial septal defect may also occasionally produce

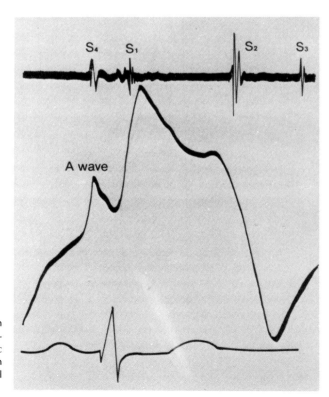

FIG. 7-4. Palpable atrial or fourth heart sound. Light pressure with fingertips will often detect presystolic distention of the left ventricle when the patient is turned to the left lateral decubitus position.

a palpable RV S_3. In severe RV dysfunction an S_3 may be heard and felt. Classically, RV events are marked by inspiratory augmentation and expiratory attenuation or disappearance.

OTHER CAUSES OF PALPABLE CARDIOVASCULAR ACTIVITY

In addition to the tactile precordial phenomena related to LV and RV systolic and diastolic events, palpable precordial activity is occasionally detectable as a result of vascular pulsations or ectopic LV wall-motion abnormalities.[4,8]

Palpable Cardiovascular Events

AORTA. When either the ascending aorta or the aortic arch is enlarged or dilated, palpable systolic pulsations may be detected. Thus, with aortic aneurysms, diffuse aortic dilatation, or aortic dissection, a systolic impulse may be felt in the right first or second intercostal space, in the right or left sternoclavicular junction, or in the suprasternal areas. Dilatation or enlargement of the brachiocephalic vessels may also cause prominent vascular pulsations at the suprasternal notch or above the clavicles.

PULMONARY ARTERY. Dilatation or enlargement of the pulmonary artery is usually associated with pulmonary hypertension, which itself may result from hyperkinetic (high flow) states or from increased pulmonary vascular resistance. Idiopathic dilatation of the pulmonary artery results in an enlarged proximal pulmonary artery segment. All these conditions may produce a palpable systolic impulse in the second to third left intercostal space just to the left of the sternal edge. This is easily detectable in thin subjects.

LEFT VENTRICULAR ECTOPIC IMPULSE. Focal wall-motion abnormalities or an overt LV aneurysm may produce systolic impulses that are detectable at sites away from the LV apical beat, usually medial and superior to the apical area.[6,7] With anteroseptal LV scarring or dyskinesis, the ectopic impulse may be found at the lower parasternal edge and thus may simulate RV activity.

PALPABLE HEART SOUNDS AND MURMURS. Loud sound transients (such as an increased S_1, A_2, or P_2) are often readily palpable. An opening snap is commonly palpable in mitral stenosis, as is a loud S_1; on occasion the diagnosis of this valve lesion can be made prior to using the stethoscope. Ejection clicks may be easily felt; the aortic ejection sound is detected at the LV apex, while a pulmonic ejection sound is palpable at the upper left sternal border.

THRILLS. Any loud murmur may be transmitted to the chest wall, where it can produce a vibratory sensation to the examining hand. These palpable murmurs or thrills correlate with a murmur intensity of Grade IV/VI or greater. Such murmurs may be felt at the apex (mitral regurgitation, obstructive hypertrophic cardiomyopathy), lower left sternal border (ventricular septal defect), or cardiac base (pulmonic stenosis, aortic stenosis). Obviously, in thin subjects the likelihood of a thrill is greater than in muscular or fleshy patients. A diastolic thrill may occasionally be felt, usually at the apex with the subject in the lateral decubitus position in mitral stenosis, or at the lower left sternal border in acute aortic regurgitation secondary to a perforated or ruptured aortic cusp.

Clinical Presentation

HOW TO EXAMINE THE PRECORDIUM

For optimal precordial examination, it is important for the examiner and patient to be relaxed. The room should be comfortably warm. Clothing and undergarments must be removed to allow unobstructed visualization and palpation of the chest. Because the examiner must be prepared, for example, to count intercostal spaces, measure the distance of the precordial impulse from the sternum or axillary line, and so on, chest exposure should be maximal. The subject should be lying comfortably, in the supine position or with the thorax elevated no more than 30 degrees (Fig. 7-5). Perloff suggests that the 30-degree position is preferable because precordial examination in this position may bring out abnormalities more often than examination when the patient is supine.[8] Patients with suspected or definite cardiovascular disease should routinely be examined in the left lateral decubitus position; the subject should

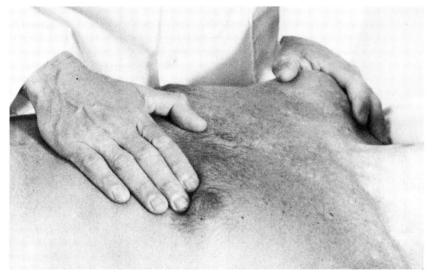

FIG. 7-5. Palpation of the apex impulse, supine position. The patient may also be examined with the thorax and head elevated 20°–30°.

be instructed to turn on his or her left side at a 45-degree to 60-degree angle with the examining table, elevating the left arm over the head so that the physician may have unobstructed access to the left precordium (Fig. 7-6).

Inspection

Careful visual observation of the chest is useful in the precordial examination, particularly after preliminary palpation has identified the site of the apical beat or any other impulses that may be present. Retraction movements, which may be more obvious than outward motion to the eye, are quite prominent in severe degrees of LV and RV enlargement. Tangential lighting with the examining lamp or a pen light may accentuate visible movements on the chest wall.

Palpation

The examiner should be standing comfortably at the patient's right side (see Fig. 7-5). Both the palm of the hand and the ventral surface of the proximal metacarpals and fingers should be used for palpation. One must learn which aspect of the hand has the best sense of touch. It is advisable to use the pads of the fingers for precise localization and assessment of LV and RV activity;

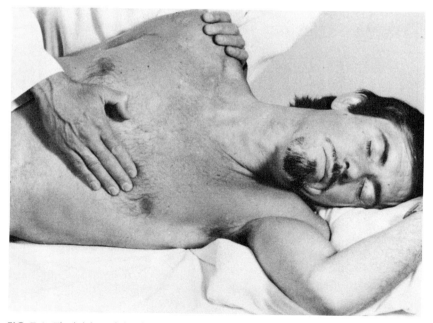

FIG. 7-6. The left lateral decubitus position. Use this maneuver in any patient with suspected LV pathology. The subject's left arm should be extended above the head.

the palm and proximal metacarpals are usually best used to localize palpable cardiac motion as well as to detect precordial thrills.

Varying pressure with the hand should be applied once a precordial impulse is identified. High-frequency sounds, such as an increased S_1, an opening snap, or a transmitted thrill, are best detected with the hand firmly applied to the chest. However, the subtle, low-frequency motion of a palpable S_3 or S_4 or double systolic apical impulse will be felt only with light pressure of the fingers and may be totally obscured if the examination is not performed correctly.

Timing of precordial events is best carried out by simultaneously palpating the carotid arterial pulse with the left hand. Some find that concomitant auscultation of S_1 and S_2 is useful for timing purposes. Actual observation of the stethoscope head positioned directly on the apical impulse can help identify systole.

It is desirable to use held end-expiration for the RV examination. Firm pressure, using the heel of the hand with the wrist cocked upward, is advisable (Fig. 7-7). The lower sternum and adjacent third through fifth ribs and left interspaces should be examined in this manner. The examining hand and fingers should be carefully observed, as low-amplitude RV activity is often seen rather than felt. Some experts also suggest exploring the subxiphoid or epigastric region with the extended fingers oriented superiorly; the patient should be instructed to hold his breath in end-inspiration as careful palpation for the descending right ventricle is performed (Fig. 7-8). This technique is particularly useful in patients with an increased anteroposterior diameter, obesity, or chronic obstructive pulmonary disease (COPD).

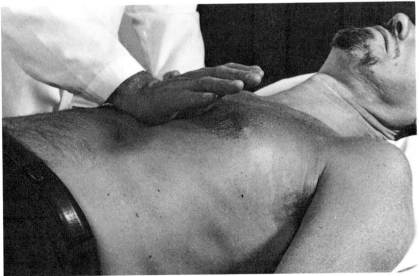

FIG. 7-7. Detection of parasternal or RV activity. Instruct the subject to hold his breath in end-expiration and use firm downward pressure with the heel of the hand.

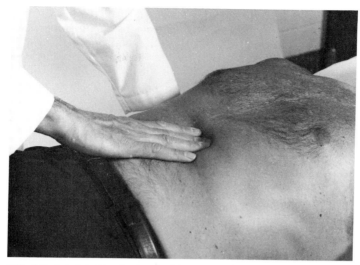

FIG. 7-8. Subxiphoid palpation for RV activity. This technique can be useful for subjects with large chests, obesity, or COPD. Instruct the patient to hold his breath in end-inspiration. Do not mistake abdominal aortic pulsations for inferior cardiac motion.

Characteristics of the Normal Apical Impulse

In normal subjects the apical impulse in the supine position produces a gentle outward motion that is usually felt in only one intercostal space (see Fig. 7-1, Fig. 7-2A). This anterior movement is brief and nonsustained, pulling away from the examining fingers by mid-systole. It occupies a maximal area of 2 cm² to 2.5 cm² (no larger than a quarter) and is found in the fourth or fifth left intercostal space at or inside the midclavicular line. It should not be located more than 10 cm to the left of the midsternal line. There may be respiratory alterations in the amplitude of the apical beat; focus on end-expiration if the impulse is hard to locate.

The characteristics of the normal apical impulse are summarized in Table 7–1.

Table 7–1.   The Normal Apical Impulse

A gentle, nonsustained tap
An early systolic anterior motion that ends before the last third of systole
Location within 10 cm of the midsternal line in the fourth or fifth left intercostal space
A palpable area less than 2 cm² to 2.5 cm² and detectable in only 1 intercostal space
RV motion that is not normally palpable
Diastolic events that are not normally palpable
Complete absence in some older individuals

In the left lateral decubitus position, the apical beat may contact the chest wall slightly more laterally and inferiorly than in the supine position. There is considerable controversy as to whether the contour of the apical impulse becomes altered in the left lateral position (see below). A recent study suggested that an apical impulse with an area of 3 cm^2 or more in the left lateral position is specific for LV enlargement.[12]

Right Ventricular Activity

In most normal subjects, parasternal activity is not usually detectable. However, in young or thin people, a gentle shock or tap at the lower left sternal border may be felt, and, occasionally, a pulmonary artery impulse in the second to third left intercostal space adjacent to the sternum may be detected. Forceful, sustained, or high-amplitude parasternal motion is always an abnormal finding.

Point of Maximum Impulse (PMI)

Many textbooks and articles in the literature use the term *PMI* to denote the apical beat. Although not ideal, this expression is so commonly used that it has become acceptable. Nevertheless, it should be recognized that the terms *PMI* and *apical impulse* are not necessarily synonymous. In some patients, the most prominent, or "maximal," impulse may actually reflect ectopic LV motion, RV activity, or a vascular impulse.

Other Palpable Events

In a subject with suspected cardiac disease, the examiner should explore the entire precordium with firm pressure of the hand and proximal fingers, analyzing the aortic, pulmonic, lower sternal, and apical regions. In this way, the unexpected vascular impulse, such as a dilated or aneurysmal ascending aorta or pulmonary artery, may be detected. Particular attention should be given to the upper sternal area, to the manubrium, and to the adjacent first to second intercostal spaces below the medial aspect of the clavicles. Aortic pulsations and systolic thrills are often found here.

If a patient has coronary artery disease, particularly with a prior myocardial infarction, careful examination for ectopic impulse should be carried out. These typically occur medial and superior to the apical impulse. The use of the entire palm and proximal metacarpals will help detect the diffuse lift of a very large left or right ventricle. On occasion, the entire anterior precordium will move in systole. This technique is also suited for the detection of thrills and palpable heart sounds.

Percussion

Under ordinary circumstances, percussion is neither necessary nor useful. When a PMI cannot be identified, however, the technique may help establish the presence or absence of cardiomegaly and will identify the approximate left border of the heart. In patients with a large pericardial effusion, the apex beat may actually be detected inside the lateral border of the cardiac silhouette, as determined by percussion.

Variations of the Apical Beat

ABSENT APICAL IMPULSE. It is not commonly realized that many older subjects (over age 50) do not have palpable cardiac activity when examined in the supine position. This may be due to an increase in the anteroposterior thoracic diameter, an increase of muscle or fat on the chest wall, or a physiologic decrease in the force of LV contraction with age. Whenever an apical impulse cannot be felt in the supine position, the left heart border should be percussed, and the patient should be carefully examined in the left lateral decubitus position (see Fig. 7-6). The latter is a much more valuable maneuver than percussion. In most adults, LV activity can be felt when the subject is turned onto the left side, particularly in expiration; often the PMI will then be identifiable after the patient is again turned supine. In some normal adults, an apex impulse will not be detectable in either position.

LATERAL DISPLACEMENT WITHOUT CARDIOMEGALY. In some people the apical beat or PMI may be displaced to the left although the cardiac and LV chamber sizes are actually normal. This displacement may occur in conjunction with skeletal abnormalities such as scoliosis, the straight-back syndrome (narrow anteroposterior diameter, loss of normal thoracic kyphosis, marked pectus excavatum), or intrathoracic pathology.[13] A large right pleural effusion, pneumothorax, atelectasis, or extensive pulmonary fibrosis may distort the heart's position in the chest and result in a displaced cardiac impulse without actual cardiomegaly.

ASSESSMENT OF THE APICAL CARDIAC IMPULSE

The assessment of the apical cardiac impulse should include analysis of the following parameters:

Location
Size
Force
Duration
Contour

In addition, there should be visual inspection of the chest for the presence of prominent retraction waves as well as for systolic and diastolic events. As already mentioned, a complete precordial examination consists of a systematic evaluation of the lower sternal area, pulmonary and aortic regions, and sternoclavicular sites.

Characteristics

LOCATION.   Identify the site of the apical impulse on the thorax with respect to both the longitudinal and horizontal axes of the patient. Note in which intercostal space the PMI or apical beat is located; occasionally a large heart will result in detectable precordial activity in 2 or even 3 intercostal spaces. Localize the apical impulse with reference to the midclavicular line, distance from the midsternum, or relationship to the left anterior axillary line.

SIZE.   If the apical impulse is larger than normal, it is useful to note the area of contact with the chest. Any area greater than 2 cm² to 2.5 cm² in the supine position, or greater than 3 cm² in the left decubitus position, represents cardiac enlargement.[12]

FORCE OR AMPLITUDE.   Is the apical beat a soft, unimpressive impulse or does it lift the examining fingers off the chest wall? Is the anterior or outward excursion greater than normal, consistent with a hyperdynamic or hyperkinetic PMI? An increase in force is consistent with LV hypertrophy and preserved systolic function. Assessment of the force of contraction is the most subjective and least quantifiable aspect of precordial examination.

DURATION.   The duration of the systolic outward motion is probably the most important feature of the precordial exam. Although cardiomegaly or hypertrophy can exist in the presence of a brief "normal" outward movement, or even when the PMI is absent, a truly sustained LV impulse in the supine or 30-degree elevation position is distinctly abnormal (see Fig. 7-2C). Such findings suggest a pressure-overloaded ventricle (*e.g.*, aortic stenosis, hypertension) or an LV chamber with a depressed ejection fraction and a substantially dilated cavity. A study by Conn demonstrated that a *sustained* apex impulse in the supine position was highly correlated with an increase in angiographically determined LV mass, and this observation was actually more sensitive than the electrocardiogram (ECG) in the diagnosis of LV hypertrophy.[14]

The critical point to assess is whether or not the impulse "stays up" into the second half of systole. Timing that uses simultaneous auscultation of S_1 and S_2 is essential in making this observation. With practice, one can be quite accurate in assessing the actual duration of the apical impulse. Simple observation of movement of the head of the stethoscope resting on the PMI may be helpful.

LEFT LATERAL DECUBITUS POSITION.   It is unclear whether an LV impulse that becomes sustained when the patient is turned into the left lateral position but is of normal duration in the supine position has the same specificity for LV enlargement as a sustained impulse (LV heave) that is present when the patient is lying flat. Because the left decubitus position causes the heart to approximate the chest wall more closely, many experts feel that the observation of a prolonged impulse in this position has little diagnostic value. I believe that a definite *sustained* impulse in the left lateral position is highly suggestive of true LV dilatation. False positives may occur, however, and echocardiography is recommended in equivocal cases.

CONTOUR. The normal apical impulse is a brief, nonsustained anterior motion in early systole (see Fig. 7-2A). A sustained LV beat is the commonest abnormality of contour (see above), but occasionally other patterns are noted.

A double systolic impulse may be seen in hypertrophic obstructive cardiomyopathy (IHSS) and occasionally in some patients with severe LV dyssynergy or LV aneurysm in coronary artery disease. Presystolic distention is commonly found in the left lateral position in patients who have decreased LV compliance, such as that stemming from coronary artery disease, hypertensive heart disease, or aortic valve disease (see below). Palpable diastolic events, such as an S_3 or a pericardial knock, also fall into the general category of contour changes.

PALPABLE A WAVE (PRESYSTOLIC DISTENTION). Palpable A waves are usually detected in the left decubitus position.[11] The apical beat is carefully identified, and varying pressure is applied with the pads of the fingers at the site of the LV impulse. A double early systolic impulse is noted, feeling like a "shelf" or ridge on the upstroke of the beat (see Fig. 7-4). Usually, this low-amplitude finding will best be felt when finger pressure is light; firm pressure with the fingers may make the finding more difficult or impossible to feel. On occasion, this presystolic distention can be quite prominent.

The palpable A wave reflects a high LV end-diastolic pressure and decreased LV compliance. It is an important observation because it documents a definite abnormality that usually implies LV hypertrophy and increased chamber stiffness. The audibility of the S_4 does not correlate with palpability; presystolic distention may be detectable when the S_4 is quite soft. Occasionally, one may not be able to hear an S_4 at all, even though it is palpable; this is because the frequency of the diastolic filling event is extremely low (usually less than 50 cycles per second).

PALPABLE S_3. The S_3 is less often palpable than an S_4. It is most often observed in severe mitral regurgitation or in a markedly dilated cardiomyopathic ventricle. As with the S_4, palpation is greatly enhanced in the left decubitus position. The S_3 appears as a brief outward motion in early diastole, gently tapping the examining finger pads but not displacing the fingers, since it is usually not forceful.

Parasternal or Right Ventricular Impulses

All of the above also applies to the evaluation of RV or parasternal activity. However, the low-amplitude impulse produced by RV hypertrophy or dilatation is usually more difficult to evaluate than apical LV activity. Nevertheless, an increased amplitude or sustained parasternal motion is usually discernible on careful examination.

Palpable diastolic events are often best detected using held-inspiration and the subxiphoid or epigastric approach, with the fingers extended to identify these low-frequency and low-amplitude motion abnormalities (see Fig. 7-8).

PRECORDIAL MOTION ABNORMALITIES IN SPECIFIC CARDIOVASCULAR DISORDERS

The following section summarizes the major palpable findings in a variety of common adult cardiovascular conditions (Table 7-2).

Aortic Stenosis

In mild aortic stenosis the PMI may be normal. The typical apical impulse in hemodynamically significant valve aortic stenosis is sustained, with outward motion palpable in late systole (see Fig. 7-2C). It is typically forceful and readily displaces the examining fingers. Unless LV function is impaired and LV dilatation has occurred, the apical impulse is usually not displaced laterally more than 1 cm to 2 cm. In severe aortic stenosis, the impulse may be felt in more than one intercostal space. Presystolic distention of the left ventricle (palpable A wave) is common in such situations, particularly in the left lateral position (see Fig. 7-4). When present, the palpable S_4 indicates that there is a large LV–aortic pressure gradient (unless there is coexisting coronary or hypertensive heart disease).

A systolic thrill at the second right intercostal space is often found in aortic stenosis. Palpable sound vibrations may radiate upward toward the clavicle

Table 7–2.   Major Types of Precordial Impulses

Impulse	Hyperdynamic	Sustained	Late Systolic
Left ventricular impulse (apical beat)	Hyperkinetic circulatory states Thin chest wall	Pressure overload Hypertension Aortic stenosis	LV dyssynergy Hypertrophic cardiomyopathy Mitral valve prolapse (rare)
	Pectus excavatum	Chronic or severe volume overload states	
	Volume overload Aortic regurgitation Mitral regurgitation Ventricular setpal defect	LV dilatation, especially with decreased ejection fraction LV dysfunction LV aneurysm	
Right ventricular impulse (parasternal area)	Hyperkinetic circulatory state in young subjects Volume overload Atrial septal defect Tricuspid regurgitation	Pressure overload Pulmonary stenosis Pulmonary hypertension Cor pulmonale Mitral stenosis Pulmonary emboli Cardiomyopathy	Severe mitral regurgitation

(Abrams J: Precordial motion in health and disease. Mod Concepts Cardiovasc Dis 49:55–60, 1980. By permission of the American Heart Association, Inc.)

and also may be present over the manubrium or in the second left intercostal space. Occasionally, in older patients or those with an increased thoracic diameter, a systolic thrill is detected at the apex. An aortic thrill is usually best felt when the subject is upright and leaning forward with the breath held in end-expiration.

A palpable aortic ejection sound is commonly found in subjects with a congenitally bicuspid aortic valve. This sound is typically felt only at the apex, and can be differentiated from the LV impulse itself as a discrete, high-frequency transient. A detectable thrill or ejection sound correlates less well with the hemodynamic severity of the valve obstruction than does a sustained apical impulse or presystolic distention of the left ventricle.

Aortic Regurgitation

With moderate aortic regurgitation, the apex impulse may not be displaced but will typically be hyperdynamic and unsustained (see Fig. 7-2B). As the LV cavity dilates, the PMI is displaced laterally and downward and often takes up 2 or more intercostal spaces. Marked medial retraction may be seen. With a major volume overload, a sustained apical impulse is often felt. This impulse indicates severe LV cavity dilatation, even without significant depression of LV systolic function. The palpable area of the apical beat will be increased. In the left lateral position presystolic distention (palpable S_4) is often felt but an S_4 may not be heard. If an S_4 is audible or palpable, one can exclude the diagnosis of coexisting mitral stenosis, which may be suggested by the presence of a diastolic rumbling murmur (Austin Flint murmur). If coexisting aortic stenosis is present, the apical impulse will be sustained, large, forceful, and displaced inferolaterally.

It is rare to detect a palpable diastolic thrill in aortic regurgitation unless there is perforation or eversion of an aortic cusp resulting in an extremely loud diastolic murmur.

Mitral Regurgitation

The apical impulse is normal to hyperdynamic in mild to moderate mitral regurgitation. In severe mitral regurgitation, particularly when chronic, the LV impulse is displaced laterally and has an increased force and amplitude. A sustained PMI suggests that LV systolic function has decreased and that the ejection fraction is abnormal, or that major LV dilatation has occurred. The impulse may be quite large, being felt in 2 or more intercostal spaces. It is common to feel a systolic apical thrill in severe mitral regurgitation; with the onset of congestive heart failure or marked depression of LV function, the thrill may disappear as the murmur attenuates.

Mitral regurgitation is the usual cause of a late systolic impulse at the parasternal area or lower left sternal border. This outward motion can be quite prominent, reflecting the systolic jet of a large volume of blood into a dilated left atrium that expands during LV ejection (see Fig. 7-3). It is critical to time this parasternal activity to assess whether it is early or holosystolic, as opposed to late systolic. Simultaneous palpation of the LV impulse is essential; if the parasternal lift is due to left atrial expansion and not to pulmonary hypertension, it will occur in the second half of systole *after* the LV impulse is felt and after S_1 is heard. If there is coexisting pulmonary hypertension, the parasternal impulse will be sustained throughout systole. In such cases, the independent effect of left atrial systole will not be detected.

A visible and palpable S_3 may be noted in severe mitral regurgitation, particularly in the left lateral position. In acute mitral regurgitation, a palpable S_4 may be noted. The finding of presystolic distention is extremely important because it indicates that the condition is of recent onset.[15] An S_4 is never heard or felt in chronic rheumatic mitral regurgitation.

Mitral Stenosis

Precordial examination in mitral stenosis is often very rewarding, and the diagnosis may be suggested even before the stethoscope is used. S_1 is typically palpable at the apex or somewhat medially. S_2 may be palpable if there is pulmonary hypertension (increased P_2). The opening snap is often readily felt between the lower left sternal border and the apex, particularly in relatively thin patients. In the left lateral position, a diastolic thrill may be manifest at the apex but is usually palpable only over a very small area.

LV activity in pure mitral stenosis is unimpressive. However, most patients with moderate to severe degrees of mitral stenosis will have a parasternal or RV lift. Even when resting pulmonary artery pressure is not markedly elevated, pulmonary pressure typically rises with exercise and RV hypertrophy is common. Thus, a holosystolic parasternal lift is a common finding in hemodynamically significant mitral stenosis. A large left atrium will cause the right ventricle to be more anterior than usual, and this may contribute to the common finding of detectable parasternal activity in mitral stenosis. The more vigorous and sustained the RV lift, the more likely it is that one is dealing with significant pulmonary hypertension.

Obstructive Hypertrophic Cardiomyopathy (IHSS)

In obstructive hypertrophic cardiomyopathy, an unusual condition, precordial palpation may be very informative. The A wave is typically very prominent and palpable and the LV impulse is forceful and vigorous. Compliance is markedly decreased in these abnormally hypertrophied left ventricles. The heart is usually not displaced laterally. A mid- or late systolic secondary bulge may be present, resulting in a double, or bifid, precordial impulse. When the A wave is palpable, the precordial motion actually will be trifid in nature ("triple ripple").[16] The palpable A wave in this condition does not necessarily correlate with a large gradient across the LV outflow tract.

A systolic thrill, usually somewhat superior and medial to the apex, may often be felt, but, in contradistinction to aortic stenosis, it has poor radiation to the neck. Some patients have RV outflow tract obstruction, and this can result in a parasternal heave as well as a systolic thrill in the third to fourth intercostal space adjacent to the sternum.

Cardiomyopathy

The typical finding in congestive cardiomyopathy is a rather diffuse anterior precordial motion. It is often difficult to be sure if this is entirely LV in origin. The LV impulse is sustained and displaced inferolaterally. It may or may not be forceful, and it usually occupies more than one intercostal space. Presystolic distention (palpable A wave) and a palpable S_3 are common. Parasternal activity is also often noted. This activity contributes to the diffuse heaving or rocking precordial motion that may be found in such patients. Careful observation may reveal a retraction wave between the parasternal and apical regions. On rare occasions, a mid- or late systolic bulge may be observed.

Coronary Artery Disease

In patients with angina pectoris who have no history of myocardial infarction, the apical impulse is usually normal, although presystolic distention may be noted in the left lateral position.

A palpable S_4 is probably the most common abnormality of precordial motion in coronary artery disease. It is important to examine all patients with suspected or proven coronary artery disease in the left lateral decubitus position for optimal palpation and auscultation. Rarely, if a patient is examined during an episode of chest pain, a *transient* ectopic ventricular pulsation, presystolic distension, or sustained PMI may be detected.[17] In subjects with prior myocardial infarction, the apical impulse may be normal, sustained, or ectopic, or there may be a late systolic motion suggesting LV dyssynergy. Ectopic impulses are common in patients with LV aneurysms or severe LV dyssynergy.[7,17] If there is anteroseptal dyssynergy, a parasternal lift may be present, simulating RV hypertrophy.[8] A sustained apical impulse suggests either LV hypertrophy or a wall-motion abnormality.

Atrial Septal Defect

The uncomplicated atrial septal defect (ASD) causes volume overloading of the right ventricle, and this usually results in an easily detectable, nonsustained left lower sternal pulsation (hyperdynamic right ventricle). A pulmonary artery lift is common in the second or third left intercostal space. If coexisting pulmonary hypertension is present, the parasternal or RV impulse is sustained and "heaving" in quality. Even without significant pulmonary hypertension, a high flow ASD with a large volume overload may produce a sustained RV lift. The pulmonic second sound (and the pulmonary artery itself) may be palpable in patients with an ASD and this does not necessarily imply pulmonary hypertension.

Tricuspid Regurgitation

Tricuspid regurgitation in an adult usually results from acquired pulmonary hypertension and RV hypertrophy. In such instances, an RV or parasternal heave is likely to be found. Systolic retraction is commonly seen medial to the apical (LV) beat. Subxiphoid palpation may be necessary to detect RV activity in patients with COPD or obesity (see Fig. 7-8). Rarely, severe tricuspid regurgitation can produce right lower anterior chest pulsations that are palpable and visible, reflecting expansion of the right atrium during systole. Careful examination of the liver during held-inspiration will usually reveal pulsations with each cardiac systole. These are undulant, low-pressure impulses, and visual observation of the examining hand and fingers is often more helpful than palpation itself.

Summary

Careful precordial examination can be very rewarding to the skilled physician. Although many patients with overt cardiac dilatation and hypertrophy may have a normal apical impulse or even undetectable precordial activity, one can usually obtain clues of LV or RV enlargement from precordial palpation. Percussion is rarely necessary but should be performed whenever palpable LV activity cannot be identified. Physicians should routinely use the left lateral decubitus position, particularly in patients with coronary, hypertensive, or aortic valve disease. The detection of a palpable A wave or presystolic distention is consistent with decreased compliance caused by LV wall hypertrophy or fibrosis. A sustained LV impulse is a most useful finding and suggests either a chronic pressure overload or LV dilatation with a depressed ejection fraction. An apical impulse that is felt in two or more interspaces or is greater than 2.5 cm^2 to 3 cm^2 in area in the supine or left lateral position is highly suggestive of LV dilatation.

Careful examination of the lower left sternal area is also rewarding and will often detect pulmonary hypertension or left atrial expansion in mitral regurgitation. Palpable cardiac events, such as an ejection sound, opening snap, or a loud S$_1$ or S$_2$, are common, although frequently missed by the casual observer. Such clues are very useful in the assessment of a suspected cardiovascular lesion. Patients should be examined in the supine, left lateral, 30-degree, and even in the sitting positions for a total exploration of the precordium. Little is known about the factors relating to the contact of the heart with the anterior chest wall, but it is clear that different body positions can enhance or diminish the information from precordial palpation.[10] When performed with care and intelligence, the precordial examination can be extremely rewarding.

References

1. Basta LL, Bettinger JJ: The cardiac impulse: A new look at an old art. Am Heart J 97:96, 1979
2. Mounsey JPD: Inspection and palpation of the cardiac impulse. Prog Cardiovasc Dis 10:187, 1967

3. Constant J: Inspection and palpation of the chest. In Bedside Cardiology, 2nd ed, pp 100. Boston, Little, Brown & Co., 1976

4. Abrams J: Precordial motion in health and disease. Mod Concepts Cardiovasc Dis 49:55, 1980

5. Stapleton JF, Groves BM: Precordial palpation. Am Heart J 81:409, 1971

6. Chizner MA: Bedside diagnosis of the acute myocardial infarction and its complications. Curr Probl Cardiol 7:14, 1982

7. McGinn FX, Gould L, Lyon AF: The phonocardiogram and apexcardiogram in patients with ventricular aneurysm. Am J Cardiol 21:467, 1968

8. Perloff JK: The movements of the heart—observation, palpation, and percussion. In Physical Examination of the Heart and Circulation, pp 130–170. Philadelphia, WB Saunders, 1982

9. Basta LL, Wolfson P, Eckberg D, et al: The value of left parasternal impulse recordings in the assessment of mitral regurgitation. Circulation 48:1055, 1973

10. Reddy PS, Meno F, Curtiss EF, et al: The genesis of gallop sounds: Investigation by quantitative phono- and apexcardiography. Circulation 63:922, 1981

11. Bethell HJN, Nixon PGF: Examination of the heart in supine and left lateral positions. Br Heart J 9:902, 1973

12. Ellen SD, Crawford MH, O'Rourke RA: How accurate is precordial palpation for detecting increased left ventricular size? Circulation 66:II–266, 1982

13. DeLeon A, Perloff JK, Twigg H, et al: The straight back syndrome: Clinical cardiovascular manifestations. Circulation 32:193, 1965

14. Conn RD, Cole JS: The cardiac apex impulse: Clinical and angiographic correlations. Ann Intern Med 75:185, 1971

15. Ronan JA, Steelman RB, DeLeon AC, et al: The clinical diagnosis of acute severe mitral insufficiency. Am J Cardiol 27:284, 1971

16. Shah PM: Newer concepts in hypertrophic obstructive cardiomyopathy. II. JAMA 242:1771, 1979

17. Eddleman EEJ, Langley JO: Paradoxical pulsation of the precordium in myocardial infarction and angina pectoris. Am Heart J 63:579, 1962

8

FIRST AND SECOND HEART SOUNDS

Edward I. Curtiss, M.D., and P. Sudhakar Reddy, M.D.

The bedside assessment of the first heart sound (S_1) usually includes an estimate of its intensity, an assessment of the uniformity of this intensity from cycle to cycle, and a determination of whether two S_1 components are audible. Evaluation of the second heart sound (S_2) includes observations of the relative intensity of its aortic (A_2) and pulmonic (P_2) components, as well as of their separation relative to the respiratory cycle.

Physiology

GENESIS OF HEART SOUNDS

The most widely accepted theory of heart sound production is that proposed by Robert Rushmer.[1] This theory states that heart sounds are produced by the abrupt acceleration and deceleration of blood masses contained by an elastic boundary. Sudden motion imparted to the blood results in stretching of the heart walls, valves, and adjacent arteries, which, with the blood itself, constitute the *cardiohemic system*. Because these structures are elastic, they recoil, displacing blood in the opposite direction. Repetition of this stretch and recoil sequence produces vibrations of the entire, interdependent cardiohemic system. The vibrations are transmitted in all directions and will be audible on the chest wall if their intensity is sufficiently high and their frequency is within the audible range. According to this hypothesis, the deceleration of blood columns attendant upon closure of the atrioventricular (AV) and the semilunar valves results in the production of S_1 and S_2, respectively.

Using data derived from intracardiac pressure and sound studies, Stein and his colleagues have attempted to modify Rushmer's hypothesis.[2] They propose that heart sounds are produced by pressure gradients created across closed, elastic valves. The pressure gradient constitutes the net force acting on the blood mass. Because force is equal to the product of mass and acceleration, force is proportional to acceleration if mass remains constant. Thus, pressure gradients and acceleration will be closely related. We, therefore, do not find these theories to be mutually contradictory. Stein and his associates also maintain that sounds are due to valvular vibrations *per se,* in contradistinction to Rushmer's postulate that audible sounds are due to vibrations of the whole cardiohemic system. The issue is difficult to resolve because, as stated above, changes in pressure and flow are interdependent and closely related in time. However, it must be borne in mind that the sounds we perceive at the bedside represent vibrations of the chest wall. As Figure 8-1 illustrates, there may be differences between internally and externally recorded vibrations. The externally audible sound will probably relate more closely to vibrations of the cardiohemic system than to intracardiac pressure transients.

CARDIAC VIBRATIONS VERSUS HEART SOUNDS

Graphic records have been used to explain the characteristics of the cyclical vibrations that the auscultor perceives as sounds on the chest wall. These phonocardiographic displays, however, are filtered, nonquantitative re-

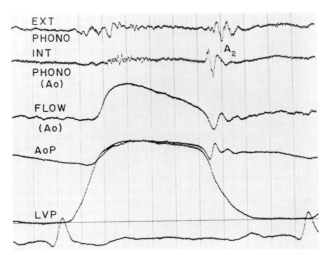

FIG. 8-1. Pressure-flow correlates of A_2 in a dog, recorded at 150 mm/sec. From the top down, the traces are an external phonocardiogram (*ext phono*), an internal phonocardiogram (*int phono*) in the aorta (*Ao*), aortic flow velocity, aortic (*AoP*) and left ventricular (*LVP*) pressure, and an electrocardiogram. The interval between heavy time lines is 50 msec. The flow trace is filtered and therefore is delayed by approximately 10 msec. Toward the end of ventricular systole, there is an abrupt decline in aortic pressure and flow. The former is abruptly arrested (the dicrotic notch) and followed by a sharp pressure rise (the dicrotic wave). A_2 begins at the time of the notch, which represents stretching of the valve. It is followed by valvular recoil, represented by the dicrotic wave. Note that the externally and internally recorded A_2 do not coincide.

cordings that can be translated only with great difficulty into terms of sound, which is the subjective interpretation of a temporally discrete vibratory event. This caveat must constantly be kept in mind when viewing the records that follow.

In these phonocardiographic records, two vibratory events may appear to be temporally separated by a visually appreciable interval. However, the human auditory system can distinguish two sounds only if their higher-frequency contents are separated by an interval exceeding 20 msec.[3] This minimal interval is significantly affected by the frequency composition and intensity of the two sets of vibrations. Lower-frequency and lower-intensity sounds require a separation greater than 30 msec in order to be audibly distinguishable. Even if two sounds are separated by the requisite interval for audibility, the second component may be masked if the first component is very loud and the second is soft. In such cases, our ability to perceive the second component is significantly diminished, especially if the level of ambient noise is high.

Our bedside appreciation of the intensity of a sound is subject to modification by vibratory characteristics other than intensity. When two sounds are of equal intensity but differ in frequency, we will perceive the higher-frequency sound as louder.[3]

Physiology of the First Heart Sound

GENESIS OF THE FIRST HEART SOUND

It has clearly been shown that S_1 consists of one or two sets of vibrations that are temporally related to closure of the AV valves. The first component is related to mitral (M_1) closure and the second is related to tricuspid (T_1) closure.[4-8] The cessation of antegrade mitral transvalvular flow and M_1 occur approximately 20 msec to 40 msec after left atrial–left ventricular (LA–LV) pressure crossover.[4] S_1 normally occurs during the rapid rise of intraventricular pressure at a time when LV pressure considerably exceeds LA pressure (Fig. 8-2). The continuation of antegrade mitral flow against this pressure gradient is due to the blood's inertia, inertia being the property of mass that resists changes in velocity. Once the blood mass has been set in motion, energy is required to stop it. This energy is derived from LV contraction and is reflected in the negative (with respect to flow) pressure gradient.

The relations between LV pressure, LA pressure, the mitral component of S_1, and mitral valve motion are shown in Figure 8-3A. At the onset of ventricular diastole, the AV valve opens so that the cusps are widely separated (*D* to *E* in the mitral valve echogram shown in Fig. 8-3A). During subsequent ventricular filling, the mitral leaflets tend to approximate but do not coapt (*E* to *F* in Fig. 8-3A). Under normal circumstances, atrial systole results in an increased displacement of blood from atrium to ventricle, causing the partially approximated cusps to move into a more divergent position (*F* to *A* in Fig. 8-3A). When atrial systole ceases, the ventricle recoils, tending to appose the

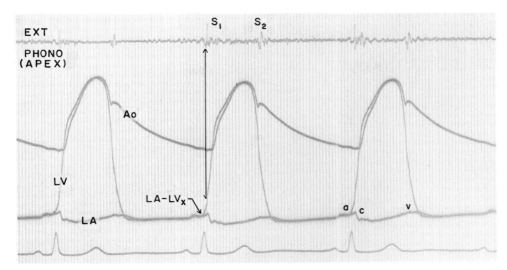

FIG. 8-2. Pressure correlates of the mitral component (M_1) of S_1 in a young woman with an atrial septal defect and a normal mitral valve. From the top down, the traces are an external phonocardiogram (*ext phono*), aortic pressure (*Ao*), left ventricular pressure (*LV*), and left atrial pressure (*LA*). Note that M_1 or S_1 occurs approximately 30 msec after LA-LV pressure crossover (*$LA-LV_x$*) during the rapid rise of intraventricular pressure. S_1 is coincident with the C wave in the left atrium. This wave begins with a sharp pressure rise (valvular stretch) followed by a rapid fall (valvular recoil).

leaflets once again (*A* to *B* in Fig. 8-3A). This presystolic portion of AV valve closure is thus *atriogenic*. However, atriogenic closure is interrupted by the onset of ventricular contraction. The force of ventricular systole displaces blood within its cavity toward the AV valve. Final AV valve closure is normally *ventriculogenic* (*B* to *C* in Fig. 8-3A).[8] Following coaptation, the elastic AV valve is stretched toward the atrium by the momentum of the ventricular blood mass. In a brief period, the AV valve reaches its greatest possible excursion or stretch capacity, and the intracavitary blood column is abruptly decelerated, or checked. This sets into motion the stretch–recoil sequence. The cardiohemic system is now vibrating, producing the discrete sonic event appreciated on the chest wall as S_1. The stretch–recoil sequence is marked in the atrial pressure trace by the C wave, an initial sharp pressure rise (*stretch*) followed by a rapid fall (*recoil*) (see Fig. 8-2).

DETERMINANTS OF FIRST HEART SOUND INTENSITY

The intensity or loudness of S_1 is determined by the momentum (the product of mass and velocity) achieved by the intracavitary blood column at the time of AV valve closure. Since the AV valve cusps constitute the

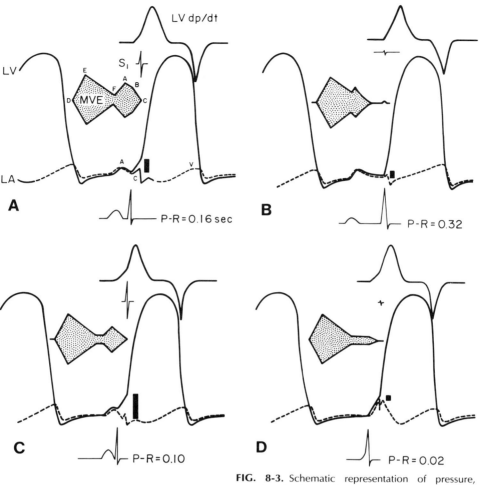

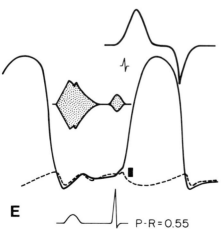

FIG. 8-3. Schematic representation of pressure, sound, and valve motion correlates of S₁. (*A*) Normal P–R interval. Left ventricular (*LV*) and left atrial (*LA; dashed lines*) pressure, the rate of change of LV pressure (*LV dp/dt*), and the mitral valve echocardiogram (*MVE*) are illustrated. In the MVE, the separation between the anterior mitral leaflet (upper line) and the posterior leaflet (lower line) is shown by the dotted area. The heavy black bar at the time of S₁ indicates the LV–LA pressure gradient. (*B*) Abnormally prolonged P–R interval. (*C*) Relatively short P–R interval. (*D*) Atrial and ventricular systoles essentially coincident. (*E*) Markedly prolonged P–R interval. Following atriogenic mitral valve closure in mid diastole, reopening occurs due to continuing blood inflow from the pulmonary arterial to venous beds. The valve is open at the onset of ventricular systole and a louder S₁ occurs than that associated with the prolonged P–R interval illustrated in (*B*).

advancing edge of the ventricular blood column being displaced toward the atrium, the velocity term can be estimated from determinations of valve closure velocity. An estimate of velocity is also provided by the net force (ventricular pressure minus atrial pressure) displacing the AV valve. The magnitude of the ventriculoatrial pressure gradient should depend most heavily on the rate at which intraventricular pressure is developed during systole. Excellent correlations have been demonstrated between M_1 intensity and the peak rate of ventricular pressure development, and also between M_1 intensity and echocardiographic estimates of peak mitral valve closure velocity.[9-11]

Following the onset of ventricular systole, there are progressive increases in ventricular pressure and in the rate at which it is being developed. In any given person, the later the AV valve closes after the onset of ventricular systole, the louder will be S_1.[8,11,12] If the time to closure is held constant and the rate of pressure development is augmented (*e.g.*, by administration of an inotropic agent), the difference between ventricular and atrial pressures will be greater than in the control state, and a louder S_1 will result.

One of the major determinants of pressure development at the time of AV valve closure is the temporal relationship between atrial and ventricular systole, or the P–R interval.[8,10-13] This relationship will tend to determine the separation of the AV valve leaflets at the onset of ventricular systole. In humans, valve closure is atriogenic at relatively long P–R intervals (180 msec–500 msec) (see Fig. 8-3B). Ventricular contraction accelerates blood toward the AV valve only during the time required to stretch the closed valve to its elastic limit. S_1 occurs with or very shortly after the onset of ventricular systole, when the rate of ventricular pressure development is negligible and an insignificant pressure gradient exists between ventricle and atrium. Thus, S_1 is soft or inaudible. At intermediate P–R intervals, some time is allowed for incomplete atriogenic valve closure prior to the onset of ventricular systole, and S_1 will be intermediate in intensity (Fig. 8-3A). At relatively short P–R intervals, the valve cusps are in their most divergent position when ventricular contraction begins. There is negligible atriogenic closure following leaflet separation by atrial systole. Final coaptation of the AV valve is delayed, so that the ventriculoatrial pressure gradient will be greater than in the intermediate position, leading to a louder S_1 (Fig. 8-3C). At very short P–R or R–P intervals, atrial systole coincides with ventricular systole, diminishing the ventriculoatrial gradient at the time of AV valve closure, and S_1 is again soft or inaudible (Fig. 8-3D). When the P–R interval is markedly prolonged following atriogenic mitral valve closure in mid-diastole, reopening occurs due to continuing blood inflow from the pulmonary arterial bed to the pulmonary venous bed (Fig. 8-3E). The valve is open at the onset of ventricular systole, and the S_1 is louder than that associated with the prolonged P–R interval illustrated in Figure 8-3B.

The interval between echocardiographic mitral and tricuspid valve closure has been found to average 25 msec to 35 msec, which is considerably longer than the average 10-msec interval between the onsets of rapid pressure rise in the left and right ventricles.[6,14,15] The relatively delayed closure of the tricuspid valve may explain the similarity in intensity of M_1 and T_1 despite the very different rates of peak pressure development in the two ventricles.

Clinical Presentation

INCREASED FIRST HEART SOUND INTENSITY

Mitral Stenosis

A loud S_1 is one of the salient physical findings in rheumatic mitral stenosis. Numerous studies have documented a delayed onset of S_1.[16,17] Figure 8-4 (*Top*) shows the correlation between pressures in the left ventricle and left atrium, a mitral valve echogram (MVE), and internal and external sound traces recorded in a patient with mitral stenosis and sinus rhythm. In normal individuals, LV–LA pressure crossover occurs at the onset of ventricular systole (*i.e.*, the onset of rapid ventricular pressure rise). Note that in patients with mitral stenosis, the crossover is delayed because of the elevated LA pressure. However, the interval from LV–LA pressure crossover to mitral valve closure and S_1 is the same as in the normal state (see Fig. 8-2 and Fig. 8-4).[18,19]

Figure 8-4 (*Bottom*) shows the correlation between pressure and mitral valve motion in a patient with mitral stenosis and atrial fibrillation. The rate of LV pressure development (LV dp/dt) is also shown. Following the onset of ventricular systole, LV dp/dt progressively increases until the onset of ejection. Due to the delay in mitral valve closure imposed by the elevated LA pressure, at the time of mitral valve closure, LV dp/dt will be greater than in unaffected persons. Because the interval from LV–LA pressure crossover to mitral valve closure is the same as in the normal state but the rate of pressure development during this period is greater, a larger ventriculoatrial pressure gradient will exist at the time of AV valve closure, resulting in a louder S_1 than normal.

Even in the absence of an end-diastolic gradient, a fibrotic stenotic mitral valve probably requires a greater than normal force (LV–LA pressure gradient at the time of S_1) for displacement. Thus, a loud S_1 may be present with minor degrees of stenosis. However, in order to produce an M_1, the mitral valve must be capable of stretch and recoil. When the valve is essentially noncompliant, as, for example, when it is heavily calcified and densely fibrotic, M_1 may be absent. Since the mechanism that produces an opening snap resembles that which produces M_1, the absent S_1 will tend to be accompanied by absence of the snap. Hence, at the bedside, two of the salient auscultatory features of mitral stenosis will be lacking.

Tachycardia

Although S_1 tends to become louder with tachycardia, the degree to which it does so depends on the mechanism of heart rate augmentation and the degree of P–R interval shortening. The increase in heart rate associated with dynamic exercise is adrenergically mediated. Increased inotropy is associated wtih an augmented rate of ventricular pressure development and an appreciably louder S_1.[20] An increase in heart rate mediated by cholinergic or vagal withdrawal does not significantly affect ventricular pressure development, and the increase in S_1 intensity is difficult to appreciate.[9]

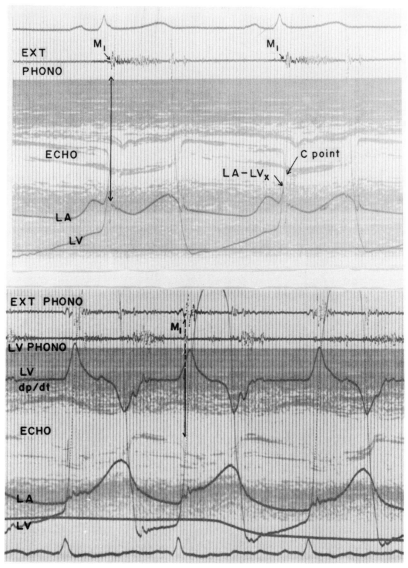

FIG. 8-4. (*Top*) Pressure–mitral valve motion correlates in a patient with mitral stenosis and sinus rhythm. An external phonocardiogram (*ext phono*) is recorded at the cardiac apex. Mitral valve motion is shown above and below the trace labeled *echo*. The C *point* of this trace represents mitral valve closure. Pressures are recorded simultaneously with the echocardiogram by equisensitive micromanometer catheters in the left atrium (*LA*) and left ventricle (*LV*). The first heart sound (M_1), the C point of the echo, and the C wave of the LA are coincident. As compared to Fig. 8-2, S_1 lags behind the onset of rapid LV pressure rise. This is due to the elevated LA pressure, which delays LV–LA pressure crossover ($LA–LV_x$). The delay causes M_1 to occur at a higher LV-LA pressure gradient than normal. (*Bottom*) Pressure–mitral valve motion correlates in a patient with mitral stenosis and atrial fibrillation. The rate of LV pressure development (*LV dp/dt*) is shown in addition to the traces shown in the upper panel. Note that M_1 occurs relatively close to peak LV *dp/dt* because of the delay described above. The higher *dp/dt* results in a louder S_1 than normal.

Hyperkinetic States

Hyperkinetic states are associated with an increased cardiac output that may (as in thyrotoxicosis, hyperadrenergic stimulation, or idiopathic hyperkinetic heart syndrome) or may not (as with AV fistulae or pregnancy) be associated with an increase in myocardial contractility.[21] Hyperkinetic states tend to be associated with a loud S_1 and an increase in stroke volume. In the absence of increased contractility, increased ventricular end-diastolic volume must be present. In such cases, the momentum will be greater at AV valve closure because of the increase in the mass (volume) being accelerated toward the atria. When contractility is enhanced, velocity will be increased, which also will contribute to an increased momentum at AV valve closure.

Mitral Valve Prolapse

In patients with holosystolic mitral valve prolapse, an increase in S_1 intensity has been reported to accompany the almost pansystolic murmur that tends to distinguish this group from those with mitral regurgitation of other etiologies (Fig. 8-5).[22] Patients with mid to late systolic prolapse manifest normal

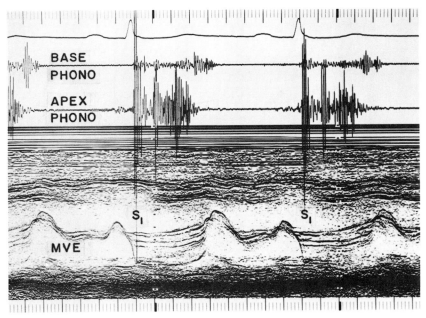

FIG. 8-5. Phonocardiogram and mitral valve echocardiogram (*MVE*) in a patient with severe mitral regurgitation and holosystolic mitral valve prolapse. Note the loud S_1 introducing the systolic murmur. It occurs at the nadir of posterior movement of the anterior mitral leaflet, identifying it as M_1. The loud S_1 tends to identify the etiology of mitral regurgitation as prolapse.

S_1 intensity. In some, however, Valsalva strain may induce holosystolic prolapse accompanied by an increase in S_1 intensity and apparent loss of the click. The increase in S_1 intensity in patients with holosystolic prolapse may be due to a delay in the checking action of the mitral valve caused by increased valve displacement.

DECREASED FIRST HEART SOUND INTENSITY

A uniform decrease in S_1 intensity should be expected in clinical conditions that lead to preclosure (*i.e.*, closure prior to ventricular systole) of the AV valve or to a reduced rate of intraventricular pressure development.

First Degree Atrioventricular Block

When AV conduction times are prolonged (*i.e.*, greater than 180 msec), S_1 is either reduced in intensity or absent (see Fig. 8-2). Valve closure tends to be purely atriogenic, causing checking of the intraventricular blood mass to occur at the onset of ventricular systole, when there is a negligible pressure gradient between ventricle and atrium.[8,10]

Valvular Regurgitation

S_1 intensity is diminished both in pansystolic mitral regurgitation and in severe aortic regurgitation. Maintenance of the integrity of isovolumic systole appears to be an important requirement for generation of an S_1. In pansystolic mitral regurgitation, M_1 is not discernible. It is not clear if M_1 is absent or is masked by the mitral regurgitant murmur, the onset of which may precede checking of the mitral valve. Theoretically, M_1 intensity may be decreased for two reasons. First, some of the energy of ventricular contraction may be spent developing the kinetic energy responsible for regurgitant flow, thereby diminishing the rate of rise of intraventricular pressure. Second, the rise in LA pressure caused by regurgitation may decrease the ventriculoatrial pressure gradient at the time of valve checking.

In acute massive aortic regurgitation, aortic diastolic pressure can be markedly reduced and LV pressure markedly elevated, leading to equilibration of these pressures at the onset of LV systole.[22] Since the energy of ventricular contraction is immediately converted into kinetic energy in the form of aortic transvalvular flow, the energy producing mitral valve displacement is reduced, and M_1 is soft or inaudible. A more common cause of the diminished S_1 amplitude in aortic regurgitation, however, is preclosure of the mitral valve as a result of a rapid increase in LV filling pressure. At end diastole, LV pressure exceeds LA pressure. Since the ventriculoatrial pressure gradient is extremely low, S_1 will be decreased in intensity or absent. The absence of S_1 in acute aortic regurgitation may lead to confusion in the identification of systole and diastole (Fig. 8-6). At the bedside, one generally identifies the shorter phase of the cardiac cycle as systole and the longer one as diastole. In acute aortic regurgitation, especially when due to infective endocarditis, the accompanying

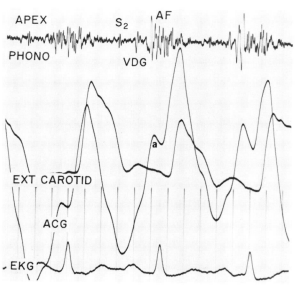

FIG. 8-6. Phonocardiographic findings in a patient with acute aortic regurgitation. An external indirect carotid pulse tracing (*ext carotid*) and an apexcardiogram (*ACG*) are also recorded. The sinus rate is 113 cycles/min. Despite a normal P–R interval, no discrete vibration corresponding to S_1 can be identified. S_2 is diminished in amplitude. A prominent ventricular diastolic gallop (*VDG*) and a presystolic Austin Flint murmur (*AF*) are present. (Reddy PS, Leon DF, Krishnaswami V, et al: Syndrome of acute aortic regurgitation. In Leon DF, Shaver JA (eds): Physiologic Principles of Heart Sounds and Murmurs. American Heart Association Monograph 46 Dallas, American Heart Association, 1975. By permission of the American Heart Association, Inc.)

tachycardia tends to equalize the durations of systole and diastole. The interval defined by a prominent ventricular gallop sound (mistaken for S_1) and an aortic ejection sound (mistaken for S_2) will be shorter than the ensuing interval and may be incorrectly identified as systole. To preclude this error, carotid palpation during auscultation is essential.

Ventricular Dysfunction

Any congestive cardiomyopathic condition will tend to diminish S_1 intensity because the rate of intraventricular pressure development is diminished in these states. During the early course of acute myocardial infarction, decreased S_1 amplitude is accompanied by prolongation of the pre-ejection period, an indirect reflection of a diminished rate of LV pressure development.[23] The diminished S_1 intensity in left bundle branch block is usually a result of associated myocardial disease.[24,25]

VARIABLE FIRST HEART SOUND INTENSITY

High-grade Atrioventricular Block and Atrioventricular Dissociation

Second degree AV nodal or Wenckebach AV block is associated with varying P–R intervals. However, many of the P–R intervals exceed 180 msec. Thus, S_1, if it is perceptible, will generally be heard only with the cardiac cycle terminating the long pause, that is, the cycle associated with the shortest P–R interval.

Complete heart block results in gross variation of the P–R intervals and, therefore, marked cycle-to-cycle variation in S_1 intensity (Fig. 8-7). Shah and his colleagues, in their study of patients with this dysrhythmia, found no recordable S_1 when the P–R interval exceeded 0.20 sec.[10] Most of the observed P–R intervals did not exceed 0.50 sec. Burgraaf and Craige, however, found S_1 to reappear when the P–R interval was greater than this value.[11] The finding was associated with diastolic reopening of the mitral valve following atriogenic preclosure. Reopening is probably caused by rising LA pressure due to continued inflow of blood from the pulmonary arterial bed into the pulmonary venous bed (see Fig. 8-3E).

Striking variation in S_1 intensity accompanied by a slow, regular ventricular rate suggests the presence of AV dissociation but does not give information regarding the atrial rate. This may be determined from inspection of the jugular venous pulse. If the atrial rate is significantly faster than the ventricular rate, AV block is present. If the patient was known not to have bundle branch block prior to the examination, then the discovery of audible expiratory splitting of S_2 (see Abnormal Second Heart Sound Splitting , below) suggests a ventricular escape mechanism. Striking variation of S_1 intensity associated with a rapid but regular ventricular rate suggests junctional or ventricular tachycardia.

Atrial Fibrillation

Varying S_1 intensity is an oft-cited physical finding in the presence of atrial fibrillation. However, there is no direct linear relationship between S_1 intensity and P–R interval. Mills and Craige have demonstrated a close relation between S_1 intensity and echocardiographic estimates of mitral valve closure velocity in atrial fibrillation.[26] The relation between closure velocity and cycle length is complex. With short ventricular cycle lengths, ventriculogenic AV valve closure may begin during the rapid filling phase of the immediately preceding diastole, during which the AV valve leaflets are rela-

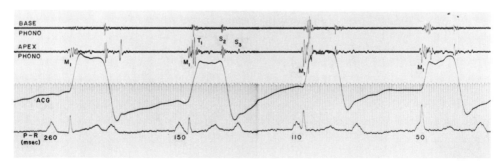

FIG. 8-7. Dependence of S_1 amplitude on P–R interval in a patient with congenital complete heart block. An apexcardiogram (*ACG*) is recorded with the phonocardiogram (*phono*). There is a progressive shortening of the P–R interval. The amplitudes of M_1 and T_1 vary as the P–R interval varies. There is a progressive increase in S_1 amplitude as the P–R interval shortens from 260 to 110 msec. At a very short P–R interval (50 msec), amplitude decreases. Refer to Fig. 8-3 for an explanation of these findings.

tively divergent, leading to a loud S_1. If S_1 occurs after the rapid ventricular filling phase, then intensity is likely to be related to changes in the rate of ventricular pressure development that depend on cycle length. This relationship is curvilinear.[27] S_1 amplitude and the rate of pressure development tend to increase with increasing cycle length until a critical cycle length is reached; thereafter, there is little change as the preceding diastole prolongs. In addition, the rate of pressure development is influenced not only by the length of the immediate R–R cycle but by the penultimate one as well. Thus, at the bedside, we can expect to hear varying S_1 intensity in atrial fibrillation, but it will be difficult to relate the observed intensity to cycle length.

Pulsus Alternans and Electrical Alternans

Pulsus alternans and electrical alternans produce an alternating S_1 intensity despite a constant cardiac cycle length and P–R interval. Pulsus alternans is a regular alternation in the force of LV contraction that leads to a palpable alternation in pulse amplitude as perceived at the bedside. It is usually associated with cardiomyopathic conditions. The mechanism for this phenomenon is unclear, but the regular alternation in the rate of intraventricular pressure development is responsible for the alternating intensity of S_1.[28]

Electrical alternans is a regular alternation in the configuration or amplitude of the electrocardiographic wave forms. This finding is generally associated with large pericardial effusions. The heart is suspended by the great vessels in a large fluid volume, rendering it almost weightless. This permits the heart to swing in a pendular arc whose period is twice the heart rate. Ventricular systole occurs at each end of the pendular arc. The alternation in S_1 intensity is due to the alternating distance and fluid volume between the source of sound production and the chest wall.[29]

SPLITTING OF THE FIRST HEART SOUND

Audible splitting of S_1 occurs both in the normal state and in pathologic conditions.[6] Thus, the mere presence of the finding is not a useful sign of cardiac disease. When splitting of S_1 is present, M_1 may be assumed to be the first component (Fig. 8-8). With the possible exceptions of right bundle branch block and Ebstein's anomaly, M_1–T_1 intervals exceeding 60 msec are unusual. Even in the former entity, very wide splitting is unusual. This is probably related to the difficulty in electrocardiographically determining the site of bundle branch block (*i.e.*, proximal or distal) and distinguishing a true intraventricular conduction defect from RV hypertrophy. We could detect no delay in the onset of rapid pressure rise in the right ventricle in atrial septal defect despite the presence of the electrocardiographic pattern of complete right bundle branch block.[30]

In mitral stenosis and left bundle branch block, the normal M_1–T_1 sequence may be reversed due to an abnormally delayed M_1.[5,25] However, the T_1–M_1 interval usually does not reach the range for audibility, and only a single sound will be heard at the bedside.

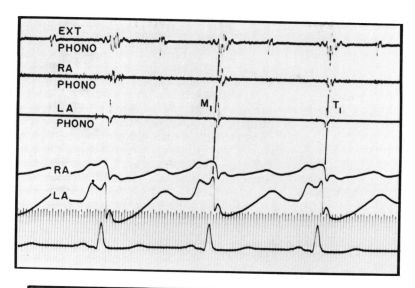

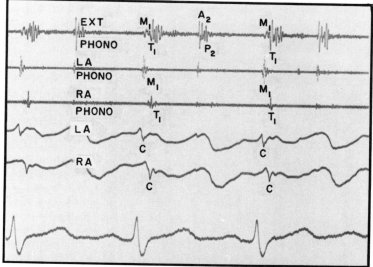

FIG. 8-8. The two components of S_1, mitral (M_1) and tricuspid (T_1). (*Top*) External sound, internal sound (*phono*) and pressure are recorded from the right (*RA*) and left (*LA*) atria in a patient with hypertrophic cardiomyopathy. The individual components of S_1 are separately recorded from their respective atria. They are coincident with the C waves (at the bottom of the solid vertical line) in the respective pressure traces. M_1 occurs first. T_1 occurs 20 msec later, a separation that is insufficient for human discrimination of two sounds. S_1 will be audibly single. (*Bottom*) The same traces as above in a patient with an atrial septal defect. In this instance, the interval between M_1 and T_1 approaches 30 msec, so two S_1 components may be audible at the bedside.

DIFFERENTIAL DIAGNOSIS OF THE FIRST HEART SOUND COMPLEX

Sounds occurring around the time of S_1 include an atrial gallop (S_4), M_1, T_1, an aortic ejection sound, and a mitral click. Under conditions where S_1 is inaudible, S_4 can be mistaken for S_1. Maneuvers designed to decrease venous return, such as assumption of the standing position, will tend to decrease the intensity of S_4, whereas S_1 intensity should remain the same or increase (Fig. 8-9).[31] If such a maneuver is not possible, application of tourniquets or inflation of blood pressure cuffs around the extremities may be attempted. In addition, advantage may be taken of the fact that the characteristic frequency of S_4 is generally lower than S_1, and it is less widely transmitted than S_1. If the patient is ausculted at the apex, using the diaphragm and an S_1 is present, the sound will persist as the site of auscultation proceeds up the left sternal border to the cardiac base.

A more common auscultatory problem is differentiation of an S_4–S_1 from an M_1–T_1 or an S_1–ejection sound sequence. Since S_4 is a low-frequency vibration, it is frequently palpable as a presystolic bulge at the apex. Palpation of this wave tends to establish the first component as S_4. Further evidence suggesting

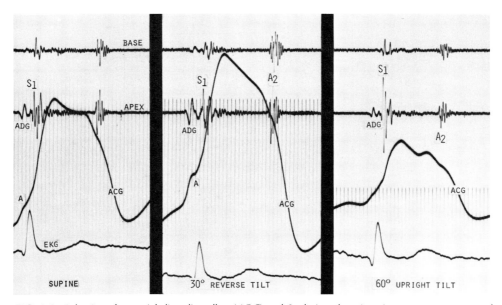

FIG. 8-9. Behavior of an atrial diastolic gallop (*ADG*) and S_1 during alterations in venous return caused by tilting. As compared to the supine position, the ADG increases in amplitude with an increase in venous return (30-degree reverse tilt). During a decrease in venous return (60-degree upright tilt), the ADG decreases in intensity, while S_1 shows the opposite change. (Shaver JA, Griff FW, Leonard JJ: Ejection sounds of left sided origin. In Leon DF, Shaver JA (eds): Physiologic Principles of Heart Sounds and Murmurs, p. 27. American Heart Association Monograph No. 46, Dallas, American Heart Association, 1975. By permission of the American Heart Association, Inc.)

that the first component is S_4 includes localization to the apex and disappearance or marked diminution in intensity of the sound upon standing.

When two high-pitched sounds are identified around the time of S_1, the first of these is generally M_1. The second may be T_1, an aortic ejection sound, or an early systolic click. Exclusion of an aortic ejection sound depends upon excluding aortic disease, both vessel and valve, on other grounds. When such disease is present and a basal systolic ejection murmur is absent, bedside differentiation of S_1–aortic ejection sound from M_1–T_1 is not possible.

The differentiation of T_1 from an early systolic mitral click depends upon interventions that will cause the click, if present, to occur in mid-or late diastole. The maneuvers include squatting, elevation of the legs in the supine position, and Valsalva release. Positive identification of an early systolic click and consequent exclusion of T_1 should not be made unless these maneuvers cause a significant delay in the timing of the second high-frequency component.

Physiology of the Second Heart Sound

GENESIS OF THE SECOND HEART SOUND

Figure 8-1 shows the pressure–flow correlates of A_2 (aortic component of S_2) as recorded by equisensitive micromanometric catheters in the left ventricle and aorta of a dog. The aortic flow trace is delayed by approximately 10 msec. During the early portion of ejection, ventricular pressure is greater than arterial pressure, while the reverse is true toward the conclusion of this systolic phase. These gradients are related in part to acceleration and deceleration of blood flow. During early systole, when forward flow velocity is increasing, there is a positive gradient in favor of the ventricle. After peak flow velocity is achieved, the positive gradient tends to disappear, and it eventually becomes negative. Toward the conclusion of ejection, resistive and other forces oppose the inertial force maintaining forward flow and the negative pressure gradient increases in magnitude.[32] When the gradient reaches a critical level, the semilunar valve closes.

There is general agreement that aortic valve closure is a silent event.[33,34] Following valve closure, the cusps are distended toward the ventricle by the greater pressure in the aorta. This distention is associated with an abrupt fall in aortic pressure and an abrupt deceleration of flow. The direction of flow at this juncture is negative, or, in other words, toward the ventricle. The fall in aortic pressure and the negative flow are arrested when the aortic valve reaches its maximum distensibility. The arrest of the pressure fall constitutes the dicrotic notch or incisura (Fig. 8-1). The subsequent recoil of the valve toward the aorta produces the postincisural pressure wave, or dicrotic wave, and a return of the aortic flow curve to the baseline, or zero flow.

The pressure oscillations generated by the valvular stretch–recoil sequence are identified as A_2 in intracardiac phonocardiograms. The simultaneous abrupt deceleration of the blood column causes the heart and great vessels to vibrate. These vibrations of the cardiohemic system are perceived on the chest wall as S_2.

DETERMINANTS OF SECOND HEART SOUND INTENSITY

The intensity of A_2 is related to the arterioventricular pressure gradient across the closed semilunar valve during production of the sound. Both Kusukawa and associates and Stein and associates found a positive correlation between the magnitude of the aortic–LV pressure gradient at the time of the incisural notch and the intensity of A_2.[35–37] However, both groups reported a much better correlation between intensity and the peak rate of change of the gradient $(d\Delta p/dt_{max})$. Stein and associates have also demonstrated a similar excellent correlation between right heart $d\Delta p/dt_{max}$ and P_2 (pulmonic component of S_2) intensity.[37] On theoretical grounds, these authors have suggested that the intracardiac sound pressure (intensity) produced by a vibrating elastic membrane is related to its rate of deflection. They predicted that the amplitude and rate of valve distention would be more closely related to the rate of change of diastolic pressure gradient than to its absolute value (Fig. 8-10).[36,38] In the normal state, the $d\Delta p/dt_{max}$ of the right heart is significantly less than that of the left.[37] This difference results in a P_2 that is significantly softer than A_2.

There is a good direct correlation between $d\Delta p/dt_{max}$ and peak negative LV dp/dt (which reflects the rate of fall in ventricular pressure during early dias-

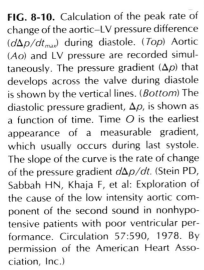
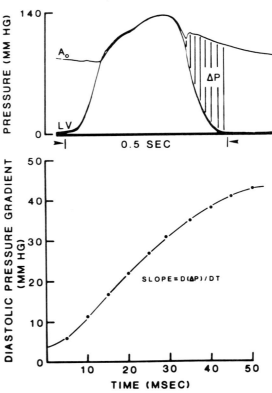

FIG. 8-10. Calculation of the peak rate of change of the aortic–LV pressure difference $(d\Delta p/dt_{max})$ during diastole. (*Top*) Aortic (*Ao*) and LV pressure are recorded simultaneously. The pressure gradient (Δp) that develops across the valve during diastole is shown by the vertical lines. (*Bottom*) The diastolic pressure gradient, Δp, is shown as a function of time. Time *O* is the earliest appearance of a measurable gradient, which usually occurs during last systole. The slope of the curve is the rate of change of the pressure gradient $d\Delta p/dt$. (Stein PD, Sabbah HN, Khaja F, et al: Exploration of the cause of the low intensity aortic component of the second sound in nonhypotensive patients with poor ventricular performance. Circulation 57:590, 1978. By permission of the American Heart Association, Inc.)

tole.)[36] The latter parameter may be affected by the development of heart disease.[39] Although it has been shown that depression of LV performance tends to diminish the intensity of A_2, it remains to be proven that augmenting LV contractility will cause an increase in the intensity of S_2.[36]

SPLITTING OF THE SECOND HEART SOUND

Physiologic splitting of S_2 consists of an inspiratory movement toward a wider separation of its two components, A_2 and P_2; A_2 always precedes P_2 (Fig. 8-11). As mentioned above, the human auditory system can usually distinguish two sounds only if they are separated by more than 20 msec. A separation of this magnitude is normally attained only during inspiration. Hence, at the bedside, S_2 is audibly single during expiration and splits into two audible components during inspiration. The audibility of S_2 splitting will be significantly affected by the frequency composition and intensity of the components. In normal subjects, audible splitting probably requires a separation closer to 30 msec than to 20 msec. In pulmonary hypertension, on the other hand, splitting of less than 30 msec may be evident to the ear because of the increased intensity and higher characteristic frequency of P_2.

Normal physiologic splitting is primarily due to an inspiratory delay in P_2 (Fig. 8-12). During inspiration, the RV pre-ejection period shortens, the ejection

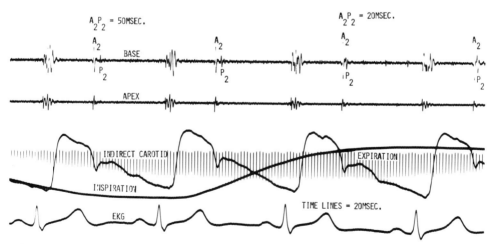

FIG. 8-11. Physiologic splitting of S_2 in a normal young male. During inspiration, the A_2–P_2 interval is 50 msec and both components are easily audible. As compared to expiration, the A_2–P_2 interval is wider, primarily due to a later occurrence of P_2. During expiration, the A_2–P_2 interval narrows to 20 msec, which is below the 30 msec required for human discrimination of two sounds. At the bedside, only a single S_2 is perceived. (Curtiss EI: Newer concepts in physiologic splitting of the second heart sound. In Leon DF, Shaver JA (eds): Physiologic Principles of Heart Sounds and Murmurs, p. 68. American Heart Association Monograph No. 46. Dallas, American Heart Association, 1975. By permission of the American Heart Association, Inc.)

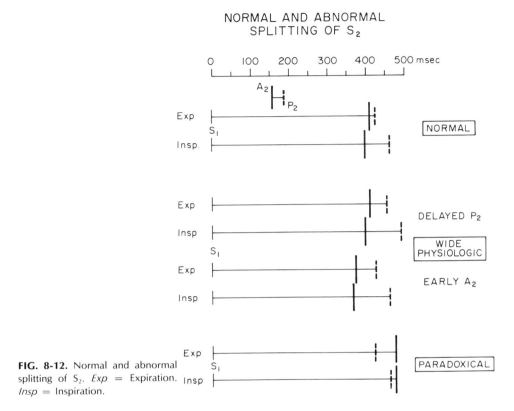

FIG. 8-12. Normal and abnormal splitting of S₂. *Exp* = Expiration. *Insp* = Inspiration.

time prolongs, and there is a net increase in the Q–P₂ interval.[40] A decrease in the Q–A₂ interval also occurs, but it accounts for only 20% of the inspiratory augmentation of the A₂–P₂ interval.[41] The later occurrence of P₂ during this respiratory phase has been attributed to an increase in systemic venous return to the right heart that selectively prolongs the duration of RV mechanical systole. Although inspiratory prolongation of this interval undoubtedly occurs, it may not be the sole or even the most important determinant. Figure 8-13 shows the pressure–sound correlates of S₂ as obtained from simultaneous micromanometric pressure tracings in two young individuals without heart disease. The incisurae of the aortic and pulmonary arterial pressure traces are temporally separated from their ventricular pressure traces. This interval, descriptively termed "hangout" by Shaver and associates, is rarely longer than 15 msec in the left heart.[42] In the right heart, however, the hangout interval may vary from 33 msec to 120 msec, contributing significantly to the duration of RV ejection. Note that, in Figure 8-13B, the pulmonary artery incisura occurs when RV pressure is almost equal to ventricular end-diastolic pressure, which suggests that P₂ occurs well after the right ventricle has begun to relax. Flow continues into the pulmonary artery despite RV relaxation because of the inertia of the stroke volume.

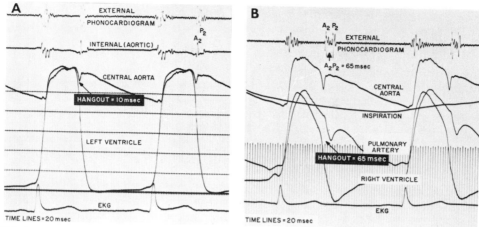

FIG. 8-13. Simultaneous manometric recordings from the artery and ventricle of (A) the left and (B) the righthearts in two subjects without heart disease. The sounds related to semilunar closure (A_2 and P_2) are coincident with the incisurae of the respective arterial pressure traces. These incisurae are separated by a finite interval, termed the "hangout" interval, from the ventricular pressure traces. This interval is brief in the normal left heart and much longer in the right heart. Note in (B) that P_2 and the pulmonary incisura occur when RV pressure is less than the end-diastolic pressure, *i.e.*, at or after the onset of RV relaxation. (Curtiss EI, Matthews RG, Shaver JA: Mechanism of normal splitting of the second heart sound. Circulation 51:157, 1975. By permission of the American Heart Association, Inc.)

The right-sided hangout interval has been found to correlate closely with the inspiratory A_2–P_2 interval; its duration appears to be inversely related to vascular impedance (*i.e.*, the total opposition to flow, which includes not only a resistance term but also the compliance or capacitance of the vascular bed).[32] Curtiss and associates have presented evidence, that in normal physiologic splitting, an inspiratory decrease in pulmonary vascular impedance may be a primary factor prolonging RV ejection.

Since most of the respiratory movement of A_2–P_2 depends on changes in the Q–P_2 interval, alterations in the right-sided circulation may cause less-than-normal Q–P_2 movement, resulting in "fixed" splitting of S_2. Two possible mechanisms are involved: either the right heart stroke volume is fixed—that is, it does not vary significantly with respiration—or respiratory modulation of pulmonary vascular impedance is markedly diminished.[41]

Clinical Presentation of the Second Heart Sound

CLINICAL EVALUATION OF INTENSITY

Since heart sounds are widely distributed over the chest surface, the relative intensity of semilunar closure sounds cannot be estimated solely by relying upon the loudness of a single S_2 in the traditional "aortic" (second intercostal space, left sternal border) and "pulmonic" (second intercostal space, right sternal border) auscultatory areas. Obviously, a reliable estimate will depend on identification of separated aortic and pulmonic components. In order to separate these two components, the patient can be requested to increase the depth of respiration, but in a continuous fashion. If asked to hold his breath during a respiratory phase, the patient will probably perform a Valsalva maneuver, negating the purpose of the respiratory maneuver. When relative estimates of intensity are used, it must be borne in mind that the intensities of A_2 and P_2 can be affected independently.

INCREASED INTENSITY OF SEMILUNAR CLOSURE SOUNDS

The major cause of a significant increase in the loudness of semilunar closure sounds is hypertension. In systemic hypertension, the quality of the A_2 has been described as "tambour." The intensity of A_2 may subsequently decrease independent of changes in aortic diastolic pressure when ventricular decompensation occurs during the course of hypertensive heart disease. This decrease results from a diminished rate of isovolumic LV relaxation, which decreases the rate of change of the arterio-ventricular diastolic pressure gradient.[36]

In pulmonary hypertension, the intensity of P_2 increases. Part of the apparent increase may be due to the higher characteristic frequency of the sound. However, increased intensity is always associated with an increase in $d\Delta p/dt_{max}$.[37] Unfortunately, it is not possible to estimate the degree of pulmonary hypertension from the intensity of P_2.[16] The fact that after the age of approximately 30 years P_2 is generally not audible at the apical auscultatory area is of some clinical aid in identifying an abnormally loud P_2.[43] Thus, a discretely identifiable P_2 at the apex after this age signifies an increase in intensity of this sound.

DECREASED SECOND HEART SOUND INTENSITY

Valve Disease

In calcific aortic stenosis, there is a direct relation between the degree of cusp calcification and the severity of LV outflow tract obstruction.[44] Since the leaflets are noncompliant, stretch and recoil of the aortic valve are diminished, reducing the amplitude of A_2 (Fig. 8-14B). Thus, a loud A_2 is evidence against significant valvular calcification. However, in congenital aortic stenosis, prior to calcification in the later years, the aortic valve is thin and pliable, and A_2 is normal in intensity (Fig. 8-14A). In the older age group, normal A_2 intensity does not exclude significant LV outflow tract obstruction, since the level of obstruction may be below the level of the aortic valve.

Decreased intensity of P_2 is found in association with both infundibular and valvular pulmonic stenosis. In mild RV outflow tract obstruction, pulmonary arterial pressure and P_2 intensity may be normal. As the severity of stenosis increases, pulmonary artery pressure falls, which probably results in a decrease in $d\Delta p/dt_{max}$ and, thus, diminished P_2 intensity (Fig. 8-15).

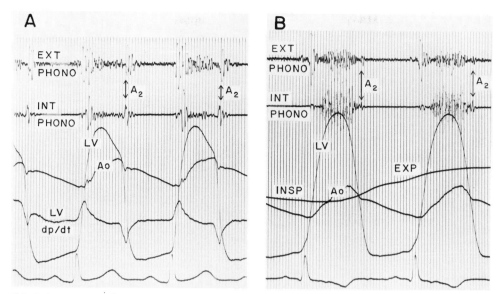

FIG. 8-14. Intensity of A_2 in (A) congenital noncalcific and (B) in calcific acquired aortic stenosis. Simultaneous pressures in the left ventricle (LV) and aorta (Ao) are shown in addition to the phonocardiogram. Relative to the intensity of S_1, the intensity of A_2 is markedly decreased in calcific aortic stenosis due to loss of valvular mobility. In the congenital form, however, the valve retains its mobility: despite stenosis, A_2 intensity is normal.

A_2 tends to be diminished in pure aortic regurgitation. The mechanism for this decrease has not been directly investigated but the following factors have been suggested: (1) the diminished aortic diastolic pressure may be associated with a diminished rate of change of the early diastolic pressure gradient; (2) the regurgitation does not permit the aortic valve to tense upon closure; and (3) the cross-sectional valvular area capable of vibration may be diminished.[45]

Ventricular Dysfunction

In patients with acute myocardial infarction, A_2 intensity is lower than normal during the early phase but tends to increase during the convalescent phase as LV function improves.[23] Stein and colleagues demonstrated that A_2 amplitude was diminished in patients with chronic LV dysfunction and found a good correlation between peak negative LV dp/dt and A_2 amplitude. They attributed the reduction in A_2 amplitude to an impaired rate of isovolumic LV relaxation.

ASSESSMENT OF SECOND HEART SOUND SPLITTING

The clinical assessment of S_2 splitting is best performed with the patient lying comfortably in the supine position and breathing continuously. The respiratory rate may be controlled by instructing the patient to inspire and expire as the examiner raises and lowers his hand. Respiratory changes in S_2 splitting will occur during the first one or two cardiac cycles, occurring at

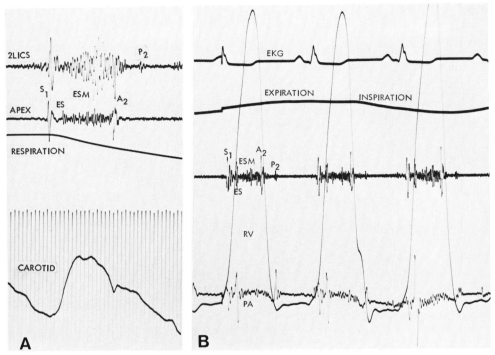

FIG. 8-15. Wide splitting of S_2 in valvular pulmonic stenosis. (*A*) Phonocardiographic traces from the base and apex; inspiration is a downward deflection in the respiratory trace. (*B*) Simultaneous RV and pulmonary pressures (*PA*). *ES* = pulmonic ejection sound. *ESM* = ejection systolic murmur.

the beginning of each respiratory phase. The changes are most easily detected along the left sternal border in the second or third intercostal space. Following examination in the supine position, the examination should be repeated in the sitting position.

In the bedside assessment of S_2 splitting, the patient's age must be taken into consideration. In a phonocardiographic study of 162 normal subjects, Harris and Sutton found inspiratory splitting of S_2 to be 20 msec or less in 45% of those over 40 years of age; in the 5 to 40 age group this finding was present in only 8%.[43] Hence, as patient age increases, the likelihood of hearing single S_2 during both respiratory phases also increases.

In younger people, the maximum inspiratory split has been found to average 40 msec to 50 msec; during quiet respiration, it may be further widened by increasing the depth of respiration. The absolute magnitude of the inspiratory separation is of little clinical importance.

Abnormal Second Heart Sound Splitting

The key to the bedside detection of abnormal splitting of S_2 is the absence of audible fusion of A_2 and P_2 during expiration (Fig. 8-12). This may occur even though directional movement of the two sounds is physiologic—

that is, there is perceptible widening of the A_2–P_2 interval during inspiration. Adolph and Fowler found audible expiratory splitting in only 22 of 200 normal adults in the recumbent position; assumption of the sitting position resulted in expiratory fusion in 20 of the 22 (Fig. 8-16).[46] Audible expiratory splitting in the supine position was virtually absent in normal adults over 50 years of age. The mechanism responsible for the postural behavior of A_2–P_2 in some normal young adults has not been elucidated. However, when audible expiratory splitting is found, the need for evaluation in the sitting position is underscored.

In the past, attention has been called to fixed splitting of S_2 as a useful sign of an underlying cardiac abnormality, but this must be qualified. If the inspiratory augmentation of the A_2–P_2 interval is less than 20 msec, splitting is said

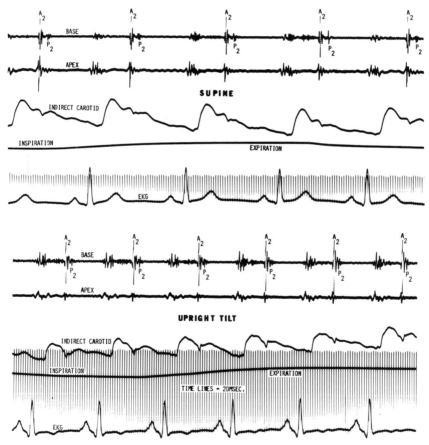

FIG. 8-16. Effect of posture on audible expiratory splitting of S_2 in a normal young male. In the supine position (upper panel), A_2 and P_2 are separated by at least 60 msec during both respiratory phases. With assumption of the upright position, S_2 closes (A_2–P_2 interval ≤ 30 msec) during expiration. (Shaver JA: Phonocardiography in Clinical Practice. In Rapoport E (ed): Cardiology Update, 1981, p 325. Amsterdam, Elsevier/North-Holland, 1981)

to be *fixed*. This finding is present in most people over 50 years of age. In these people, however, expiratory splitting is generally 20 msec; therefore, inspiratory splitting is *narrow*—that is, ≤ 40 msec. Fixed splitting is held to be clinically significant when it is associated with *wide* (≥ 40 msec) expiratory splitting.

When the respiratory behavior of the A_2–P_2 interval is the reverse of physiologic splitting, the splitting is said to be *paradoxic* (Fig. 8-12). This type reveals itself by narrowing of the A_2–P_2 interval during inspiration and widening during expiration. Such behavior is due to an abnormally delayed A_2; A_2 occurs after P_2 in both respiratory phases. The Q–A_2 interval does not change significantly with respiration. As in the normal state, P_2 occurs earlier during expiration, leading to an audible separation between P_2 and A_2. During inspiration, P_2 moves closer to A_2, tending to produce an audibly single second sound.

CAUSES OF ABNORMAL PHYSIOLOGIC SPLITTING (A_2 PRECEDES P_2)

Right Ventricular Electromechanical Delay

The electrocardiographic pattern of right bundle branch block can be associated with wide expiratory splitting of S_2 due to a selective delay in electrical activation of the right ventricle. However, the electrocardiographic abnormality may be due to a peripheral site of block with no detectable abnormality of splitting. When the electrocardiographic pattern is due to RV hypertrophy, the splitting abnormality will be of the type associated with the etiology of the hypertrophy. In uncomplicated right bundle branch block with audible expiratory splitting, there may be perceptible inspiratory widening of the split (Fig. 8-17); when pulmonary hypertension or congestive heart failure supervenes, this inspiratory widening frequently disappears.

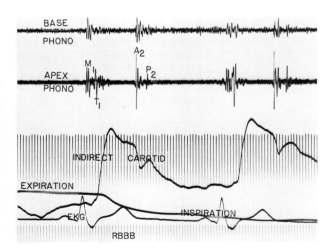

FIG. 8-17. Splitting of S_2 in right bundle branch block (*RBBB*). Although audible expiratory splitting was present, there is significant physiologic respiratory movement of the A_2–P_2 interval. During expiration, this interval is 65 msec, and it widens to 100 msec during inspiration. (Shaver JA: Phonocardiography in Clinical Practice. In Rapoport E (ed): Cardiology Update, 1981, p 325. Amsterdam, Elsevier/North-Holland, 1981)

Prolongation of Right Ventricular Mechanical Systole

PULMONARY HYPERTENSION.   In chronic pulmonary hypertension due to pulmonary vascular disease, the $Q-P_2$ interval is generally within the normal range. The RV ejection time is abnormally decreased and the hangout interval is abbreviated as compared to the systemic circulation.[30] These decreases are accompanied by prolongation of the isovolumic contraction time, leading to a relatively normal $Q-P_2$ interval. The audible expiratory split generally tends to be narrow—that is, within the range of 20 msec to 40 msec (Fig. 8-18). P_2 can be audibly detected during expiration more easily than usual because its frequency and intensity are increased. Respiratory variation in the A_2-P_2 interval is reduced, either because of the inability of the compromised right ventricle to accept an inspiratory augmentation of venous return or because of loss of the normal respiratory modulation of pulmonary vascular impedance.[41]

Wide rather than narrow expiratory splitting is reported to be typical of acute pulmonary hypertension due to massive, but not segmental, pulmonary embolism.[47] The $Q-A_2$ interval decreases because stroke volume is low, but there is no proportional shortening of the $Q-P_2$ interval.[47] The reason for the

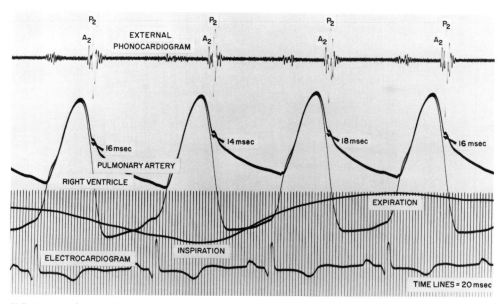

FIG. 8-18. Splitting of S_2 in moderately severe (mean pulmonary pressure = 54 mm Hg) pulmonary hypertension. Pressure tracings were obtained by micromanometer catheters. There is fixed splitting of S_2. Although the A_2-P_2 interval is not wide (≤ 40 msec), audible expiratory splitting was present due to the increased intensity and higher characteristic frequency of P_2. Note that, in contrast to Figure 8-14B, the hangout interval (indicated by the arrows) is abbreviated to 14 msec to 18 msec, comparable to that in the systemic arterial circulation. (Curtiss EI, Matthews RG, Shaver JA: Mechanism of normal splitting of the second heart sound. Circulation 51:157, 1975. By permission of the American Heart Association, Inc.)

latter finding is conjectural, but it is probable that the acute selective increase in afterload significantly prolongs RV isovolumic contraction time—perhaps to a greater degree than in chronic pulmonary hypertension. After three to six days of convalescence, expiratory splitting returns to normal.

SEVERE PULMONIC STENOSIS. In moderate to severe pulmonic stenosis with intact ventricular septum, prolongation of the RV ejection phase increases linearly with the degree of obstruction. As a result, the width of the expiratory split correlates fairly well with the transvalvular gradient (see Fig. 8-15).[48]

DECREASED IMPEDANCE OF THE PULMONARY VASCULAR BED

Decreased impedance of the pulmonary vascular bed is characterized by a prolonged $Q-P_2$ interval, a normal RV pre-ejection period (electromechanical and isovolumic contraction times), a prolonged ejection time, and a widened hangout interval.

Atrial Septal Defect

Audible expiratory splitting of S_2 is the essential auscultatory finding in atrial septal defect (Fig. 8-19). Its absence tends to exclude the diagnosis.[46,49] Expiratory splitting is wide (40 msec–120 msec) and respiratory variation in the A_2-P_2 interval is less than 20 msec. In atrial septal defect, audible expiratory splitting uniformly persists in the sitting position, which tends to distinguish it from the splitting encountered in normal young people. Even when the split is associated with complete right bundle branch block, the lack of perceptible

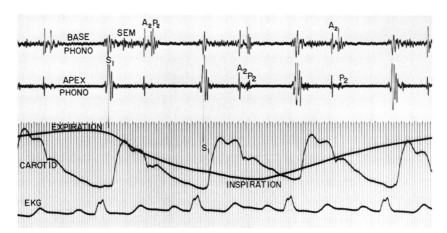

FIG. 8-19. Wide, physiologic splitting of S_2 in atrial septal defect. Splitting is "fixed," *i.e.*, respiratory movement is less than 20 msec. The A_2-P_2 interval during expiration is 60 msec, *i.e.*, widely split (>40 msec). (Shaver JA: Phonocardiography in Clinical Practice. In Rapoport E (ed): Cardiology Update, 1981, p 325. Amsterdam, Elsevier/North-Holland, 1981)

respiratory variation in its width should raise the possibility of atrial septal defect.

The width of the A_2–P_2 split does not correlate with the degree of left-to-right shunting. In addition, audible expiratory splitting of S_2 frequently persists following surgical repair of the defect.[45] These findings are difficult to explain if the wide splitting is attributed to prolongation of RV mechanical systole due to selective volume overloading. O'Toole and associates found the A_2–P_2 interval to correlate closely with the right-sided hangout interval in patients with atrial septal defect. They interpreted this finding to mean that the durations of RV and LV mechanical systoles are approximately equal and attributed the delayed P_2 to increased capacitance (decreased impedance) of the pulmonary vascular bed.[49]

In addition to wide expiratory splitting of S_2, another cardinal physical finding in atrial septal defect is marked attenuation or failure of the Q–P_2 interval to increase during inspiration, which leads to fixed splitting of S_2. In the normal state, an increase in pulmonary capacitance and a decrease in impedance appears to be one of the major reasons for inspiratory prolongation of RV ejection. In atrial septal defect, the pulmonary vascular bed is markedly expanded because of the hyperkinetic circulation. With inspiration, the capacitance of the already expanded vascular bed may fail to increase any further. Therefore, inspiratory prolongation of RV ejection time will be significantly less than normal. Inspiratory widening of the A_2–P_2 interval related to increased systemic venous return and decreased pulmonary venous return may also be absent in atrial septal defect. The respiratory changes in venous return still occur in this condition. However, the inspiratory increase in systemic return is balanced by the diminutions in left-to-right shunting and pulmonary venous return, and there is no change in either RV or LV stroke volume.[50] If the decrease in pulmonary venous return is smaller than the augmentation in systemic return, there may be an increase in *both* right-sided and left-sided output. For instance, during inspiration, if systemic venous return increases by 20 ml, pulmonary venous return decreases by 10 ml, and the left-to-right shunt decreases by 15 ml, then left and right heart volumes will increase by 5 ml each. Without the shunt, the net difference between left and right returns would have been 30 ml. Thus, the atrial septal defect prevents selective increases or decreases in right heart output during respiration.

Mild Pulmonic Stenosis and Idiopathic Dilatation of the Pulmonary Artery

Both mild pulmonic stenosis and idiopathic dilatation of the pulmonary artery may be associated with very wide (> 80 msec) expiratory splitting and a P_2 of normal intensity (Figs. 8-20 and 8-21).[42] These conditions share the finding of significant main pulmonary artery dilatation. However, in idiopathic dilatation, no pulmonary valve abnormality is present; rather, there is an elastic tissue deficiency in the arterial wall.[51] In both conditions, there is an increase in capacitance of the pulmonary vascular bed, which widens the hangout interval.

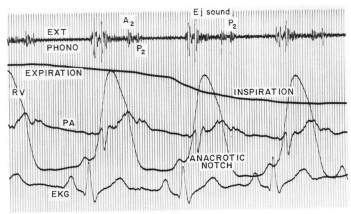

FIG. 8-20. Wide splitting of S_2 in mild pulmonic stenosis. Pressures from the right ventricle (*RV*) and pulmonary artery (*PA*) are recorded simultaneously. Although the systolic gradient was less than 30 mm Hg, there is wide expiratory splitting of S_2 *Ej*=ejection. (Shaver JA, Nadolny RA, O'Toole JD, et al: Sound pressure correlates of the second heart sound: An intracardiac sound study. Circulation 39:316, 1974. By permission of the American Heart Association, Inc.)

SHORTENED DURATION OF LEFT VENTRICULAR SYSTOLE (EARLY A$_2$)

Wide physiologic splitting of S_2 may occur as a consequence of selective shortening of the LV ejection period, which results in a relatively early A_2 (see Fig. 8-12). This can occur in mitral regurgitation and ventricular septal defect.[46] In these conditions, there is a low-impedance pathway for LV outflow.

PARADOXIC SPLITTING OF THE SECOND HEART SOUND

Paradoxic splitting of S_2 is almost always due to a delayed A_2 (see Fig. 8-12).

Left-Sided Electromechanical Delay

Left bundle branch block is the most common cause of paradoxic splitting in the adult population. The Q–A_2 interval is prolonged because the duration of the pre-ejection period is increased. This can be the result of electromechanical delay or of a prolonged isovolumic contraction time; both intervals are generally prolonged in patients with audible expiratory splitting and left bundle branch block (Fig. 8-22).[24,25]

In patients with ventricular pacemakers that use an endocardial RV electrode, paradoxic splitting is due to a relative delay in LV activation. A shift

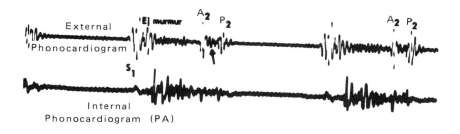

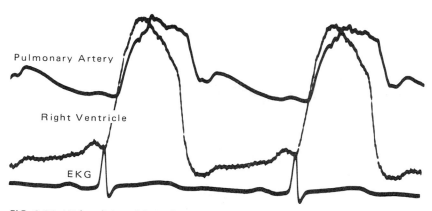

FIG. 8-21. Wide splitting of S_2 in idiopathic dilatation of the pulmonary artery. (Shaver JA, Nadolny RA, O'Toole JD, et al: Sound pressure correlates of the second heart sound: An intracardiac sound study. Circulation 39:316, 1974. By permission of the American Heart Association, Inc.)

from paradoxic to physiologic splitting is a valuable bedside finding that may indicate trans-septal perforation.

A rare cause of paradoxic splitting is early activation of the right ventricle due to a RV bypass tract.[52] Type B Wolff–Parkinson–White syndrome should be suspected when paradoxic splitting is encountered in an otherwise healthy young person without a cardiac murmur.

Other Causes

Although paradoxic splitting is said to be a valuable sign of a prolonged ejection period in LV outflow tract obstruction and, thus, evidence of a hemodynamically significant lesion, the audibility of this phenomenon has never been determined on a systematic basis. From phonocardiographic tracings, Harris and associates identified reversed splitting of S_2 in 20% of patients with hypertrophic subaortic stenosis and in 5% of those with valvular aortic

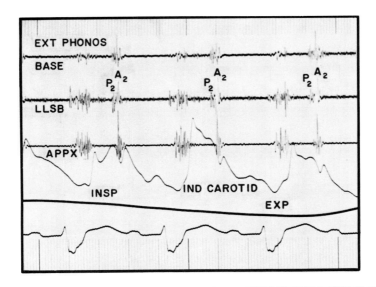

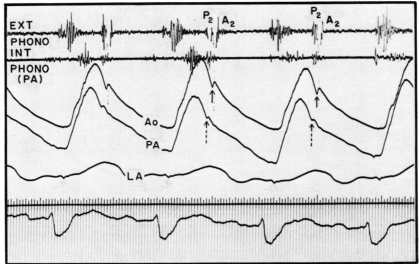

FIG. 8-22. Paradoxic splitting of S_2 in a patient with aortic valve disease and left bundle branch block. The latter delays A_2 so that it occurs after P_2 during both phases of respiration. (*Top*) External phonocardiograms are recorded at the base and lower left sternal border (*LLSB*). The Q–A_2 interval does not change during respiration but the Q–P_2 interval shortens during expiration and lengthens during inspiration. The P_2–A_2 interval tends to narrow during inspiration—this behavior is the reverse of normal physiologic splitting. (*Bottom*) Micromanometer pressures are recorded from the aorta (*Ao*) and pulmonary artery (*PA*) in the same patient. The incisurae of the aortic (*solid arrow*) and pulmonary artery (*dashed arrow*) are temporally the reverse of normal.

stenosis.[53] However, we believe paradoxic splitting to be a rare finding at the bedside. In hemodynamically significant obstruction, the systolic murmur tends to persist up to the aortic component, burying P_2 if it occurs prior to A_2.

In chronic systemic hypertension, the $Q–A_2$ interval tends to be normal, and paradoxic splitting, although reported, is very rare. However, paradoxic splitting due to prolongation of the LV ejection period has been demonstrated in normal subjects with acute systemic hypertension induced by methoxamine.[54] Reversed splitting may be clinically etectable during acute hypertensive crises.

Paradoxic splitting is also said to occur during anginal attacks.[55] In our experience, reversed splitting is an unusually rare manifestation of ischemic heart disease. If evanescent paradoxic splitting is detectable with angina, it probably represents transient left bundle branch block.

DIFFERENTIAL DIAGNOSIS OF AUDIBLE EXPIRATORY SPLITTING

When S_2 is not audibly split, other sounds occurring around the time of S_2 may be mistaken for audible expiratory splitting. These include a late systolic click, an opening snap due to AV valve stenosis, a third heart sound, (S_3), and a pericardial knock.

An S_3 is lower in frequency than S_2 and is usually not heard at the basal auscultatory area. It occurs 120 msec to 160 msec after A_2, an unusually wide split for $A_2–P_2$.

If a late systolic click is unassociated with a late systolic murmur in the recumbent position, assumption of the standing position will cause the click to become louder and to occur earlier and will possibly cause a murmur to emerge. The shortness of the S_1–"S_2A" interval relative to the heart rate and the increase in loudness of "A_2" (an unusual finding when arterial pressure falls in the standing position) should alert one to the correct identification of the click or false "A_2."

An opening snap of the mitral valve (acquired tricuspid stenosis is almost always associated with mitral stenosis) may be exceptionally difficult to distinguish from P_2. Both are high-pitched and audible along the left sternal border. An apical diastolic murmur, atrial fibrillation, and a left lower parasternal heave are not confirmatory of an opening snap, since these same findings can be present in atrial septal defect with a large left-to-right shunt. When the underlying rhythm is sinus, the auscultatory changes associated with a change from the recumbent to the standing position may be of value.[56] In mitral stenosis, the A_2–OS interval widens upon standing, presumably due to the fall in left atrial pressure; in normals and patients with atrial septal defect, the A_2–P_2 interval tends to narrow upon standing.

A pericardial knock occurs in constrictive pericarditis during early diastole. The sound is generally high-pitched and may occur earlier than the usual ventricular gallop sound. However, the A_2–pericardial knock interval usually approximates 120 msec. Such wide "splitting" should suggest that the second high-frequency component may not be P_2.

Summary

S_1 and S_2 are temporally related to closure of the AV and semilunar valves, respectively. The act of closure is believed to produce abrupt deceleration of blood columns, which, in turn, causes vibrations of the valves and cardiohemic system. Heart sound intensity is related to the momentum achieved by the blood column at the time of closure. In the normal state, pressure gradients are established across the closed valve. The velocity term of momentum can be indirectly estimated by the magnitude of the pressure gradient, which is heavily dependent on the rate of change of ventricular pressure (dp/dt).

S_1 has two components, the mitral and the tricuspid, which may not be audibly distinguishable. Valve closure normally occurs after the onset of ventricular systole during the rapid rise of pressure. Sound intensity is closely related to the magnitude of the gradient from ventricle to atrium at the time of closure, which, in turn, is closely related to ventricular dp/dt. Conditions that increase myocardial contractility, such as hyperadrenergic states and thyrotoxicosis, increase S_1 intensity, whereas myocardial depression, as encountered in cardiomyopathic states, decreases intensity. In mitral stenosis, valve closure is delayed; it occurs when ventricular dp/dt is greater than normal, which results in a greater ventriculoatrial pressure gradient and, therefore, a louder S_1. When a period of isovolumic systole is absent, as, for example, in pansystolic mitral regurgitation and severe acute aortic regurgitation, S_1 is absent or markedly diminished.

The temporal relation between atrial and ventricular systoles, or the P–R interval, is a major determinant of S_1 intensity. This relation tends to determine the position of the AV valve leaflets at the onset of ventricular systole. A long P–R interval results in atriogenic closure of the AV valve (*i.e.,* closure prior to ventricular systole) and S_1 is soft or absent. A short P–R interval results in widely separated AV valve leaflets at the onset of LV systole. This results in delayed AV valve closure; a loud sound occurs at a higher rate of pressure development.

Variable S_1 intensity is encountered in conditions characterized by variable P–R intervals, such as complete heart block, or by variable rates of ventricular pressure development, such as pulsus alternans and, probably, atrial fibrillation.

The two components of S_2, A_2 and P_2, are related to aortic and pulmonic valve closure, respectively. Physiologic splitting of S_2 consists of an audibly single sound during expiration with separation into two audible components during inspiration, A_2 being followed by P_2. During expiration, the A_2–P_2 interval is < 30 msec, below the minimum interval for human discrimination of two sounds. The inspiratory widening of the A_2–P_2 interval is due to a delay in the occurrence of P_2. In the normal state, the delay in P_2 is due to inspiratory augmentation of systemic venous return and a fall in pulmonary vascular impedance that prolongs the duration of ejection.

The essential auscultatory finding in abnormal splitting of S_2 is audible expiratory splitting. The major causes are ventricular electromechanical delay (*e.g.,* right bundle branch block), prolonged duration of RV mechanical systole (*e.g.*, severe pulmonic stenosis), and decreased pulmonary vascular impedance (*e.g.*, atrial septal defect). In paradoxic splitting of S_2, A_2 follows P_2. A_2 is abnormally delayed, and the respiratory behavior of P_2 is normal. Consequently, the P_2–A_2 interval narrows during inspiration and widens during expiration. The major cause of this finding is LV electromechanical delay, for example, left bundle branch block.

Reduced respiratory variation of A_2–P_2 results from respiratory fixation of RV stroke volume or from failure of respiration to effect changes in pulmonary vascular impedance. Both mechanisms are probably operative in atrial septal efect.

The intensity of semilunar closure sounds is closely related to the peak rate of change in the arterioventricular pressure gradient that begins during the terminal phase of systolic ejection. The peak rate of ventricular pressure fall during diastole is also related to the peak rate of change in the arterioventricular pressure gradient. S_2 intensity is increased in hypertension. It decreases when ventricular contractility is depressed. Anatomical changes, such as aortic stenosis, that reduce the ability of the semilunar valves to stretch and recoil also result in diminution of S_2 intensity.

References

1. Rushmer RF (ed): Cardiovascular Dynamics, p 293. Philadelphia, WB Saunders, 1976
2. Stein PD, Stein HN: Origin of the second heart sound: Clinical relevance of new observations. Am J Cardiol 41:108, 1978
3. Feigen LP: Physical characteristics of sound and hearing. Am J Cardiol 28:130, 1971
4. Laniado S, Yellin EL, Miller H, et al: Temporal relation of the first heart sound to closure of the mitral valve. Circulation 47:1006, 1973
5. O'Toole JD, Reddy PS, Curtiss EI, et al: The contribution of tricuspid valve closure to the first heart sound: An intracardiac micromanometer study. Circulation 53:752, 1976
6. Waider W, Craige E: First heart sound and ejection sounds. Echocardiographic and phonocardiographic correlation with valvular events. Am J Cardiol 35:346, 1975
7. Mills PG, Chamusco RF, Moos S, et al: Echophonocardiographic studies of the contribution of the atrioventricular valves to the first heart sound. Circulation 54:944, 1976
8. Wexler LF, Pohost GM, Rubenstein JJ, et al: The relationship of the first heart sound to mitral valve closure in dogs. Circulation 66:235, 1982
9. Sakamoto T, Kusukawa R, MacCanon DM, et al: Hemodynamic determinants of the amplitude of the first heart sound. Circ Res 16:45, 1965
10. Shah PM, Kramer DH, Gramiak R: Influence of the timing of atrial systole on mitral valve closure and on the first heart sound in man. Am J Cardiol 26:231, 1970
11. Burgraaf GW, Craige E: The first heart sound in complete heart block. Circulation 50:17, 1974
12. Leech G, Brooks N, Green–Wilkinson A, et al: Mechanism of influence of PR interval on loudness of first heart sound. Br Heart J 138, 1980

13. Stept ME, Heid CE, Shaver JA, et al: Effects of altering P–R interval on the amplitude of the first heart sound in the anesthetized dog. Circ Res 25:255, 1969
14. Brooks N, Leech G, Leatham A: Factors responsible for normal splitting of first heart sound: High speed echophonocardiographic study of valve movement. Br Heart J 24:695, 1979
15. Milner S, Moyer RA, Venables AW, et al: Mitral and tricuspid valve closure in congenital heart disease. Circulation 53:513, 1976
16. Surawicz B, Mercer C, Chlebus H, et al: Role of the phonocardiogram in evaluation of the severity of mitral stenosis and detection of associated valvular lesions. Circulation 34:195, 1966
17. Oreshkov V: Q-1 or C1 interval in the diagnosis of mitral stenosis. Br Heart J 29:778, 1967
18. Thompson ME, Shaver JA, Heidenreich FP, et al: Sound, pressure and motion correlates in mitral stenosis. Am J Med 49:436, 1970
19. Salerni R, Reddy PS, Sherman E, et al: Pressure and sound correlates of the mitral valve echocardiogram in mitral stenosis. Circulation 58:118, 1978
20. Hume L, Reuben SR: The effect of exercise on the amplitude of the first heart sound in normal subjects. Am Heart J 95:4, 1978
21. Gorlin R: The hyperkinetic heart syndrome. JAMA 182:823, 1962
22. Reddy PS, Leon DF, Krishnaswami V, et al: Syndrome of acute aortic regurgitation. In Leon DF, Shaver JA (eds): Physiologic Principles of Heart Sounds and Murmurs, p 166. American Heart Association Monograph 46. Dallas, American Heart Association, 1975
23. Stein PD, Sabbah HN, Barr I: Intensity of heart sounds in the evaluation of patients following myocardial infarction. Chest 75:679, 1979
24. Adolph RJ, Fowler NO, Tanaka K: Prolongation of isovolumic contraction time in left bundle branch block. Am Heart J 78:585, 1969
25. Burgraaf GW: The first heart sound in left bundle branch block: An echophonocardiographic study. Circulation 63:429, 1981
26. Mills, P, Craige E: Echophonocardiography. Progr Cardiovasc Dis 20:337, 1978
27. Sakamoto T, Jusukawa R, MacCanon DM, et al: The amplitude of the first heart sound in experimentally induced atrial fibrillation. Dis Chest 48:401, 1976
28. Sakamoto T, Kusukawa R, MacCanon DM, et al: First heart sound amplitude in experimentally induced alternans. Dis Chest 50:470, 1966
29. Costeas FX, Poulias G, Louvros N, et al: Acoustic, mechanical and electrical alternans in hemopericardium of occult leukemic origin. Chest 60:460, 1971
30. Curtiss EI, Reddy PS, O'Toole JD, et al: Alternations of right ventricular systolic time intervals by chronic pressure and volume overloading. Circulation 53:997, 1976
31. Leonard JJ, Weissler AM, Warren ZV: Observations on the mechanism of atrial gallop rhythm. Circulation 17:1007, 1958
32. Murgo JP, Altobelli SA, Dorethy JF, et al: Normal ventricular ejection dynamics in man during rest and exercise. In Leon DF, Shaver JA (eds): Physiologic Principles of Heart Sounds and Murmurs, p 92. American Heart Association Monograph 46. Dallas, American Heart Association, 1975
33. MacCanon D, Arevalo F, Meyer EC: Direct detection and timing of aortic valve closure. Circ Res 14:387, 1964
34. Sabbah HN, Stein PD: Investigation of the theory and mechanism of the origin of the second heart sound. Circ Res 39:874, 1976
35. Kusukawa R, Bruce DW, Sakamoto T, et al: Hemodynamic determinants of the amplitude of the second heart sound. J Appl Physiol 21:938, 1966
36. Stein PD, Sabbah HN, Khaja F, et al: Exploration of the cause of the low intensity aortic component of the second sound in nonhypotensive patients with poor ventricular performance. Circulation 57:590, 1978

37. Stein PD, Sabbah HN, Anbe DT, et al: Hemodynamic and anatomic determinants of relative differences in amplitude of the aortic and pulmonary components of the second heart sound. Am J Cardiol 42:539, 1978

38. Sabbah HN, Stein PD: Relation of the second sound to diastolic vibration of the closed aortic valve. Heart Circ Physiol 3:H696, 1978

39. Papapieto SE, Coghlan C, Zisserman D, et al: Impaired maximal rate of left ventricular relaxation in patients with coronary artery disease and left ventricular dysfunction. Circulation 59:984, 1979

40. Leighton RF, Weissler AM, Weinstein PB, et al: Right and left ventricular systolic time intervals: Effects of heart rate, respiration and atrial pacing. Am J Cardiol 27:66, 1971

41. Curtiss EI, Matthews RG, Shaver JA: Mechanism of normal splitting of the second heart sound. Circulation 51:157, 1975

42. Shaver JA, Nadolny Ra, O'Toole JD, et al: Sound pressure correlates of the second heart sound: An intracardiac sound study. Circulation 39:316, 1974

43. Harris A, Sutton: Second heart sound in normal subjects. Br Heart J 30:739, 1968

44. Glancy DL, Freed TA, O'Brien KP, et al: Calcium in the aortic valve: Roentgenologic and hemodynamic correlations in 148 patients. Ann Intern Med 71:245, 1969.

45. Sabbah HN, Khaja F, Anbe DT, et al: The aortic closure sound in pure aortic insufficiency. Circulation 56:859, 1977

46. Adolph RJ, Fowler NO: The second heart sound: A screening test for heart disease. Mod Concepts Cardiovasc Dis 39:91, 1970

47. Logue RB, Cobbs BW, Barney ER: The second heart sound in pulmonary embolism and pulmonary hypertension. Trans Am Clin Climatol Assoc 78:38, 1966

48. Leatham A, Weitzman D: Auscultatory and phonocardiographic signs of pulmonary stenosis. Br Heart J 19:303, 1957

49. O'Toole JD, Reddy PS,Curtiss EI, et al: The mechanism of splitting of the second heart sound in atrial septal defect. Circulation 56:1047, 1977

50. Higgen MM, Braunwald E: The splitting of the second heart sound in normal subjects and in patients with congenital heart disease. Circulation 25:328, 1962

51. Schrine V, Vogelpoel L: Role of the dilated pulmonary artery in abnormal splitting of the second heart sound. Am Heart J 63:501, 1962

52. Zuberbuhler JR, Bauersfeld SR: Paradoxical splitting of the second heart sound in the Wolff-Parkinson-White syndrome. Am Heart J 70:595, 1965

53. Harris A, Donmoyer T, Leatham A: Physical signs in differential diagnosis of left ventricular obstructive cardiomyopathy. Br Heart J 31:501, 1969

54. Shaver JA, Kroetz FW, Leonard JJ, et al: Effect of steady-state increases in systemic arterial pressure on the duration of left ventricular ejection time. J Clin Invest 47:217, 1968

55. Yurchak PM, Gorlin R: Paradoxical splitting of the second heart sound in coronary heart disease. N Engl J Med 269:741, 1963

56. Surawicz B: Effect of respiration and upright position in the interval between the two components of the second heart sound and that between the second sound and mitral opening snap. Circulation 16:422, 1957

9

THIRD AND FOURTH HEART SOUNDS

John F. Stapleton, M.D.

Definition

In 1838, twenty years after Laennec introduced the stethoscope, another French physician, Charcellay, described presystolic sounds.[1,2] Bouillaud coined the term "gallop rhythm" in 1847, according to his pupil and colleague Pierre-Carl Potain (Fig. 8-1) who described gallop rhythm in 1875.[3,4] The perceptive observations of these early French clinicians (Fig. 9-1) are best appreciated by those who have ausculted the heart with a 19th-century stethoscope.

As the term is used today, *gallop rhythm* refers to the cadence created by diastolic heart sounds, usually when associated with rapid heart rates. There are two diastolic heart sounds: one associated with atrial contraction, the other occurring with rapid ventricular filling in early diastole. Patients may have either or both sounds. Although the rhythm of a galloping horse is a four-sound sequence (cantering causes three sounds), medical gallop rhythm can have either three or four sounds. The term gallop rhythm implies abnormality, even though healthy persons may also have diastolic sounds.

The extra heart sound associated with early diastolic ventricular rapid filling is known as *the third heart sound*. It is also called a *ventricular filling sound*, or simply S_3. This sound occurs in most healthy children, and in many young adults; it is then called a *physiologic third heart sound*.[5,6] A similar ventricular filling sound may accompany heart disease; in this setting the cadence is called *ventricular gallop rhythm*, and the sound itself is often loosely labeled a *ventricular gallop sound*, or simply a *ventricular gallop*.[7-9]

S_3 occurs 0.12 sec to 0.18 sec after the onset of the second heart sound (S_2), as the rapid filling phase of early diastole merges with the longer period of

214

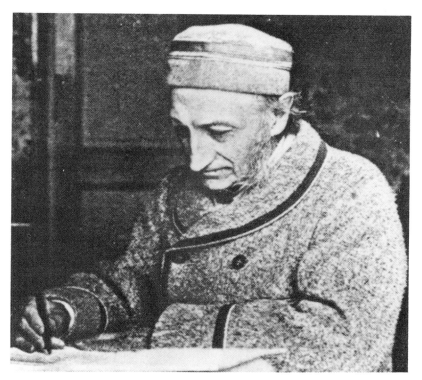

FIG. 9-1. Pierre-Carl Potain (1825–1901), who described diastolic gallop sounds in 1875, proposed that they originated in abrupt deceleration of the ventricular wall—a hypothesis supported by modern technology. He also described the extra diastolic sound of constrictive pericarditis, systolic clicks, and inspiratory splitting of the second heart sound (S_2). (McKusick VA: Cardiovascular Sound in Health and Disease, p 21. Baltimore, Williams and Wilkins, 1958)

slow diastolic filling (diastasis). Recordings of the apex impulse best demonstrate this timing; S_3 coincides with the peak of the initial diastolic ascent caused by quick outward movement of the ventricular wall as blood rapidly enters the left ventricle (Fig. 9-2).

The sound associated with atrial contraction is called *the fourth heart sound.* It is also known as the *atrial sound,* or simply S_4. This sound is best identified by its relationship to the electrocardiographic P wave (Fig. 9-3). Left atrial (LA) sounds occur 0.14 sec to 0.24 sec after the onset of P, coinciding with the peak of the atrial precordial thrust.[10] Right atrial (RA) sounds occur 0.09 sec to 0.16 sec after the onset of P.[10] S_4 can be heard in normal persons but often accompanies heart disease. In the latter case, S_4 may impart a cadence known as *presystolic* or *atrial gallop rhythm;* the sound in these instances is often called an *atrial gallop sound,* or simply an *atrial gallop.*

When both S_3 and S_4 are present, the expression *quadruple rhythm* is often employed (Fig. 9-4). When tachycardia or atrioventricular (AV) block causes both sounds to fuse into a single sound, the term *summation gallop* applies.

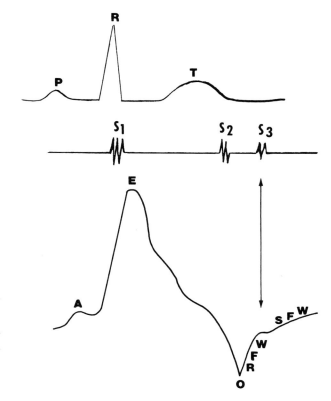

FIG. 9-2. Early ventricular filling sound (*S₃*) with apex cardiogram (*lower curve*). *S₃* coincides with completion of rapid filling wave (*RFW*) and beginning of slow filling wave (*SFW*) or diastasis. *E*=Early systolic apical impulse. *O*=Mitral valve opening.

Physiology

Over a century has passed since Potain related S_3 to rapid ventricular filling. The mechanism of production still cannot be stated with certainty. There are three hypotheses, each with notable adherents. Potain's original concept is still viable: "If the cardiac muscle loses its tone, the ventricle, in dilating, arrives rapidly at the point where resistance of the fibers of its wall limits its distention; then, suddenly arrested, it produces a tension, shock and gallop sound."[4] The preponderance of evidence supports this view today. Continuance or reappearance of the left ventricular (LV) S_3 after installation of a mitral valve prosthesis has been cited as confirming a myocardial source of

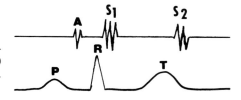

FIG. 9-3. Sketch of atrial sound (*A*), or *S₄*, with electrocardiogram. *S₄* follows the atrial depolarization (*P*) wave of the electrocardiogram. S_1=First heart sound. S_2=Second heart sound.

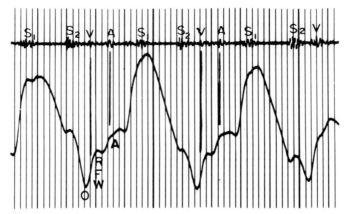

FIG. 9-4. Phonocardiogram recorded with apex cardiogram. Both ventricular filling sound (*V*), or S_3, and atrial sound (*A*), or S_4, are present, constituting quadruple rhythm. Vertical time lines are 0.04 sec apart. (Stapleton JF: The extra heart sound. Am Fam Physician 9:79, 1974. By permission of American Academy of Family Physicians.)

this sound.[11] Moreover, S_3 has been demonstrated to coincide exactly with the abrupt deceleration of ventricular expansion that occurs as diastolic rapid filling ends.[12] However, other investigators report disappearance of S_3 after mitral valve replacement and propose that S_3 arises from vibration of the mitral valve structure, including leaflets, chordae tendineae, and papillary muscles, during early diastolic ventricular filling.[13] This hypothesis attributes S_3 to sudden tensing of the valve leaflets in response to the initial diastolic surge of blood into the left ventricle.[14-16] A third hypothesis ascribes the sound to the impact of the heart against the chest wall, pointing to the fact that S_3 is of greater intensity when recorded over the precordium than when recorded within the heart by intracardiac sound tracings.[17]

Since S_4 also occurs during a period of vigorous ventricular filling—due to atrial contraction—and since S_4 is acoustically similar to S_3, it probably arises from the myocardium when the ventricular wall abruptly decelerates after expanding to accommodate atrial systole. The timing of atrial contraction normally would place this sound within S_1.[18,19] When atrial systole is separated from ventricular systole by conduction delay, S_4 often becomes audible even though the heart is otherwise normal. When caused by heart disease, S_4 will move toward S_1 as the underlying disorder improves.[18] This phenomenon has been demonstrated by reducing the venous return of hypertensive patients with tourniquets; this maneuver will cause S_4 to migrate into S_1 (Fig. 9-5).[19]

Although the production of S_3 and S_4 has been studied in many interesting ways, the precise source and meaning of these sounds continue to intrigue investigators. Although the etiologic mechanism is not certain, important hemodynamic correlations have been made with both S_3 and S_4. The physiologic S_3 of healthy children and young adults is associated with normal cardiovascular pressures and flow. The S_3 of heart disease usually signifies ventricular dilatation and myocardial failure with high diastolic pressure and

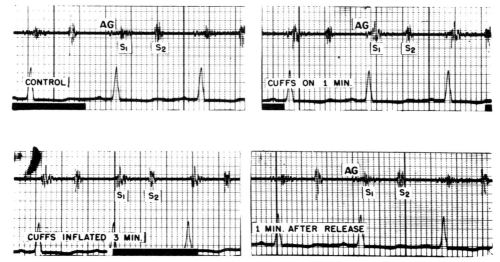

FIG. 9-5. Migration of S_4 or atrial gallop (AG) sound into S_1, when venous return is reduced by applying tourniquets to the extremities. After 3 min of cuff compression the atrial sound is no longer seen, but it returns within one min after release. (Leonard J, Weissler A, Warren J: Observations on the mechanism of atrial gallop rhythm. Circulation 17:1007, 1958. By permission of the American Heart Association.)

volume and reduced ejection fraction; cardiac output may be low.[20] S_3 also accompanies severe valvular regurgitant lesions, indicating diastolic volume overloading with excessive early diastolic ventricular filling; myocardial contractility is usually depressed when S_3 accompanies left heart regurgitant lesions in patients over 40 years of age.[20,21]

S_4 often occurs in persons with normal cardiovascular dynamics.[20,22] When associated with heart disease, S_4 usually denotes diminished ventricular compliance due to hypertrophy, ischemia, or fibrosis.[22] Wall thickening is more prominent than is cavity dilatation. Diastolic atrial and ventricular pressures and cardiac output are often normal even when S_4 accompanies heart disease, an important contrast with S_3.[20,22]

Clinical Presentation

THIRD HEART SOUND

S_3 is a low-pitched vibration, occurring 0.12 sec to 0.18 sec after the onset of S_2 (Fig. 9-4). It is best heard at the cardiac apex by ausculting with the stethoscope bell held gently to the skin, with the patient recumbent. The sound may be more audible when the patient is in the left lateral posture. S_3 sometimes waxes and wanes, becoming loud and then almost disappearing a few beats later (Fig. 9-6). It is often faint but can be heard in most children if carefully sought. Healthy young adults frequently present with this sound,

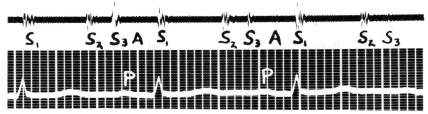

FIG. 9-6. Prominent physiologic S_3 in 17-year-old nursing student without heart disease. Note striking variations in intensity. Very faint S_4 (*A*) and innocent systolic murmur are also present.

which then gradually disappears during the third decade. It is seldom heard in normal individuals over 30 years of age.

Pathophysiologic Significance

Early diastolic S_3 may accompany conditions associated with increased blood flow, such as thyrotoxicosis, severe anemia, pregnancy, or vigorous exercise; underlying cardiac function may be normal.

Like the physiologic S_3, the S_3 of heart disease, commonly called a ventricular gallop, consists of low-frequency vibrations best heard at the apex with the stethoscope bell and augmented by left lateral recumbency. It is often faint and easily overlooked, requiring intent listening in a quiet room. The S_3 of heart disease occurs 0.12 sec to 0.20 sec after the onset of S_2, coinciding with the peak of the rapid filling wave of precordial movement tracings (Fig. 9-2).

When tachycardia accompanies the S_3 of heart disease, the cadence of a galloping (or cantering) horse is created, giving rise to the expression *gallop rhythm.* The term "gallop rhythm," however, is commonly used whether or not tachycardia is present. Ventricular gallop rhythm is a finding of serious import. It usually accompanies myocardial failure and may be a subtle forerunner of clinical decompensation. It is a regular concomitant of pulsus alternans and is louder with the stronger beats. Its intensity often relates to the severity of failure, growing fainter as compensation is restored and becoming louder as the patient worsens. It is, therefore, a reliable and inexpensive tool for evaluating response to therapy. When S_3 accompanies heart failure, a favorable effect of digitalis can be anticipated.[23] A loud, persistent S_3 with cardiomyopathy or myocardial infarction is an ominous sign associated with high mortality.[24,25] Prompt subsidence of S_3 suggests a more favorable outlook.

The ventricular gallop of RV failure is heard at the lower left sternal edge. It may augment with inspiration. RV gallop rhythm is uncommon.

Ventricular gallop sounds can be induced or enhanced by measures that promote venous return. The simplest of these is to elevate the recumbent patient's lower extremities. Sustained hand grip will augment S_3, as will amyl nitrite inhalation.[26,27] The beat following an extrasystole may contain a previously unheard S_3—the postextrasystolic gallop.

Conversely, reducing venous return as with the tourniquets about the extremities, may eliminate S_3.[28] Cardiac slowing, as with carotid sinus pressure, often diminishes or eliminates S_3; this maneuver may also clarify the early diastolic timing of S_3 when the basic rate is too rapid for accurate timing.[29,30]

Although in adults with heart disease S_3 often means heart failure, patients with mitral or aortic regurgitation, or with significant left-to-right shunting due to ventricular septal defect or patent ductus arteriosus, may have a prominent early diastolic S_3 without heart failure (Fig. 9-7). These diastolic overloading disorders are characterized by vigorous and excessive early diastolic ventricular filling, which may generate not only an S_3 but also a short, rapid, rumbling, filling murmur. Atrial septal defect or tricuspid regurgitation may cause early diastolic RV sounds by the same mechanism. Individuals with overloading of either ventricle may maintain normal myocardial contractility for years after S_3 is detected.

Since most children have a physiologic S_3, this finding is less specific in pediatric heart disease than among adults. However, the ventricular gallop rhythm of heart failure does occur in children. Although it may soften or intensify as decompensation improves or worsens and does not vary as much from cycle to cycle as the physiologic S_3 often does, the diagnosis of ventricular gallop rhythm in children must be made with caution.

Distinction from Other Sounds

Ventricular gallop sounds must be distinguished from the opening snap of mitral stenosis. The latter is high-pitched, closer to S_2 (0.04 sec–0.12 sec after S_2) and often transmits well to the left sternal edge and to the base of the heart. Pressing down firmly with the stethoscope diaphragm will usually eliminate gallop sounds but does not affect the audibility of the mitral opening snap. The cadence of the sounds of mitral stenosis, featuring an accentuated S_1 and a high-pitched opening snap occurring quickly after S_2, differs from the rhythm created by a low-pitched ventricular gallop sound, heard later in diastole and usually associated with a normal or even diminished S_1 (Fig. 9-8).

S_3 seldom accompanies severe mitral stenosis, presumably because rapid LV filling is prevented by mitral obstruction. Occasionally, RV gallop sound may

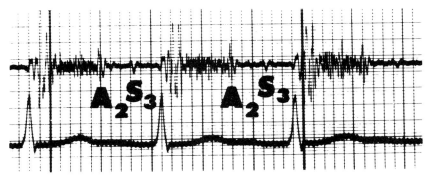

FIG. 9-7. Prominent ventricular filling sound (S_3) in ventricular septal defect. A_2=Aortic closure sound. (Stapleton JF: Essentials of Clinical Cardiology, p 155. Philadelphia, FA Davis, 1983)

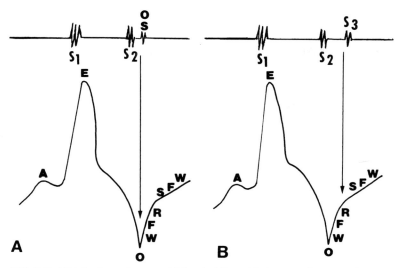

FIG. 9-8. (A) Mitral opening snap (OS) coinciding with O point of apex cardiogram, preceding rapid filling wave (RFW) in early diastole. (B) Onset of ventricular filling sound (S_3) coinciding with completion of rapid filling and beginning of slow filling wave (SFW) or diastasis. E = Early systolic peak of apex cardiogram, A = Atrial precordial movement.

accompany the chronic RV failure of long-standing pulmonary hypertensive mitral stenosis. Young patients with mitral stenosis may present with an audible S_3 that is distinct from the mitral opening snap.[31]

Patients with constrictive pericarditis often present with an early diastolic sound that can be mistaken for S_3. The pericardial sound—sometimes called the pericardial knock—occurs 0.06 sec to 0.16 sec after S_2. Like the mitral opening snap, it is high-pitched, may transmit well along the left sternal edge, and does not disappear with stethoscope pressure.

FOURTH HEART SOUND

Pathophysiologic Significance

The atrial or fourth heart sound (S_4) is a ubiquitous sound heard under many circumstances.[10,16,18,22] While often signifying heart disease, S_4 also occurs without it. It may accompany the physiologic S_3 in some young persons; it is less common as a physiologic sound of youth and generally fainter than S_3 when these two sounds occur together in healthy children (see Fig. 9-6). Elderly individuals may present with S_4 without demonstrable heart disease, perhaps as a result of the reduced myocardial compliance of age.

Audible vibrations caused by atrial systole may contribute to the normal S_1 or to faint, low-pitched vibrations at the beginning of S_1.[18] When the P–R interval lengthens, these atrial vibrations may then constitute a discrete sound.

When complete AV block affects an otherwise normal heart, S_4 is clearly heard apart from S_1 and S_2 (Fig. 9-9). S_4 is loudest when atrial systole happens to coincide with early diastolic rapid ventricular filling. Occasionally, S_4 during complete block is a split sound, perhaps arising from both atria.

The commonly heard S_4 is a left atrial event. It is a low-pitched sound, best heard at the cardiac apex with the stethoscope bell held gently to the skin.[32] Left lateral recumbency provides maximal audibility. The sound is often well heard over the lower left parasternal area and, like S_3, may transmit to the right supraclavicular fossa.[33] Right atrial gallop sounds are best heard along the lower left sternal edge; these often increase with inspiration.

Sympathetic stimulation enhances the force of atrial contraction. Therefore, excitement, apprehension, exercise, cold pressor tests, sympathomimetic drugs, or thyrotoxicosis will produce or exaggerate S_4. Increased venous return will also increase the intensity of S_4; this is the mechanism by which amyl nitrite augments S_4, both in the presence of heart disease and in its absence.[27] However, this agent may leave unaffected or may even diminish S_4 in severe hypertension, when the lowered atrial pressure and reduced LV afterload produced by amyl nitrite apparently outweigh the effect of increased venous return. Reducing venous return can lessen or eliminate S_4. Sitting, standing, or breath holding may abolish S_4, as may carotid sinus pressure.[29,30]

The significance of S_4 can often be judged by concomitant findings—that is, by the "company it keeps." It commonly accompanies cardiac disorders that reduce myocardial compliance. Aortic stenosis, myocardial infarction, hypertension, and cardiomyopathy (both hypertrophic and dilated) are the diseases most commonly associated with abnormal LA sounds. When heard in young patients with aortic stenosis, S_4 usually indicates serious obstruction with a significant transvalvular gradient.[34] Atrial sounds so commonly accompany myocardial infarction that their absence should suggest inadequate auscultation.[35,36] The sound often persists as a chronic finding after the infarct has healed. S_4 may occur transiently during angina pectoris. When associated with hypertension, S_4 suggests that hypertrophy has reduced myocardial distensibility.[36,37] Successful therapy may lengthen the interval between the electrocardiographic P wave and S_4, thus shortening the interval between S_4 and S_1. Progression of disease may cause S_4 to occur earlier in presystole.

Abnormal S_4 is regularly accompanied by increased atrial deflections on precordial movement tracings.[17,32,38] A presystolic impulse from atrial contraction is sometimes palpable (Fig. 9-10). Such concomitant pulsatile abnormalities confirm the abnormal nature of the S_4 since the S_4 heard in normal individuals is not associated with increased precordial movement during atrial systole.[39]

As might be expected, the atrial sound disappears when atrial fibrillation develops (Fig. 9-11). If sinus rhythm is restored after prolonged fibrillation, S_4

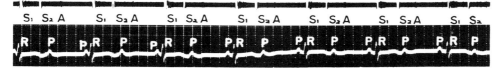

FIG. 9-9. Complete AV block unmasks independent atrial sounds (A).

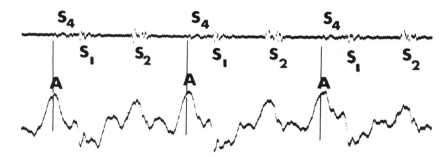

FIG. 9-10. Atrial thrust and gallop in hyperthyroidism with CHF. Lower curve is precordial movement tracing that presents a prominent presystolic impulse (*A*) that was readily palpable and that corresponds with the timing of S₄ on the phonocardiogram.

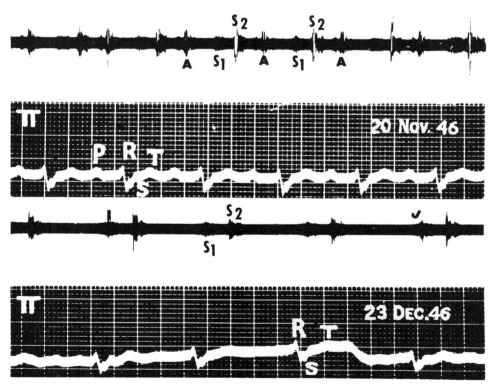

FIG. 9-11. Sound created by atrial systole (*A*) disappears when atrial fibrillation develops (upper tracings, 20 Nov; lower tracings, 23 Dec). (Levine S, Harvey WP: Clinical Auscultation of the Heart p 91. Philadelphia, WB Saunders, 1959)

may not develop until several days after reversion. This observation suggests that the atria do not function effectively after prolonged fibrillation and require time to recover contractility.[40] S_4 is seldom heard when long-standing atrial distention has diminished the force of atrial contraction. Therefore, chronic mitral regurgitation does not cause an audible S_4, whereas acute mitral regurgitation usually does.

Distinction from Other Sounds

An S_4 that closely precedes the S_1 causes a double sound complex resembling a split S_1. The differentiation is usually easy, since S_4 is usually maximal over the cardiac apex whereas splitting of S_1 is loudest along the lower left sternal border. The simplest distinction is achieved by pressing firmly with the stethoscopic diaphragm; S_4 is eliminated by this maneuver, whereas the audibility of a split S_1 is unaffected. Another double sound complex involving S_1 is that created by an aortic or pulmonic ejection sound. These sounds closely follow S_1 and simulate splitting. The high-pitched character and basal prominence of ejection sounds serve to separate this double complex from those caused by S_4 or splitting of S_1 (Fig. 9-12).

SUMMATION GALLOP SOUND

Summation gallop sound is a single, and often loud, diastolic sound that ocurs when atrial systole happens to coincide with early diastolic rapid filling (see Fig. 9-4). It usually appears when tachycardia or a long P–R interval causes early diastolic and presystolic filling to fuse into a single, over-vigorous rapid filling period. The clinical significance of the summation gallop lies in the auscultatory confusion it may create, particularly when the sound is louder than S_1 or S_2. Otherwise, it has the clinical meaning of the S_3 and S_4 that have fused to generate it.

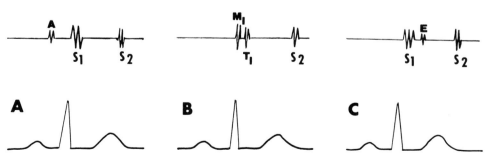

FIG. 9-12. Three double sound complexes involving S_1. (A) Atrial sound (A) follows electrocardiographic P wave and precedes S_1. (B) S_1 splits into mitral closure sound (M_I) and triscuspid closure sound (T_1). (C) S_1 followed by early systolic ejection sound (E).

Summary

The presence of S_3 in a young person or patient with increased blood flow secondary to pregnancy, anemia, or thyrotoxicosis may be interpreted as a physiologic event that does not indicate cardiac disease. However, in most adult patients with cardiac disease, a prominent S_3 usually reflects impending or overt heart failure. With effective therapy, the S_3 can be expected to decrease in amplitude or disappear. An S_3 may also accompany aortic or mitral regurgitation in the absence of heart failure.

An audible S_4, heard best at the cardiac apex in the left lateral decubitus position, reflects decreased compliance of the left ventricle and preservation of atrial contractility. In adults, the most common conditions altering LV compliance are systemic hypertension, ischemic heart disease, valvular heart disease, and cardiomyopathy. An S_4 is common in normal people, particularly the elderly.

Inspiratory augmentation of an S_3 or S_4 that is heard best along the left lower sternal border suggests an RV origin.

When both S_3 and S_4 are audible, an increase in heart rate causes the two sounds to overlap and a summation gallop sound may be heard in mid-diastole.

Bibliography

1. Laennec RTA: Auscultation Mediate. American edition, 1832
2. Charcellay A: Memoire sur plusieurs cas, remarquables de defaut de synchronisme des battements et des bruits des ventricules du coeur. Archives Générales de Médecine 68:393, 1838
3. Potain PC: Du rythme cardiaque appelébruit de galop, de son mecanisme et de sa valeur séméilogique. Bulletins et Mémoires du Société Medicale des Hôpitaux 12:137, 1875
4. Potain PC: Du bruit de galop. Gazette des Hôpitaux Civiles et Militaires 53:529, 1880
5. Dock W, Grandell F, Taubman F: The physiologic third heart sound: Its mechanism and relation to protodiastolic gallop. Am Heart J 50:449, 1955
6. Levine SA, Harvey WP: Clinical Auscultation of the Heart, 2nd ed. Philadelphia, WB Saunders, 1959
7. Harvey WP, Stapleton J: Clinical aspects of gallop rhythm with particular reference to diastolic gallops. Circulation 18:1017, 1958
8. Sloan AW: Cardiac gallop rhythm. Medicine 37:197, 1958
9. Warren JV, Leonard JJ, Weissler AM: Gallop rhythm. Ann Intern Med 48:580, 1958
10. Weitzman D: The mechanism and significance of the auricular sound. Br Heart J 17:70, 1955
11. Coulshed N, Epstein EJ: Third heart sound after mitral valve replacement. Br Heart J 34:301, 1972
12. Ozawa Y, Smith D, Craige E: Origin of the third heart sound. Circulation 67:393, 1983
13. Fleming J: Evidence for a mitral valve origin of the left ventricular third heart sound. Br Heart J 31:192, 1969
14. Nixon PGF: The genesis of the third heart sound. Am Heart J 65:712, 1963
15. Kuo PT, Schnabel TG Jr, Blakemore WS, et al: Diastolic gallop sounds: The mechanism of production. J Clin Invest 36:1035, 1957

16. Crevasse L, Wheat M, Wilson J, et al: The mechanism of the generation of the third and fourth heart sounds. Circulation 25:635, 1962
17. Reddy P, Meno F, Curtiss E, et al: The genesis of gallop sounds: Investigation by quantitative phono- and apexcardiography. Circulation 63:922, 1981
18. Kincaid–Smith P, Barlow J: Atrial sound and component of the first heart sound. Br Heart J 21:479, 1959
19. Leonard J, Weissler A, Warren J: Observations on the mechanism of atrial gallop rhythm. Circulation 17:1007, 1958
20. Shah P, Yu P: Gallop rhythm, hemodynamic and clinical correlation. Am Heart J 78:823, 1969
21. Abdulla A, Frank M, Erdin R Jr, et al: Clinical significance and hemodynamic correlates of the third heart sound gallop in aortic regurgitation. Circulation 64:464, 1981
22. Bethell H, Nixon P: Understanding the atrial sound. Br Heart J 35:229, 1973
23. Lee D, Johnson R, Bingham J, et al: Heart failure in outpatients. N Engl J Med 306:699, 1982
24. Riley C, Russell R, Rackley C: Left ventricular gallop sound and acute myocardial infarction. Am Heart J 86:598, 1973
25. Shah P, Gramiak R, Kramer D, Yu P: Determinants of atrial (S_4) and ventricular (S_3) gallop sounds in primary myocardial disease. N Engl J Med 278:753, 1968
26. Cohn P, Thompson P, Strauss W, et al: Diastolic heart sounds during static (handgrip) exercise in patients with chest pain. Circulation 47:1217, 1973
27. Sawayama T, Marumoto S, Niki I, et al: The clinical usefulness of the amyl nitrite inhalation test in the assessment of the third and atrial heart sounds in ischemic heart disease. Am Heart J 76:746, 1968
28. Leonard J, Weissler A, Warren J: Modification of ventricular gallop rhythm induced by pooling of blood in the extremities. Br Heart J 20:502, 1958
29. Harris W, Rodin P, Tabatznik B: Modification of the atrial sound by the cold pressor test, carotid sinus massage, and the Valsalva maneuver. Circulation 27:1128, 1963
30. Read J, Porter W: The efficacy of carotid sinus pressure in the differential diagnosis of triple rhythms. Am J Med 19:177, 1955
31. Gamble W, Reddy P: Preservation of the third heart sound in mitral stenosis. N Engl J Med 308:498, 1983
32. Bethell H, Nixon P: Some aspects of the left atrial sound. Am Heart J 88:399, 1974
33. DiDonna G, O'Rourke R, Peterson K, et al: Transmission of audible praecordial gallop sounds to right supraclavicular fossa. Br Heart J 37:1277, 1975
34. Caulfield W, de Leon A Jr, Perloff J, et al: The clinical significance of the fourth heart sound in aortic stenosis. Am J Cardiol 28:179, 1971
35. Turner P, Hunter J: The atrial sound in ischaemic heart disease. Br Heart J 35:657, 1973
36. Kincaid–Smith P, Barlow J: The atrial sound in hypertension and ischemic heart disease. Br Heart J 20:502, 1958
37. Kontos H, Shapiro W, Kemp V: Observations on the atrial sound in hypertension. Circulation 27:877, 1963
38. Cohn P, Vokonas P, Williams R, et al: Diastolic heart sounds and filling waves in coronary artery disease. Circulation 44:196, 1971
39. Denef B, Geest H, Kesteloot H: The clinical value of the calibrated apical A Wave and its relationship to the fourth heart sound. Circulation 60:1414, 1979
40. O'Rourke R: Appearance of atrial sound after reversion of atrial fibrillation. Br Heart J 32:597, 1970

10

MURMURS

Joseph K. Perloff, M.D.

Definition

A cardiovascular murmur is a relatively prolonged series of auditory vibrations that can be characterized according to intensity (loudness), frequency (pitch), configuration (shape), quality, duration, direction of radiation, and timing in the cardiac cycle. Correct assessment of these features in murmurs of a given description sets the stage for the correct diagnostic conclusions. The intensity or loudness of a murmur is graded I to VI, in a scale based on recommendations made by Freeman and Levine in 1933.[1] A Grade I murmur is so faint that it is heard only with special effort. A Grade II murmur is faint but readily detected; Grade III is prominent but not loud; a Grade IV murmur is loud; and a Grade V murmur is very loud. A Grade VI murmur is loud enough to be heard with the stethoscope just removed from contact with the chest.

Physiology of Systolic Murmurs

A loud murmur generally radiates from its site of maximal intensity, and the direction of radiation sometimes provides useful information about the murmur's origin. Frequency, or pitch, varies from high to low. The configuration, or shape, of a systolic murmur can be crescendo, decrescendo,

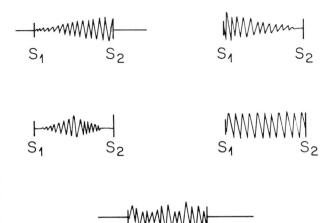

FIG. 10-1. The five basic shapes or configurations of systolic murmurs are schematically illustrated as crescendo, decrescendo, crescendo-decrescendo, plateau (even), or variable (uneven).

crescendo-decrescendo (diamond-shaped), plateau (even), or variable (uneven) (Fig. 10-1). A crescendo murmur increases progressively in intensity during the course of systole, whereas a decrescendo murmur does the opposite. A crescendo-descrescendo murmur increases to a peak and then declines. A plateau murmur has a relatively constant intensity throughout its course, whereas an uneven murmur is variable in intensity. The quality of murmurs is characterized by descriptive terms such as harsh, rough, rumbling, scratchy, buzzing, grunting, blowing, musical, whooping, squeaking, and so on. A murmur can be long or short in duration, with all gradations in between. Long murmurs occupy all or almost all of systole.

Murmurs are best classified according to their location (timing) in the cardiac cycle, using the first and second heart sounds, (S_1 and S_2) as a framework.[2] *Systolic* murmurs are classified, according to their time of onset and termination, as midsystolic, holosystolic, early systolic, or late systolic (Fig. 10-2). A midsystolic murmur begins after S_1 and ends before S_2. The termination of the midsystolic murmur must be related to the component of S_2 on its side of origin (See Fig. 10-2). Accordingly, midsystolic murmurs originating in the *left* heart end before the aortic component of S_2 (A_2); midsystolic murmurs originating in the *right* heart end before the pulmonic component (P_2). A holosystolic murmur begins with S_1, occupies all of systole and ends with S_2 on its side of origin. Thus, holosystolic murmurs originating in the *left* heart end with A_2, while those originating in the *right* heart end with P_2. The term *regurgitant systolic murmur,* originally applied to a murmur that occupied all of systole, has fallen into disuse because regurgitation can also be accompanied by mid-systolic, early systolic, or late systolic murmurs. The term *ejection systolic murmur,* originally applied to crescendo–decrescendo (midsystolic) murmurs, should also fall into disuse, since midsystolic murmurs are not necessarily due to ejection.

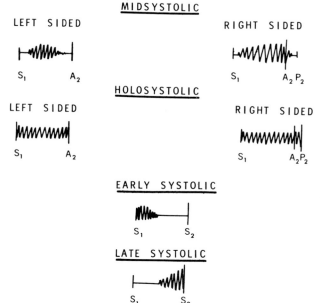

FIG. 10-2. Systolic murmurs are descriptively classified according to their time of onset and termination as midsystolic, holosystolic, early systolic, and late systolic. The termination of the murmur must be related to the appropriate component of S_2 on its side of origin, that is, the aortic component (A_2) for systolic murmurs originating in the left heart (left-sided) and the pulmonic component (P_2) for systolic murmurs originating in the right heart (right-sided).

Clinical Manifestations of Systolic Murmurs

MIDSYSTOLIC MURMURS

There are five principal settings in which midsystolic murmurs occur (see Fig. 10-2):

1. Some forms of mitral regurgitation, especially papillary muscle dysfunction
2. Accelerated ejection into the great arteries
3. Dilatation of the aortic root or pulmonary trunk
4. Morphologic changes in the semilunar valves or their lines of attachment without obstruction
5. Obstruction to ventricular outflow

The physiologic mechanisms responsible for the midsystolic murmur of mitral regurgitation (as a rule, papillary muscle dysfunction) entail early systolic competence of the valve followed by midsystolic incompetence and a late systolic decrease in regurgitant flow. The physiologic mechanism of *outflow* midsystolic murmurs reflects the patterns of phasic flow across the left ventricular (LV) or right ventricular (RV) outflow tract, as originally described by Leatham (Fig. 10-3).[3] Following S_1 (isovolumetric contraction), ventricular pressure rises sufficiently to open the relevant semilunar valve (aortic or pulmonic). It is not until then that ejection commences and the murmur begins. As ejection proceeds, the murmur increases (crescendo); as ejection declines, the murmur

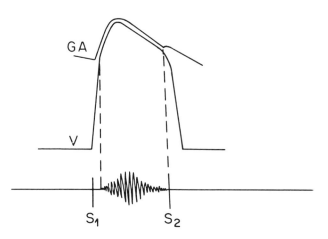

FIG. 10-3. Schematic illustration of the physiologic mechanism of an outflow midsystolic murmur generated by phasic flow (ejection) into aortic root or pulmonary trunk. The ventricular (*V*) and great arterial (*GA*) pressure pulses are shown with schematic phonocardiogram. The mumur begins after S₁ as ventricular pressure exceeds the pressure in the relevant great artery. The murmur rises in crescendo to a peak as flow proceeds, then declines in decrescendo as flow diminishes, ending just before S₂ when ventricular pressure falls below the pressure in the great artery.

declines (decrescendo). Forward flow then ceases, and the murmur ends before ventricular pressure drops below central arterial pressure with closure of the aortic or pulmonic valve and generation of A_2 or P_2.

The murmur of aortic stenosis is the prototype of the outflow midsystolic murmur. It begins after S_1 or with an ejection sound, rises in crescendo to a systolic peak, and declines in decrescendo to end before A_2. The quality of the murmur at the right base is typically harsh, rough, and grunting, especially when loud. The murmur may have an early systolic peak and a short duration; a relatively late peak and a prolonged duration, or any gradation in between, but whether it is long or short, the murmur remains symmetrical (diamond-shaped). Intensity varies from bare audibility to Grade VI. The location and radiation of the murmur of aortic stenosis are influenced largely, but not exclusively, by the direction of the high-velocity jet within the aortic root. In typical valvular aortic stenosis, the murmur is maximal in the second right intercostal space, with radiation upward, to the right, and into the neck. In supravalvular aortic stenosis, the murmur occasionally is loudest even higher (first right intercostal space), with disproportionate radiation into the right carotid artery.[4] In older patients (men or women, generally over 65 years of age) aortic sclerosis (no obstruction) or stenosis is commonly caused by calcification of previously normal trileaflet aortic valves (Fig. 10-4).[5] The accompanying murmur in the second right intercostal space is harsh, noisy, and impure, whereas the murmur at the cardiac apex is typically pure, often musical. The noisy, impure murmur (right base) originates within the aortic root because of turbulence caused by the high-velocity jet. The pure musical murmur at the apex is ascribed to periodic high-frequency vibrations of fibrocalcific cusps without commissural fusion (Figs. 10-4 and 10-5). This murmur is best recorded within the cavity of the left ventricle and, accordingly, is best heard at the apex over the LV impulse. The dissociation of these two aortic systolic murmurs—the noisy right basal and the musical apical—is sometimes called the *Gallavardin phenomenon.*[6]

The apical midsystolic murmur of aortic sclerosis or stenosis must be distinguished from an apical midsystolic or holosystolic murmur caused by mitral

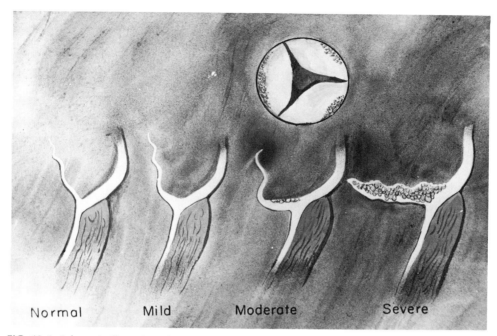

FIG. 10-4. Schematic illustration of aortic valve variations, beginning on the left with normal attachment of an aortic cusp to its sinus. The mildest alteration consists of a ridgelike, fibrous thickening at the base of the three cusps as they insert into the sinuses of Valsalva. Calcium can subsequently be deposited on the aortic surface of the fibrous ridge (*moderate*) and can ultimately extend to the free edges of the leaflets (*severe*) converting a previously normal trileaflet valve into one with severe calcific aortic stenosis. (Perloff JK: The Clinical Recognition of Congenital Heart Disease. Philadelphia, WB Saunders, 1979)

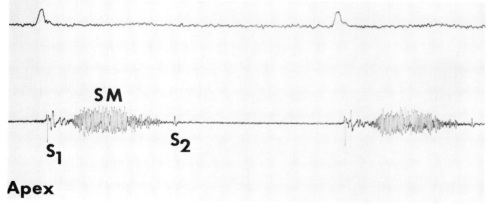

FIG. 10-5. A high-frequency, musical, relatively long midsystolic murmur at the apex in a 76-year-old woman with moderate calcification of a trileaflet aortic valve.

regurgitation.[7] Clear audibility of S_2 at the apex generally means that the murmur finishes before A_2 and is likely to be midsystolic. Conversely, if A_2 is well heard at the base but is inaudible at the apex, the sound is probably buried in late systolic vibrations of an apical holosystolic murmur. When the aortic valve is immobile (densely calcified), the closure sound is soft or inaudible, so that the length and configuration of the murmur are difficult, if not impossible, to establish by auscultation. Registration of a simultaneous phonocardiogram from the second right intercostal space and the apex with a synchronous carotid arterial pulse sometimes establishes the timing of A_2 (with the aortic incisura), and therefore serves to establish both the configuration and the timing of the apical murmur. When premature ventricular beats are followed by pauses longer than the dominant cycle length, the intensity of the apical midsystolic murmur of aortic sclerosis or stenosis typically increases in the beat following the premature contraction, whereas the intensity of the midsystolic or holosystolic murmur of mitral regurgitation remains unchanged. The same pattern holds in atrial fibrillation.

The murmur of valvular pulmonic stenosis can be taken as the prototype of an outflow midsystolic murmur originating in the right heart.[4] The murmur is typically maximal in the second left intercostal space, beginning after the first heart sound or with an ejection sound, rising in crescendo to a systolic peak, and declining in decrescendo to end before a delayed P_2 (Fig. 10-6).

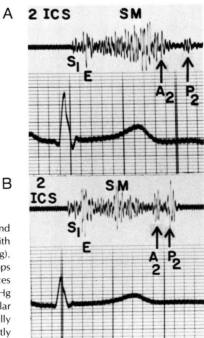

FIG. 10-6. *(A)* Preoperative phonocardiogram in the second left intercostal space *(2 ICS)* from a 21-year-old woman with congenital valvular pulmonic stenosis (gradient 80 mm Hg). An asymmetric midsystolic murmur peaks late and envelops A_2. P_2 is delayed and soft. An ejection sound *(E)* introduces the murmur. *(B)* The postoperative gradient was 20 mm Hg and the phonocardiogram now resembles that of mild valvular pulmonic stenosis (symmetric midsystolic murmur virtually ending before A_2, with P_2 clearly evident and only slightly delayed).

Radiation is characteristically upward and to the left, and when loud the murmur is heard in the suprasternal notch and at the base of the neck, particularly on the left. The length and configuration of the murmur are useful signs of the degree of pulmonic obstruction. The greater the obstruction, the longer the duration of RV ejection and the longer the murmur (see Fig. 10-6A). The lengths of RV and LV ejection can be compared by relating the end of the pulmonic stenotic murmur (a right-sided event) to the timing of A_2 (a left-sided event).[4] A soft, symmetric midsystolic murmur that ends before both A_2 and P_2 is a feature of mild pulmonic stenosis (see Fig. 10-6B). A loud, asymmetric, kite-shaped murmur that peaks in late systole and extends well beyond A_2 but finishes before a delayed, soft P_2 is a feature of severe pulmonic stenosis. All gradations in between can occur. The long, asymmetric midsystolic murmur of severe pulmonic stenosis is sometimes mistaken for the holosystolic murmur of ventricular septal defect, especially when P_2 is inaudible and when A_2 is buried in the murmur. These features are especially misleading when the murmur is maximal in the third left intercostal space. Careful attention to S_2 can resolve this problem if inspiration renders P_2 audible by moving it away from the end of the holosystolic murmur of ventricular septal defect.

Dilatation of the aortic root or pulmonary trunk is often accompanied by soft, short, midsystolic murmurs. Such murmurs occur, for example, with the aortic root dilatation of Marfan's syndrome or of syphilis in the left heart, and with idiopathic dilatation of the pulmonary trunk or pulmonary hypertension in the right. In ostium secundum atrial septal defect, rapid flow across the pulmonic valve into a dilated pulmonary trunk generates a typical midsystolic murmur. Midsystolic murmurs are also generated by rapid ejection into a normal aortic root or pulmonary trunk, as in anemia, pregnancy, fever, or thyrotoxicosis. Accelerated LV ejection in pure aortic regurgitation results in a midsystolic murmur that may be surprisingly loud (see Fig. 10-18).

Most people, if not all, have innocent or normal murmurs at some time during their lives. A list of these follows:

INNOCENT SYSTOLIC MURMURS
Vibratory systolic murmur (Still's murmur)
Pulmonic systolic murmur (pulmonary trunk)
Peripheral pulmonic systolic murmur (pulmonary branches)
Supraclavicular or brachiocephalic systolic murmur
Systolic mammary souffle
Aortic systolic murmur

INNOCENT CONTINUOUS MURMURS
Venous hum
Continuous mammary souffle

All of the six systolic murmurs except the mammary souffle are midsystolic.[4] A common form of innocent, normal midsystolic murmur is the vibratory murmur described in 1909 by George Still: a short, buzzing, pure, medium-frequency murmur that probably originates from periodic vibrations of the pulmonic leaflets at their attachments (Fig. 10-7).[8] A second innocent pulmonic midsystolic murmur that occurs in older children, adolescents, and young adults represents an exaggeration of normal ejection vibrations within the pulmonary

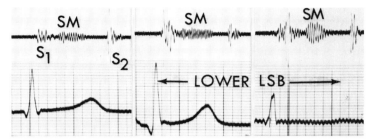

FIG. 10-7. Three innocent vibratory midsystolic murmurs (*SM*) from healthy children. The murmurs are pure in frequency, relatively brief in duration, and maximal along the lower left sternal border (*LSB*). (Perloff JK: The Clinical Recognition of Congenital Heart Disease. Philadelphia, WB Saunders, 1979)

trunk.[4] In contrast to the vibratory midsystolic murmur of Still, the pulmonic midsystolic murmur is relatively impure (Fig. 10-8). A similar innocent midsystolic murmur occurs in thin patients with diminished anteroposterior chest dimensions (loss of thoracic kyphosis, for example) because of the proximity of the pulmonary trunk to the chest wall.[9] Innocent supraclavicular systolic murmurs originate in the proximal brachiocephalic arteries. They may radiate to below the clavicles but are always louder above the clavicles (Fig. 10-9).[4] The

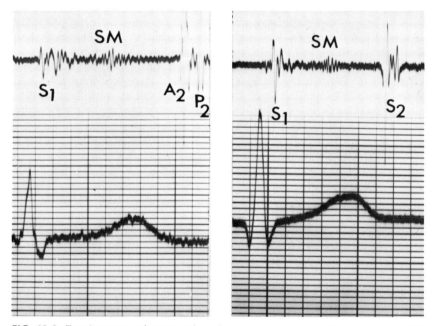

FIG. 10-8. Two innocent pulmonic midsystolic murmurs in normal children age 8 and 11 years. The tracings were recorded from the second left intercostal space. The murmurs are brief in duration, midsystolic, and relatively impure in frequency. (Perloff JK: The Clinical Recognition of Congenital Heart Disease. Philadelphia, WB Saunders, 1979)

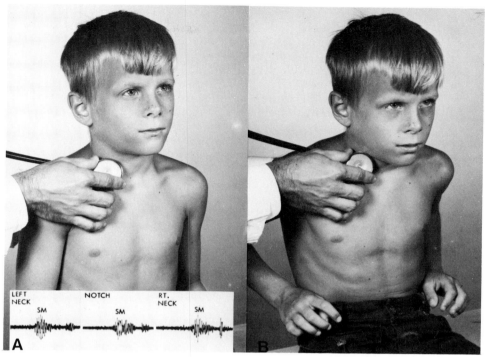

FIG. 10-9. (*A*) The phonocardiographic insert records innocent supraclavicular systolic murmurs in the left neck, suprasternal notch, and the right neck. The photograph shows the stethoscopic bell applied to the right supraclavicular fossa while the patient sits with shoulders relaxed and arms in front of the chest. (*B*) When the elbows are brought well behind the back (hyperextension of the shoulders), the murmur typically disappears or diminishes. (Perloff JK: The Physical Examination of the Heart and Circulation. Philadelphia, WB Saunders, 1982)

commonest form of innocent midsystolic murmur in adults beyond middle age is the aortic sclerotic murmur, which is at the benign end of a spectrum that has dense calcific aortic stenosis at the other end (see Fig. 10-4).

HOLOSYSTOLIC MURMURS

Holosystolic murmurs are generated by flow from a chamber or vessel whose pressure or resistance throughout systole is higher than the pressure or resistance of the chamber or vessel receiving the flow (see Fig. 10-2). Prototypical holosystolic murmurs in the left heart are caused by mitral regurgitation,[10] in the right heart by tricuspid regurgitation,[3] between the ventricles by ventricular septal defects,[4] and between aortic root and pulmonary trunk by aorticopulmonary window or, less commonly, by pulmonary hypertensive patent ductus.[4] The timing of holosystolic murmurs within the framework established by S_1 and S_2 reflects the physiologic and anatomical mechanisms responsible for their production (Fig. 10-10). LV pressure exceeds left atrial (LA) pressure at the very onset of systole, so that in some forms of mitral incompetence, regurgitant flow and murmur commence with S_1. The murmur then persists up to or slightly beyond A_2, provided the mitral valve remains incompetent and the LV pressure at end-systole exceeds LA pressure. When the regurgitant stream is directed posterolaterally within the LA cavity, the murmur radiates into the axilla, to the angle of the left scapula and, occasionally, to the vertebral column, with bone conduction from the cervical to the lumbar spine.[10] When the regurgitant stream is directed forward and medially against the atrial septum (near the base of the aorta), the murmur radiates to the left sternal edge and base, and even into the neck.[10] It is important to underscore that the murmur of mitral regurgitation is not always holosystolic, but can be midsystolic (see above), early systolic, or late systolic (see below).

The holosystolic murmur of high-pressure tricuspid regurgitation (elevated RV systolic pressure) occurs for reasons analogous to those just described for the holosystolic murmur of mitral regurgitation.[11] An inspiratory increase in loudness (Carvallo's sign) is a feature of recognized diagnostic importance. Occasionally, the tricuspid murmur is audible *only* during inspiration. Amplification occurs because the inspiratory increase in RV volume is converted into an increase in the stroke volume and velocity of regurgitant flow. When the right ventricle fails, this capacity is lost, so Carvallo's sign vanishes.

The murmur of simple, uncomplicated ventricular septal defect is holosystolic because the defect remains patent while LV systolic pressure and systemic resistance exceed RV systolic pressure and pulmonary resistance from the onset to the end of systole. A holosystolic murmur is perceived by auscultation in some patients with large aortopulmonary connections, especially aortopul-

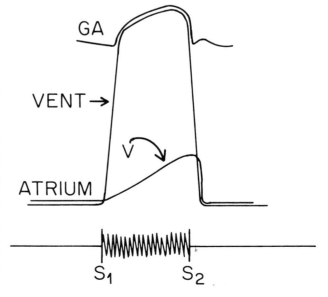

FIG. 10-10. Schematic illustration of a great arterial (*GA*), ventricular (*vent*), and atrial pressure pulse together with phonocardiogram illustrating the physiologic mechanism of holosystolic murmurs heard in some forms of mitral and tricuspid regurgitation. Ventricular pressure exceeds atrial pressure at the very onset of systole, so regurgitant flow and murmur commence with S_1. The murmur persists up to or slightly beyond S_2 since regurgitant flow persists to the end of systole (LV pressure still far exceeds left atrial pressure).

monary window, and, less commonly, large patent ductus arteriosus.[4] In these disorders, a progressive rise in pulmonary vascular resistance abolishes the diastolic portion of the continuous murmur, leaving a murmur that is holo-systolic or nearly so. There may be a short gap between S_1 and the onset of the murmur, since flow through the aortopulmonary window or ductus does not begin until after the aortic valve opens (Fig. 10-11). However, this gap tends to be imperceptible on auscultation because rapid early flow is generated by brisk LV ejection in the face of a low aortic diastolic pressure.

EARLY SYSTOLIC MURMURS

Early systolic murmurs begin with S_1, diminish in decrescendo, and end well before the subsequent S_2, generally at or before the middle of systole (see Fig. 10-2). Such murmurs are associated with certain types of mitral regurgitation, with tricuspid regurgitation and, with ventricular septal defect. Acute severe mitral regurgitation is typically accompanied by an early systolic murmur or a holosystolic decrescendo murmur that diminishes or ends before S_2 (Fig. 10-12).[12] This timing and configuration occur because regurgitation into a normal-sized and, therefore, relatively nondistensible left atrium pro-

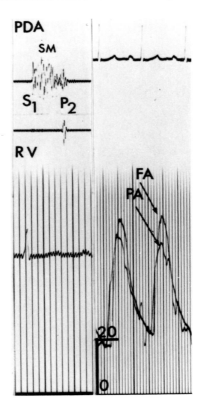

FIG. 10-11. Tracings from a 3-year-old girl with a pulmonary hypertensive patent ductus arteriosus and a 2.7 to 1, left-to-right shunt. The intracardiac microphone records a decrescendo holosystolic murmur within the lumen of the ductus (*PDA*). The right ventricle (*RV*) is silent except for P_2. The femoral arterial (*FA*) and pulmonary arterial (*PA*) pulses separate in systole but are identical in diastole. (Perloff JK: The Clinical Recognition of Congenital Heart Disease. Philadelphia, WB Saunders, 1979)

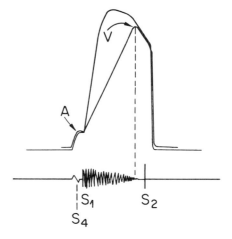

FIG. 10-12. Ventricular (*V*) and atrial (*A*) pressure pulses with schematic phonocardiogram illustrating the mechanism of the early systolic murmur of acute severe mitral regurgitation or low-pressure tricuspid regurgitation. The large V wave reaches ventricular pressure at end-systole (*upper curved arrow*), so significant regurgitant flow diminishes or ceases. Accordingly, the murmur is early systolic, decrescendo, paralleling the hemodynamic pattern of regurgitant flow.

duces a large V wave that tends to approach LV pressure in late systole; a late systolic decline in LV pressure favors this tendency. Accordingly, regurgitant flow is maximal in early systole and minimal in late systole. The murmur parallels this pattern, declining or vanishing before S_2 (see Fig. 10-12).

An early systolic murmur is also a feature of low-pressure tricuspid regurgitation—that is, tricuspid regurgitation with normal RV systolic pressure. Tricuspid valve infective endocarditis (which is associated with drug abuse) is a case in point. The mechanism responsible for the timing and configuration of this murmur is analogous to that described above for acute severe mitral regurgitation (see Fig. 10-12). Tall right atrial (RA) V waves readily reach the level of normal RV pressure in late systole, so both regurgitation and murmur are chiefly, if not exclusively, *early* systolic. Furthermore, because normal RV systolic pressure results in a comparatively low rate of regurgitant flow, the resulting murmurs are usually medium- or low-frequency murmurs, in contrast to the high-frequency holosystolic murmur of tricuspid regurgitation with *elevated* RV systolic pressure (see above).

An early systolic murmur occurs in the presence of a large ventricular septal defect when the pulmonary vascular resistance rises enough to decrease or abolish late systolic shunting. A murmur of similar timing and configuration occurs with a very small nonpulmonary hypertensive ventricular septal defect in which the communication is functionally abolished in late systole, confining the shunt to early systole (Fig. 10-13). The latter murmur is typically soft, pure, high in frequency, and sharply localized to the mid- or lower left sternal edge (see Fig. 10-13). As time goes on, this early systolic murmur may disappear altogether (spontaneous closure of the defect).

LATE SYSTOLIC MURMURS

The late systolic murmur is a hallmark of mitral valve prolapse (Fig. 10-14).[14] Typically, the leaflets are competent during early ventricular contraction but overshoot in late systole. The murmur begins in mid- to late systole,

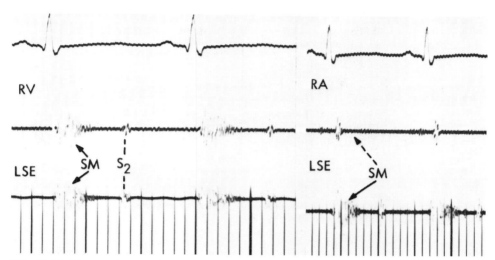

FIG. 10-13. Phonocardiograms from a 4-year-old girl with a very small ventricular septal defect and a trivial left-to-right shunt. A soft, pure, high-frequency early systolic decrescendo murmur (*SM*) is recorded within the right ventricle (*RV*) and along the lower left sternal edge (*LSE*). When the intracardiac microphone was withdrawn into the right atrium (*RA*) the murmur vanished. (Perloff JK: The Clinical Recognition of Congenital Heart Disease. Philadelphia, WB Saunders, 1979)

and rises in crescendo to A_2. One or more mid- to late systolic clicks often precede the murmur. Mitral regurgitation occurs because prolapse is sufficient to disrupt leaflet apposition in late systole. Physical maneuvers that diminish LV volume (prompt standing after squatting or Valsalva's maneuver, for example) increase the degree of prolapse, enhance the audibility of the murmur, and result in earlier prolapse and a murmur of earlier onset (Fig. 10-15). Physical maneuvers that increase LV volume (squatting or sustained hand grip, for example) have the opposite effects.[14] Pharmacologic interventions that variably alter LV volume produce analogous results but are less practical at the bedside than simple physical maneuvers. In an occasional patient with mitral valve prolapse, a striking late systolic whoop or honk is intermittently heard, either spontaneously or in response to physical or pharmacologic interventions.[14] The murmur is high in frequency, musical, widely transmitted, and occasionally loud enough to be sensed by the patient. The musical whoop is thought to

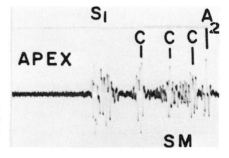

FIG. 10-14. Phonocardiogram from the cardiac apex in a patient with mid- to late systolic clicks (*C*) and a late systolic murmur (*SM*) of mitral valve prolapse. A_2 = aortic component of S_2.

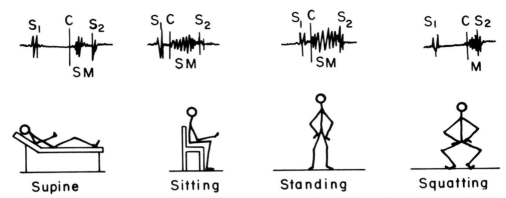

FIG. 10-15. Postural changes affecting the auscultatory signs of mitral valve prolapse. Sitting or standing causes the systolic click to move closer to S_1, so the murmur is prolonged. On squatting, the click moves toward S_2 and the murmur becomes shorter though later. The converse is the case with prompt standing. (Devereux RB, Perloff JK, Reichek N, et al: Mitral valve prolapse. Circulation 54:3, 1976. By permission of the American Heart Association, Inc.)

arise from mitral leaflets and chordae set into high-frequency vibration. Maneuvers as simple as sitting, leaning forward, or prompt standing may convert a simple late systolic murmur into the distinctive, and sometimes disconcerting, whoop.

SYSTOLIC ARTERIAL MURMURS

Extracardiac systolic arterial murmurs originate in either systemic or pulmonary arteries. Detection requires careful auscultation at nonprecordial sites, although such murmurs are occasionally heard over the precordium as well. Systolic arterial murmurs are due to such anatomic abnormalities in an artery as tortuosity or luminal narrowing or to increased flow through normal arteries.[15,16] The rise and decline of pulsatile flow generally imparts a crescendo-descrescendo shape to the murmur. Although configuration and duration are important, timing with S_1 and S_2 is necessarily imprecise, since the murmurs originate at variable distances downstream from the heart.

The most common cause of a systolic arterial murmur is peripheral vascular disease (narrowing) of carotid, subclavian, or ileofemoral arteries. The systolic murmur over the site of coarctation of the aortic isthmus (midthoracic spine between the scapulae) is another case in point.[4] An example of a systolic arterial murmur caused by increased flow through normal, nonobstructed vessels is the systolic "mammary souffle," an innocent murmur heard during late pregnancy and in the early postpartal period.[17] Such murmurs may be systolic or continuous. Another innocent systolic arterial murmur is the "supraclavicular murmur," which is heard in normal children and adolescents (see Fig. 10-9).[18] The configuration is crescendo-decrescendo, the onset abrupt, and the duration brief. At times, the intensity is disconcertingly loud. These murmurs originate within major brachiocephalic arteries, probably near their aortic origins. Loud supraclavicular systolic murmurs radiate below the clavicles, but invariably with attenuation. The murmurs can be made to decrease or vanish by simple hyperextension of the shoulders, that is, by bringing the elbows behind the back until the muscles of the shoulder girdle are taut (see Fig. 10-9).[4]

In the lesser circulation, systolic arterial murmurs are caused by congenital stenosis of the pulmonary artery and its branches or, more rarely, by luminal narrowing following pulmonary embolism.[15] In addition, innocent pulmonic arterial systolic murmurs are sometimes heard in newborn infants because the anatomical arrangements at birth set the stage for turbulence caused by a temporary drop in systolic pressure from the pulmonary trunk to its branches.[19] These pulmonary arterial systolic murmurs disappear with maturation of the pulmonary bed within the first few weeks or months of life.

MANEUVERS TO DIAGNOSE SYSTOLIC MURMURS

Physical maneuvers are routinely used during auscultation of systolic murmurs.[20] Respiration is employed in the form of normal breathing; exaggerated excursions; full held expiration; occasionally, full held inspiration; and Valsalva's maneuver. Normal breathing or exaggerated excursions improve analysis of both the early systolic and holosystolic murmurs of tricuspid regurgitation. These murmurs increase during inspiration, provided that the right ventricle can increase its stroke volume and regurgitant flow. Full held expiration with firm pressure of the diaphragm applied to the second left intercostal space dramatically reinforces the pulmonic midsystolic murmur associated with loss of thoracic kyphosis (straight back). Valsalva's maneuver is, in many respects, an exaggeration of expiration and inspiration. Straining, by reducing LV volume, serves to exaggerate the degree of mitral valve prolapse, causing the click(s) to come earlier and the murmur to be longer. In hypertrophic obstructive cardiomyopathy, the decrease in LV volume during straining exaggerates the LV–aortic gradient and the systolic murmur, whereas release of the Valsalva maneuver has the opposite effect.

Positions that are useful in the analysis of systolic murmurs include the left lateral decubitus, sitting upright, sitting and leaning forward, squatting followed by prompt standing, supine with passive elevation of the legs, prone with the trunk elevated on elbows and knees, and certain special positions of the head and neck and of the shoulders and arms. A few examples suffice. The presence of premature ventricular beats in the left lateral decubitus may assist in distinguishing an apical midsystolic murmur caused by LV outflow from a murmur of the same configuration caused by mitral regurgitation (in the first case, the beat following the compensatory pause is amplified, in the second, it remains unchanged). Squatting and prompt standing are done together and in that sequence. Squatting, by increasing resistance to LV discharge, increases the loudness of most murmurs of mitral regurgitation; prompt standing has the opposite effect. Squatting also results in a transient increase in LV volume, so that mitral valve prolapse lessens in degree and the click(s) are delayed; the late systolic murmur shortens and may vanish, but what remains is louder (Fig. 10-15).Prompt standing causes prolapse to increase, so that the click(s) and late systolic murmur occur earlier, are generally more obvious, and are occasionally converted into a prominent systolic whoop or honk. Other maneuvers that reduce LV volume may provoke the systolic whoop, but none is more effective than prompt standing. In hypertrophic obstructive cardiomyopathy, the increase in LV volume with squatting serves to reduce the gradient and decrease the loudness of the systolic murmur, while prompt standing has the opposite effect. A pericardial rub is sometimes best heard when auscultation is performed with the patient supine and resting on elbows and knees to raise the trunk comfortably above the bed or examining table. Pericardial rubs occasionally are mistaken for intracardiac murmurs, generally systolic, and especially midsystolic murmurs. Diagnosis is simplest when all three phases are present (systolic, mid-diastolic and late diastolic (presystolic). The elbow-knee position is designed to promote apposition between visceral and parietal pericardium and may improve audibility of the diastolic components of a rub, thus allowing an isolated systolic component to be distinguished from a midsystolic murmur. The shoulder and arm maneuvers useful in assessing supraclavicular systolic murmurs are illustrated in Figure 10-9.

Exercise, both isotonic and isometric, serves a useful purpose in the evaluation of systolic murmurs. Isotonic exercise, by increasing the heart rate and the volume and rate of flow, improves the audibility of outflow systolic murmurs (aortic or pulmonic). Isometric exercise (sustained hand grip) provokes an increase in resistance to LV discharge by increasing systemic vascular resistance and arterial pressure. Accordingly, mitral valve prolapse lessens, and the systolic click(s) and murmur appear later. The murmur may become louder, as in other forms of mitral regurgitation. In hypertrophic obstructive cardiomyopathy, the gradient and murmur lessen in response to hand grip.

Physiology and Clinical Manifestations of Diastolic Murmurs

Diastolic murmurs are descriptively classified according to their time of onset as early diastolic, mid-diastolic, or late diastolic (presystolic) (Fig. 10-16). An early diastolic murmur starts with A_2 or P_2, depending on its site of origin. A mid-diastolic murmur begins at a clear interval after S_2. A late diastolic murmur is located immediately before S_1 (presystolic).

EARLY DIASTOLIC MURMERS

The prototype of the early diastolic murmur originating in the left heart is aortic regurgitation. The murmur begins at the time of A_2, that is, as soon as LV systolic pressure falls below aortic root pressure. The murmur is generally decrescendo, mirroring the progressive decline in volume and rate from regurgitant flow during the course of diastole. The high velocity of regurgitation generates a high-frequency blowing murmur that is occasionally musical when incompetence results from an everted cusp (Fig. 10-17). In some

EARLY DIASTOLIC

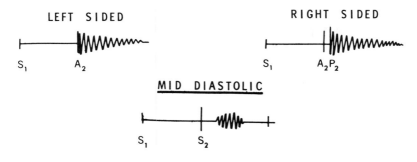

LEFT SIDED   RIGHT SIDED

MID DIASTOLIC

LATE DIASTOLIC (PRESYSTOLIC)

LEFT SIDED   RIGHT SIDED

FIG. 10-16. Diastolic murmurs classified according to their time of onset as early diastolic, mid-diastolic, or late diastolic (presystolic). Diastolic murmurs originate in the left heart (left-sided) or right heart (right-sided).

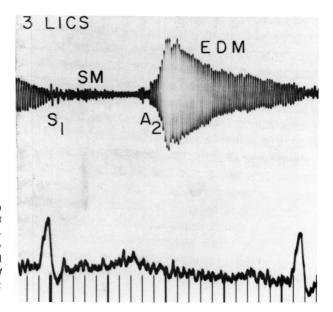

FIG. 10-17. Phonocardiogram in the third left intercostal space (*3 LICS*) records a pure, high-frequency musical decrescendo early diastolic murmur (*EDM*) associated with eversion of an aortic cusp. *SM* = midsystolic murmur. A_2 = aortic component of S_2.

patients with chronic free aortic regurgitation, the murmur begins with a short crescendo followed by a longer decrescendo (Fig. 10-18). The murmur tends to diminish or end before the next S_1, especially when aortic diastolic pressure is low enough to approach LV pressure toward the end of diastole. However, in mild to moderate chronic aortic regurgitation, the aortic diastolic pressure consistently exceeds LV pressure, so the murmur, though decrescendo, tends to last throughout diastole. Faint, high-frequency murmurs of aortic regurgitation are difficult to hear and must be specifically sought by applying firm pressure of the stethoscopic diaphragm at the midleft sternal border while the patient sits, relaxes, leans forward, and holds the breath in full exhalation. Soft or equivocal murmurs increase in intensity when squatting or a sustained hand grip temporarily raises aortic root pressure. Direction and radiation of the diastolic murmur of aortic regurgitation should be determined by comparative auscultation along the left and right sternal borders, especially at the level of the third intercostal space.[21] Selective radiation of the murmur to the right sternal edge suggests aortic root dilatation.

The murmur of acute severe aortic regurgitation (biscuspid valve infective endocarditis, dissecting aneurysm, etc.) differs in important respects from the murmur of chronic severe aortic regurgitation.[22] The length (duration) of the murmur is relatively short because of early equilibrium of aortic diastolic pressure with the steeply rising diastolic pressure in the left ventricle. The pitch or frequency of the murmur is generally medium and impure because the velocity of regurgitant flow is less rapid than in chronic severe aortic regurgitation. In addition, this short, medium-frequency diastolic murmur may be surprisingly soft (Grade II/VI). These features are in contrast to the conspic-

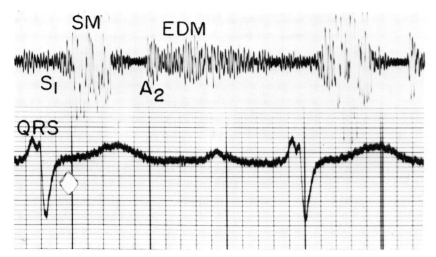

FIG. 10-18. Phonocardiogram in the second right intercostal space in a patient with pure chronic severe aortic regurgitation. S_1 is soft because the P–R interval is long. There is a relatively loud but short midsystolic murmur (*SM*) due to rapid ejection across the aortic valve. The early diastolic murmur (*EDM*) of aortic regurgitation begins with the aortic component (A_2) of S_2, commencing with a short crescendo followed by a longer decrescendo.

uous, long, pure, high-frequency blowing diastolic murmur of chronic severe aortic regurgitation (Fig. 10-18).

The prototypical early diastolic murmur in the *right* heart is generated by pulmonary regurgitation due to pulmonary hypertension.[11] The Graham Steell murmur begins with a loud P_2 because the elevated pressure exerted on the incompetent valve begins at the moment that RV pressure drops below the pressure in the pulmonary trunk. Steell observed, "When the second sound is reduplicated, the murmur proceeds from its latter part"[23] (Fig. 10-19). The increased diastolic pressure causes high-velocity regurgitant flow and results in a high-frequency blowing murmur that may last throughout diastole. The basic configuration of the murmur is decrescendo, although, occasionally, the amplitude may be relatively uniform throughout diastole. At times, the murmur may begin with a short crescendo. The problem of how the murmur may be distinguished from that of aortic regurgitation was underscored by Steell. Even today, differentiation may be difficult or impossible when the murmur is soft and the systemic arterial pulse is normal.[23] Differentiation, if made, depends upon the clinical setting rather than on auscultation.

MID-DIASTOLIC MURMURS

Mid-diastolic murmurs typically occur across mitral or tricuspid valves because of atrioventricular (AV) valve obstruction or abnormal patterns of AV flow, or across an incompetent pulmonic valve in the presence of normal

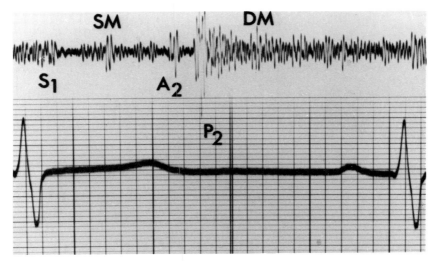

FIG. 10-19. Phonocardiogram in the second left intercostal space from a 26-year-old woman with patent ductus arteriosus, suprasystemic pulmonary vascular resistance, and reversed shunt. There is a midsystolic murmur (*SM*) into a dilated pulmonary trunk. An early diastolic Graham Steell murmur (*DM*) begins with a loud, delayed pulmonic component (*P₂*) of S₂. (Perloff JK: The Clinical Recognition of Congenital Heart Disease. Philadelphia, WB Saunders, 1979)

pulmonary arterial pressure (see Fig. 10-16). The mid-diastolic murmur of mitral stenosis provides a useful point of departure.[24] This murmur may be present with atrial fibrillation or sinus rhythm and characteristically follows the opening snap (Fig. 10-20). The murmur must be deliberately sought by placing the bell of the stethoscope lightly against the skin over the LV impulse with the patient in the left lateral decubitus position. Because the murmur originates in the cavity of the left ventricle, transmission to the chest is maximal at the site where the left ventricle is palpated. The duration of the mid-diastolic murmur in atrial fibrillation is a useful sign of the degree of mitral stenosis because a murmur that lasts up to S_1 implies a persistent gradient at the end of diastole.[25] A faint or doubtful murmur can be reinforced when the heart rate is transiently increased by a maneuver as simple as several vigorous coughs. In tricuspid stenosis, a mid-diastolic murmur typically occurs with atrial fibrillation but not, as a rule, with sinus rhythm.[26] This tricuspid murmur differs from the mitral mid-diastolic murmur in two important respects: Loudness selectively increases during inspiration, and the sound is localized to a relatively limited area along the left sternal edge. The tricuspid murmur originates within the RV cavity and is transmitted to the overlying left sternal border. The inspiratory increase in loudness occurs because inspiration results in augmented RA volume, a fall in RV diastolic pressure, and a parallel increase in the gradient and flow rate across the tricuspid valve.[26]

Mid-diastolic murmurs also occur across normal AV valves in the presence of increases in the volume and velocity of flow. Such murmurs are generated

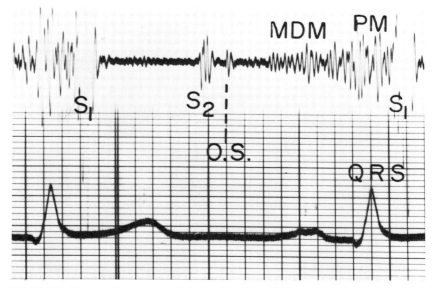

FIG. 10-20. Phonocardiogram recorded over the LV impulse in a patient with pure, severe, rheumatic mitral stenosis. S_1 is very loud. There is no murmur in systole. S_2 is followed by a close opening snap (*OS*) after which a mid-diastolic murmur (*MDM*) and a presystolic murmur (*PM*) occur.

across the mitral valve in patients with ventricular septal defect, patent ductus arteriosus, or pure mitral regurgitation, for example, and across the tricuspid valve in ostium secundum atrial septal defect or tricuspid regurgitation (Fig. 10-21).[4,27] These mid-diastolic murmurs are typically short and medium-pitched, tend to occur with large shunts or marked AV valve incompetence, and are often preceded by an S_3, especially in the presence of mitral or tricuspid regurgitation. When atrial contraction coincides with the phase of rapid diastolic filling, as in complete heart block, flow is augmented, so short, mid-diastolic murmurs sometimes occur. Mid-diastolic AV murmurs are believed to result from antegrade flow across a valve that is closing rapidly because of simultaneous filling of the recipient ventricle. A similar mechanism has been proposed for the Austin Flint murmur, which may be mid-diastolic, or pre-systolic as Flint originally described (see below).[28,29]

The mid-diastolic murmur of low-pressure pulmonary regurgitation (*i.e.*, without pulmonary hypertension) occurs when there is a congenital or acquired anatomical derangement of the valve itself. The congenital derangement varies from a minor structural fault to complete absence of the valve.[4] Acquired defects most commonly follow pulmonic valve infective endocarditis (Fig. 10-22) or surgical repair of an obstructed RV outflow tract. A low diastolic pressure in the pulmonary trunk results in a low rate of regurgitant flow so that the accompanying murmur is low- to medium-pitched. The murmur typically begins at a perceptible interval after P_2, is crescendo-decrescendo in configuration, and ends well before the subsequent S_1.[4] The timing can be understood when simultaneous pulmonary arterial and RV pressure pulses are examined

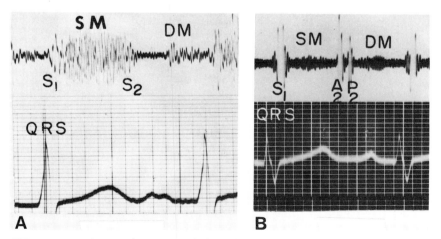

FIG. 10-21. (A) Phonocardiogram recorded over the LV impulse in a patient with a ventricular septal defect with large left-to-right shunt holosystolic murmur (*SM*) and augmented flow across the mitral valve generating a mid-diastolic (*DM*) murmur. (B) Phonocardiogram from the fourth left intercostal space, left sternal edge in a patient with a large left-to-right shunt ostium secundum atrial septal defect. After a relatively loud S_1, there is a soft midsystolic murmur (*SM*) followed by fixed splitting of S_2 (A_2, P_2). Augmented flow across the tricuspid valve generates a soft but distinct mid-diastolic murmur *DM*).

FIG.   10-22. Phonocardiogram
from the third left intercostal space
in a 21-year-old woman with pulmonic valve infective endocarditis
as a result of heroin abuse. A medium-frequency mid-diastolic murmur (*DM*) follows S_2 by a clear interval. The murmur ends well before
the subsequent S_1.

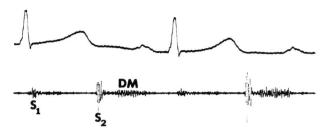

(Fig. 10-23). The onset of the murmur is delayed because regurgitant flow is minimal at the time of P_2, the diastolic pressure exerted on the incompetent valve at that instant is negligible. Regurgitation then accelerates as RV pressure dips below the diastolic pressure in the pulmonary trunk, and, at that point, the murmur reaches its maximum (see Fig. 10-23). Equilibration of pulmonary arterial and RV pressures in diastole eliminates regurgitant flow and abolishes the murmur prior to the next S_1. When P_2 is late, soft, or absent, an even more conspicuous gap exists between A_2 and the onset of the pulmonary diastolic murmur. Thus, the murmur of low-pressure pulmonary regurgitation is mid-diastolic and medium in frequency.

LATE DIASTOLIC MURMURS

Late diastolic or presystolic murmurs occur during the period of late (active) ventricular filling that follows atrial contraction (see Fig. 10-16). At normal heart rates, the murmurs are therefore presystolic and imply sinus rhythm. They originate at either the mitral or tricuspid orifice, usually because of obstruction, but occasionally because of abnormal patterns of presystolic AV flow.

The most representative presystolic murmur accompanies mitral stenosis in sinus rhythm because AV flow is augmented by atrial systole (see Figs. 10-20 and 10-24A).[24] However, a significant contributory cause of the presystolic crescendo is contraction of the left ventricle in the face of end-diastolic flow across the stenotic mitral valve. Therefore, such a murmur is sometimes heard in atrial fibrillation, especially during short cycle lengths. The technique for eliciting or reinforcing the presystolic murmur is the same as that for the mitral mid-diastolic murmur described above. In tricuspid stenosis with sinus rhythm, the presystolic murmur characteristically occurs with absent or trivial mid-diastolic vibrations (see Fig. 10-24B). The presystolic timing of the murmur corresponds with maximal antegrade flow and gradient, which may be negligible until the moment of RA contraction. The murmur is crescendo-decrescendo in shape, usually rather discrete, fading in decrescendo toward S_1, in contrast to the presystolic murmur of mitral stenosis, which tends to rise in crescendo to S_1 (see Fig. 10-24A). The most valuable auscultatory sign of tricuspid stenosis in sinus rhythm is the effect of respiration on the loudness of the presystolic murmur. During inspiration, RA volume increases, provoking an increase in RA contractile force while RV end-diastolic pressure falls. The

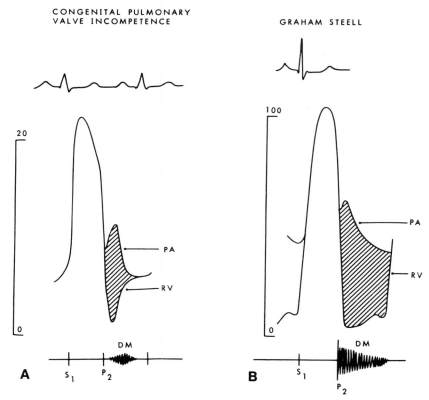

FIG. 10-23. (*A*) In congenital pulmonary valve regurgitation, a relatively low pressure is exerted against the incompetent valve; the murmur (*DM*) begins shortly after the RV and pulmonary arterial (*PA*) pressure pulses diverge and is loudest when the diastolic gradient (*crosshatched area*) is maximal (note the early diastolic dip in the RV pulse). Equilibration of the pulmonary arterial and RV pressures in latter diastole eliminates the regurgitant gradient and abolishes the murmur. (*B*) In the presence of pulmonary hypertension, a relatively high pressure is exerted against the incompetent pulmonic valve. The large regurgitant gradient (*crosshatched area*) diminishes during the course of diastole, but the PA and RV pressure pulses do not equilibrate. The accompanying murmur begins early (with P_2) and is high in frequency, decrescendo, and holodiastolic. (Perloff JK: The Clinical Recognition of Congenital Heart Disease. Philadelphia, WB Saunders, 1979)

result is a larger gradient, a more rapid velocity of flow, and an increase in the intensity of the presystolic murmur (see Fig. 10-24B).

Obstruction at the mitral or tricuspid orifice generally implies previous rheumatic fever, or, less commonly, congenital stenosis. Myxomas of either right or left atrium occasionally cause both mid-diastolic and presystolic murmurs that resemble mitral or tricuspid stenosis. In this setting, the "tumor plop" may be mistaken for an opening snap.

Late diastolic murmurs that occur because of abnormal patterns of presystolic AV flow occasionally result from large left-to-right shunts. Ostium secundum

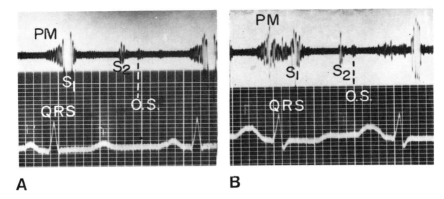

A   **B**

FIG. 10-24. (A) Phonocardiogram recorded over the LV impulse in a patient with mitral stenosis. There is a typical crescendo presystolic murmur (*PM*) maximal just before a loud S$_1$. After the opening snap (*OS*) there is virtually no mid-diastolic murmur. (*B*) Phonocardiogram recorded at the fourth left intercostal space in a patient with rheumatic tricuspid stenosis. The presystolic murmur (*PM*) is crescendo-decrescendo, fading before S$_1$. The first cycle is during inspiration, so the presystolic murmur is prominent. During expiration (*second cycle*) the murmur is soft. The OS is mitral.

atrial septal defect with increased tricuspid valve flow is an example, although the murmurs associated with this defect are usually mid-diastolic (see above).[4] Short, crescendo-decrescendo diastolic murmurs may follow atrial contraction in complete heart block, appearing sometimes in presystole but generally in middiastole, when flow during the passive filling phase is augmented by atrial contraction. The Austin Flint murmur was described in 1862 as "presystolic blubbering."[29]

Since late diastolic (presystolic) murmurs tend to be relatively low or medium in frequency, auscultation should be conducted with light pressure of the bell of the stethoscope. Presystolic murmurs originating across the mitral valve are best detected over the LV impulse when the patient turns into the left lateral decubitus position. Presystolic murmurs across the tricuspid valve are best detected with the patient supine while the examiner applies the stethoscope to the lower left sternal edge, moving the bell locally in search of the murmur.

The classic pericardial rub in sinus rhythm is triple-phased, that is, midsystolic, mid-diastolic, and late diastolic (presystolic). The systolic component of the rub is the most consistent, followed by the presystolic. In atrial fibrillation, the rub is, at best, double-phased (systolic and mid-diastolic); the presystolic component vanishes. The diagnosis of a rub is least secure (and is often impossible) when only a single phase remains—generally the midsystolic but occasionally the presystolic.

MANEUVERS TO AID IN DIAGNOSING DIASTOLIC MURMURS

Physical maneuvers are routinely used during auscultation of diastolic murmurs.[20] Respiration employs normal breathing or exaggerated excursions. The mid-diastolic and presystolic murmurs of tricuspid stenosis (right-sided) are augmented during inspiration. The soft, early diastolic murmur of aortic regurgitation or pulmonary hypertensive pulmonary regurgitation is enhanced with full held expiration or with sitting or leaning forward. Changing to the left lateral decubitus not only permits identification of an LV impulse as an important site for auscultation, but also serves transiently to accelerate the heart rate. Light pressure of the bell of the stethoscope over the LV impulse just after the patient turns into the left lateral position improves audibility of the mid-diastolic and presystolic murmurs of mitral stenosis. Repeated vigorous coughing reinforces this augmentation. Squatting, by increasing resistance to LV discharge, increases the intensity of the diastolic murmur of aortic regurgitation.

Isotonic exercise accelerates the heart rate and the volume and rate of flow and improves audibility of inflow diastolic murmurs (mitral or tricuspid). Isometric exercise (sustained hand grip), by provoking an increase in resistance to LV discharge, reinforces the soft, early diastolic murmur of aortic regurgitation.

Physiology and Clinical Manifestations of Continuous Murmurs

The term "continuous" is best applied to murmurs that begin in systole and continue without interruption through the timing of S_2 into all or part of diastole (Fig. 10-25). Accordingly, a murmur need not fill both phases of the cardiac cycle to merit the term. A systolic murmur that extends into

CONTINOUS MURMURS

AORTO-PULMONARY (P.D.A.)	ARTERIAL	VENOUS

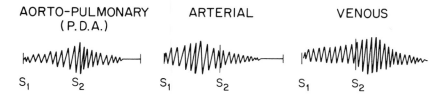

HOLOSYSTOLIC, EARLY DIASTOLIC MURMURS

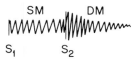

FIG. 10-25. Continuous murmurs begin in systole and continue without interruption through the timing of S_2 into all or part of diastole. Such murmurs are aortopulmonary, (such as patent ductus arteriosus [*PDA*]), arterial, or venous. Holosystolic (*SM*) plus early diastolic (*DM*) murmurs occupy all of the cardiac cycle but are two separate murmurs rather than one continuous murmur.

diastole without stopping at S_2 is also continuous, even if the murmur fades completely before the subsequent S_1. Continuous murmurs occur as blood flows from systole into diastole, without phasic interruption, from a higher to a lower pressure or resistance zone. Such murmurs are due chiefly to aortopulmonary connections, arteriovenous connections, disturbances of flow patterns in arteries, and disturbances of flow patterns in veins.

PATENT DUCTUS ARTERIOSUS

The aortopulmonary continuous murmur that first comes to mind is the typical murmur of patent ductus arteriosus. The murmur characteristically peaks just before and after S_2 and is soft or absent before and after S_1 (Figure 10-26). In 1900, George Anderson Gibson provided an accurate, meticulous description. The ductus murmur, he wrote, "persists through the second heart sound and dies away gradually during the long pause. The murmur is rough and thrilling. It begins softly and increases in intensity so as to reach its acme just about or immediately after the incidence of the second sound, and from that point gradually wanes until its termination."[30] Alterations in the differences in vascular resistance between greater and lesser circulations influence the length of the continuous murmur of patent ductus arteriosus.[11] An

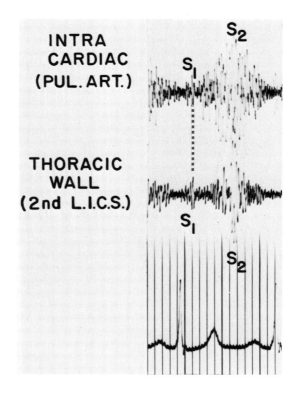

FIG. 10-26. Simultaneous intrapulmonary and thoracic wall phonocardiograms from a 7-year-old girl with patent ductus arteriosus, normal pulmonary arterial pressure, and a 2-to-1, left-to-right shunt. In the words of Gibson, the murmur "begins softly and increases in intensity so as to reach its acme just about, or immediately after the incidence of the second heart sound, and from that point gradually wanes until its termination."[1] (Perloff JK: The Clinical Recognition of Congenital Heart Disease, Philadelphia, WB Saunders, 1979)

increase in pulmonary vascular resistance causes the diastolic pressure in the pulmonary artery to approach and then to reach systemic levels, diminishing and finally abolishing diastolic flow. The diastolic portion of the continuous murmur shortens and finally disappears altogether, leaving the murmur confined to systole (see Fig. 10-11). As systolic flow across the ductus diminishes and is ultimately abolished, the systolic portion of the murmur shortens and finally disappears, leaving the ductus silent. It is noteworthy that because aortopulmonary septal defect is generally associated with pulmonary vascular resistance that is high enough to eliminate the diastolic component of the continuous murmur, a continuous murmur is relatively uncommon. Surgically produced aortopulmonary connections (Blalock, Waterston, or Pott's shunts) result in murmurs resembling those of patent ductus arteriosus (see Fig. 10-27), and the effect of pulmonary hypertension on their lengths is analogous.

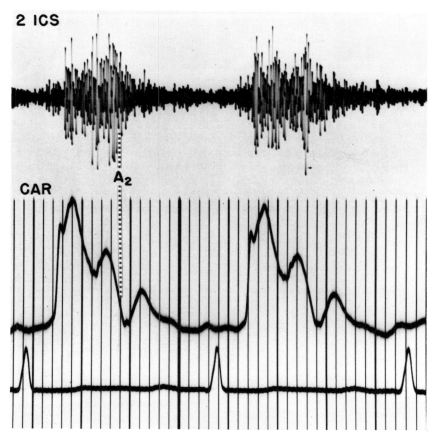

FIG. 10-27. Phonocardiogram in the second left intercostal space (*2 ICS*) in a patient with a left Blalock-Taussig anastomosis. The continuous murmur begins in systole, rises to a peak just before A₂ and diminishes during the course of diastole. The murmur is punctuated by eddy sounds. *CAR* = carotid pulse showing a bisferiens contour.

ARTERIOVENOUS FISTULAE

Continuous murmurs due to arteriovenous connections can stem from such congenital or acquired disorders as systemic arteriovenous fistulae, coronary arterial fistulae (Fig. 10-28), anomalous origin of the left coronary artery from the pulmonary trunk, communication from a sinus of Valsalva aneurysm to the right heart (Fig. 10-29) and so on.[4] The configuration, location, and intensity of continuous murmurs such as these vary considerably. For example, when a congenital coronary arterial fistula enters the right ventricle, contraction of that chamber may compress the fistula, causing the murmur to become either softer or louder in systole, depending upon the degree of compression (see Fig. 10-28). With ruptured aneurysm of a sinus of Valsalva, the continuous murmur does not peak before and after S_2, but tends to be louder in either systole or diastole, sometimes creating a to-and-fro impression (see Fig. 10-29). The continuous murmur of a systemic arteriovenous fistula can be obliterated by local compression (when the fistula is small) or by selective compression of the afferent artery. A common cause of such a murmur is the surgically produced forearm arteriovenous connection used for chronic renal dialysis.

OTHER CAUSES OF CONTINUOUS MURMURS

Continuous murmurs are occasionally due to disturbances of flow patterns in constricted systemic or pulmonary arteries when a significant continuous difference in pressure exists between the two sides of the narrowed segment. A common cause is critical obstruction of a large brachiocephalic or ileofemoral artery in a patient with atherosclerotic peripheral vascular disease. A less common cause is coarctation of the aorta with a critically reduced lumen associated with a continuous murmur in the back over the zone of constriction

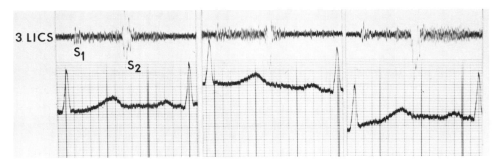

FIG. 10-28. Phonocardiograms from a 37-year-old woman with a coronary arteriovenous fistula between the right coronary artery and the outflow tract of the right ventricle. The continuous murmur is maximal in the second and third left intercostal spaces (*3 LICS*); the configuration of the murmur varies from beat to beat. (*A*) the murmur is symmetrical in shape and peaks around S_2. (*B*) The murmur is louder in systole. (*C*) The murmur is louder in diastole. (Perloff JK: The Clinical Recognition of Congenital Heart Disease. Philadelphia, W B Saunders 1979)

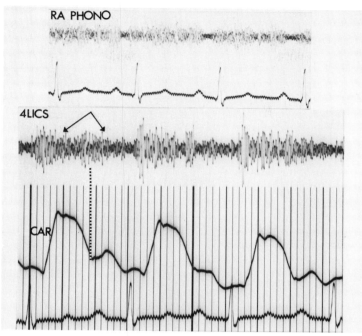

FIG. 10-29. Phonocardiograms from the right atrial cavity (*RA*) and the fourth left intercostal space (*4 LICS*) in a 17-year-old boy with ruptured sinus of Valsalva aneurysm into the right atrium. There is a continuous murmur that does *not* peak around S_2 but tends to be maximal in systole. In the thoracic wall tracing (*bottom*) the continuous murmur (*arrows*) exhibits either systolic *or* diastolic accentuation from beat to beat. *CAR* = carotid pulse. (Perloff JK: The Clinical Recognition of Congenital Heart Disease. Philadelphia, WB Saunders, 1979)

(Fig. 10-30).[4] It is well to remember that arterial continuous murmurs, especially those arising in constricted arteries, are characteristically louder in systole.

Disturbances of flow patterns in nonconstricted arteries sometimes produce continuous murmurs. Witness the continuous murmur of systemic arterial collaterals found in certain types of cyanotic congenital heart disease, such as, for example, pulmonary atresia with ventricular septal defect (Fig. 10-31).[4] These continuous murmurs must be diligently sought, since they are randomly located throughout the thorax. The *mammary souffle*, an innocent systolic murmur heard during late pregnancy and early in the postpartal period, is sometimes continuous.[17] Since this continuous murmur is arterial, it is typically louder in systole (Fig. 10-32). Maximal intensity is anywhere over either lactating breast, but there is a tendency for the murmur to be somewhat louder in the second or third right or left intercostal space. There is generally a distinct gap between S_1 and the onset of the murmur, that is, before blood ejected from the left ventricle arrives at the artery of origin. A relatively loud systolic murmur

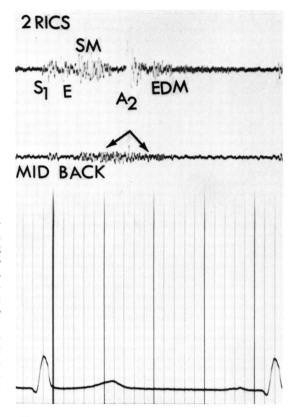

FIG. 10-30. Phonocardiograms from a 10-year-old boy with coarctation of the aorta and a bicuspid aortic valve. The tracing from midback was recorded over the site of coarctation and shows a murmur that is delayed in onset and extends well into diastole (*arrows*). In the second right intercostal space (*2 RICS*) the auscultatory signs of the bicuspid aortic valve are shown, namely, an aortic ejection sound (*E*), a short midsystolic murmur (*SM*) and an early diastolic murmur (*EDM*) of aortic regurgitation. (Perloff JK: The Clinical Recognition of Congenital Heart Disease. Philadelphia, WB Saunders, 1979)

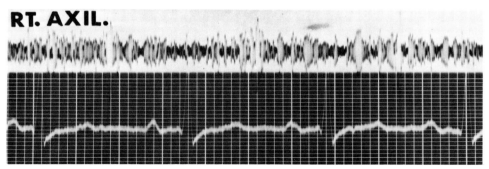

FIG. 10-31. Phonocardiogram recorded from the right axilla in a cyanotic child with pulmonary atresia and ventricular septal defect. The continuous murmur varies in intensity from beat to beat, sometimes louder in systole (*first cycle*), sometimes louder in diastole (*second cycle*).

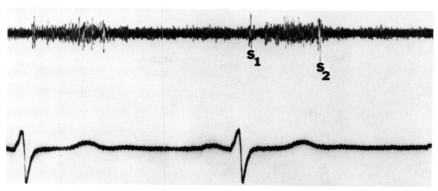

FIG. 10-32. Continuous mammary souffle at the upper left chest in a normal 26-year-old lactating woman. The murmur is continuous but louder in systole, and does *not* peak around S$_2$. (Perloff JK: The Clinical Recognition of Congenital Heart Disease. Philadelphia, W B Saunders, 1979)

continues through S$_2$ with the diastolic portion attenuated. It often fades completely before the subsequent S$_1$. The mammary souffle is best heard with the patient supine and may vanish altogether when she is in the upright position. Light pressure with the stethoscope tends to augment the murmur and bring out its continuous features, while firm pressure with the stethoscope or digital pressure peripheral to the site of auscultation serves to abolish the murmur. The loudness of the mammary souffle may vary spontaneously from day to day, from hour to hour, or from beat to beat.

A continuous murmur due to altered flow patterns in normal veins is epitomized by the cervical *venous hum* (Fig. 10-33). The hum is far and away the commonest type of innocent continuous murmur. It is probably universal in normal children and is frequently elicited in healthy young adults even in the absence of thyrotoxicosis, anemia, or pregnancy.[31] Carl Potain described the venous hum in 1867: "The thrill, which is felt by placing the finger lightly above the clavicle over the course of the vessel of the neck, is sometimes continuous and frequently intermittent; it is this last case which interests us above all here. . . . A light pressure exerted above the point of exploration can make it appear or reinforce it, while a stronger pressure extinguishes it completely, proofs positive . . . that we are concerned with a venous phenomenon and that this thrill does not arise at all from an artery."[32] To elicit the hum, the patient should be examined in the sitting position (see Fig. 10-33); the stethoscopic bell is applied to the medial aspect of the right supraclavicular fossa while the examiner's left hand grasps the patient's chin from behind and pulls it rather tautly to the left and up. The hum should then reach is maximal intensity. Occasionally, the hum may appear or increase when the chin is simply tilted up, and, at times, it is prominent without neck maneuvers and irrespective of position. Deep inspiration causes augmentation in some subjects. The hum can be reduced or abolished by a number of simple maneuvers, especially by digital compression of the ipsilateral internal jugular vein, by removing the "stretch" on the neck as the head is returned to the neutral position, by the Valsalva maneuver, or by recumbency. The simplest and most useful procedure is application of pressure to the deep jugular vein with the

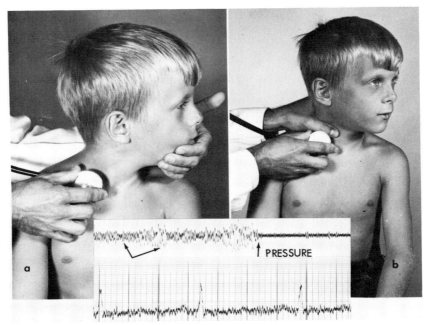

FIG. 10-33. The insert shows a typical cervical venous hum (*arrows*). The continuous murmur is louder in diastole. Digital pressure on the right internal jugular vein (*vertical arrow*) obliterates the murmur. (A) The bell of the stethoscope is applied to the medial aspect of the right supraclavicular fossa. The left hand grasps the patient's chin from behind and pulls it tautly to the left and upward. The hum is elicited. (B) This illustrates digital compression of the right internal jugular vein for obliteration of the hum. The head has returned to a more neutral position. (Perloff JK: The Clinical Recognition of Congenital Heart Disease. Philadelphia, W B Saunders, 1979)

thumb of the free hand (see Fig. 10-33B). Compression typically causes instantaneous disappearance of the hum, which suddenly but transiently intensifies as pressure is released. The term "hum" does not necessarily describe the quality of these cervical venous continuous murmurs, which may be rough, noisy, or accompanied by a high-pitched whine. Like venous continuous murmurs in general, the hum is truly continuous, though typically louder in diastole. Radiation of a loud venous hum below the clavicle invites a mistaken diagnosis of an intracardiac continuous murmur. Obliteration by digital pressure abolishes the transmitted hum and precludes error.

References

1. Freeman AR, Levine SA: The clinical significance of the systolic murmur. Ann Intern Med 6:1371, 1933
2. Soffer A, Feinstein AR, Luisada AA, et al: Glossary of cardiologic terms related to

physical diagnosis and history. I. Heart murmurs. (Bethesda Conference, Committee on Standardized Terminology). JAMA 200:1041, 1967

3. Leatham A: Auscultation of the heart. Lancet 2:703–757, 1958
4. Perloff JK: The Clinical Recognition of Congenital Heart Disease. Philadelphia, WB Saunders, 1979
5. Roberts WC, Perloff JK, Constantino T: Severe valvular aortic stenosis in patients over 65 years of age. Am J Cardiol 27:497, 1971
6. McKusick VA: Cardiovascular Sound in Health and Disease. Baltimore, Williams & Wilkins, 1958
7. Reichek N, Shelbourne JC, Perloff JK: Clinical aspects of rheumatic valvular disease. Progr Cardiovasc Dis 15:491, 1973
8. Still GF: Common Disorders and Diseases of Childhood. London, Frowde, 1909
9. De Leon AC, Perloff JK, Twigg H, et al: The straight back syndrome: clinical cardiovascular manifestations. Circulation 32:193, 1965
10. Perloff JK, Harvey WP: Auscultatory and phonocardiographic manifestations of pure mitral regurgitation. Progr Cardiovasc Dis 5:172, 1962
11. Perloff JK: Auscultatory and phonocardiographic manifestations of pulmonary hypertension. Progr Cardiovasc Dis 9:303, 1967
12. Ronan JA, Steelman RB, de Leon AC, et al: The clinical diagnosis of acute severe mitral insufficiency. Am J Cardiol 27:284, 1971
13. Rios JC, Massumi RA, Breesman WT, et al: Auscultatory features of acute tricuspid regurgitation. Am J Cardiol 23:4, 1969
14. Devereux RB, Perloff JK, Reichek N, et al: Mitral valve prolapse. Circulation 54:3, 1976
15. Perloff JK, Lebauer EJ: Auscultatory and phonocardiographic manifestations of isolated stenosis of the pulmonary artery and its branches. Br Heart J 31:314, 1969
16. Perloff JK, Caulfield WH, de Leon AC: Peripheral pulmonary artery murmur of atrial septal defect. Br Heart J 29:411, 1967
17. Tabatznik B, Randall TW, Hersch C: The mammary souffle of pregnancy and lactation. Circulation 22:1069, 1960
18. Stapleton JF, El-Hajj MM: Heart murmurs simulated by arterial bruits in the neck. Am Heart J 61:178, 1961
19. Danilowitz DA, Rudolph AM, Hoffman JIE, et al: Physiologic pressure differences between main and branch pulmonary arteries in infants. Circulation 45:410, 1972
20. Dohan MC, Criscitiello MG: Physiological and pharmacological manipulations of heart sounds and murmurs. Mod Concepts Cardiovasc Dis 39:121, 1970
21. Harvey WP, Corrado MA, Perloff JK: Right-sided murmurs of aortic insufficiency. Am J Med Sci 245:533, 1963
22. Morganroth J, Perloff JK, Zeldis SM, et al: Acute severe aortic regurgitation. Ann Intern Med 87:223, 1977
23. Steell G: Physical Signs of Cardiac Disease, 2nd Edition. Edinburgh, 1881
24. Wood P: An appreciation of mitral stenosis. Br Med J 1:1051–1113, 1954
25. Reichek N, Shelbourne JC, Perloff JK: Clinical aspects of rheumatic valvular disease. Prog Cardiovasc Dis 15:491, 1973
26. Perloff JK, Harvey WP: Clinical recognition of tricuspid stenosis. Circulation 20:346, 1960
27. Perloff JK, Harvey WP: Auscultatory and phonocardiographic manifestations of pure mitral regurgitation. Prog Cardiovasc Dis 5:172, 1962
28. Fortuin N, Craige E: On the mechanism of the Austin Flint murmur. Circulation 45:558, 1972

29. Flint A: On cardiac murmurs. Am J Med Sci 44:29, 1862
30. Gibson GA: Persistence of the arterial duct and its diagnosis. Edinburgh Medical
     Journal 8:1, 1900
31. Jones FL: Frequency, characteristics and importance of the cervical venous hum
     in adults. N Engl J Med 267:658, 1962
32. Potain PC: Des mouvements et des bruits qui se passent dans les veines juglaires.
     Bull Mem Soc Med d'hop de Paris 4:3, 1867

11

CONGESTIVE HEART FAILURE

Lawrence D. Horwitz, M.D., and E. Wayne Grogan, M.D.

Definition

Heart failure is a condition in which the ability of the heart to pump blood is inadequate to meet the metabolic needs of the body. This may reflect an abnormality of contractile function of the heart or may be due to excessive pressure or volume loads that cannot be overcome despite initially normal contractile function. Heart failure can also occur because of inadequate cardiac filling: this appears to be the major abnormality in hypertrophic cardiomyopathy. Although heart failure is usually accompanied by low cardiac output, situations can exist in which output is actually normal or higher than normal. For example, in the presence of extremely high metabolic demands, as occurs in hyperthyroidism, the output may be high but still inadequate.

In addition to an inadequate cardiac output, heart failure is often characterized by congestion caused by excessive accumulation of blood behind either of the two ventricles. Traditional hypotheses of heart failure have focused on one or other of these manifestations of heart failure. The *backward failure hypothesis* describes heart failure as an accumulation of blood in the lungs in conjunction with elevated pulmonary venous, left atrial (LA), and left ventricular (LV) diastolic pressures due to failure of the left ventricle or as an accumulation of systemic venous blood in conjunction with elevated systemic venous, right atrial (RA), and right ventricular (RV) diastolic pressures due to failure of the right ventricle.[1] Such typical symptoms or signs of heart failure as dyspnea or edema are due to the resultant increase in interstitial fluid in the lungs or systemic organs. In contrast, the *forward failure hypothesis* stresses the inadequate delivery of blood to the systemic organs and the resultant retention of fluid due to inadequate renal blood flow, which, in turn, leads to pulmonary or systemic congestion.[2] Both these theories have considerable descriptive value in explaining most cases of heart failure, but distinguishing between them is of limited practical value. In the clinical setting, the concept, derived from the backward failure hypothesis, that relates congestion to the right or left side of the heart is useful for diagnosis. When fluid accumulation is primarily behind the left heart ("left-sided failure"), interstitial fluid in the lungs is increased and typical symptoms are dyspnea, orthopnea, and paroxysmal nocturnal dyspnea. When fluid accumulation is primarily behind the right heart ("right-sided failure"), edema, ascites, and hepatic congestion are likely to result. Although, in many cases, pulmonary and systemic venous congestion coexist, the distinction between them can be useful clinically in patients in whom one or the other predominates. Congestion can occur without heart failure after excessive administration of intravenous fluids or in patients with volume overload due to renal failure or anemia.

Physiology

The typical alteration in heart failure is an abnormal diminution in myocardial contractile function that is due to myocardial damage or volume or pressure overload. A variety of circulatory adjustments are then invoked that may or may not compensate to some degree for the congestion and relatively low cardiac output that are generally present. These adjustments include myocardial dilatation or hypertrophy, alterations in autonomic control of the circulation, increased activity of the renin-angiotensin-aldosterone system, increased vasopressin activity, and changes in the affinity of hemoglobin for oxygen. Other alterations, such as redistribution of blood flow in the lung and systemic circulation, may be related to humoral or neural phenomena.

DEPRESSED MYOCARDIAL FUNCTION

Diminished myocardial contractile function is characteristic of most types of heart failure. This is demonstrable in isolated cardiac muscle as a decrease in the magnitude or rate of myocardial force development with isometric contraction and as an abnormality in the estimated myocardial force–velocity relationships with isotonic contractions.[3,4] In patients with heart disease, diminished myocardial contractile function is usually detectable as a decreased ventricular ejection fraction, abnormal ventricular function curves, a diminished rate of increase in ventricular pressure, or a diminished rate of ventricular shortening.

Ejection fraction is the volume of blood ejected per beat (stroke volume) divided by the ventricular end-diastolic volume. If stroke volume = SV; end-diastolic ventricular volume = EDV; and end-systolic ventricular volume = ESV; then

$$\text{Ejection fraction} = \frac{SV}{EDV} = \frac{EDV\text{-}ESV}{EDV}$$

LV ejection fraction can be readily obtained from radiographic ventricular angiograms with injection of angiographic contrast material or with radionuclide first pass or gated ventriculography. Estimates can also be made by echocardiography. Normal LV ejection fractions exceed 0.50. In heart failure, ejection fraction tends to fall, because either stroke volume cannot be maintained at normal levels even at rest or, if it is maintained, it is associated with ventricular dilatation and an increased end-diastolic volume. Although RV ejection fractions can also be obtained by these techniques, normal values have not been defined. LV ejection fractions below 0.40 are common in heart failure, with severe cases usually being below 0.30. In clinical practice, ejection fraction has proven to be easily and reliably obtainable. It is the most commonly used estimate of ventricular function.

Ventricular function curves that use the Frank–Starling relationship are occasionally employed to evaluate patients with heart disease.[5-8] Normally, as ventricular end-diastolic myocardial fiber length is increased, stroke volume and stroke work (the product of stroke volume and arterial pressure during ejection) increase. When ventricular function is impaired, stroke volume or stroke work rise less or do not rise at all as ventricular end-diastolic fiber length increases. Function curves can be obtained by increasing ventricular filling with infusions of fluids, isometric exercise, or drugs, such as angiotensin, that elevate arterial pressure.[7-9] Clinically, both end-diastolic ventricular volume and pressure are used as indices of ventricular end-diastolic fiber length. Ventricular diastolic volumes are superior to pressures for this purpose because some conditions, such as coronary artery disease, alter ventricular pressure–volume relationships by decreasing compliance, so that a high end-diastolic pressure may be associated with a normal end-diastolic volume and fiber length.

Myocardial contractile function can also be estimated by measuring maximum rates of pressure generation or maximum rates of myocardial shortening. Pressure generation is generally estimated as the maximum first derivative of ventricular pressure during the early isovolumic phase of ventricular contraction (dp/dt_{max}). Myocardial shortening can be estimated from angiographic ventriculograms or echocardiograms as maximum decreases during ejection of ventricular circumference, volume, or diameter. Overlap between normal and abnormal values has limited the usefulness of these techniques in detecting abnormal myocardial contractile function. However, the techniques are useful for serial studies of myocardial function in humans and in animal studies.[10]

Systolic time intervals are estimates of ventricular function during ejection derived from simultaneous electrocardiogram, phonocardiogram, and indirect carotid pressure measurements.[11] These measurements have not been reliable indices of inotropic state in clinical practice. Efforts to derive the theoretical maximum velocity of shortening of the contractile element of ventricular muscle fibers from clinical data have also not been useful clinically.

BIOCHEMICAL ALTERATIONS IN THE MYOCARDIUM

Many investigators have attempted to relate biochemical abnormalities to the diminished myocardial contractile function usually present in heart failure. A very limited amount of knowledge has been accrued. Myocardial oxygen consumption and inotropic state are diminished in the failing heart, and, presumably, less chemical energy is utilized for the contractile process.[12] The myocardial stores of high-energy phosphates that are the chief sources of chemical energy for the contractile process do not appear to be deficient. In early stages of heart failure, levels of glycogen, adenosine triphosphate (ATP), and phosphocreatine are decreased, but in chronic failure they are generally normal.[13] However, abnormally low levels of myosin ATPase and other forms of myocardial ATPase enzymes that control hydrolysis of ATP to release high-energy phosphates have been reported in human and animal models of chronic heart failure.[14-16] As a result of these low levels, the energy available to contractile proteins during shortening and the rate or extent of fiber shortening may be reduced. Abnormalities of calcium transport in the sarcoplasmic reticulum have been suspected in failing hearts. Reduced calcium uptake in the sarcoplasmic reticulum has been reported in chronically failing calf hearts.[17] Abnormalities of the myocardial action potential suggestive of abnormal intracellular electrolyte concentrations have been reported in other animal models.[18] High potassium levels and other electrolyte changes are known to depress the activity of contractile proteins *in vitro*.[19] In early stages of heart failure, there is evidence of increased rates of protein synthesis with high ribonucleic acid (RNA) levels. Presumably these changes are associated with the development of myocardial hypertrophy. In late stages of heart failure, protein synthesis is not increased.[13]

MYOCARDIAL HYPERTROPHY AND DILATATION

Dilatation of the heart in response to diminished myocardial contractile function or abnormal pressure or volume loads is a fundamental physiologic response. As initially described by Frank and Starling, increases in end-diastolic fiber length result in an increased strength of contraction and augmented stroke volume.[5,6] Although the utility of this response for acute and chronic compensation is well established, there are potential disadvantages. As described by the Laplace's Law wall tension varies with the square of the radius. Thus, dilatation of the heart can substantially increase the tension that must be generated with each systole. The resultant increase in myocardial energy expenditure increases myocardial oxygen need, an often deleterious alteration. There is also a possibility that excessive lengthening of the myocardial fibers beyond a critical length may place the heart on a descending limb of the Starling curve, where strength of contraction and stroke volume begin to diminish.[6] Certainly, with chronic dilatation myocardial function frequently is diminished and stroke volume is low. This may, in part, be related to distortions in muscle fiber orientation.

Heart failure due to chronic exposure to excessive pressure or volume loads, leads to myocardial hypertrophy, which is characterized by increased myocardial fiber size or number.[13,20] Although some animal studies have found myocardial contractile force in hypertrophied hearts to be enhanced,[21] more commonly it is diminished.[3,22,23] Usually in such circumstances the blood supply to the myocardium does not increase in proportion to the increase in muscle mass.[24] Ischemia and scarring may result and contribute to the diminution in function. There is reason to believe that pathological hypertrophy due to pressure or volume loading may differ in important ways from hypertrophy seen in athletes or others who have undergone exercise training. Hearts with pathological hypertrophy typically have diminished capillary density, low concentrations of contractile protein ATPase (an enzyme important to contractile function), areas of scarring, abnormalities in contractile function, and increased capillary permeability.[14-16,22,25] In contrast, "physiologic" hypertrophy due to exercise training is associated with increases in capillary density, normal myocardial ATPase, and absence of scarring or evidence of ischemia.[26,27] In general, contractile function is normal in hearts with physiologic hypertrophy but is reduced with pathologic hypertrophy.

Hypertrophy tends to differ according to whether a pressure or a volume load predominates. When the systolic load is due to high pressures, as in valvular aortic stenosis, there is a substantial, fairly uniform increase in wall thickness without dilatation, a situation termed *concentric hypertrophy*.[28] With diastolic overload due to high volumes of blood, as in aortic valve insufficiency, the heart tends to dilate, but the thickness of the wall is usually unchanged. In the volume overload cases, the total mass of ventricular muscle is increased because ventricular volume is increased, but wall thickness is maintained rather than reduced, as would occur with dilatation without hypertrophy. The hypertrophy in volume overload states is termed *eccentric* because it tends not to be uniform but rather to result in a change to a more spherical ventricular configuration.

SYMPATHETIC NERVOUS SYSTEM ALTERATIONS

Usually, in heart failure, circulating norepinephrine and epinephrine levels are excessive, and cardiac norepinephrine is depleted.[4,29,30] Despite the high levels of norepinephrine, blood dopamine beta hydroxylase, an enzyme usually released together with norepinephrine from sympathetic nerves, is low in patients with heart failure.[31] The significance of these changes is unclear, but high levels of sympathetic stimulation seem to be necessary for maintenance of myocardial function in the failing heart.[32] It has recently been reported that failing human hearts have decreased sensitivity to catecholamine because of decreased beta adrenergic receptor density.[33] This may be an adaptive response to continued high levels of catecholamine release. Alpha adrenergic receptor stimulation is probably a major mechanism causing peripheral circulatory vasoconstriction in patients with heart failure.[34]

Parasympathetic nervous system activity may also be decreased in heart failure. Decreases in sensitivity to atropine and in baroreceptor-mediated responses to pressors have been reported in humans and animals with heart failure.[35,36]

RENIN-ANGIOTENSIN SYSTEM AND ALDOSTERONE ACTIVITY

In patients with chronic heart failure, high plasma renin, angiotensin, and aldosterone levels have been demonstrated.[37–39] Whereas sodium restriction normally stimulates increases in angiotensin and aldosterone levels, in patients with heart failure it has opposite effects.[40] Angiotensin may contribute to generalized and regional vasoconstriction in heart failure patients.[41] The high aldosterone levels, which appear to be induced by angiotensin, probably contribute to the sodium retention that is characteristic of this condition.[29]

VASOPRESSIN ACTIVITY

Evidence is growing that in patients with heart failure there is an increase in the levels of circulating vasopressin.[42] Whether this hormone plays a role in edema formation through its renal effects or on regional vascular tone through its effects on vascular smooth muscle is not clear.

INCREASED OXYGEN EXTRACTION

The low cardiac output usually present in heart failure results in diminished delivery of oxygen to the tissues. This is partly compensated for by increased oxygen extraction by the tissues. The arteriovenous oxygen difference is increased due to a low mixed venous oxygen concentration. The oxygen–hemoglobin dissociation curve is shifted to the right in heart failure, and 2,3 diphosphoglycerate is increased.[43] This may enhance oxygen transport to the tissues.

REDISTRIBUTION OF BLOOD FLOW

In heart failure associated with elevated pulmonary venous pressures, blood flow is redistributed from the lower or dependent lobes of the lung to the upper lobes of the lung as a result of increased pulmonary vascular resistance in the lower lobes.[44,45] Whether the mechanism is vasoconstriction due to humoral or neural effects, or a mechanical phenomenon due to dependent extracellular fluid accumulation and decreased compliance is unknown. Redistribution of pulmonary blood flow is a valuable compensatory mechanism, since blood is diverted away from poorly ventilated edematous lower lobes to better-ventilated upper lobes, allowing higher systemic arterial oxygen saturations than would otherwise occur.

A high systemic vascular resistance is characteristic of heart failure associated with a low cardiac output.[35] Regional vasoconstriction is particularly marked in the splanchnic bed and kidneys. In general, blood flow to the heart and brain tends to be preserved at the expense of flow to the less vital organs, such as the splanchnic bed, skin, and skeletal muscles. Sympathetic stimulation, and possibly such humoral mechanisms as angiotensin or vasopressin release, may cause the systemic vasoconstriction. Although regional vasoconstriction in the systemic bed may be helpful in maintaining a near-normal flow to the heart and brain in the face of a low cardiac output, it also has detrimental aspects. Renal vasoconstriction tends to result in expansion of extracellular fluid, which often causes edema of the pulmonary or systemic circulation. In addition, the increase in total systemic vascular resistance due to varying degrees of the regional vasoconstriction results in a relative increase in mean arterial pressure, which increases cardiac work and energy expenditure. As a result, the relative increase in arterial pressure often causes a reduction in cardiac output. There is considerable evidence that reduction of systemic vasoconstriction increases cardiac output while preserving flow to the heart and brain and also increases urinary output through increased renal blood flow.[46,47] This is an important principle of therapy for heart failure.

Clinical Presentation

SYMPTOMS

Most symptoms of heart failure may be considered to be due to one of two causes: congestion of the pulmonary or systemic circulation, or inadequate regional blood flow due to low cardiac output (Table 11-1). Congestion occurs when the filling pressure or end-diastolic pressure of either ventricle

Table 11–1.   Causes of Major Findings in Heart Failure

Increased RV Filling Pressure	Increased LV Filling Pressure	Low Cardiac Output
Distended neck veins	Dyspnea	Fatigue
Edema	Orthopnea	Mental confusion
Ascites	Paroxysmal nocturnal dyspnea	Cool skin
Hepatomegaly		Peripheral cyanosis
	Rales, rhonchi, or wheezing	
	Pleural effusion	
	X-ray signs of congestion	

is elevated, whether because of decreased compliance, inadequate ventricular emptying, or volume overload of the entire vascular compartment. Elevated LV end-diastolic pressures result in elevated LA and pulmonary venous pressures, causing pulmonary congestion. Elevated RV filling pressures cause elevated RA and systemic venous pressures, and result in systemic congestion.

Pulmonary Congestion

Pulmonary congestion may range in severity from a modest increase in pulmonary venous pressure to frank alveolor pulmonary edema. Congestion of any significant degree is usually experienced by the patient as dyspnea. Dyspnea occurs when one becomes aware of discomfort or difficulty in breathing. It may occur in normal persons when, as a result of exercise, greater minute ventilation is required and the faster respiratory rate, increased tidal volume, and increased work of breathing become noticeable.

Normal persons are unaware of their breathing during quiet respiration. However, patients with congestive heart failure may experience dyspnea at rest because of the greater effort required to expand the congested, less compliant lungs.[48] In noncompliant lungs, the same minute ventilation can be achieved at a lower energy cost by breathing more rapidly at lower tidal volumes. This is because, at equivalent tidal volumes, in the presence of pulmonary congestion, breathing is being performed on a steep portion of the compliance curve of the lungs, where a greater negative inspiratory force is required to achieve the same increase in lung volume. More rapid, shallow breaths ensure that breathing is being performed on the flat portion of the compliance curve, where less inspiratory force is required to produce a given change in volume. Although these rapid, shallow breaths require less effort, they are perceived by the patient as dyspnea. Actual reductions in tidal volume may occur in patients with large pleural effusions, which reduce lung volumes and tend to cause severe dyspnea.

With exercise and the need for even greater minute ventilation, the sensation of breathlessness becomes more pronounced. The patient with congestive heart failure must attempt to increase both respiratory rate and tidal volume to maintain adequate gas exchange. Consequently, the work and the oxygen cost of breathing are increased significantly. In addition, the patient with elevated LV filling pressure at rest may develop further increases in LV end-diastolic and pulmonary venous pressures during exercise if the left ventricle is limited in its ability to increase its performance at higher work loads. This rise in pulmonary venous and pulmonary capillary pressure with exercise may further decrease lung compliance and further contribute to the development of dyspnea with exercise.

Orthopnea and paroxysmal nocturnal dyspnea are related symptoms. Patients with congestive heart failure may have edema fluid in the interstitium of the lower extremities while they are upright. Paroxysmal nocturnal dyspnea occurs when, upon reclining, the edema fluid is redistributed centrally and the increase in central blood volume causes pulmonary congestion.[49] The patient then awakens with the sensation of dyspnea and must sit or stand to gain relief. Often, the patient notices a suffocating feeling, as if he or she were not getting enough air, and sits or stands before an open window. Nocturnal cough may be a clinical equivalent of paroxysmal nocturnal dyspnea. Central redistribution of edema fluid may result in engorgement of bronchial vessels and bronchial mucosal edema and may stimulate the afferent arc of the cough reflex. Paroxysmal nocturnal dyspnea requires time for the edema fluid to redistribute and usually occurs 2 hours to 5 hours after the patient retires. Patients with bronchitis may begin to have a productive cough with or without dyspnea after lying down to sleep, but coughing usually occurs about 30 minutes after retiring, when mucus shifts position within the bronchi and stimulates coughing.

Orthopnea is inability to lie in the recumbent position without becoming short of breath. Patients may use several pillows or may even sleep upright in a chair. The number of pillows required is often a useful clinical index of the severity of the patient's symptoms. Orthopnea results in part from the same mechanism as paroxysmal nocturnal dyspnea; that is, central redistribution of edema fluid. In addition, however, the congested, poorly compliant lungs are easier to inflate when total thoracic compliance is maximal, in the upright position. Lying supine, the pressure of the abdominal contents is partly brought to bear upon the diaphragm. The diaphragms are elevated, and total thoracic compliance is decreased. The work of breathing may then be increased enough to contribute to dyspnea. Some patients who customarily sleep on their left side or in a prone position may have little or no orthopnea although they have orthopnea in the supine position. In such cases, relatively small portions of the lungs may be in dependent positions where they are subject to congestion.

Cardiac asthma occurs when severe pulmonary congestion due to LV failure results in bronchospasm. The precise mechanisms by which bronchospasm is triggered remain unclear. However, it is thought that bronchial venous congestion, bronchial mucosal edema, and resulting increases in bronchial secretions may play a role. Patients who are subject to bronchospasm as a result of chronic obstructive airways disease appear to be more likely to develop cardiac asthma as a result of LV failure.

Cardiogenic pulmonary edema occurs when hydrostatic pulmonary capillary pressure exceeds plasma oncotic pressure and fluid begins to exude into the pulmonary interstitium and, ultimately, into the alveoli.[50,51] This pressure excess may result from LV failure or, as in mitral stenosis, from obstruction to LV inflow. It is most often seen in the setting of an acute rise in LV filling pressure, as in acute myocardial infarction. The interstitial fluid causes a decrease in total lung compliance, and the alveolar fluid causes a decrease in the total alveolar capillary membrane surface area available for gas exchange. Marked abnormalities of gas exchange result, with hypoxemia, compensatory hyperventilation, hypocapnia, and a characteristic clinical syndrome that may include severe dyspnea; tachypnea; anxiety; cyanosis; and frothy, blood-tinged sputum.

Systemic Congestion

Elevated venous pressure from RV failure, tricuspid valve disease, or constrictive pericarditis results in congestive hepatomegaly. This may cause symptoms of right upper quadrant pain and fullness, particularly if right heart failure develops acutely. Chronically elevated hepatic venous pressure may lead to portal hypertension and mesenteric congestion, with nausea, abdominal fullness, and even malabsorption and protein-losing enteropathy. However, it must be remembered that a common cause of nausea and other gastrointestinal symptoms in patients with congestive heart failure is digitalis toxicity.

Edema is the major manifestation of systemic congestion. The most important cause of edema is an increase in the total body content of salt and water. Congestive heart failure results in a decrease in arterial blood volume, which is detected by the kidney at the juxtaglomerular apparatus. Activation of the renin-angiotensin-aldosterone system causes subsequent retention of salt and water by the kidney. This is an adaptive mechanism, in that the increase in blood volume increases the diastolic volume in the ventricles and, hence, increases stroke volume by the Frank–Starling mechanism. However, once circulating blood volume is increased substantially, much of the added volume no longer remains within the intravascular space but passes into the interstitial fluid. With increases in interstitial fluid of more than 5 liters, edema becomes apparent, usually in dependent portions of the body. In the early stages, ankle edema may appear only at the end of the day, after the legs have been dependent for many hours. With more fluid accumulation, however, edema becomes apparent throughout the day and may eventually impair mobility and cause discomfort. Venous disease can also cause posturally dependent edema and must be distinguished from heart failure as a cause of this finding.

Nocturia may develop early in the course of congestive heart failure. This symptom is related to the mobilization and central redistribution of dependent edema fluid during recumbency. This increase in central blood volume results in a higher glomerular filtration rate, and the rate of urine flow may require the patient to urinate several times during the night.

Low Output Symptoms

A cardiac output that is inadequate to meet the needs of the peripheral tissues is characteristic of congestive heart failure. In less severe cases of congestive heart failure, cardiac output may be adequate at rest but may not rise sufficiently to meet the increased metabolic requirements of the tissues during exercise. The inadequate oxygen delivery to skeletal muscle during exercise leads to local accumulation of metabolites, progressively more anaerobic metabolism, and the early onset of muscle fatigue and exhaustion. In patients with severe congestive failure, cardiac output may be inadequate even at rest. Such patients have persistent symptoms of fatigue and exhaustion even without exercising.

Symptoms may result from inadequate perfusion of other organ beds as well. Mental confusion, disorientation, and disruption of the normal sleep-wake cycle may result from cerebral hypoperfusion, particularly in the elderly. These symptoms may be exacerbated by the prerenal azotemia that is seen in congestive heart failure as a result of renal hypoperfusion, due either to inadequate cardiac output or to inadequate circulatory blood volume from over-vigorous diuresis. Cool skin may be reported due to low cutaneous blood flow.

PHYSICAL FINDINGS

Careful physical examination of the patient in congestive heart failure may elicit cardiac, pulmonary, and peripheral findings. Those findings may result from congestion, from inadequate cardiac output, or from compensatory mechanisms that are activated in response to heart failure.

Cardiac Findings

Patients with congestive heart failure may have resting tachycardia if their heart failure is severe and usually have inappropriately rapid increases in heart rate in response to mild exercise. The tachycardia is due in part to the increase in sympathetic nervous system activity that occurs in patients with heart failure. Reflex parasympathetic withdrawal and stretch of the sinoatrial node due to cardiac dilatation are other possible contributing factors.

In severe congestive heart failure, there may be obvious cardiomegaly, detectable by palpation. The apex impulse may be displaced well to the left of its usual position, at or near the midclavicular line, and may be diffuse. Percussion is less helpful than palpation in detecting cardiomegaly because the left cardiac border may be difficult to define.

A third heart sound (S_3) may be audible in patients with congestive heart failure. Although this finding is normal in children, in adults it is a reliable sign of ventricular decompensation. S_3 is a low-pitched filling sound that is heard during the rapid filling phase of early diastole and may originate from either the right or the left ventricle. The most reliable means of distinguishing RV S_3 from LV S_3 is its behavior during respiration. Like most right-sided cardiac events, RV S_3 increases with inspiration, when the drop in intrathoracic pressure causes an increase in venous return to the right ventricle. LV S_3 does not change with respiration.

Systolic murmurs from atrioventricular (AV) valvular regurgitation due to either mitral or tricuspid papillary dysfunction may be present during decompensated congestive heart failure and absent when heart failure has improved. During decompensated congestive heart failure, dilatation of the ventricle may lead to an abnormal distorted relationship of the valve leaflets with the chordae, papillary muscles, and underlying ventricular wall and interfere with function of the mitral or tricuspid valve. After treatment the ventricle may return to its former size, and the AV valvular apparatus resumes its normal geometry and competence.

The intensity of the first heart sound (S_1) may be diminished in severe congestive heart failure due to the decreased rate of pressure rise in the ventricle. In patients with aortic or mitral valvular insufficiency this tendency may be exaggerated by premature closure of the valve.[52] In patients with long-standing LV failure or mitral stenosis resulting in significant pulmonary hypertension, the intensity of the pulmonic component of the second heart sound (P_2) may be increased.

Signs Resulting From Congestion

Pulmonary congestion resulting in dyspnea may be detected by the patient's rapid, shallow respirations. Percussion of the chest may reveal dullness at the bases suggesting pleural effusion in patients with long-standing congestive heart failure. Pleural effusions due to congestive heart failure are more commonly right-sided than left-sided, and are seen more frequently when RV failure is present in addition to LV failure.

Auscultation of the chest may reveal moist inspiratory rales. These are thought to occur when collapsed, fluid-filled alveoli open suddenly during inspiration. Rales are most often heard at the bases in patients who have been upright but are heard in the most dependent portions of the lungs in patients who, for example, have been lying on their side for several hours. The height to which rales are heard over the thorax is an indication of the severity of pulmonary congestion.

With severe, acute LV failure, for example after extensive myocardial infarction, the patient may present with pulmonary edema. This dramatic syndrome is very characteristic. The patient often sits bold upright, with severe tachypnea and air hunger and must use the accessory muscles of respiration in order to adequately ventilate his stiff, noncompliant lungs. He may appear agitated and fearful, with diaphoresis and even piloerection, or "goose flesh," caused by the intense compensatory sympathetic discharge. Impairment of oxygenation and sympathetically mediated peripheral vasoconstriction may lead to central cyanosis, peripheral cyanosis, or both.

Occasionally, the patient with severe LV failure will develop diffuse bronchospasm, or *cardiac asthma.* Inspiratory and expiratory wheezes may be heard over the entire thorax, the expiratory phase of respiration may be prolonged, and pulsus paradoxus may be detected. Cardiac asthma may initially be difficult to distinguish from asthma due to obstructive airways disease.

Systemic congestion results from a combination of an excess of intravascular and extravascular fluid due to renal salt and water retention and high systemic venous pressure. High systemic venous pressure can be detected by examining the jugular veins, preferably the right internal jugular vein. The mean RA pressure in cm H_2O can be estimated by measuring the vertical height of the jugular venous blood column above the sternal angle, and adding 5 cm, the distance of the sternal angle from the mid right atrium. Pressures above 10 cm H_2O are abnormal and suggest right heart failure.

A more subtle sign of right heart failure is the hepatojugular reflux. In early heart failure, the circulating blood volume may be increased, but the capacity of the systemic venous bed is adequate to prevent a rise in systemic venous pressure. However, the application of firm pressure to the abdomen, usually over the right upper quadrant, decreases the volume of the hepatic and splanchnic venous beds and causes *hepatojugular reflux,* a sustained rise in jugular venous pressure in response to this maneuver. Chronic RV failure may lead to hepatomegaly and ascites. Prolonged hepatic congestion may ultimately result in cardiac cirrhosis with all the other attendant signs of portal hypertension. In addition to a variety of liver diseases, other causes of hepatomegaly and ascites include constrictive pericarditis and systemic venous obstruction due to tumor or thrombosis.

Dependent edema is a common sign of congestive heart failure. Edema may not be detectable until 5 liters or more of excess extravascular fluid have accumulated, and then may only appear as mild pitting edema over the tibias or ankles. Edema of recent onset is distinguished by its spongy, pitting quality and the lack of overlying skin changes. Edema of long standing, however, may result in thickening and brawny induration of the overlying skin, that may not resolve even after diuresis.

Signs Resulting From Inadequate Cardiac Output

Peripheral circulatory adjustments to inadequate cardiac output are responsible for many of the physical findings of congestive heart failure. Congestive heart failure leads to an increase in levels of circulating norepinephrine as well as to activation of the renal renin-angiotensin system. Both norepinephrine and angiotensin II cause peripheral vasoconstriction, and, when congestive heart failure is severe, blood flow to the heart and brain is preserved at the expense of blood flow to less vital areas such as skin and skeletal muscle. This central diversion of blood flow is manifested by the cool, pale or sometimes cyanotic, extremities of the patient. In addition, the patient with severe congestive heart failure may have mild fever because of inability to radiate heat through peripheral vasodilation.

Patients with inadequate cardiac output may develop signs and symptoms of a diffuse or toxic-metabolic encephalopathy. Confusion, disorientation, and restlessness may be seen during an exacerbation of heart failure, only to remit after treatment. More severe degrees of congestive heart failure may lead to a severely depressed level of consciousness. These cerebral symptoms are thought to be related to a combination of several factors: a decline in cerebral blood flow due to inadequate cardiac output, associated atherosclerotic cerebral vascular disease, and impaired autoregulation with inadequate reduction of cerebral vascular resistance in response to decreased flow.

Cheyne–Stokes respirations are seen occasionally in congestive failure. This pattern of periodic breathing, in which periods of hyperpnea alternate with periods of apnea, is thought to result from a prolongation of the circulation time between the pulmonary venous bed and the medullary chemoreceptors that regulate breathing. Hyperpnea results in well-oxygenated, hypocapnic pulmonary venous blood that may, because of the slow circulation time, take many seconds to reach the medulla. When it does, ventilatory drive is markedly decreased, resulting in apnea, which in turn causes hypercapnia and, eventually, hyperpnea again.

In long-standing severe congestive heart failure, patients may lose significant amounts of weight, resulting in cardiac cachexia. This end-stage picture results from a combination of many factors, including anorexia due to splanchnic congestion; occasionally, protein-losing enteropathy; poor appetite, perhaps due to the mental disturbances of congestive heart failure; and underperfusion of end organs.

Summary

Heart failure is a condition in which cardiac output is inadequate to meet the metabolic needs of the body. Most commonly, it is related to abnormal myocardial contractile function. Dilatation of the heart, which through the Frank–Starling mechanism increases stroke volume, and tachycardia and activation of various neural and hormonal mechanisms are fundamental responses to an abnormally low cardiac output. Myocardial hypertrophy is a chronic adaptation to some forms of heart failure, but its value in enhancing ventricular function is dubious. Redistribution of blood flow away from dependent, edematous regions of the lungs is beneficial because it improves systemic arterial oxygen saturation. Redistribution also occurs in the systemic vasculature due to vasoconstriction in the splanchnic bed, skin, and skeletal muscle. This tends to preserve flow to the heart and brain, but the vasoconstriction is often harmful because it further depresses cardiac output by increasing aortic impedance. Reversal of systemic vasoconstriction by vasodilators is the basis of a highly effective form of treatment of low-output heart failure.

Symptoms and signs of heart failure are due primarily either to congestion of the pulmonary or systemic beds or to low cardiac output. Symptoms related to pulmonary congestion are dyspnea, orthopnea, and paroxysmal nocturnal dyspnea. Symptoms related to systemic congestion are swelling of the feet or abdomen, and discomfort due to liver congestion. Symptoms of low cardiac output are easy fatigability, mental confusion, and insomnia.

Typical findings on examination of the heart in heart failure are cardiomegaly, an S_3, and murmurs of AV valve regurgitation. Pulmonary congestion may be associated with rales, rhonchi, wheezes, or dullness at the bases if pleural effusions are present. Systemic congestion is associated with edema, ascites, hepatomegaly in early stages, and jugular venous distention. Low cardiac output results in cool, pale or cyanotic skin, decreased levels of consciousness, and, rarely, fever. Other findings may include nocturia, Cheyne–Stokes respirations, and cardiac cachexia.

References

1. Hope JA: Treatise on the Diseases of the Heart and Great Vessels. London, Williams-Kidd, 1832
2. Mackenzie J: Disease of the Heart, 3rd ed. London, Oxford University Press, 1913
3. Spann JF Jr, Buccino RA, Sonnenblick EH, et al: Contractile state of cardiac muscle obtained from cats with experimentally produced ventricular hypertrophy and heart failure. Circ Res 21:341, 1967
4. Chidsey CA, Sonnenblick EH, Morrow AG, et al: Norepinephrine stores and contractile force of papillary muscle from the failing human heart. Circulation 33:43, 1966
5. Frank O: Zur Dynamik des Herzmuskels. 2. Biol 32:370, 1895. Translated in Am Heart J 58:282, 1959
6. Patterson SW, Starling EH: On the mechanical factors which determine the output of the ventricles. J Physiol (Lond) 48:357, 1914

7. Ross J Jr, Braunwald E: The study of left ventricular function in man by increasing resistance to ventricular ejection with angiotensin. Circulation 29:739, 1964
8. Payne RM, Horwitz LD, Mullins CB: Comparison of isometric exercise and angiotensin infusion as stress test for evaluation of left ventricular function. Am J Cardiol 31:428, 1973
9. Bishop VS, Horwitz LD: Quantitative assessment of cardiac pump performance. J Physiol 269:355, 1977
10. Barnes GE, Bishop VS, Horwitz LD, et al: The maximum derivatives of left ventricular pressure and transverse internal diameter as indices of the inotropic state of the left ventricle in conscious dogs. J Physiol (Lond) 235:571, 1973
11. Weissler AM, Harris WS, Schoenfield CD: Bedside techniques for the evaluation of ventricular function in man. Am J Cardiol 23:577, 1969
12. Henry PD, Eckberg D, Gault JH, et al: Depressed inotropic state and reduced myocardial oxygen consumption in the human heart. Am J Cardiol 31:300, 1973
13. Meerson FZ: The myocardium in hyperfunction, hypertrophy and heart failure. American Heart Association Monograph No. 26. New York, American Heart Association, 1969
14. Alpert NR, Gordon MS: Myofibrillar adenosine triphosphate activity in congestive heart failure. Am J Physiol 202:940, 1962
15. Gordon MS, Brown AL: Myofibrillar adenosine triphosphate activity of human heart tissue and congestive heart failure: Effects of ouabain and calcium. Circ Res 19:534, 1966
16. Luchi RJ, Kritcher EM, Thyrum PT: Reduced cardiac myosin adenosine triphosphate activity in dogs with spontaneously occurring heart failure. Circ Res 24:513, 1969
17. Suko J, Vogel JHK, Chidsey CA: Intracellular calcium and myocardial contractility III. Reduced calcium uptake and ATPase of the sarcoplasmic reticular fraction prepared from chronically failing calf hearts. Circ Res 27:235, 1970
18. Gelband H, Bassett AL: Depressed transmembrane potentials during experimentally induced ventricular failure in cats. Circ Res 32:625, 1973
19. Szent–Gyorgi AG: Protein of the myofibril. In GH Bourne (ed): The Structure and Function of Muscle, vol 2. Academic Press, New York, 1960
20. Massa N: Liber introductorius anatomiae. 1534
21. Williams JF Jr, Potter RD: Normal contractile state of hypertrophied myocardium following pulmonary artery constriction in the cat. J Clin Invest 54:1266, 1974
22. McCullagh WH, Covell JW, Ross J Jr: Left ventricular dilation and diastolic compliance changes during chronic volume overloading. Circulation 45:943, 1972
23. Meerson F, Kapelko VI: The significance of the interrelationships between the intensity of the contractile state and the velocity of relaxation in adapting cardiac muscle to function at high work loads. J Mol Cell Cardiol 7:293, 1975
24. Katz L: The mechanism of heart failure. Circulation 10:663, 1954
25. Laughlin MH, Diana JN: Myocardial transcapillary exchange in the hypertrophied heart of the dog. Am J Physiol 229:838, 1975
26. Malhotra A, Pempargkul S, Schaible T, et al: Contractile proteins and sarcoplasmic reticulum in physiologic cardiac hypertrophy. Am J Physiol 241:H263, 1981
27. Oscai LB, Mole PA, Holloszy JO: Effects of exercise on cardiac weight and mitochondria in male and female rats. Am J Physiol 220:1944, 1971
28. Linzbach AJ: Heart failure from the point of view of quantitative anatomy. Am J Cardiol 5:370, 1960
29. Chidsey CH, Braunwald E, Morrow AG: Catecholamine excretion and cardiac stores of norepinephrine in congestive heart failure. Am J Med 39:442, 1965

30. Thomas JA, Marks BH: Plasma norepinephrine in congestive heart failure. Am J Cardiol 41:233, 1978
31. Horwitz LD, Travis VS: Low serum dopamine-β-hydroxylase activity: a marker of congestive heart failure. J Clin Invest 62:899, 1978
32. Gaffney TE, Braunwald E: Importance of the adrenergic nervous system in the support of circulatory function in patients with congestive heart failure. Am J Med 34:320, 1963
33. Bristow MR, Ginsburg R, Minobe W, et al: Decreased catecholamine sensitivity and B-adrenergic receptor density in failing human hearts. New Engl J Med 307:205, 1982
34. Kramer RS, Mason DT, Braunwald E: Augmented sympathetic neurotransmitter activity in the peripheral vascular bed of patients with congestive heart failure and cardiac norepinephrine depletion. Circulation 38:629, 1968
35. Eckberg DL, Drabinsky M, Braunwald E: Defective cardiac sympathetic control in patients with heart disease. New Engl J Med 285:877, 1971
36. Higgins CB, Vatner SF, Eckberg DL, et al: Alterations in the baroreceptor reflex in conscious dogs with heart failure. J Clin Invest 51:715, 1972
37. Merrill AJ, Morrison JL, Brannon ES: Concentration of renin in renal venous blood in patients with chronic heart failure. Am J Med 1:468, 1946
38. de Champlain J, Boucher R, Genest J: Arterial angiotensin levels in edematous patients. Proc Soc Exp Biol Med 113:932, 1963
39. Camargo CA, Dowdy AJ, Hancock EW, et al: Decreased plasma clearance and hepatic extraction of aldosterone in patients with heart failure. J Clin Invest 44:356, 1965
40. Genest J, Granger P, de Champlain J, et al: Endocrine factors in congestive heart failure. Am J Cardiol 22:35, 1968
41. Davis JO, Freeman RH, Johnson JA, et al: Agents which block the action of the renin-angiotensin system. Circ Res 34:279, 1974
42. Szatalowicz VL, Arnold PE, Chaimovitz C, et al: Radioimmunoassay of plasma arginine vasopressin in hyponatremic patients with congestive heart failure. New Engl J Med 305:263, 1981
43. Woodson RD, Torrance JD, Shappell SD, et al: The effect of cardiac disease on hemoglobin-oxygen binding. J Clin Invest 49:1349, 1970
44. West JB, Dollery CT, Heard BE: Increased pulmonary vascular resistance in the dependent zone of the isolated dog lung caused by perivascular edema. Circ Res 17:191, 1965
45. Simon M: The pulmonary veins in mitral stenosis. J Fac Radiol 9:25, 1958
46. Miller RR, Vismara LA, Williams DO, et al: Pharmacological mechanisms for left ventricular unloading in clinical congestive heart failure: Differential effects of nitroprusside, phentolamine, and nitroglycerin on cardiac function and peripheral circulation. Circ Res 39:127, 1976
47. Parmley WW, Chatterjee K: Vasodilator therapy. Curr Probl Cardiol 2:1, 1978
48. Collins JV, Clark TJH, Brown DU: Airway function in healthy subjects and in patients with left heart disease. Clin Sci Molec Med 49:217, 1975
49. Perera FA, Berlinen RW: The relation of postural hemodilution to paroxysmal dyspnea. J Clin Invest 22:25, 1943
50. Visscher MD, Haddy FJ, Stephens G: The physiology and pharmacology of lung edema. Pharmacol Rev 8:389, 1956
51. Robin ED, Cross CE, Zelis R: Pulmonary edema. N Engl J Med 288:239, 1973
52. Meadows WR, Sharp JT, Zachariudakis S: Premature mitral valve closure: A hemodynamic explanation for absence of the first sound in aortic insufficiency. Circulation 28:251, 1963

12

PULMONARY EMBOLISM

Joseph R. Benotti, M.D., and James E. Dalen, M.D.

Definition

Pulmonary embolism (PE) is defined as the acute partial or total occlusion of one or more pulmonary arterial branches by emboli, which form as thrombi in the venous system and migrate to the pulmonary circulation. In addition to embolism of the pulmonary circulation by venous thrombi, the subject to which this discussion is confined, a variety of other tissues and materials including fat, bone marrow, amniotic fluid, malignant tumors, feces, numerous foreign bodies, and injected substances may embolize the pulmonary circulation.[1-7]

It is estimated that approximately 630,000 cases of PE occur annually in the USA. Approximately 67,000 of these cases (11%) sustain massive PE causing death within 1 hour. The remaining 567,000 patients (90%) survive for longer than 1 hour and are likely to come to medical attention. Of these 567,000 patients with PE, the correct diagnosis is established in only 163,000 cases (29%), and the diagnosis is not made in 400,000 (71%). In the undiagnosed and untreated group, approximately 280,000 patients (70%) survive and 120,000 (30%) die as a result of PE. In the approximately 163,000 patients (29%) in whom the diagnosis of PE is established and therapy is instituted, about 150,000 patients (92%) survive and 13,000 patients (8%) die with PE as the primary cause or a major contributing factor.[8] The salient features concerning these estimates are that:

1. PE is a fairly common disease, with an incidence of approximately 0.32% (630,000 cases annually/in a U.S. population of approximately 200,000,000 people)

277

2. Approximately 90% of patients with acute PE survive and may come to medical attention

3. Appropriate therapy demands clinical suspicion leading to rapid diagnosis

4. The mortality of untreated PE is approximately 30%. This can be reduced to 8% with prompt diagnosis and therapy[8]

Pathophysiology

In over 90% of cases, thrombi that embolize to the lungs originate in the deep venous system of the lower extremities above the popliteal veins.[9] Conditions predisposing to deep venous thrombosis (DVT) were intially described by Virchow in 1860. These include stasis of blood in the lower extremities, injury to the blood vessel wall, and any condition that predisposes to a hypercoagulable state.[10] The diseases associated with a hypercoagulable state include such rare conditions as polycythemia vera and primary thrombocytosis but also many very common illnesses, such as occult or overt malignancy and myocardial infarction.[11] The risk factors that predispose to the development of venous thrombosis are prolonged medical or surgical illness, lower extremity trauma, and overt or occult malignancy. It is clear that any medical or surgical illness that places the patient at bed rest for more than a few days promotes stasis of blood in the lower extremities and may lead to DVT and PE.

The consequences of embolic occlusion of one or more pulmonary arterial branches are directly related to the magnitude of pulmonary vascular obstruction and to the patient's underlying cardiopulmonary status.[12] PE always affects regional perfusion and secondarily affects regional ventilation in the lungs. Depending on the magnitude of the PE and the presence of underlying cardiopulmonary disease, acute PE may cause a variety of hemodynamic and pulmonary derangements. PE causing minimal obstruction of the pulmonary circulation in a healthy individual is hemodynamically inconsequential and may only cause respiratory alkalosis, with little or no arterial hypoxemia.[13–15] More significant PE causes arterial hypoxemia and pulmonary hypertension of increasing severity. As the magnitude of embolic obstruction and pulmonary hypertension increases, the right ventricle fails and cardiac output declines.[14] In the extreme case, massive or saddle PE obstructing the main pulmonary artery can cause acute cardiogenic shock with cardiac arrest within minutes of the event.[16] Patients with underlying cardiopulmonary disease and previous pulmonary hypertension are likely to develop more severe pulmonary hypertension in response to PE. However, they can tolerate more severe pulmonary hypertension without developing right ventricular (RV) failure, presumably because of antecedent RV hypertrophy in response to prior pulmonary hypertension.[17,18]

Acute obstruction of a segmental pulmonary artery results in abrupt total or near-total loss of perfusion to that lung segment. The release of vasoactive substances (serotonin) by degranulating platelets as they aggregate on the surface of the thrombus may elevate pulmonary vascular resistance and compound the perfusion abnormality.[19,20] This phenomenon may, in part, account for the fact that pulmonary hypertension can develop in response to PE whereas mechanical obstruction of a similar magnitude due to balloon catheter occlusion is not associated with pulmonary hypertension. As alveolar perfusion falls in the face of continued ventilation, the alveolar O_2 tension (P_AO_2) rises and the CO_2 tension (P_ACO_2) falls. Alveolar hypocarbia or regional alkalosis may elicit bronchial smooth muscle contraction and narrowing of the airways to the embolized lung segment. Regional bronchoconstriction may be aggravated by serotonin released from platelets as they aggregate and degranulate on the surface of the embolus.[21] The net result is some reduction in regional ventilation in conjunction with the reduction in regional perfusion. Pneumoconstriction reduces ventilation to the embolized lung segment. In conjunction with reduced alveolar perfusion, this tends to restore ventilation–perfusion (V/Q) balance and lessen the degree of arterial hypoxemia stemming from the PE. Airway narrowing may give rise to increased airway resistance and localized inspiratory wheezing over the embolized lung segment.[22–24] Acute alveolar hypoperfusion as a consequence of PE compromises the capability of Type III alveolar macrophages to synthesize and secrete alveolar surfactant.[25] Loss of surfactant increases the alveolar wall tension opposing the transmural pressure responsible for alveolar distention, thereby promoting loss of lung volume and collapse of the embolized and underperfused lung segment. In the extreme, this may result in a decrease in regional ventilation to the point of segmental or lobar atelectasis.[26] As regional pulmonary perfusion falls in the embolized segment, pulmonary blood flow to other, nonembolized regions of the lung increases. Yet the remaining normal lung tissue may already be overinflated in compensation for volume loss in the embolized segments. Consequently, regional pulmonary compliance may be so reduced that no net increase in ventilation to these segments occurs. Increased perfusion to other lung regions where ventilation does not increase proportionately results in areas where blood transit time is reduced and perfusion is somewhat increased in relation to ventilation. These regions of excessive perfusion relative to ventilation in nonembolized pulmonary segments may significantly contribute to the development of arterial hypoxemia as a result of PE. The impact of PE on pulmonary function include compensatory pneumoconstriction, sometimes with wheezing; atelectasis, resulting in intrapulmonary right-to-left shunting; and V/Q imbalance. These mechanisms, to a variable degree in each patient, are important in the development of arterial hypoxemia in response to PE.

The mechanisms by which PE results in dyspnea are much less clearly understood. PE of any consequence causes the lung to become stiffer and more difficult to ventilate. This may be a result of surfactant loss and atelectasis in embolized segments and compensatory overexpansion (reduced regional compliance) in normal lung tissue. If mean pulmonary artery pressure is elevated, fluid transudation and lung lymphatic flow increase. These elevations in vascular pressure and interstitial fluid content also tend to make the lung stiffer and more difficult to ventilate.

Dyspnea does not seem to be closely related to the severity of arterial hypoxemia. Approximately 14% of patients with PE maintain an arterial oxygen tension (P_aO_2) in excess of 89 mm Hg, yet nearly all patients with PE are dyspneic or tachypneic early in their clinical course.[26,27] Almost 75% of patients with PE have a P_aO_2 exceeding 60 mm Hg: that is, the arterial hypoxemia is mild in severity and insufficient to activate the aortic and carotid chemoreceptors to augment ventilatory frequency.[26] Nonetheless, dyspnea and tachypnea are the most frequent clinical manifestations of PE. The mechanism of dyspnea in PE is not well understood. However, the consequence of stiff or noncompliant lungs, whether a result of PE, pneumonia, pulmonary edema, or adult respiratory distress syndrome, is that the patient must generate an excessive amount of inspiratory force (negative pleural pressure) to effect physiologic lung expansion and alveolar ventilation. The uncomfortable awareness of breathing characteristic of these syndromes appears to be in no small part related to this disproportionate respiratory effort required for lung expansion. As the lungs become stiffer, the normal inspiratory drop in transmural pressure can maintain adequate ventilation only when inspiration both commences at lower lung volumes and is characterized by increased respiratory excursions. The increased work of breathing is mitigated by ventilating the lung more frequently with a smaller volume. Consequently, the patient with PE ventilates from a lower functional residual capacity while breathing a smaller tidal volume at a more rapid rate (tachypnea). Associated chest pain due to pleurisy also causes the patient to take more shallow breaths.

The effect of PE on the pulmonary circulation is determined by the magnitude of obstruction, the adequacy of RV compensation and the presence of pre-existing cardiopulmonary disease.[14] A small pulmonary embolus may lodge in a third- or fourth-order pulmonary artery branch, abolishing flow to one or more lung segments and initiating loss of lung volume, significantly disordered gas exchange, dyspnea, and tachypnea by the mechanisms previously outlined. However, the embolic arterial occlusion is not extensive enough to increase pulmonary vascular resistance and mean pulmonary artery pressure.

Larger PEs reduce the total pulmonary vascular cross-sectional area enough to elevate pulmonary vascular resistance. RV work and mean pulmonary artery pressure then increase to maintain cardiac output. However, because pulmonary vascular reserve in a patient previously free of cardiopulmonary disease is extensive, PE must be large enough to occlude 30% to 50% of the vascular cross-sectional area as estimated angiographically before the increase in pulmonary vascular resistance is sufficient to provoke the development of pulmonary hypertension.[14] Patients with pre-existing cardiopulmonary disease, whose pulmonary vascular reserve has already been compromised, tend to develop more severe pulmonary hypertension in response to PE of a lesser magnitude. Yet these patients often tolerate more severe pulmonary hypertension without developing a decline in cardiac output and RV failure, presumably because of antecedent RV hypertrophy.[17,18] Common pulmonary conditions that reduce the reserve capacity of the pulmonary vasculature include chronic bronchitis and emphysema, bullous lung disease, pulmonary fibrosis of any etiology, and pulmonary resection. Similarly, any cardiac disease associated with pulmonary venous hypertension results in passive pulmonary hypertension. Passive pulmonary hypertension similarly reduces the ability of the pulmonary circuit to accommodate increased regional flow by distention and recruitment in response to embolic occlusion. Passive pulmonary hypertension may lead to pulmonary arteriolar constriction (reactive pulmonary hypertension). This commonly occurs in cases of advanced mitral valve disease but is less common in response to severe and long-standing LV failure of any etiology.[29] The net effect of passive and reactive pulmonary hypertension is a reduction in pulmonary vascular reserve. The consequence is that any further increase in pulmonary vascular resistance resulting from even a small PE (well tolerated in an otherwise normal patient) elevates pulmonary artery pressure. Clearly, a small PE in a normal patient would not be expected to elicit significant pulmonary hypertension, although it may elicit mild pulmonary hypertension as a result of hypoxemia.[34] PE of similar magnitude in a patient with reduced pulmonary vascular reserve might be expected to result in more severe pulmonary hypertension, even if there had been no resting pulmonary hypertension prior to the embolic event.

Acute obstruction of 30% to 50% of the pulmonary vascular cross-section area elevates pulmonary vascular resistance enough to result in pulmonary hypertension if cardiac output is maintained.[18] The magnitude of the elevation in pulmonary vascular resistance, in part, determines the overall impact of the PE on the patient's cardiovascular status. The previously normal right ventricle remains compensated and able to eject into the pulmonary circuit against the increased afterload until the mean pulmonary artery pressure exceeds 35 mm Hg to 45 mm Hg.[14] At that point the right ventricle cannot generate sufficient systolic tension to empty completely against a further increase in afterload, the right ventricle dilates, RV diastolic and RA pressures rise above 10 mm Hg, and RV failure occurs.[14] Despite the reduced stroke volume, cardiac output is maintained by compensatory tachycardia. With massive PE (obstruction of 75% or more of the pulmonary vascular cross-sectional area) the extreme elevation in RV afterload so drastically reduces the RV stroke volume that the cardiac output cannot be maintained despite tachycardia, and shock develops. The reduction in cardiac output due to active massive PE may be so severe that arterial hypotension persists despite maximal reflex augmentation of systemic vascular resistance.

In massive PE with cardiogenic shock, arterial hypoxemia may initially be relatively mild. Presumably, the embolized segments undergo regional airway constriction, volume loss, and atelectasis, which minimizes the impact on overall V/Q balance. Paradoxically, however, medical therapy that improves RV performance and cardiac output (inotropic drugs or fluid resuscitation or both) may worsen arterial hypoxemia. This is presumably a result of the reestablishment of flow through previously poorly perfused and poorly ventilated lung segments. Though regional flow readily increases with therapy, improvement in regional ventilation lags behind. The regional V/Q ratio falls and worsening arterial hypoxemia may ensue despite hemodynamic improvement.[30]

PULMONARY INFARCTION

Circulation to the lungs arrives from two sources. The low-pressure pulmonary arteries deliver a large volume of relatively desaturated blood to the alveoli. Bronchial arteries originating from the aorta or intercostal arteries carry a much smaller volume of saturated blood at systemic pressure to the pulmonary parenchyma. The bronchial arteries anastomose with the pulmonary arteries distally. Pathologic pulmonary infarction, defined as necrosis of interalveolar septae, alveolar hemorrhage, and healing with scar formation over several weeks to months, is more likely to occur if there is pre-existing compromise of blood flow through the pulmonary or bronchial circulations.[32] In advanced congestive heart failure, flow through these circulations is severely compromised. Pulmonary arterial flow, pulmonary blood oxygen content, bronchial arterial flow, and systemic arterial oxygen content are all reduced. The lungs are congested, and the diffusion distance for oxygen delivery to the pulmonary tissues is increased. The relative importance of each of these factors in predisposing the cardiac patient to the development of true pulmonary infarction as a consequence of PE is unclear. Nonetheless, autopsy evidence of true pulmonary infarction is much more likely to be found when PE occurs in the patient with underlying cardiopulmonary disease. However, a syndrome of incomplete pulmonary infarction, often occurs in patients without prior cardiopulmonary disease.[33] As a consequence of pulmonary infarction, patients develop fever, hemoptysis, pleuritic chest pain, and, as shown by chest x-ray, one or more pulmonary infiltrates often associated with a small exudative pleural effusion. The explanation for the occurrence of the pulmonary infarction syndrome in the absence of previous cardiopulmonary disease relates to the location of the embolism in relation to entrance of the bronchial arteries into the pulmonary arterial circuit. With proximal embolic pulmonary artery occlusion, bronchial collateral inflow at systemic pressure is dissipated through the large and very compliant pulmonary artery circuit at very low pressure distal to the occlusion. Conversely, if a large embolus fragments proximally and migrates distally, or if smaller emboli occur, smaller, medium-sized pulmonary arteries are occluded nearer the site of bronchial artery–pulmonary artery anastomoses. The bronchial collateral inflow at systemic pressure is conducted and dissipated through a much smaller and less compliant distal pulmonary artery circuit at a higher pressure. The consequence is traumatic disruption of alveolar capillary integrity and alveolar hemorrhage. Similarly, this inflammatory response may elicit an exudative and often hemorrhagic pleural effusion. If resolution is complete, the followup chest x-ray several weeks after the PE has no evidence of scarring. Presumably, the amount of irreversable alveolar septal and pulmonary interstitial destruction is insufficient to disrupt the structural framework of the lung and its reparative capabilities— hence the term "incomplete" pulmonary infarction or pulmonary hemorrhage.[33]

Clinical Presentation

PE usually presents as one of three rather clearly defined syndromes in patients free of underlying cardiac pulmonary disease: acute unexplained dyspnea; pulmonary infarction; or cor pulmonale, with or without cardiogenic shock.[27] In patients with underlying heart disease, PE may also manifest itself as worsening congestive heart failure.

ACUTE DYSPNEA

PE almost always causes dyspnea; the severity is not related to the size of the PE or to the severity of the resultant arterial hypoxemia. Rather, dyspnea is related to stimulation of pulmonary stretch receptors as a result of the excessive inspiratory effort required to ventilate the noncompliant lung. Approximately 84% of patients with PE complain of dyspnea and 96% demonstrate dyspnea or tachypnea or both.[27] Dyspnea in association with PE is almost always of abrupt onset. Consequently, patients can often rather precisely specify the time at which dyspnea first appeared. The differential diagnosis of acute unexplained dyspnea (after cardiopulmonary conditions such as congestive heart failure, pneumonia, atelectasis, pleural effusion, or pneumothorax have been excluded) includes the hyperventilation syndrome and PE. The historical consideration of greatest importance in differentiating between PE and the hyperventilation syndrome is whether or not the patient has a predisposition to venous thromboembolism. In a patient with acute unexplained dyspnea and a predisposition to PE, the physician should make the presumptive diagnosis of PE and proceed to obtain further studies to confirm or rule out this diagnosis. The finding of normal arterial blood gases in the patient on room air is especially helpful in excluding PE.

In the patient presenting with PE manifest by acute unexplained dyspnea, the most important physical finding is tachypnea. This is defined as a respiratory rate in excess of 18 breaths/min measured by the examining physician over a full minute. Nearly all patients with PE presenting as acute unexplained dyspnea manifest tachypnea early in the course, and its absence makes the diagnosis of PE extremely unlikely.

PULMONARY INFARCTION SYNDROME

The clinical hallmark of the pulmonary infarction syndrome is pleuritic chest pain. This is sharp and invariably confined to the thorax; that is, it does not radiate to the arm, neck, or jaw as does the pain of myocardial ischemic syndromes. However, it may radiate to the shoulder because of diaphragmatic irritation. Chest pain in association with the pulmonary infarction syndrome is often aggravated by coughing, deep breathing, or any significant motion of the chest; that is, it clearly has a pleuritic component.

Other symptoms in the pulmonary infarction syndrome include dyspnea, cough, and sometimes hemoptysis of a small to moderate amount of blood. Since injury severe enough to involve a major blood vessel is uncommon, hemoptysis is mild or moderate. It is usually characterized by pink to frankly red sputum with the red blood cells distributed homogeneously throughout.

Physical findings in the pulmonary infarction syndrome may include tachypnea, evidence of pulmonary consolidation, pleural effusion, and possibly a pleural friction rub.[27,33] Since the PE is rarely of sufficient magnitude to elevate the pulmonary artery pressure substantially, there are usually no physical findings suggestive of RV hypertension (increased pulmonic component of the second sound (P_2), left parasternal lift) or RV failure. The principal differential diagnosis of pulmonary infarction is pneumonia. Bacterial pneumonia is suggested by the presence of a high spiking fever, leukocytosis with a total white blood cell count in excess of 15,000/mm³ and a left shift in the differential. Purulent sputum increases the probability of bacterial pneumonia. Viral pneumonia is suggested by an antecedent history of symptoms compatible with upper respiratory tract infection, constitutional symptoms including diffuse myalgias, malaise, fever, and gastrointestinal distress and a mild to moderate leukocytosis with lymphocytosis and little or no left shift in the differential. It must be emphasized that patients with pulmonary infarction almost always have an identifiable predisposition to deep venous thrombosis.

ACUTE COR PULMONALE AND CARDIOGENIC SHOCK

When PE presents as cor pulmonale, acute RV failure, and cardiogenic shock, it reflects massive embolic occlusion with obstruction of at least 60% to 75% of the pulmonary arterial cross-sectional area. When the pulmonary artery occlusion approaches 50% to 75% of total pulmonary vascular cross-sectional area, the right ventricle must generate a systolic pressure exceeding 50 mm Hg to 60 mm Hg to elevate mean pulmonary arterial pressure to above 40 mm Hg, the level required to maintain the pressure gradient for normal pulmonary blood flow and cardiac output. The previously normal right ventricle, lacking any time to develop hypertrophy, cannot accommodate to such an acute severe pressure overload state. The consequence is dilatation and failure of the right ventricle, an elevation in RV diastolic and central venous pressure and a fall in stroke volume. If the compensatory tachycardia cannot maintain the cardiac output above a critical level, progressive peripheral organ hypoperfusion, arterial hypotension, and cardiogenic shock ensue.

The patient with acute cor pulmonale and RV failure due to massive pulmonary embolism presents with severe dyspnea and air hunger. Oppressive midsternal and anterior chest discomfort may occur in 25% of patients.[35] Clearly lacking a pleuritic component, this chest pressure is quite different from the sharp chest pain due to pleuritis accompanying PE presenting as pulmonary infarction. This more ominous chest discomfort may relate to acute RV distention or to subendocardial ischemia involving the right ventricle as a consequence of the acute severe pressure overload state.[36] In conjunction with this pain, there is often a profound degree of restlessness and anxiety associated with a fear of impending doom. Massive PE not uncommonly may initially manifest itself as syncope. In fact, over 90% of patients with syncope as a major manifestation of PE have acute cor pulmonale by hemodynamic or electrocardiographic criteria.[37] Syncope results from massive embolic occlusion of the pulmonary artery with a critical reduction in cardiac output, arterial pressure, and cerebral perfusion. If the emboli fragment or migrate distally, allowing some improvement in pulmonary perfusion, cardiac output and arterial pressure may suddenly spontaneously recover to the point that cerebral perfusion and consciousness are restored. If spontaneous improvement in pulmonary perfusion does not occur, syncope may progress to cardiac arrest. This is often characterized by electromechanical dissociation. External cardiac massage sometimes results in prompt and dramatic restoration of blood pressure and consciousness because the embolus fragments and migrates distally, permitting improved pulmonary blood flow and cardiac output.[38-40] Unfortunately, it is more often ineffective.

The patient with cor pulmonale and RV failure due to cardiogenic shock usually displays tachypnea. Tachycardia occurs in approximately 50% of cases of massive PE.[27,28,41] Hypotension, cyanosis, cool moist extremities, mental clouding, and oliguria (urine output less than 20 cc/hr) in the presence of distended neck veins define the presence of cardiogenic shock.

The cardiovascular examination is critical in identifying the patient with acute cor pulmonale and RV failure due to massive PE. The neck veins are distended above the clavicle with the patient upright. The *sine qua non* of RV failure is elevation of the central venous pressure in excess of 8 mm Hg. The corollary is that in the patient with hypotension and shock of unclear etiology, a normal or low central venous pressure rules out PE as the cause of hypotension unless the patient is simultaneously profoundly volume depleted—an unlikely coincidence. It cannot be overemphasized that accurate measurement of the central venous pressure is a critically important diagnostic intervention. In many patients, a very obese or muscular neck precludes satisfactory visualization of the jugular venous meniscus. In this circumstance, the central venous pressure must be accurately measured through a central line, with the position of the tip radiologically confirmed in the superior vena cava or right atrium prior to the institution of major therapeutic interventions.

Reflecting the acute elevation in RV afterload and pulmonary artery pressure, the patient with massive PE may demonstrate an intensified P_2. Because of the resistance to emptying, RV ejection is delayed and P_2 may split widely on inspiration and move toward, but not be superimposed on, the aortic second sound (A_2) on expiration. A systolic murmur best heard over the RV outflow tract and pulmonary valve may reflect acute dilatation of the main pulmonary trunk due to pulmonary hypertension. A left parasternal lift may be present, reflecting acute pressure overload and dilatation of the right ventricle.

The electrocardiogram (ECG) in patients with massive PE and acute RV strain usually demonstrates right axis deviation, incomplete right bundle branch block, and ST segment depression and T wave inversion in the right precordial leads.[42] These changes are respectively due to RV pressure overload, acute RV dilatation, and, possibly, subendocardial ischemia of the right ventricle.[31] The acute right axis shift in response to massive PE may manifest itself as a deep S wave in lead I, a deep Q wave in lead III and a deeply inverted T wave in lead III—the "$S_1Q_3T_3$" pattern first described by McGinn and White in 1935.[35]

The differential diagnosis of acute RV failure and shock due to PE includes cardiac tamponade and myocardial infarction with involvement of the right ventricle. The central venous pressure is elevated in all of these conditions unless there is coincident profound volume depletion. Pulsus paradoxus (an inspiratory decline in arterial systolic pressure in excess of 10 mm Hg), absence of precordial pulsations, and muffled heart sounds are suggestive of cardiac tamponade. The ECG finding of diffuse low voltage suggests pericardial effusion, whereas electrical alternans is almost diagnostic of pericardial tamponade. In tamponade the echocardiogram is very helpful. It characteristically reveals, posterior to the left ventricle and anterior to the right ventricle, a "clear" pericardial space that is characteristic of posterior and anterior pericardial effusion. It also demonstrates an exaggerated inspiratory increase in RV end-diastolic dimension and decrease in LV end-diastolic dimension in conjunction with an elevation in pericardial pressure, sometimes before the clinical findings suggestive of tamponade, are demonstrable.[43] Though pulsus paradoxus is characteristic of cardiac tamponade it and Kussmaul's sign have been found occasionally in cases of massive pulmonary embolism.[44]

RV infarction as a cause of RV failure and cardiogenic shock is differentiated from massive pulmonary embolism on the basis of clinical, electrocardiographic, and hemodynamic characteristics.[45,46] In massive PE, dyspnea is the most common symptom, while in myocardial infarction, severe chest pain is most prominent. In massive PE, there may be an RV lift and accentuation of the intensity of the sound of pulmonic valve closure. In the patient with myocardial infarction with or without RV infarction, the precordial impulse is usually rather quiet and the heart sounds are of reduced intensity. Similarly, the ECG characteristically reveals the evolutionary pattern of acute transmural or subendocardial infarction. In the patient with cardiogenic shock due to either PE or RV infarction, the central venous pressure is elevated. However, in massive PE there is invariably pulmonary hypertension of at least moderate severity. The pulmonary artery systolic pressure usually exceeds 40 mm Hg to 50 mm Hg. Pulmonary vascular resistance is elevated due to embolic occlusion of the pulmonary arteries such that the mean pulmonary artery pressure exceeds the mean pulmonary capillary wedge or LA pressure by at least 20 mm Hg.

In the patient with cardiogenic shock due to RV infarction, the fundamental derangement is a severe reduction in the contractile function of the right ventricle.[47,48] Despite an elevation in ventricular diastolic and central venous pressure, the intrinsically damaged right ventricle cannot generate sufficient systolic pressure to adequately perfuse the pulmonary circulation and fill the left ventricle. Accordingly, the pulmonary systolic and mean pressures are normal or reduced, and the pulse pressure in the pulmonary artery is usually narrow. The pressure gradient between the pulmonary artery and left atrium is invariably less than 10 mm Hg, sometimes less than 5 mm Hg, reflecting a normal to low pulmonary vascular resistance and a reduced cardiac output. In both syndromes, the cardiac output is reduced.

CONGESTIVE HEART FAILURE

PE may present as worsening congestive heart failure in a patient with previously evident cardiac disease. Because activities are restricted and cardiac output is reduced, venous return from the deep veins of the lower extremities is sluggish and the risk of deep venous thrombosis is increased. In such patients, PE of any magnitude is likely to elicit a substantial rise in mean pulmonary artery pressure because the pulmonary circulatory reserve has already been compromised by passive congestion and, possibly, by precapillary pulmonary hypertension. The acute increase in pulmonary artery pressure raises perfusion pressure to the remaining patent and well-perfused pulmonary arterial segments. The consequence is an increase in fluid transdution, a reduction in lung compliance, worsening dyspnea, and, in the extreme case, acute pulmonary edema. As a consequence of PE, more severe arterial hypoxemia and, possibly, hypotension with a reduction in coronary perfusion pressure further impair ventricular systolic performance. This reduces cardiac output and elevates mean LV diastolic and pulmonary capillary pressures to aggravate the pre-existing congestive heart failure state. Because of prior compromise in nutritive pulmonary blood flow, these patients are at a great risk for developing true pulmonary infarction as a consequence of PE.

The most common clinical manifestations of PE in the patient with cardiac disease are the nonspecific symptoms and signs of worsening congestive heart failure: dyspnea, orthopnea, paroxysmal nocturnal dyspnea, tachpnea, pulmonary rales, tachycardia, an LV S_3, and evidence of right heart failure. Findings more specific for PE include clinical evidence of deep venous thrombosis.

LABORATORY FINDINGS

PE is not a difficult clinical diagnosis in the previously healthy patient with obvious predisposition to venous thromboembolism (VTE) who develops acute unexplained dyspnea, the pulmonary infarction syndrome, or acute cor pulmonale with RV failure. The difficult problem is that many patients obviously predisposed to VTE have chronic cardiac or pulmonary disorders whose exacerbations often are clinically similar or identical to those of PE.

Various laboratory tests have been advocated and have subsequently fallen into disfavor as reliable screening tests facilitating the clinical diagnosis of pulmonary embolism. Of all the radiological and biochemical tests available, the perfusion lung scan and the P_aO_2 test are the most sensitive in detecting PE.[47]

Arterial Blood Gases

Approximately 85% of patients with acute PE demonstrate arterial hypoxemia (P_aO_2 <80 mm Hg while breathing room air). The remaining 15%, who have normal arterial blood gases while breathing room air despite acute PE, are usually young, previously healthy individuals without previous cardiopulmonary disease who have sustained small pulmonary emboli and who usually present with pleuritic pain. Despite the absence of arterial hypoxemia, these patients invariably demonstrate at least moderate arterial hypocarbia. Thus, in previously healthy patients, arterial hypocarbia and respiratory alkalosis may be a more sensitive marker of acute PE than arterial hypoxemia. However, it is also nonspecific, since a normal P_aO_2 and respiratory alkalosis are also characteristic of the anxiety–hyperventilation syndrome. Some patients with underlying chronic obstructive lung disease (COLD) may be incapable of significant hyperventilation in response to acute PE. In such chronic CO_2

retainers, PE may manifest itself as hypoxemia with a restoration of relative eucapnea. The paradox of worsening dyspnea unresponsive to bronchodilators despite "improved" ventilation, as manifest by a reduction in a chronically elevated P_aO_2, suggests PE in the patient with COLD.[48]

The severity of arterial hypoxemia correlates to some degree with the magnitude of PE. Nonetheless, patients with circulatory failure due to massive PE may display only mild arterial hypoxemia, which may paradoxically worsen with successful treatment of the shock state.[30]

Chest X-ray

Chest x-ray films lack sensitivity and specificity in the diagnosis of acute PE. However, new and subtle abnormalities on chest x-ray films of the patient with a predisposition to thromboembolic disease may direct the astute clinician to consider PE in the differential diagnosis and, therefore, to obtain more definitive diagnostic studies. In 50 patients with angiographically confirmed PE, approximately 70% had an abnormal chest x-ray with one or more of the following findings: pulmonary infiltrate (51%), pleural effusion (35%), and elevated diaphragm (27%).[47] Infiltrate and pleural effusion result from the pulmonary infarction syndrome. Diaphragmatic elevation represents atelectasis, most likely due to surfactant loss, pleurisy, and splinting of respirations. Other radiologic findings include abrupt cutoff of a pulmonary vascular shadow and regional hyperlucency of the lung resulting from embolic occlusion and regional oligemia. These findings are subtle, relatively infrequent, and extremely subject to interobserver variation. The chest x-ray is not nearly as sensitive as the perfusion lung scan in screening for PE.

Deep Venous Thrombosis

In all patients with suspected PE, evaluation of the deep venous system is extremely valuable. The clinical assessment of deep venous thrombosis is unreliable. The findings of erythema, warmth, localized tenderness, and, particularly, unilateral leg swelling are suggestive. However, approximately 50% of patients with deep venous thrombosis of the lower extremities neither experience symptoms nor demonstrate abnormalities on physical examination.[49,50] Nevertheless, excluding patients at risk for pelvic thrombophlebitis following gynecologic, colorectal, or prostatic surgery, over 90% of patients presenting with acute PE have deep venous thrombosis involving the veins of the thigh (above the popliteal vein).[9] Therefore, the presence of deep venous thrombosis of the thigh established by an objective diagnostic technique, such as impedance plethysmography (IPG) or contrast venography in a patient with suspected PE makes the diagnosis of PE much more likely. Conversely, the absence of deep venous thrombosis in a patient suspected of PE makes the diagnosis much less likely unless there is reason to suspect pelvic thrombophlebitis.

Routine ventilation/perfusion lung scans in all patients with deep venous thrombosis of the thigh confirmed by venography or IPG reveal that approximately 50% have abnormality suggestive of PE.[9] The implication is that PE, as well as deep venous thrombosis of the thigh, is frequently an asymptomatic event in patients at risk.

Contrast Venography

Contrast venography is the most accurate method for detecting deep venous thrombosis of the lower extremity.[50] However, an experienced radiologist is needed to perform and interpret it. It is expensive, time-consuming, and somewhat painful, and it carries some morbidity. Postvenography phlebitis, in fact, is not an infrequent complication. A variety of noninvasive procedures have been developed to screen patients for deep venous thrombosis. Contrast venography remains the standard by which all other methods are evaluated.

[125]I Fibrinogen Scanning

[125]I fibrinogen scanning relies upon radioactive labeling of the patients' circulating fibrinogen pool followed by interval serial scanning of the legs with a scintillation detector. A localized increase in radioactivity over the lower extremity indicates augmented fibrinogen turnover, a characteristic of any active thrombotic process.

[125]I fibrinogen scanning is very sensitive in detecting active thrombophlebitis in the soleal veins of the calf and has been invaluable as a research tool in defining the epidemiology and pathogenesis of venous thromboembolic disease.[9] It appears that in patients at risk for VTE, the clots initially form within the cusps of the soleal veins. In the majority of patients, these thrombi remain confined to the deep venous system of the calf. However, the presence of thrombosis below the level of the popliteal vein does not place the patient at significant risk for PE unless the thrombotic process propagates to involve the deep veins of the thighs.[49] [125]I screening is exquisitely sensitive in detecting calf vein thrombosis. It is much less reliable, however, in detecting proximal deep venous thrombosis of the thigh—a potentially lethal, but relatively infrequent, sequel. Consequently, ^{125}I fibrinogen scanning has been most useful as a sensitive research tool in studying the pathogenesis of VTE and evaluating the efficacy of a variety of prophylactic measures.

Impedance Plethysmography

Electrical IPG records changes in blood volume brought on by respiration and cuff-induced venous hypertension.[9,51] Inflation of a blood pressure cuff about the proximal thigh to a pressure of 45 mm Hg occludes venous return. Arterial inflow continues, and the venous volume of the thigh increases. As the cuff is deflated, blood rapidly exits through patent deep veins and the volume of the thigh rapidly decreases. These volume changes are measured as fluctuations in the resistance to the constant passage of a small electric current between electrodes positioned on the thigh distal to the occluding cuff. If the deep venous system of the thigh is patent, thigh volume and conductance to current flow rapidly decline as the cuff is deflated and blood promptly exits. If the deep venous system is occluded by thrombi above the popliteal level, the egress of blood is retarded. Consequently, the decline in venous volume as recorded by a decline in conductance (increase in resistance to current flow) is very gradual. A normal IPG reliably excludes thrombi in the deep venous system of the thigh with a specificity exceeding 90% in comparison studies using contrast venography.[9] This provides very useful information because the majority of pulmonary emboli originate in the capacious veins of the thigh. Unfortunately, a positive test is not specific (13% false positives in one study); its value, therefore is greatest when taken in the total clinical context. Negative IPGs help in excluding the diagnosis of PE, except in the patient at risk of PE from pelvic thrombophlebitis following gynecologic, colorectal, or prostatic surgery.

Lung Scans

A firm diagnosis of PE requires documentation by a perfusion lung scan (PLS). The PLS detects any macroscopic abnormality in pulmonary perfusion and is the most sensitive indicator of PE. The PLS is abnormal in all cases of PE, and a normal PLS in multiple projections rules out PE with the highest available diagnostic certainty.[52–54]

However, the PLS is almost as nonspecific as it is sensitive for PE. It detects *any* regional abnormality in pulmonary blood flow, whether due to PE, COLD, or any other pulmonary parenchymal abnormality.[55–57] A regional reduction in perfusion on the PLS consequently is not specific for pulmonary embolism and may be due to chronic airway or interstitial (pulmonary parenchymal) disease in the absence of PE. The specificity of the PLS in the diagnosis of PE is significantly increased if pulmonary parenchymal disease can be excluded as a cause of any regional perfusion abnormalities. Since the specific pathophysiologic hallmark of PE is impaired-to-absent perfusion to one or more lung segments with relative preservation of ventilation, the most specific noninvasive way to establish the diagnosis is by the coexistent demonstration of these abnormalities. Ventilation is assessed by having the patient inhale radioactive xenon. Pulmonary parenchymal disease compromises pulmonary ventilation (V) and perfusion (Q) in such a way that the PLS usually reveals an abnormality in ventilation and perfusion in the same lung segments—a *matched V/Q defect.* This matched defect, if of sufficient magnitude, often corresponds to an abnormality on the chest x-ray. An isolated matched V/Q abnormality, especially in conjunction with an abnormality on the plain chest x-ray, is likely to be due to an acute process (pneumonia, atelectasis, etc.) or chronic lung disease (bullous emphysema, etc.) that primarily affects the pulmonary parenchyma: that is, it is very unlikely that it is due to PE.

The other important feature of PLS in the diagnosis of pulmonary embolism is the character of the perfusion defect. If due to PE, it should be segmental; that is, it should have a perimeter similar to the perfusion distribution of one or more proximal pulmonary arteries. Pulmonary emboli occlude large pulmonary arteries and are usually of sufficient size even after fragmentation on initial impact to be caught in arteries no smaller than third-order (segmental) pulmonary arteries. Perfusion defects of a subsegmental nature are more likely to reflect impaired regional flow due to the parenchymal vascular and air space destruction associated with panacinar or centrilobular emphysema. Impaired regional flow is also suggested by an abnormally prolonged washout time for xenon from the affected area as determined by serial ventilation lung scans.

Though a PLS showing matched V/Q defects usually has a low probability of representing PE, there are exceptions. Since a pulmonary embolus is likely to fragment upon impacting on the pulmonary arterial bifurcation, the PLS will usually reveal more than one segmental perfusion defect in addition to the matched defect characteristic of pulmonary infarction.

Clinical pulmonary infarction often results from alveolar hemorrhage and atelectasis. Consequently, ventilation as well as perfusion to the affected segment is impaired, resulting in a matched defect. However, there are usually several segmental perfusion defects that ventilate normally in conjunction with the matched V/Q defect in pulmonary infarction.

In the case of a matched defect in ventilation and perfusion, the size of the ventilation defect relative to the perfusion defect bears some relation to the likelihood of pulmonary embolism. If, on xenon scanning or chest x-ray, the ventilation abnormality is substantially larger than the perfusion defect, the problem is more likely to be related to pulmonary parenchymal disease, and the likelihood of pulmonary embolism is low. If the perfusion abnormality is significantly larger than the ventilation abnormality, the process is more likely to be related to pulmonary vascular occlusion; that is, the likelihood of PE is greater. The PLS in the patient with suspected pulmonary embolism should be interpreted according to the following guidelines:[58,59]

1. A completely normal PLS in multiple views reliably rules out the presence of PE.
2. Perfusion defects of a nonsegmental or subsegmental nature with regionally matched abnormalities on the ventilation scan (decreased ventilation or delayed xenon washout) or chest x-ray film are unlikely to represent PE (probability <10%).
3. Multiple segmental or lobar perfusion defects in regions of the lung that are radiologically normal and ventilate normally suggest PE with a probability of 90%.
4. One or more segmental or subsegmental perfusion abnormalities with matching ventilation defects may or may not be due to PE. In this circumstance, pulmonary angiography is required to establish the diagnosis with certainty.

Pulmonary Angiography

INDICATIONS.   When the clinical findings and the results of the PLS and IPG are inconclusive, pulmonary angiography may be indicated to confirm or exclude the presence of PE.[58-60] Specific indications include the patient in whom anticoagulation is contraindicated, and the patient who develops bleeding as a result of anticoagulant therapy. The young, otherwise healthy patient with suspected PE should almost always undergo pulmonary angiography for diagnostic confirmation unless there is a contraindication to this procedure. Similarly, the diagnosis of PE should be confirmed by pulmonary angiography if surgical therapy (venous interruption or embolectomy) is contemplated.

CONTRAINDICATIONS. The only absolute contraindication to pulmonary arteriography is a known major systemic allergy to angiographic contrast medium. The presence of primary pulmonary hypertension greatly increases the risk of this procedure. However, pulmonary angiography can be safely performed if small volumes of contrast medium are used to selectively visualize second- and third-order pulmonary arteries. Mainstream pulmonary angiography with a large volume of contrast medium is contraindicated in patients with primary pulmonary hypertension. The PLS findings should be used to choose the sites for selective injections.

TECHNIQUE. Selective pulmonary angiography is preferably performed by cutdown in the antecubital fossa.[61] The femoral venous approach should be avoided because of the risk of delayed hemorrhage from the femoral venous puncture site even if heparinization is delayed for several hours after completion of the procedure. This risk is magnified if fibrinolytic therapy is used to promote more rapid resolution of pulmonary emboli.

RA and RV pressures are recorded during passage of the catheter through the right heart. Pulmonary artery pressure is recorded. Cardiac output can be measured by a variety of methods. If the patient with previously known cardiopulmonary disease or suspected PE manifests an apparent worsening of congestive heart failure, the pulmonary artery wedge pressure should also be measured.

If massive PE is suspected, mainstream pulmonary angiography is performed. Otherwise selective pulmonary angiography is usually adequate. The regions of interest are selected according to the location of perfusion abnormalities on the PLS. Traditionally, the serial cut film technique has been used. This is because cut film is the only technique by which both entire lung fields can be visualized during mainstream pulmonary angiography. Furthermore serial cut film provided better image resolution then the first-generation cineangiographic equipment.

Over the past several years, cineangiography has become increasingly popular in the performance of pulmonary angiography.[62] It allows dynamic detection of the emboli as they are silhouetted by contrast medium in the proximal pulmonary arteries. Artifacts due to vessel overlap, streaming of contrast, and inadequate filling of otherwise patent arterial branches by nonselective injections are more readily detected. Another method that is likely to increase the sensitivity of this diagnostic procedure is balloon occlusion pulmonary angiography.[63,64] The pulmonary arterial segment in question is selectively catheterized with a balloon-tipped flow-directed catheter. The balloon is then inflated to occlude flow to the artery, and several milliliters of contrast medium are injected through the distal port of the catheter beyond the site of balloon occlusion. This allows visualization of single second- and third-order pulmonary arterial branches while avoiding the injection of a large volume of contrast medium, which could cause artifacts due to vessel overlap or possibly a false negative study, since a small embolus could be obscured by being totally enveloped by the contrast medium. Controlled deflation of the balloon then allows the embolus to be dynamically imaged as the contrast stream flows past and slowly washes out from around it.

INTERPRETATION. Only two angiographic findings are definitive for pulmonary embolism: intravascular filling defects and arterial cutoffs.[65] Though intravascular filling defects are the most specific sign of PE, they are not always present. A large, incompletely obstructing embolus may not be seen because it is obscured by contrast medium flowing around it. Abrupt cutoff of a pulmonary artery occurs only if the embolus causes complete arterial occlusion. More commonly, an embolus straddles a bifurcation and partially occludes each branch. If an artery is flush-occluded at its origin, the angiographic cutoff may not be detected unless the absence of the specific arterial branch is noticed.

Two pulmonary angiographic findings that are suggestive but not diagnostic of PE are areas of oligemia and asymmetry of flow. Oligemia occurs whenever the pulmonary vasculature distal to an embolus fails to fill with contrast medium and hence appears underperfused in the x-ray study. If the embolus itself is totally obscured by contrast or is not visualized because it totally occludes an arterial branch at its takeoff, the only angiographic abnormality may be an area of regional oligemia. Oligemia may also result from occlusion of multiple small peripheral arterial branches in a regional lung zone. Occlusion gives a "pruned" appearance to the embolized segment; that is, the arterial tree in that area appears like a tree pruned of its small branches. However, regional oligemia due to lung disease may be present in the absence of PE.

Incomplete embolic occlusion causes a delay in filling of the arterial tree beyond the site of obstruction. The delay causes asymmetry of flow on the angiogram.

Though oligemia and asymmetry of flow are usually seen in patients with PE, they may occur in the absence of PE in patients with chronic cardiopulmonary disease. Oligemia may appear in areas that are relatively avascular due to emphysematous blebs or other pulmonary parenchymal pathology. Conditions such as LV failure or mitral stenosis, which cause pulmonary venous hypertension, may cause asymmetry of flow, particularly to the lower lobes.

The presence of oligemia and asymmetry of flow in the absence of intraluminal filling defects or vessel cutoffs warrants further angiographic evaluation. Techniques that are often helpful include selective pulmonary arterial catheterization and balloon occlusion angiography using cineangiographic filming techniques.

Employing these criteria, pulmonary angiograms can be categorized as follows:

1. Definite pulmonary embolism: intraluminal filling defects or cutoff of arteries
2. Equivocal: oligemia and/or asymmetry of flow without filling defects or cutoffs
3. Negative: no angiographic abnormalities consistent with PE

In the early years of pulmonary angiography, in one center 20% of studies were interpreted as equivocal. As a result of the technical advances outlined above, however the number has fallen to below 5%.[61] An equivocal study, too, provides valuable information. Major pulmonary embolism has been ruled out, and clinically important hemodynamic data have been obtained.

COMPLICATIONS. Complications associated with pulmonary angiography can occur secondary to traumatic passage of the catheter or as a reaction to the contrast medium. The mortality of this procedure in large series is approximately 0.4%, which is not surprisingly high, since this invasive procedure is frequently performed as an emergency procedure in unstable patients. Recognizing that pulmonary angiography is associated with a lower morbidity than anticoagulant or surgical therapy, and that the clinical and noninvasive diagnosis of PE can be fraught with error, it is prudent to study all patients suspected of pulmonary embolism with angiography whenever the clinical and noninvasive evaluation is inconclusive.

Summary

Over 90% of pulmonary emboli originate as deep venous thromboses of the lower extremities. Common predisposing factors are prolonged bed rest due to illness, lower extremity trauma, and malignancy. Minimal pulmonary vascular obstruction may cause respiratory alkalosis but no hypoxemia. More extensive obstruction, particularly in the presence of underlying cardiopulmonary disease, causes hypoxemia and pulmonary hypertension. When 75% or more of the pulmonary vascular cross-sectional area is obstructed, cardiac output is so drastically reduced that systemic hypotension ensues. Pulmonary infarction is particularly likely to occur in patients with pre-existing congestive heart failure.

Pulmonary embolism presents as acute dyspnea, pulmonary infarction, acute pulmonary hypertension with or without cardiogenic shock, or worsening congestive heart failure. Of the various laboratory tests relevant to diagnosis of pulmonary embolism, PLS and the measurement of arterial blood gases are the most sensitive and useful. Detection of deep vein thrombosis by contrast venography, radioactive fibrinogen scanning, or IPG is often helpful. When other tests are inconclusive, or surgical therapy is contemplated, pulmonary angiography is the definitive diagnostic test that should be employed.

References

1. Guenter CA, Braun TE: Fat embolism syndrome. Chest 79:143, 1981
2. Janower ML, Blennerhassett JB: Lymphangitic spread of metastatic cancer to the lung: a radiologic-pathologic classification. Radiology 101:167, 1971
3. Smith RRL, Hutchins GM: Pulmonary fecal embolization complicating the Budd-Chiari syndrome. N Engl J Med 298:1069, 1978
4. Dhingra RC, Rosen KM, Rhamtoola SH: Transvenous removal of catheter fragments from the heart and pulmonary artery. Arch Intern Med 132:419, 1973
5. Weingarten J, Kauffman SL: Teflon embolization to pulmonary arteries. Ann Thorac Surg 23:371, 1977
6. Celli B, Khan MA: Mercury embolization of the lung. N Engl J Med 295:883, 1976
7. Byers JM III, Soir JS, Fisher RS, et al: Acute pulmonary alveolitis in narcotics abuse. Arch Pathol 99:273, 1975

8. Dalen JE, Alpert JS: Natural history of pulmonary embolism. Prog Cardiovasc Dis 17:259, 1975

9. Sasahara AA, Shaman GVRK, Parisi AF: New developments in the detection and prevention of venous thromboembolism. Am J Cardiol 43:1214, 1979

10. Virchow R: Cellular Pathology. London:Churchill, 1860

11. Gore JM, Applebaum JS, Green HL, et al: Occult cancer in patients with acute pulmonary embolism. Ann Intern Med 96:556, 1982

12. McIntyre KM, Sasahara AA: Determinates of right ventricular function and hemodynamics in pulmonary embolism. Chest 65:534, 1974

13. Wilson JE, Pierce AK, Johnson RL, et al: Hypoxemia in pulmonary embolism, a clinical study. J Clin Invest 50:481, 1971

14. McIntyre KM, Sasahara AA: The hemodynamic response to pulmonary embolism in patients without prior cardio-pulmonary disease. Am J Cardiol 28:288, 1971

15. Stanek V, Ridel M, Widimsky J: Hemodynamic monitoring in acute pulmonary embolism. Bull Eur Physiopathol Respir 14:561, 1978

16. Alpert JS, Smith R, Carlson CJ, et al: Mortality in patients treated for pulmonary embolism. JAMA 236:1477, 1976

17. McIntyre KM, Sasahara AA: Determination of the cardiovascular responses to pulmonary embolism, in Moser KM, Stein M (eds): Pulmonary Thromboembolism, p 144. Chicago, Year Book Medical Publishers, 1973

18. McIntyre KM, Sasahara AA: Pulmonary angiography, scanning, and hemodynamics in pulmonary embolism: Critical review and correlations. CRC Crit Rev Radiol Sci 489, 1972

19. Thomas DP, Gurewich V, Ashford TP: Platelet adherence to thromboemboli in relation to the pathogenesis and treatment of pulmonary embolism. N Engl J Med 274:953, 1966

20. Rosoff CB, Salzman EW, Gurewich V: Release of platelet serotonin and the response to pulmonary emboli. Surgery 70:12, 1971

21. Stein M, Levy SE: Reflex and humoral responses to pulmonary embolism. Prog Cardiovasc Dis 17:167, 1974

22. Ureleste JR Jr, Saadek AB, Eggesen PF, et al: Wheezing due to pulmonary embolism: Treatment with heparin. N Engl J Med 274:231, 1966

23. Olazubal F, Roman T, Irizary LA, et al: Pulmonary emboli masquerading as asthma. N Engl J Med 278:199, 1968

24. Widenbauk WJ, Boyd A, Moran F: Pulmonary thromboembolism presenting as asthma. Br Med J 1:90, 1973

25. Chesnik V, Hodson WH, Greenfield LJ: Effects of chronic pulmonary ligation on pulmonary mechanics and surfactant. J Appl Physiol 21:1315, 1966

26. Dantzker DR, Bower JS: Alterations in gas exchange following pulmonary thromboembolism. Chest 81:495, 1982

27. Stein PD, Willis PW III, DeMeto DL: History and physical examination in acute pulmonary embolism in patients without preexisting cardiac or pulmonary disease. Am J Cardiol 47:218, 1981

28. Grossman W (ed): Cardiac Catheterization and Angiography. Philadelphia, Lea & Febinger, 1974

29. Dalen, JE, Dexter L, Ockene IS, et al: Precapillary pulmonary hypertension: Its relationship to pulmonary venous hypertension. Trans Am Clin Climatol Assoc 86:207, 1974

30. Jarden F, Gurdjian F, Desfounds P, et al: Hemodynamic factors influencing hypoxemia in massive pulmonary embolism with circulatory failure. Circulation 59:909, 1978

31. Stein PD, Dalen JE, McIntyre KM, et al: The electrocardiogram in acute pulmonary embolism. Prog Cardiovasc Dis 17:247, 1975

32. Parker BM, Smith JR: Pulmonary embolism and infarction. Amer J Med 24:402, 1958
33. Dalen JE, Haffajee CI, Alpert JS, et al: Pulmonary embolism, pulmonary hemorrhage and pulmonary infarction. N Engl J Med 296:1431, 1977
34. Alpert JS, Godtfredsen J, Ockene IS: Pulmonary hypertension secondary to minor pulmonary embolism. Chest 73:745, 1978
35. McGinn S, White PD: Acute cor pulmonale resulting from pulmonary embolism. JAMA 104:1473, 1935
36. Horn H, Dach S, Friedburg CK: Cardiac sequelae of embolism of the pulmonary artery. Arch Intern Med 64:196, 1938
37. Thames MD, Alpert JS, Dalen JE: Syncope in patients with pulmonary embolism. JAMA 238:250, 1977
38. Dalen JE, Alpert JS: Natural history of pulmonary embolism. Prog Cardiovasc Dis 17:175, 1974
39. Oakley CM: Conservative management of pulmonary embolism. Br J Surg 55:801, 1968
40. Heimbecher PO, Keon WJ, Richards KO: Massive pulmonary embolism: a new look at surgical management. Arch Surg 107:740, 1973
41. Bell WR: The clinical features of submassive and massive pulmonary emboli. Am J Med 62:355, 1977
42. Smith M, Ray CT: Electrocardiographic signs of early right ventricular enlargement in acute pulmonary embolism. Chest 58:205, 1970
43. D'Eruz IA, Cohen HC, Prabbu R, et al: Diagnosis of cardiac tamponade by echocardiography. Circulation 52:460, 1975
44. Cohen SI, Kupersmith J, Aroesty J, et al: Pulsus paradox and Kussmaul's sign in acute pulmonary embolism. Am J Cardiol 32:271, 1973
45. Szucs MM, Brooks HL, Grossman W, et al: Diagnostic sensitivity of laboratory findings in acute pulmonary embolism. Ann Intern Med 74:161, 1971
46. Lippman M, Fein A: Pulmonary embolism in the patient with chronic obstructive pulmonary disease. Chest 79:39, 1981
47. Cohn JN, Guiha NH, Broder MI, et al: Right ventricular infarction. Am J Cardiol 33:209, 1974
48. Lorell B, Seinbach RC, Pohost GM et al: Right ventricular infarction: clinical diagnosis and differentiation from pericardial tamponade and constriction. Am J Cardiol 43:465, 1979
49. Moses KM, Lemoine JR: Is embolic risk conditioned by location of deep venous thrombosis? Ann Intern Med 94:439, 1981
50. Jeffrey PC, Immelman EJ, Benator SR: Deep venous thrombosis and pulmonary embolism: An assessment of the accuracy of clinical results. S Afr Med J 57:643, 1980
51. Wheeler HB, O'Donnell JA, Anderson FA, et al: Occlusive impedance phlebography: A diagnostic procedure for venous thrombosis and pulmonary embolism. Prog Cardiovasc Dis 17:199, 1974
52. Gilday DL, Poulose KP, DeLand F: Accuracy of detection of pulmonary emboli by lung scanning correlated with pulmonary angiography. Am J Roentgenology, Radium Therapy and Nuclear Medicine 115:732, 1972
53. Guidotti TL, Fries LF, Bell WR, et al: Accuracy of screening for pulmonary embolism in an emergency room. Respiration 37:309, 1979
54. McNeil BJ, Hessel SJ, Branch WT, et al: The value of the lung scan in the evaluation of young patients with pleuritic chest pain. J Nucl Med 17:163, 1976
55. Brello DR, Matear AG, Osei–Wasu A, et al: Interpretation of indeterminant lung scintograms. Radiology 133:189, 1978

56. McNeil BJ: Ventilation-perfusion studies in the diagnosis of pulmonary embolism: Concise communication. J Nucl Med 21:319, 1980
57. Cheely R, McCarthy WH, Perry JR, et al: The role of noninvasive tests versus pulmonary angiography in the diagnosis of pulmonary embolism. Am J Med 70:17, 1981
58. Robies E: Overdiagnosis and overtreatment of pulmonary embolism: The emperor may have no clothes. Ann Intern Med 87:775, 1977
59. Menzoian JO, Williams LF: Is pulmonary angiography essential for the diagnosis of acute pulmonary embolism? Am J Surg 137:543, 1979
60. Stein PD, Willis PW III, Dalen JE: Importance of clinical assessment in selecting patients for pulmonary arteriography. Am J Cardiol 43:669, 1979
61. Alpert JS, Dalen JE: Pulmonary angiography in the diagnosis of pulmonary embolism. Internal Medicine Digest 9:17, 1974
62. Meister SG, Brooks HL, Szucs MM, et al: Pulmonary cineangiography in acute pulmonary embolism. Am Heart J 84:33, 1972
63. Bynum LJ, Wilson JE, Christensen EE, et al. Tech note: Radiographic technique for balloon-occlusion pulmonary angiography. Radiology 133:518, 1979
64. Dougherty JE, LaSala AF, Feldman H: Bedside pulmonary angiography using an existing Swan-Ganz catheter. Chest 77:43, 1980
65. Dalen JE, Brooks HL, Johnson LW, et al: Pulmonary arteriography in acute pulmonary embolism: Indications, techniques and results in 367 patients. Am Heart J 81:175, 1971

13

CARDIAC TAMPONADE AND CONSTRICTION

Ralph Shabetai, M.D., F.R.C.P., Edin

Cardiac Tamponade

Definition

Cardiac tamponade is a syndrome that develops as a result of accumulation of fluid under abnormally increased pressure in the pericardial sac. The normal intrapericardial pressure is subatmospheric.[1] Pericardial fluid accumulations that raise the intrapericardial pressure above normal but to a value lower than the right atrial (RA) pressure do not cause cardiac tamponade. Cardiac tamponade may be said to exist when the intrapericardial pressure has risen to the level of the RA pressure. When this equalization has occurred, further increases in intrapericardial pressure induce equal increases in RA pressure, with the important hemodynamic consequence that the determinant of RA pressure, and hence of systemic venous pressure, becomes the intrapericardial pressure.

In subjects without pre-existing heart disease, left atrial (LA) pressure is only a few mm Hg higher than RA pressure. When the intrapericardial pressure increases 5 mm Hg or 6 mm Hg above its normal subatmospheric pressure of -2 mm Hg to -3 mm Hg, it becomes equal to the RA pressure; a further increase of a few mm Hg brings the intrapericardial pressure to the same level as the LA pressure. When this occurs, RA, LA, and intrapericardial pressures become exactly equal to one another, and hence to the diastolic pressure in both ventricles, the pulmonary artery diastolic pressure, and the pulmonary arterial wedge pressure.[2] This state of equalized diastolic pressures with pericardial effusion or hemorrhage has been defined as cardiac tamponade.

That definition, while commonly applicable, suffers from the shortcoming that it does not take into consideration patients with pre-existing heart disease. For example, if a patient has left ventricular (LV) failure or hypertrophy with a high LV end-diastolic pressure—for example, 20 mm Hg—cardiac tamponade occurs when the intrapericardial pressure has increased to the level of the RA pressure but remains substantially below LA and LV diastolic pressures.[3] The reason that cardiac tamponade can be said to be present under these circumstances is that once intrapericardial pressure has risen to the level of the RA pressure, it influences cardiac performance, especially cardiac output. Cardiac tamponade, then, can usefully be defined as a syndrome of cardiac compression in which the accumulation of a fluid in the pericardial space raises intrapericardial pressure to the level of the venous pressure and in which intrapericardial pressure consequently influences the hemodynamic state of the patient.

TYPES OF CARDIAC TAMPONADE

The types of cardiac tamponade that are encountered clinically are enumerated here for convenience, but discussion of the significance of this classification will be deferred to the following section on physiology, which will make the basis of the classification apparent.

Surgical Cardiac Tamponade

The term *surgical cardiac tamponade* is used to describe acute cardiac tamponade occurring suddenly in persons who do not have pre-existing cardiac or pericardial disease. It is caused by the sudden introduction of blood or fluid into a small space around the heart bounded by the unyielding, inelastic pericardium. Severe compression of the heart under these circumstances gives rise to the classic triad of Beck: a small, quiet heart; raised jugular venous pressure; and hypotension with pulsus paradoxus.[4] This form of cardiac tamponade is termed *surgical* because it is commonly encountered in patients who have suffered trauma of the heart or aorta.

Medical Tamponade

By the term *medical tamponade* is meant cardiac tamponade occurring in patients who are usually on a medical service with pericardial disorders.[5] These disorders are diverse in nature, but the most common are infections, secondary neoplasms, idiopathic pericarditis, and radiation pericardial disease. In most of these patients, the pericardial effusion or bleeding has occurred more slowly than in the surgical patients, allowing the pericardium to stretch. Therefore, for any given increase in intrapericardial pressure above normal, the volume of intrapericardial fluid tends to be substantially greater than in the surgical patients. Beck's triad is often not present.[5] The heart may be large and may not be quiet, and the arterial blood pressure is usually normal.

However, in keeping with the definition of cardiac tamponade given above, the venous pressure in these patients is abnormally elevated.

Low-Pressure Cardiac Tamponade

Florid, full-blown cardiac tamponade with venous pressure elevated to 20 mm Hg, severe arterial hypotension, and striking pulsus paradoxus is generally quite obvious. It is important, however, to develop the skill to recognize cardiac tamponade long before this emergency situation has developed. There are many instances in which intrapericardial pressure has risen by only a few mm Hg, but has become equal to, and therefore the determinant of, venous pressure.[6] For example, a patient with neoplastic pericardial disease may develop a pericardial effusion. Over the course of days or weeks, the effusion may become large enough to elevate the intrapericardial pressure until it increases, for example, to 5 mm Hg, which might well be the patient's systemic venous pressure. Further increase in intrapericardial pressure to 7 mm Hg increases the systemic venous pressure to 7 mm Hg. Cardiac tamponade is present but is difficult to recognize. The patient is not in acute distress, the mild elevation of jugular venous pressure requires painstaking and accurate examination, and hypotension and pulsus paradoxus are absent. Low-pressure cardiac tamponade may also be encountered in persons in whom there is coexisting severe hypovolemia resulting from hemorrhage or from massive doses of diuretics.

Effusive Constrictive Pericarditis

Effusive constrictive pericarditis is a syndrome in which pericardial effusion under pressure is compressing the heart and in which the pericardium is thickened, thereby contributing to cardiac compression.[7] In these cases, a degree of cardiac compression persists even after evacuation of the offending pericardial fluid. The features of effusive constrictive pericarditis will be discussed in the section dealing with constrictive pericarditis, because an understanding of cardiac tamponade as well as of constrictive pericarditis is necessary to appreciate its pathophysiology and clinical features.

Physiology and Clinical Presentation

The basic pathophysiologic fault in cardiac tamponade is best understood in terms of the pressure–volume relations of the pericardial sac, which in turn are explained by the gross and histological anatomy of the pericardium. The pericardium invests the heart and is composed of two layers, the visceral pericardium, sometimes referred to as the epicardium, and the parietal pericardium, which is attached to the great vessels and the diaphragm. A small amount of pericardial fluid found between the two layers of the pericardium subserves a variety of functions, the most important of which, from the point of view of cardiac tamponade, is that it equalizes pressure, and pressure changes induced by rotation and acceleration, over the surface of the heart.[8]

The volume of the pericardial sac in which the heart is contained is not much greater than the volume of the intrapericardial contents, namely the blood-filled chambers of the heart and the great vessels.

Histologically, although it also contains a small number of elastic fibers, the principle tissue found in the pericardium is the collagen fiber.[9] This accounts for the low metabolic rate of the pericardium and for its inherent toughness. Inspection of the pericardium shows that the collagen bundles of which it is largely composed are wavy (Fig. 13-1).[10] When the pericardium is stretched, the waviness decreases until, at last, the collagen fibers are straight.[11] This straightening of the pericardial collagen fibers when the pericardium is stretched is the physical basis of the pressure–volume relation of the pericardium.[12] When intrapericardial volume is initially increased by a small amount—for example, in an adult human being, by 50 ml to 100 ml—only a small rise in intrapericardial pressure results. With further expansion of the intrapericardial volume, brought about by further increase in the quantity of pericardial fluid, the flat portion of the pericardial pressure–volume relation ends, and a sharp inflection point is registered (Fig. 13-2). During this portion of the pressure–volume curve, small increments in intrapericardial volume are responsible for substantial increases in intrapericardial pressure. Beyond the inflection point, the pericardial pressure–volume relationship becomes almost infinitely steep, and small increments of intrapericardial volume cause drastic increases in intrapericardial pressure.[13]

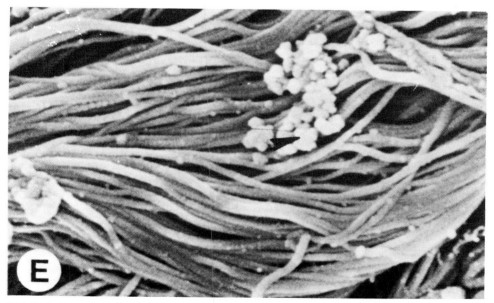

FIG. 13-1. Scanning electron micrograph of human parietal pericardium. High-magnification view showing collagen fibrils as discrete units together and cellular debris. (Ishihara T, Ferrans VJ, Jones M, et al: Histologic and ultrastructural features of normal human parietal pericardium. Am J Cardiol 46:744, 1982)

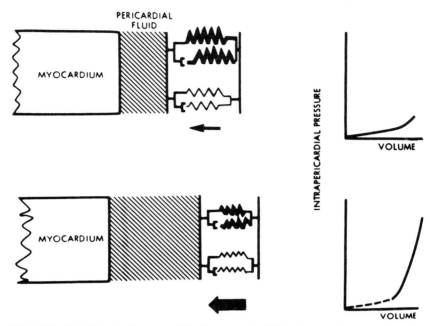

FIG. 13-2. (*Top*) Model of a pericardial effusion under slightly increased pressure, sufficient to compress the elastin springs. (*Bottom*) Model of cardiac tamponade, which compresses the heavier collagen springs (Rabkin SW, Ping Hwa Hsu: Mathematical and mechanical modeling of stress strain relationship of pericardium. Am J Physiol 229(4):896, 1975)

SUBACUTE CARDIAC TAMPONADE

It must be emphasized that the preceding description of the pericardial pressure–volume relationship applies to acute distention of the pericardium, as may occur during the induction of acute experimental cardiac tamponade in animals, or following massive trauma or rupture of the heart or great vessels, or the extraordinarily rapid development of a pericardial effusion in human subjects. The situation is altogether different when the pericardium is stretched more slowly. Any workable description of the pressure–volume relationship of the pericardium must take into account the time course over which the pericardial tissue is stretched. When the extending force on the pericardium is exerted over long periods, the pericardium can stretch; that is to say, its volume can be substantially increased with no increase in intrapericardial pressure. How else could the heart grow from its size in infancy to its size in adulthood without increasing intrapericardial pressure, and how else could pathological cardiomegaly occur without increasing intrapericardial pressure and inducing cardiac tamponade? The relative contributions of simple stretching of existing pericardial tissue, versus the growth of new pericardial tissue—that is, pericardial hypertrophy—in these circumstances has not been determined. Between the two extremes of acute, rapidly developing, cardiac tamponade at one end, and slow extension of the pericardial sac taking place over many months or years at the other, there is a whole spectrum. Acute cardiac tamponade is brought about by the sudden accumulation of a relatively small amount of fluid or blood in the pericardial space causing a substantial increase in intrapericardial pressure and greatly impeding the ability of the ventricles to fill with blood during diastole. In acute situations, the offending volume may be as little as 200 ml to 300 ml, and the intrapericardial pressure may exceed 25 mm Hg. On the other hand, a chronic pericardial effusion may amount to more than a liter in volume, and yet the associated intrapericardial pressure may be as little as 4 mm Hg, illustrating the vital importance of the time course of intrapericardial volume expansion on intrapericardial pressure and, thus on hemodynamics (Fig. 13-3). Rapid accumulation of pericardial fluid causes severe acute cardiac tamponade; effusions gathering slowly over several months may not cause cardiac tamponade at all. When the fluid accumulation is at some intermediate rate, cardiac tamponade occurs at volumes considerably larger than those encountered in acute cardiac tamponade, but usually smaller

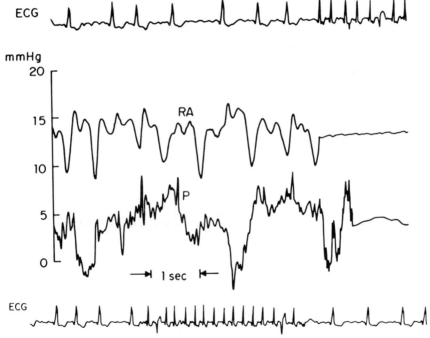

FIG. 13-3. Tracings obtained during cardiac catheterization of a patient with a massive pericardial effusion due to chronic effusive pericarditis and idiopathic congestive cardiomyopathy. Records were made before and after aspiration of more than a liter of pericardial fluid. Tracings, from top down: ECG, right atrial pressure (*RA*), and pericardial pressure (*P*). Note that the pericardial pressure is abnormally high (4 mm Hg) but consistently well below the RA pressure, which is grossly elevated because of right heart failure. Mean pressures are recorded on the right side of the figure. (Shabetai R: The Pericardium. New York, Grune and Stratton, 1981)

than those seen in chronic pericardial effusion. In some of these cases, the intrapericardial pressure elevation may be as high as in the acute cases. This occurs when the patient has not sought medical attention or when the diagnosis has been missed. In other cases, intrapericardial pressures that are distinctly abnormal but only slightly higher than the normal LA and RA pressures are found. In these cases, cardiac tamponade is less severe.

INTRAPERICARDIAL PRESSURE

In normal physiology, the intrapericardial pressure is subatmospheric. It is higher during expiration than during inspiration and is extremely close to intrapleural pressure. During the quiet phase of respiration, it is in the range of -1 mm Hg to -2 mm Hg, and during a normal inspiratory effort it falls to -3 mm Hg to -5 mm Hg.[14] With a strong inspiratory effort, intrapericardial pressure declines in proportion to the effort; for example, to -15 mm Hg to -20 mm Hg. Similarly, intrapericardial pressure is increased substantially by straining (*e.g.*, the strain phase of the Valsalva maneuver), coughing, and other interventions that increase intrathoracic pressure.[15]

Intrapericardial pressure shows fluctuations associated with the cardiac cycle superimposed on the fluctuations that are associated with the respiratory cycle. In general, intrapericardial pressure is slightly lower during systole, when the cardiac volume is reduced, than during diastole, when cardiac volume is at its maximum.[16] The precise variations of intrapericardial pressure with the cardiac cycle vary according to the location in the pericardial sac, are difficult to quantify because of hydrostatic pressure differences, and, in any case, are not really relevant to understanding the pathophysiology of cardiac tamponade. What *is* relevant is to recall that normal intrapericardial pressure is subatmospheric, that it is essentially equal to intrapleural (intrathoracic) pressure, and that these two pressures fall by an equal amount during inspiration.

Changes in Intrapericardial Pressure in Cardiac Tamponade

When cardiac tamponade occurs, intrapericardial pressure, by definition, is increased. In addition to the increase in mean intrapericardial pressure, important changes occur in the detailed morphology of intrapericardial pressure. Unfortunately, there are no clinical or noninvasive means of measuring intrapericardial pressure. Intrapericardial pressure must be obtained by inserting a catheter or needle into the pericardial space. When this is done in patients with cardiac tamponade, two changes are found: the oscillations of intrapericardial pressure related to the cardiac cycle are amplified, and intrapericardial pressure tracks intrapleural pressure less faithfully (Fig. 13-4).[17]

Respiration and Intrapericardial Pressure in Cardiac Tamponade

It has been known since 1924 that the respiratory fall in intrapericardial pressure is normally the same as that in intrapleural pressure, but that in cardiac tamponade intrapericardial pressure falls less than intrapleural pres-

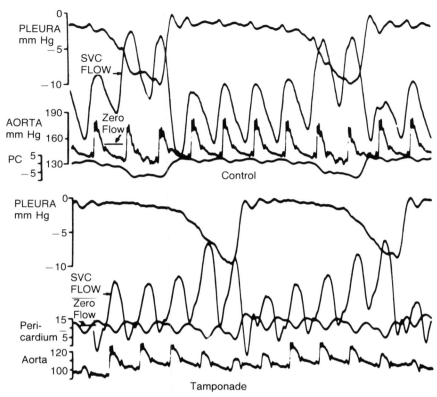

FIG. 13-4. The effect of inspiration on superior vena caval flow. (*Top*) Control. (*Bottom*) Acute cardiac tamponade. During tamponade, pulsus paradoxus is present. Superior vena caval flow is increased significantly during inspiration in the control state and almost as much in the tamponade state. Intrapericardial and intrapleural pressures each decline approximately 9 mm Hg during inspiration. *PC*=pericardium. *SVC*=superior vena cava. (Shabetai R, Fowler NO, Fenton JC, et al: Pulsus paradoxus. J Clin Invest 44:1882, 1965)

sure with inspiration.[18] Katz and Gauchat, who were among the first to record this phenomenon, thought that it was caused by failure of transmission of increased negative intrathoracic pressure to the pericardium because of the existence of a taut pericardial effusion.[18] They postulated that pericardial fluid under pressure would somehow serve as a barrier, preventing normal transmission of pressure changes across the pericardial membrane. The instruments available to them were much less sophisticated than those at hand today, which accounts for the fact that their illustrations greatly exaggerate this phenomenon, demonstrating large intrathoracic pressure swings in association with minimal or absent changes in intrapericardial pressure. These illustrations are quite different from those recorded in several subsequent studies, in which only slight differences in inspiratory fall between intrapleural and intrapericardial pressures in cardiac tamponade were present (see Fig. 13-4).[19] Furthermore, intrathroracic pressure drops occurring with inspiration are transmitted faithfully into the left ventricle and aorta, so there seems to be no *a priori* reason why this should not occur in pericardial effusion with a pressure of 20 mm Hg. Clearly, we must look elsewhere for an explanation of why the intrapleural and intrapericardial pressure drops differ in cardiac tamponade.

Intrapericardial Pressure and Systemic Venous Return

The act of inspiration lowers intrathoracic pressure, thereby creating a favorable pressure gradient from the extrathoracic veins to the intrathoracic great veins and the right atrium. This favorable filling gradient accounts for an increase of venous return to the heart that occurs with each inspiration. Following an inspiration, therefore, the volume of the right atrium and the right ventricle increases. In the absence of pericardial effusion under increased pressure, there is adequate room for this volume expansion because the pericardial volume slightly exceeds the volume of the intrapericardial contents, a difference spoken of as the *pericardial reserve volume.* In cardiac tamponade, the pericardial reserve volume has been used up, and an inspiratory increase in right heart volume within a pericardial sac that is already full causes a small increase in intrapericardial pressure.[20] This increase is considerably less than the fall in intrapericardial pressure caused by transmission of the reduced intrathoracic pressure to the pericardial sac. The net result is a drop in both intrapleural and intrapericardial pressures. When the pressures are measured using conventional techniques, that the drop in intrapericardial pressure is slightly smaller than the drop in intrapleural pressure may not be obvious. However, the phenomenon can easily be elucidated by measuring transmural intrapericardial pressure. To accomplish this, the two pressures are measured simultaneously, and the intrapleural pressure is electronically subtracted from the intrapericardial pressure. In the absence of cardiac tamponade, no change in transmural intrapericardial pressure is registered. On the other hand, when cardiac tamponade is present, a transient increase amounting to 2 mm Hg to 5 mm Hg is recorded at the peak of each inspiration.[6] This transient occurs when venous return to the right heart is increased.

SYSTEMIC VENOUS PRESSURE

Changes in RA pressure are faithfully transmitted to the superior vena cava and to the jugular veins. Details of the systemic venous pressure pulse can thus be obtained by simple inspection of a jugular venous pulse at the bedside, by placing a suitable external transducer on the jugular venous pulse, or by advancing a catheter from a systemic vein to the superior vena cava or right atrium. There is a remarkably close correspondence between wave forms obtained by the two latter techniques.

Several important features characterize a normal jugular venous pulse. The pulsations are the positive waves A, C, and V, and the negative waves X and Y. Commonly, the A and the C waves are merged. The A wave is usually dominant, but all the waves are approximately equal in amplitude and are inscribed with a similar velocity. Of great importance, the jugular venous pressure declines slightly during each inspiration. The A wave represents atrial systole. When the A and the C waves are clearly separated from one another, the nadir constituted by the downslope of the A wave and the upslope of the C wave can be distinguished and is sometimes labeled the X descent. This is a point of confusion and contention, as will be mentioned later. During iso-volumic systole, the C wave is inscribed. It has been ascribed to ascent of the closed tricuspid valve apparatus during the development of isovolumic RV tension. At the beginning of ejection, the X descent of the venous pressure is inscribed. Those who refer to the downslope of the A wave as the X descent call this new descent the X′ descent[21]. The classic literature ascribes the X (or X′) descent to descent of the tricuspid valve apparatus following the release of isovolumic tension as ventricular ejection commences. An alternative ex-planation for the X′ descent, one that is agreeable to those with an interest in the pericardium, is that during ejection the heart becomes smaller and the unoccupied intrapericardial space correspondingly larger. This causes a drop in intrapericardial pressure, promoting increased venous return. The X′ de-scent is followed by the V wave, which is associated with passive filling of the right atrium during atrial diastole. The V wave should not be confused with the systolic wave of venous pressure that occurs when the tricuspid valve is severely incompetent. The latter is generated not by passive filling of the atrium, but by regurgitant flow from the right ventricle through the incom-petent valve to the right atrium. Following the V wave, the Y descent is inscribed at about the time of opening of the tricuspid valve.

Venous Pressure and Venous Flow

There is a reciprocal relationship between venous pressure and ven-ous flow. During inspiration venous pressure declines, but venous flow in-creases (Figs. 13-5 and 13-6). Venous flow to the heart, like venous pressure, is not multiphasic. Flow is at its peak when pressure is at its lowest. The peaks of flow occur at the times of the X′ descent and the Y descent. Flow is minimal, absent, or even slightly reversed during the inscription of the A and V waves. Normal systemic venous return is thus essentially bimodal, a surge occurring during ventricular systole (X′ descent) and a second surge (Y descent) occurring early in ventricular diastole (Fig. 13-7). The systolic surge of flow is probably caused by a combination of a pistonlike movement of the tricuspid valve and the fall in intrapericardial pressure at the beginning of ventricular ejection.

At first sight, the observation that during inspiration venous pressure falls but venous return increases does not appear to make good sense. The drop in venous pressure is a reflection of transmission into the venous system of falling intrathoracic pressure. Transmural venous pressure does not fall during in-spiration, but rises. This can be ascertained by measuring the two pressures simultaneously and electronically subtracting pleural pressure from venous pressure. Thus, when one considers transmural pressure rather than absolute pressure, the paradox of a flow increasing at a time when the driving pressure appears to be falling is eliminated. Measurement of transmural pressure is not commonly available except in animal studies and in a few carefully selected patients. In the latter, esophageal pressure is frequently used as a convenient substitute for intrapleural pressure.[22]

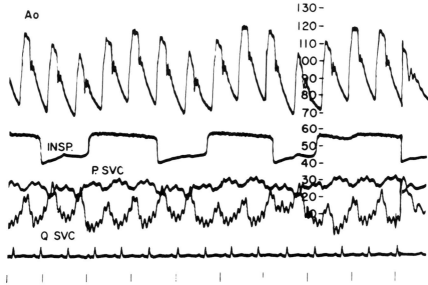

FIG. 13-5. Tracing obtained during cardiac catheterization of a patient with cardiac tamponade. The top tracing is from the ascending aorta and shows striking pulsus paradoxus. The middle tracing registers the phase of respiration. Pressure in the superior vena cava (*P. SVC*) is extremely elevated (almost 30 mm Hg). Nevertheless, the pressure drops by a few millimeters of mercury during each inspiration. With each cardiac cycle there is a single *X* descent of pressure. Below the pressure tracing is a tracing of blood flow velocity in the superior vena cava (*Q SVC*). Note that this parameter increases during each inspiration. The bottom tracing is the electrocardiogram, and the dashed lines below that denote seconds. (Shabetai R: The Pericardium. New York, Grune and Stratton, 1981)

Cardiac Tamponade and Venous Pressure and Flow

It has been established by numerous experimental and clinical measurements that cardiac tamponade, even when severe, does not prevent the normal inspiratory drop in venous pressure and the normal inspiratory increase in venous return from taking place. Many textbooks describe Kussmaul's venous sign; that is, an inspiratory increase in venous pressure in cardiac tamponade. In fact, the expected effects of inspiration on venous pressure and return are not modified by cardiac tamponade. The inspiratory increase in venous return is a cause of the inspiratory increase in transmural intrapericardial pressure in patients with cardiac tamponade. Increased venous return to the right heart during inspiration has several other important consequences, the most notable of which are interference with LV function and the generation of pulsus paradoxus.[19]

In cardiac tamponade, fluid under increased pressure compresses the heart throughout the cardiac cycle. The primary pathophysiologic alteration is inhibition of cardiac filling. In diastole, cardiac volume is at its greatest, and, therefore, compression of the heart is at its most severe. Cardiac filling cannot

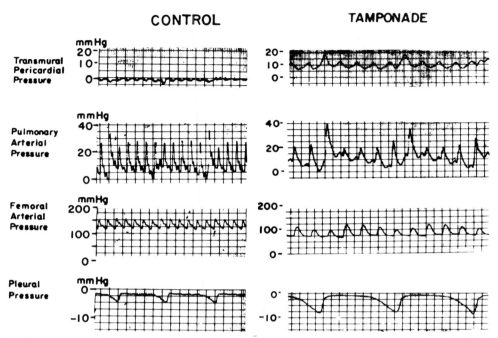

FIG. 13-6. Effect of inspiration on transmural pericardial pressure. In the control, there is no significant respiratory variation in transmural pericardial pressure. During tamponade there is a pronounced increase in transpericardial pressure with inspiration. (Shabetai R, Fowler NO, Fenton JC et al: Pulsus paradoxus. J Clin Invest 44:1882, 1965)

occur during diastole. This is the cause of one of the most dramatic and pathognomic features of the venous pulse in cardiac tamponade; absence of the Y descent.[23] In the experimental setting, it can be shown that flow through the superior vena cava and inferior vena cava occurs only during systole. During diastole, both the Y descent of venous pressure and the diastolic surge of blood toward the heart are abolished (see Fig. 13-5). The clinician does not ordinarily measure venous flow, although it can be estimated by Doppler techniques. The clinician can see and measure with a cardiac catheter, or record with an external transducing device, the absence of the Y descent of venous pressure.

It is easy at the bedside to distinguish between the X and Y waves of venous pressure. The X (or X') wave, being an event associated with ventricular systole, occurs simultaneously with the carotid pulse. The Y descent, on the other hand, is seen and recorded between the pulsations of the carotid artery. At the bedside, one need only place a finger on the carotid pulse and carefully inspect the jugular venous pulsations. A sharp inward motion occurring at the same time as the carotid pulse is an X' descent. A rapid inward motion occurring out of phase with the carotid pulse is a Y descent. Prominent Y descents are never seen in severe cardiac tamponade, and a prominent Y descent is not seen in uncomplicated mild cardiac tamponade.

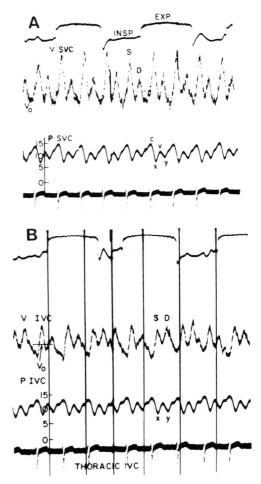

FIG. 13-7. (A) Blood flow velocity (*V SVC*) and pressure (*P SVC*) in the superior vena cava of a patient with mild congestive cardiac failure. Velocity was measured by an electromagnetic catheter-tip velocity transducer. V_I indicates zero flow. The predominant peak (*S*) is systolic and corresponds with the X descent of pressure. The second and smaller peak (*D*) corresponds with the Y trough. (*B*) Pressure and flow in the inferior vena cava of the same patient. Systolic and diastolic velocity peaks corresponding with X and Y pressure troughs are again evident.

Systemic Venous Pressure Level

When pericardial pressure is increased, reflex venoconstriction, redistribution of regional blood-flow, salt retention, and a variety of other factors combine to increase the venous pressure to the level of the intrapericardial pressure. Without this adaptation, life could not be sustained because the intrapericardial portion of the great veins would be totally occluded by the pressure of the pericardial fluid.

In cardiac tamponade, the venous pressure must therefore be evaluated for three specific features: the absolute value of the venous pressure, the occurrence of a drop of venous pressure during inspiration, and absence of the Y descent.

Right Atrial Pressure, Transmural Right Atrial Pressure, and Preload

Before leaving the subject of venous pressure, it is important once more to consider separately the absolute pressure in the great veins and right atrium and the transmural pressure. Elevation of the absolute venous and RA pressure by cardiac tamponade is, as has been discussed, obligatory for survival. The patient suffers all the consequences of raised venous pressure and the consequent passive congestion of tissues and organs. In subjects without cardiac tamponade, an increase in absolute pressure in the great veins and right atrium is accompanied by an increase of almost equal magnitude in transmural RA pressure, so that preload is high. This state of affairs does not obtain in cardiac tamponade, where the pericardial pressure and the RA and venous pressures are equal. Here, transmural RA pressure is essentially zero, and preload is greatly reduced.

CARDIAC TAMPONADE AND PULMONARY VENOUS, AND LEFT ATRIAL PRESSURES

The key difference between the pulmonary venous circulation and the systemic venous circulation is that the pulmonary venous circulation is entirely confined to the intrathoracic cage whereas the systemic venous circulation has an intrathoracic portion that is fed by an extrathoracic portion. This means that respiration exerts a primary effect on systemic venous return, but only a secondary effect on pulmonary venous return. Movement of the diaphragm and of the thoracic muscles of respiration induces a cyclical variation in the pressure of the intrathoracic portion of the systemic venous conduit, thereby causing cyclical variation in systemic venous return during the respiratory cycle.

The increase in systemic venous return, and subsequently in right heart output, that occurs with inspiration traverses the pulmonary vascular bed and eventually arrives in the pulmonary veins and left atrium, where a similar but damped respiratory variation in pulmonary venous return is recorded. The respiratory variations in systemic and pulmonary venous return are not precisely in phase with each other, the variation in pulmonary venous return being delayed by the transit time of blood traversing the pulmonary bed.[24]

The pulmonary venous circulation is not directly accessible to clinical examination. Inferences about pulmonary venous pressure and pulmonary congestion can be made from clinical and radiological examination of the lungs, and cautious deductions concerning respiratory variation in pulmonary venous return are permissible from analysis of respiratory variation in systemic arterial pressure. Direct information about pulmonary venous pressure comes from experimental observations and from observations made during cardiac catheterization of human subjects. Almost all observations concerning pulmonary venous return have been made in experimental animals, and even there the techniques are difficult and beset with pitfalls.

Most observers believe that respiratory variation in pulmonary venous return in cardiac tamponade is in the normal direction, but is exaggerated. Some observers believe that during inspiration in cardiac tamponade, retrograde blood flow occurs through the pulmonary veins. In any case, there is a distinct drop in pulmonary venous return and, therefore, in LV stroke volume. In severe cardiac tamponade, cardiac output is reduced, a factor that by itself exaggerates the respiratory variation in venous return.

In subjects without cardiac tamponade, respiratory variation in pulmonary venous return and LV stroke volume may be considered largely to reflect systemic venous return and RV stroke output. By the time the augmented RV output of inspiration appears in the aorta, the phase of respiration will have changed from inspiration to expiration, accounting in part for the normal slight reduction in inspiratory systemic arterial blood pressure and pulse pressure.

In patients with cardiac tamponade, respiratory variation in systemic venous return is responsible for more complex and graver consequences. This is because pericardial reserve volume has been exhausted, intrapericardial pressure is greatly elevated, and the pericardium is tightly stretched, thereby exerting a powerful, sometimes overwhelming, restraining influence on the heart. Under these circumstances, interaction between the chambers of the heart is greatly magnified.[25]

THE PERICARDIUM AND INTERACTION BETWEEN CARDIAC CHAMBERS

Even though human anatomy provides a small pericardial residual volume, inspection of the beating heart in the operating room uniformly shows that, under conditions of normovolemia, the pericardium is quite snugly applied to the heart. It therefore has considerable potential to restrain the volume of the heart as a whole, or that of an individual chamber when other chambers are expanded in volume. The atria are separated from each other by a septum that is common to both, and, similarly, the intraventricular septum is common to both ventricles. Muscle bundles do not respect the territory of either ventricle, but twist and turn to encompass both. The heart has a unique arrangement in that two pumps that circulate the blood in series are arranged side by side in parallel and are invested by the inelastic pericardium. When any cardiac chambers are dilatated, distortion of the shape, pressure, and compliance of the others is inevitable.[26]

Under the conditions of tamponade, right heart volume can expand during inspiration only at the expense of significant compromise of LV volume and compliance.[27] Normally, the competition for living space within the pericardial sac between the various cardiac chambers, particularly the two ventricles, is a friendly, low-key affair; in cardiac tamponade it assumes the qualities of a desperate struggle. Thus, the effect of inspiration on the relationship between systemic and pulmonary venous return is greatly exaggerated by cardiac tamponade.

NORMAL RESPIRATORY VARIATION IN ARTERIAL BLOOD PRESSURE

Many factors combine to result in a lower systemic arterial blood pressure during inspiration. The role that each plays varies from person to person, depending on such factors as the rate and depth of respiration, the ratio of the heart rate to the respiratory rate, whether posture is upright or supine, the size of the heart, and the blood volume. In patients with disease, other factors may contribute. These include obstructive airways disease; bronchospasm; cardiac enlargement, especially when acute; the state of the pericardium; and the function of the intraventricular septum.

Mechanisms

Several physiologic mechanisms contribute to lower blood pressure in normal subjects.

1. Transmission of increased negative pressure from the thorax into the left heart chambers and intrathoracic aorta, according to some authorities, creates an increased afterload on the left ventricle because the act of inspiration drops LV and intrathoracic aortic pressures but does not directly affect the extrathoracic arterial tree.[2]
2. Because a certain amount of time is required for the inspiratory increment of RV output to appear in the arterial circulation, this increment appears during expiration, which results in a higher blood pressure during expiration and, therefore, a lower one during inspiration.
3. It has been stated by some that, during inspiration, blood is pooled in the expanded pulmonary vascular bed. Most authorities, however, have concluded that this is a small or negligible factor, basing their conclusions to some extent on experiments in which venous return is held constant by a pump.[19]
4. Interaction between the left and right sides of the heart in which inspiratory increase in right heart volume decreases the compliance and volume of the left side of the heart, perhaps because of bowing of the intraventricular septum from right to left ventricle, leads to a drop in arterial blood pressure during inspiration.

PULSUS PARADOXUS IN CARDIAC TAMPONADE

Pulsus paradoxus is an important physiologic and clinical manifestation of cardiac tamponade. The usual clinical definition of pulsus paradoxus is an abnormal inspiratory decline in arterial blood pressure. Blood pressure usually declines by a few mm Hg during inspiration, but a decline of 10 mm Hg or more defines pulsus paradoxus. Experimental studies have shown that pulsus paradoxus in cardiac tamponade is associated with an inspiratory decline in LV stroke volume.[19] Pulsus paradoxus is therefore characterized not only by a fall in systolic blood pressure, but also by reduced pulse pressure: that is, the diastolic pressure falls less than the systolic pressure with inspiration. When pulsus paradoxus is pronounced, it can easily be palpated in the peripheral pulse. Thus, during inspiration the pulse weakens appreciably or actually disappears. The effect can be amplified by instructing the patient to breath slowly and deeply. When, as in surgical cardiac tamponade, the blood pressure is low, pulsus paradoxus may be difficult to elicit at the radial pulse but is usually apparent in the carotid and femoral pulses. Precise quantification of pulsus paradoxus requires measurement of intra-arterial pressure through a needle or cannula. However, an estimate can be obtained using the ordinary clinical sphygmomanometer. Specific instructions are given to the patient not to alter the pattern of respiration. When the blood pressure sounds first occur, they are heard only during expiration, but as cuff pressure continues to fall, they are heard throughout the respiratory cycle. The magnitude of the pulsus paradoxus is estimated by the difference between the pressure at which the blood pressure sounds first appear and that at which blood pressure sounds first become audible throughout the respiratory cycle.

Mechanisms

All the mechanisms that normally combine to produce a small fall in intra-arterial pressure during inspiration continue to operate in the presence of cardiac tamponade. As in normal physiology, the chief determinant of the inspiratory fall in arterial blood pressure is a decrease in venous return to the left ventricle. Two consequences of cardiac tamponade combine to greatly exaggerate inspiratory decline in arterial blood pressure; that is, to produce pulsus paradoxus. The first of these is the much stronger competition between the cardiac chambers for the now limited intrapericardial space, and the second is the reduction in overall cardiac output and stroke volume. A 10 ml reduction in a normal LV stroke volume of 90 ml has a small effect on arterial pressure, but a 10 ml reduction in a stroke volume of 30 ml greatly reduces the arterial pressure and pulse pressure.

Experimental studies in animals and patients with acute cardiac tamponade sufficient to produce obvious pulsus paradoxus have established the following:

1. Systemic venous return to the right heart increases during inspiration, just as in normal physiology, and is associated with an inspiratory increase in the dimensions of the right heart chambers.
2. If inspiratory augmentation of right heart filling is abolished by using a right heart bypass, increased intrapericardial pressure, however severe, does not induce pulsus paradoxus.
3. In cardiac tamponade, inspiration is associated with an increase in transmural pericardial pressure coincident with the increase in systemic venous return and right heart dimensions and with the fall in systemic arterial pressure.
4. The hemodynamic influence of inspiration can be mimicked in transiently apneic animals by rapidly adding a few ml of blood while they are otherwise perfused by a constant-flow right heart bypass. When the pericardial pressure is zero, this intervention does not change intrapericardial pressure but causes an increase in pulmonary arterial pressure, followed two or three beats later by an increase in arterial pressure. When the same experiment is performed after the intrapericardial pressure has been greatly elevated, the additional venous return is associated with an increase in intrapericardial pressure and a drop in aortic pressure that coincides with the increase in pulmonary arterial pressure and precedes the subsequent increase in arterial pressure (Fig. 13-8).
5. Respiratory variations in systemic arterial and pulmonary arterial pressures are neither in phase with each other nor of completely opposite phase.

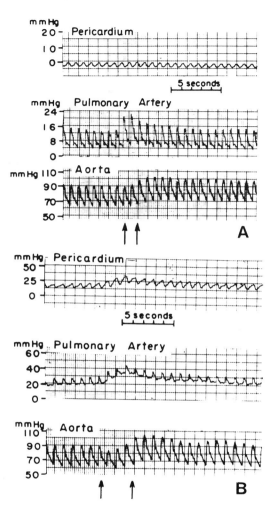

FIG. 13-8. The effect of increased venous return. (*A*) Control. The effect on pulmonary arterial and aortic pressure of an increase of approximately 15 ml in return to the right atrium during apnea after a period of steady controlled flow. Pulmonary arterial pressure rises promptly. There is no change in intrapericardial pressure. The aortic pressure rise is delayed for two cardiac cycles and is preceded by a small decline (1 mm Hg). The arrows indicate the period of addition of blood to the right atrium. (*B*) The same experiment is repeated with tamponade. The increased pulmonary arterial pressure is accompanied by a fall of 7 mm Hg in aortic pressure. Aortic pressure rise lags behind that in pulmonary arterial pressure by three cardiac cycles. The intrapericardial pressure is increased by the addition of blood to the right heart. (Shabetai R, Fowler NO, Fenton JC, et all: Pulsus paradoxus. J Clin Invest 44:1882, 1965)

That increasing intrapericardial pressure in closed-chest dogs fails to induce pulsus paradoxus during constant-flow right heart bypass does not support an earlier hypothesis that inspiratory traction by the diaphragm on the taut pericardium plays a significant role in causing pulsus paradoxus in cardiac tamponade.[28] This experiment also suggests that pooling of blood in the lungs during inspiration is an unlikely mechanism. Both the inspiratory increase in transmural pericardial pressure and the experiments in which the effects of inspiration were simulated hemodynamically indicate that, in cardiac tamponade, inspiratory increase in venous return and right heart volume exerts a deleterious effect on LV filling and emptying. Furthermore, LV end-diastolic volume is small in cardiac tamponade, an alteration that would cause it to function on a steep portion of the Frank–Starling curve, thereby exaggerating the effect of respiratory filling variations on arterial blood pressure.

The principle cause of pulsus paradoxus in cardiac tamponade is embarrassment of LV function by inspiratory increase in right heart volume. This effect is augmented by the reduced cardiac output and by the several physiologic mechanisms that normally reduce arterial blood pressure during inspiration.

THE RIGHT VENTRICLE IN CARDIAC TAMPONADE

The right ventricle is a thinner-walled chamber than the left and is, therefore, more easily compressed. It has been known for many years that LV volume is decreased in cardiac tamponade.[29] The assumption is commonly made that this is because of direct compression of the left ventricle by pericardial fluid under increased pressure. However, studies from our laboratory have shown that a major cause of reduced LV end-diastolic pressure in cardiac tamponade is reduction of pulmonary venous return, secondary to direct compression of the thin-walled right ventricle.[30] Thus, it may be that the stout-walled left ventricle is able to resist compression by pericardial fluid. Striking reduction of RV dimensions and diastolic compression of the right ventricle and right atrium are important echocardiographic findings in cardiac tamponade.[31]

Summary

Cardiac tamponade is a syndrome in which hemodynamics are strikingly altered by increased intrapericardial pressure. The most "pure" tamponade is found in surgical patients and in experimental cardiac tamponade. Tamponade in medical patients is often somewhat modified by the slower accumulation of pericardial fluid and in some cases, by pre-existing heart disease. The effects of pericardial effusion on intrapericardial pressure and thence on hemodynamics are highly dependent upon the rate of fluid accumulation.

The most important clinical sign of cardiac tamponade is increased jugular venous pressure. This pressure is characterized by a normal decline during inspiration and by absence of the Y descent. In the most acute cases, the heart is small and quiet and the blood pressure may be reduced. These features are often absent in subacute and chronic cardiac tamponade. Most cases of cardiac tamponade exhibit pulsus paradoxus, but this sign may be absent in patients with pre-existing elevation of LV diastolic pressure.

A major aid to diagnosis is to suspect cardiac tamponade in patients in whom pericardial disease or injury is a reasonable possibility. When tamponade is suspected, echocardiography should be performed to determine whether a pericardial effusion is present. If one is found, the specific signs of cardiac tamponade should be diligently sought at the bedside. In cases of doubt, or when confirmation or quantification is required, the diagnosis is established by simultaneously recording intrapericardial and RA pressure, and observing the effects on these pressures of aspirating a portion of the pericardial effusion.

Constrictive Pericarditis

Definition

Constrictive pericarditis is a condition in which filling of the heart is impeded by disease of the pericardium that decreases its compliance and obliterates the pericardial reserve volume. Constrictive pericarditis becomes significant when the volume of the scarred pericardium is less than the cardiac volume. This reduction in intrapericardial volume abnormally reduces the volume and increases the filling pressure of the cardiac chambers, thereby inducing secondary changes in ventricular emptying.

Physiology

The pericardium is a relatively inelastic membrane surrounding the heart. Pericardial volume slightly exceeds the operating cardiac volume, the difference constituting the residual volume of the pericardium. The pericardium stretches easily in the initial part of its pressure–volume relation, thereby accommodating spontaneous changes in cardiac volume. Thereafter, the pericardium becomes almost infinitely stiff, strongly resisting further stretch. In constrictive pericarditis, because of scarring, even the initial ability of the pericardium to stretch is lost.

The pericardium need not be significantly thicker than normal in constrictive pericarditis, although it often is—sometimes massively so. It is not the thickness of the pericardium *per se*, but its fixed and reduced volume that constitutes the essential pathophysiologic fault in constrictive pericarditis.

In cardiac tamponade, the heart is compressed throughout the cardiac cycle, with transient slight relief during systolic ejection, when cardiac volume is somewhat reduced. In constrictive pericarditis, the heart is surrounded by a fixed shell that compresses it little if at all during systole and the first third of diastole, but compresses it severely during the latter two-thirds of diastole. During late diastole, no cardiac filling whatever can occur. Measurement of ventricular volume throughout the cardiac cycle in patients with constrictive pericarditis shows an absolute plateau of volume lasting throughout the latter two-thirds of diastole (Fig. 13-9). This pattern is in sharp contrast to the changes in ventricular volume found in patients without constrictive pericarditis. In

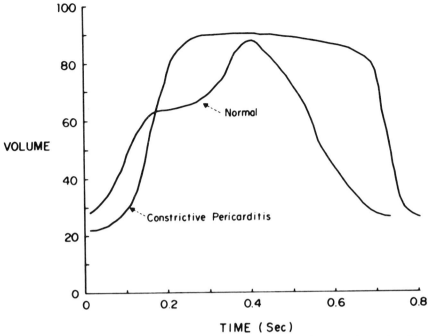

FIG. 13-9. Ventricular volume plotted against time in a patient with constrictive pericarditis. A normal LV volume curve is presented for comparison. The normal curve shows rapid filling in early diastole, followed by diastasis and a second period of rapid filling in presystole. By comparison, in constrictive pericarditis early diastolic filling is more rapid than normal, but during the rest of diastole no significant increase in the ventricular volume occurs. (Shabetai R: The Pericardium. New York, Grune and Stratton, 1981)

them, a brief period of diastasis follows early diastolic rapid filling. This is followed by a second (presystolic) period of rapid filling (Fig. 13-9). The pattern of ventricular filling in cardiac tamponade does not differ significantly from normal (Fig. 13-10).

Abnormalities of ventricular filling in constrictive pericarditis are not confined to the latter period of diastole. Early diastolic filling is more rapid than normal, probably owing to the rapid active relaxation of a ventricle with greatly reduced end-systolic volume. Thus, ventricular filling in constrictive pericarditis is characterized by abnormally rapid early diastolic filling, followed by absence of filling throughout the latter part of diastole.[32]

Corresponding to the abnormalities of ventricular filling in constrictive pericarditis, characteristic abnormalities of ventricular diastolic pressure occur. During the period of abnormally rapid ventricular diastolic filling, ventricular diastolic pressure drops precipitously, giving rise to the "early diastolic dip." During the period when the ventricle fails to fill because it has achieved the volume of the constricting pericardium, ventricular diastolic pressure is grossly

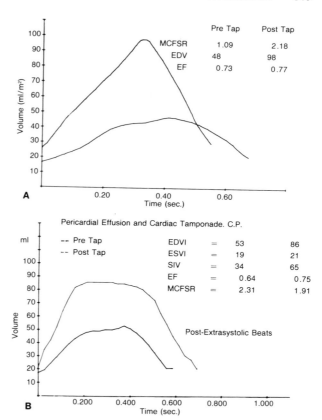

		Pre Tap	Post Tap
	MCFSR	1.09	2.18
	EDV	48	98
	EF	0.73	0.77

Pericardial Effusion and Cardiac Tamponade. C.P.

-- Pre Tap				
-- Post Tap	EDVI	=	53	86
	ESVI	=	19	21
	SIV	=	34	65
	EF	=	0.64	0.75
	MCFSR	=	2.31	1.91

Post-Extrasystolic Beats

FIG. 13-10. LV volume during the cardiac cycle in two patients with cardiac tamponade before and after removal of a portion of the pericardial fluid. Note that, following this intervention, LV diastolic volume increases. (*A*) LV pressure almost doubles after pericardiocentesis, and filling becomes much more rapid. (*B*) Postextrasystolic beats are compared in another patient. MCFSR = mean circumferential shortening rate; EDV = end diastolic volume; EF = ejection fraction. (Shabetai R: The Pericardium. New York, Grune and Stratton, 1981)

elevated and demonstrates a plateau corresponding to the plateau of volume. Together, these two abnormalities give rise to the "dip and plateau" or "square root sign" of constrictive pericarditis (see Fig. 13-11).[33] It should be said that conventional pressure measurement techniques exaggerate the dip. The dip is still present when measured with high-fidelity intracardiac transducers but is of less amplitude and seldom extends below zero, as it often does when measured with a conventional transducer and fluid-filled catheter.

VENOUS PRESSURE

For the most part, the venous pressure in constrictive pericarditis mirrors ventricular diastolic events. Thus, the LA and RA pressures show a prominent Y descent corresponding exactly with the early diastolic dips of RV and LV diastolic pressures. During the plateau of ventricular diastolic pressure, the atrial pressures have corresponding elevated plateaus of pressure. Points of similarity between the venous pressures in constrictive pericarditis and in

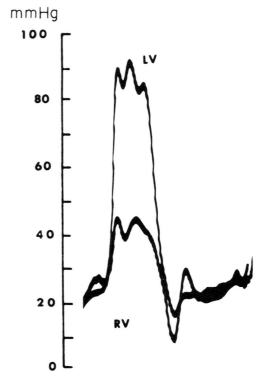

FIG. 13-11. Recording of LV and RV pressures from a patient with constrictive pericarditis. In early diastole a dip is inscribed in the pressure tracing from both ventricles, corresponding to the onset of rapid filling. Throughout the remainder of diastole, there is a plateau of pressure, which is elevated considerably above normal ventricular filling pressure and is equal for the two ventricles. (Shabetai R: The Pericardium. New York, Grune and Stratton, 1981)

cardiac tamponade are that in both the venous pressures are considerably elevated, and that, in both, left- and right-sided venous pressures are equal to one another. In cardiac tamponade, however, the X descent is prominent and the Y descent is absent. In constrictive pericarditis, a normal X descent occurs and is followed by a prominent Y descent. Another point of distinction between the venous pressures in constrictive pericarditis and cardiac tamponade is that in constrictive pericarditis, RA pressure remains constant throughout the respiratory cycle or increases during inspiration (Kussmaul's sign), whereas in cardiac tamponade, RA pressure declines during inspiration (Figs. 13-12, 13-13, and 13-14).

SYSTEMIC VENOUS RETURN

During ventricular systole in constrictive pericarditis, cardiac compression is minimal and there is no impediment to systemic venous return to the right heart. A normal X (or X[1]) descent of RA pressure with a corresponding systolic surge of blood from the vena cavae to the right atrium therefore occurs (see Fig. 13-14). During early diastole, when the ventricles are

FIG. 13-12. Pressure tracing (*P SVC*) obtained from the lower reaches of the superior vena cava in a patient with mild constrictive pericarditis. In this patient, the RA pressure is moderately elevated. Respiratory variation is absent. Note the very prominent Y descent. Above the pressure tracing is a tracing of blood flow velocity in the superior vena cava (*Q SVC*). Notice that this, too, is not influenced by respiration. Blood flow is bimodal, corresponding with the X and Y descents. The sharpest acceleration occurs simultaneously with the Y descent of pressure, which is more profound than the X descent. (Shabetai R: The Pericardium. New York, Grune and Stratton, 1981)

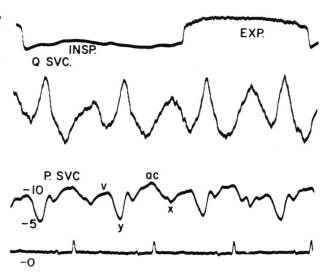

filling rapidly, the Y descent of atrial pressure occurs simultaneously with the early diastolic surge of venous return (see Fig. 13-12). The important distinction between venous return in constrictive pericarditis and that in cardiac tamponade is that in the former the normal bimodal pattern of venous return is preserved, whereas in the latter venous return is unimodal, occurring only during ventricular systole.

VENTRICULAR EJECTION, STROKE VOLUME, AND CARDIAC OUTPUT

Since in constrictive pericarditis, the ventricular end-diastolic volume is reduced and is fixed, stroke volume is reduced and cannot vary appropriately with changes in demand or in heart rate. In spite of compensatory tachycardia, cardiac output is reduced in all but the mildest cases. The response of cardiac output to exercise is greatly blunted. Tachycardia is an important adjustment in constrictive pericarditis because slow heart rates are associated with prolonged diastolic periods, during much of which no cardiac filling takes place.

The combination of increased cardiac filling pressures and reduced cardiac output results in a clinical picture resembling congestive heart failure. In reality, however, congestion in constrictive pericarditis should not be confused with heart failure because the latter implies dysfunction of the myocardium. In constrictive pericarditis, low cardiac output is a function of the reduction in the cardiac chamber size, and the raised cardiac filling pressure is a function of the abnormal external constraint on the heart.[34]

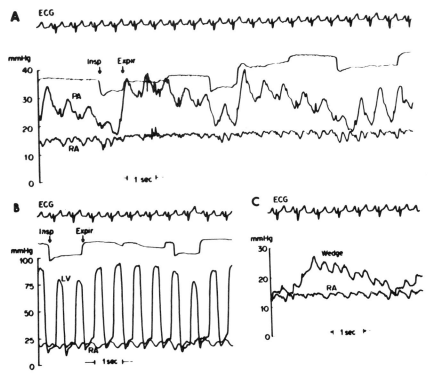

FIG. 13-13. Hemodynamics in constrictive pericarditis. (*A*) Simultaneously recorded pressures from the pulmonary artery, in which pressure falls during inspiration (presumably in response to a fall in pulmonary vascular resistance), and from the right atrium, in which respiratory variation is blocked by the pericardial scar, which prevents transmission of changing intrathoracic pressure into the right atrium. (*B*) Tracings recorded during cardiac catheterization of a patient with constrictive pericarditis, showing, from above down, electrocardiogram, phase of respiration, LV pressure, and RA pressure. The arrows mark the onset of inspiration and expiration. Note that there is close agreement between the LV diastolic pressure and the RA pressure. Simultaneous recordings of pressures from these two chambers can often very conveniently establish the diagnosis of constrictive pericarditis. Note that respiratory variation is absent from the RA pressure tracing but is present in the LV pressure tracing. An early diastolic dip of LV pressure is seen, but there is no plateau because of tachycardia. The pressures were both recorded using high-fidelity systems. (*C*) Pressure tracings recorded during cardiac catheterization of the same patient, showing, from above down, electrocardiogram, pulmonary arterial wedge pressure, and RA pressure. Note absence of respiratory variation in the RA pressure tracing. On the other hand, inspiration is associated with a profound fall in pulmonary arterial wedge pressure. These two pressures, therefore, agree only during the inspiratory phase of the respiratory cycle. (Shabetai R: The Pericardium. New York, Grune and Stratton, 1981)

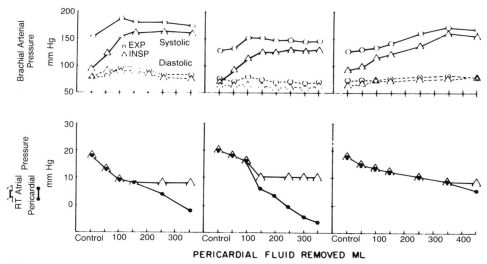

FIG. 13-14. Hemodynamic changes in three patients with cardiac tamponade during serial 50 ml withdrawals of pericardial fluid. The most significant hemodynamic changes occur during the initial aspirations while RA and intrapericardial pressures remain equilibrated. After the fall of intrapericardial pressure below RA pressure, the RA pressure shows no further change. (Reddy PS, Curtiss EI, O'Toole JD, et al: Cardiac tamponade: Hemodynamic observations in man. Circulation 58:265, 1978. By permission of the American Heart Association, Inc.)

VENTRICULAR FUNCTION

In most cases of constrictive pericarditis, the underlying myocardium is healthy and capable of normal function. The isovolumic indices of contraction based upon the instantaneous relationship between LV diastolic pressure and its first derivative are normal. These indices include peak dp/dt, V_{max}, and dp/dt at a common developed pressure of 20 mm Hg. Likewise, the ejection fraction, mean circumferential shortening rate, and other ejection phase indices of LV performance are normal. Postextrasystolic potentiation is not impaired in constrictive pericarditis.[34] These observations, derived from hemodynamic studies of patients with constrictive pericarditis, have been confirmed by noninvasive studies, in particular, by systolic time intervals showing a normal ratio of LV pre-ejection period to ejection time.

From these observations, it is concluded that reduced cardiac performance in constrictive pericarditis is caused by severe unloading of the heart and not by intrinsic or acquired disease of the myocardium. This conclusion has obvious important therapeutic implications.

ASSOCIATED MYOCARDIAL DISEASE

Disease processes that affect the pericardium may also involve the myocardium. An obvious example is radiation to the mediastinum, which may cause substantial scarring involving the myocardium as well as the pericardium.

Postoperative constrictive pericarditis may, as the name implies, be confined to the pericardium (and neighboring mediastinal structures), or may be associated with damage to the myocardium, resulting in a decrease in myocardial compliance. In severe, long-standing chronic constrictive pericarditis, especially when the pericardium is heavily calcified, the disease process commonly extends into the superficial layers of the myocardium, where it may interrupt portions of the conduction system and obliterate branches of the coronary arteries.[35] In these cases, there is true myocardial impairment associated with constrictive pericarditis. It has been shown that in chronic constrictive pericarditis, the myocardial fibers undergo a degree of atrophy.[36] If this has any functional counterpart, it must be subtle, because normal, indeed supranormal, ventricular function has frequently been demonstrated in the presence of severe constrictive pericarditis.

CARDIAC RATE AND RHYTHM

Sinus tachycardia is frequent in severe constrictive pericarditis and may be looked upon as an important compensation for reduced stroke volume. Prolonged diastasis is an obvious disadvantage when the stroke volume is low and fixed and when ventricular filling is confined to the early portion of diastole. In chronic cases, atrial fibrillation almost inevitably supervenes. For example, atrial fibrillation is almost invariable in patients with calcific constrictive pericarditis secondary to an episode of tuberculous pericarditis decades earlier. This arrhythmia has been cited as evidence of myocardial involvement in constrictive pericarditis, but measurement of ventricular function in patients with calcific constrictive pericarditis and atrial fibrillation has yielded normal results in several cases.[37] Atrial fibrillation in these cases, therefore, may be ascribed to long-standing elevation of atrial pressures.

THE GENERALIZED NATURE OF CONSTRICTIVE PERICARDITIS

In the vast majority of cases, constrictive pericarditis is a generalized process. All four cardiac chambers are invested in the pericardial scar, and all are therefore subject to the same external constraint on filling. Thus, it comes about that RA and LA pressures are equal to one another and, consequently, the ventricular diastolic pressures are also equal to one another and, of course, to the common atrial pressure.[35] Finally, the pulmonary wedge pressure and the pulmonary arterial diastolic pressure equilibrate at the level of the common atrial pressure. This finding is similar to that in cardiac tamponade, in which these same pressures also equilibrate to a common level because all cardiac chambers are surrounded by pericardial fluid exerting the same increased pressure.[2]

In constrictive pericarditis, the relationship between the LA and RA pressures is somewhat more complex than in cardiac tamponade. In cardiac tamponade, RA pressure declines in normal fashion during inspiration. The two pressures, therefore, faithfully track each other throughout the respiratory cycle. In constrictive pericarditis, the RA pressure does not fluctuate with the respiratory cycle, and therefore equilibration of the two pressures is confined to inspiration (see Fig. 13-13).

MILD CONSTRICTIVE PERICARDITIS

Much of the literature concerning constrictive pericarditis deals with severe cases in which the cardiac filling pressure is raised to 20 mm Hg or more. In mild cases, the filling pressure may be raised only to the range of 7 mm Hg to 12 mm Hg. In such cases, congestion of peripheral tissues and organs is absent or mild, and the cardiac output at rest remains within the normal range. The only clue to constriction of the heart is the somewhat elevated systemic venous pressure and the characteristic wave form of venous pressure, with abnormal prominence of the Y descent.

In some cases, constriction is so mild that it cannot be detected under basal conditions. So called "occult constrictive pericarditis" may require a large and rapid fluid challenge before it is disclosed.

EFFUSIVE CONSTRICTIVE PERICARDITIS

It is possible for disease of the pericardium to be manifested by a combination of scarring of the pericardium itself and the accumulation of pericardial effusion that may be under increased pressure. This combination, a common sequel to mediastinal radiation and to tuberculous pericarditis, gives rise to the syndrome of effusive constrictive pericarditis. The initial pathophysiology is usually dominated by tamponade. Thus, the venous and intrapericardial pressures are elevated and equal to each other. The wave form of the venous pressure is that of cardiac tamponade, showing prominence of the X descent (or X^1) and absence of the Y descent. Left and right heart filling pressures are equal.

Aspiration of pericardial fluid, as in cases of uncomplicated cardiac tamponade, results in parallel lowering of intrapericardial pressure and the venous pressures. Eventually, a point is reached at which the venous pressures level off, but the intrapericardial pressure continues to decline with further aspiration of pericardial fluid until it achieves its normal subatmospheric levels (see Fig. 13-14). In uncomplicated cardiac tamponade, from the time that intrapericardial pressure and venous pressures separate, venous pressure is normal in level, waveform, and respiratory variation. In effusive constrictive pericarditis however, the venous pressure remains abnormal after the intrapericardial pressure has been restored to normal. In these cases, the venous pressure remains higher than normal, there is absence of respiratory variation and the waveform is characterized by abnormal prominence of the Y descent (Fig. 13-15).

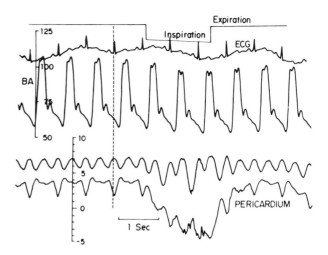

FIG. 13-15. Recording made during cardiac catheterization of a patient with effusive constrictive pericarditis owing to bronchogenic carcinoma. A considerable volume of pericardial fluid has been aspirated, and therefore the intrapericardial pressure has fallen below the RA pressure. Observe that the RA pressure shows the typical waveform of constrictive pericarditis with absence of respiratory variation. (Shabetai: The Pericardium. New York, Grune and Stratton, 1981)

Clinical Presentation

SEVERE CHRONIC CONSTRICTIVE PERICARDITIS

In severe chronic constrictive pericarditis, long-standing congestion and low cardiac output will have produced a characteristic clinical picture. Cardiac cachexia is often striking. The upper extremities are thin, the cheeks shallow and sunken. The lower extremities are swollen and the abdomen is protuberant, in striking contrast to the wasted muscle and generalized loss of subcutaneous fat. The great distention of the jugular venous system and the striking Y descent of its pulse are often obvious even when the patient is sitting up and is viewed from a distance.

Pitting edema of the lower extremities and the physical findings of ascites are present. The liver is considerably enlarged and usually is firm but is not tender. The abnormal findings in the liver are due to long-standing, severe passive congestion. Frequently, hepatic congestion in these patients results in spider angiomata.

Cardiac Examination

The great wasting of the intercostal muscles often found in severe chronic constrictive pericarditis helps to make the pulsations of the precordium more easily palpable. They are often abnormal, taking the form of systolic retraction. These retractions are also palpable. The apical beat itself may or may not be palpable but usually is not. The first and second heart sounds (S_1 and S_2) are often normal but may be diminished in intensity. The most striking, and certainly the most characteristic, auscultatory finding is a loud sound, termed the *pericardial knock*, that occurs in early diastole. It is often louder than S_1 and S_2, and derives its somewhat dramatic name from its booming character and its association with constrictive pericarditis. In actuality, it is nothing more than a loud S_3 associated with the abrupt cessation of rapid ventricular filling at the end of the early diastolic dip, near the commencement of the plateau of pressure. Its timing is somewhat later than the average opening snap of mitral stenosis, but somewhat earlier than the usual S_3 of LV dilatation and failure (Fig. 13-16).

Examination of the Neck Veins

In severe chronic constrictive pericarditis, the venous pressure is so elevated that it should be evaluated while the patient sits upright. When the patient is more supine, the venous pressure is so high that venous pulsations are damped out. With the patient in the proper posture, vigorous pulsations of the internal and external jugular systems are apparent. The dominant wave is the Y wave. This is easily recognized at the bedside both by its characteristic appearance and by its timing, which is completely out of phase with the simultaneously palpated carotid pulse (see Fig. 13-16).

Other signs of congestion in addition to hepatomegaly may be present. For example, the spleen may be palpable. Pleural effusions are common and manifest by their usual physical findings. Pulmonary congestion is often less severe than in congestive heart failure because the right ventricle is restrained by the constrictive pericarditis from flooding the lungs. Nevertheless, pulmonary venous pressure is elevated and crepitations may be heard in the lung fields.

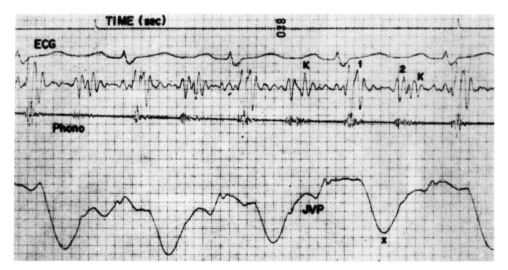

FIG. 13-16. Loud pericardial knock in a patient with severe constrictive pericarditis. Tracings, from above down, are: 1-sec time marker, electrocardiogram, two phonocardiographic channels, and the indirect jugular venous pulse. Note the loud knock sound (*K*) which occurs with the Y descent of venous pressure. (Shabetai R: The Pericardium. New York, Grune and Stratton, 1981)

Differential Diagnosis

When confronted with a patient with cachexia, anasarca, and enlargement of the liver, the differential diagnosis is rapidly narrowed to a consideration of severe right heart failure, often with associated tricuspid valve incompetence; cirrhosis of the liver; and constrictive pericarditis. The good clinician can rapidly separate cardiac and pericardial causes of the syndrome from hepatic causes because in the latter, the venous pressure is normal, whereas in both of the former, it is grossly elevated. Furthermore, in patients with cirrhosis of the liver there should not be an additional heart sound. Unfortunately, in clinical practice, this important distinction is frequently missed. Many cases of constrictive pericarditis are managed as cases of cirrhosis of the liver, sometimes for many years. Failure to observe the venous pressure is the explanation for this aberration. It is easy to see how, without adequate evaluation of the venous pressure, a patient with constrictive pericarditis may be thought to have cirrhosis. Massive edema, a greatly enlarged liver, ascites, jaundice, spider angiomata, and laboratory evidence of hepatic failure combine to deceive the physician. In some cases, they have even deceived the pathologist who, upon receiving a liver biopsy, has read "cirrhosis" instead of "cardiac cirrhosis of the liver."

In considering the differential diagnosis of heart failure, one cannot rely too extensively upon the venous pressure because with severe tricuspid incompetence, the venous pressure is greatly elevated and the Y descent is striking. However, diastolic murmurs, loud and long systolic murmurs, ventricular heaves, angina pectoris, and the history of the etiology of the disorder may point away from the pericardium and toward the heart and its valves. In most adults, severe right heart failure is caused by lung disease, LV failure, or cardiomyopathy, all of which are relatively easily recognized by symptoms and signs.

MILDER CONSTRICTIVE PERICARDITIS

It behooves the clinician to be alert to the existence of milder forms of constrictive pericarditis, as may be found in patients who have undergone cardiac surgery or radiation to the chest. Here, cachexia, fluid accumulations, and hepatomegaly are usually absent. The clue to the diagnosis often lies in a history that discloses an etiology for constrictive pericarditis. The major finding on clinical examination is the venous pressure, which is moderately elevated and shows a prominent Y descent. A pericardial knock may be present, but more often is absent. There are no signs of liver dysfunction in this group of patients. Sinus rhythm is preserved and the cardiac output is normal. These patients do not complain of fatigue and dyspnea.

RESTRICTIVE CARDIOMYOPATHY

An uncommon, but exceedingly important, differential diagnosis of constrictive pericarditis is restrictive cardiomyopathy. This is a form of cardiomyopathy, which may be either idiopathic or secondary to an infiltrative process such as amyloidosis. The diseased myocardium becomes extremely stiff from about the end of the first third of diastole onward. The hearts are not dilated and are not hypertrophied, although the ventricular myocardium may appear unduly thick by echocardiography because of the incorporation of amyloid or other infiltrates. Systolic function is usually normal. These cases, therefore, mimic constrictive pericarditis. It is frequently impossible to distinguish between constrictive pericarditis and restrictive cardiomyopathy by clinical examination alone. In both, the venous pressure is elevated and characterized by a prominent Y descent. In both, the only auscultatory abnormality is a loud S_3. Both may progress to anasarca. In both, cardiac enlargement may be absent, mild, or moderate. In both, the LV and RV diastolic pressures are characterized by the dip-and-plateau configuration.[38]

In many cases, cardiac catheterization reveals an important difference between constrictive pericarditis and restrictive cardiomyopathy: in restrictive cardiomyopathy, the LV diastolic pressure is usually greater than the RV diastolic pressure.[39] If this difference is not present at rest, it can be provoked by muscular exercise or infusion of saline. In the most obstinate cases of restrictive cardiomyopathy, the LV and RV ventricular diastolic pressures may be too close to permit diagnosis. In such cases, endomyocardial biopsy may be useful.[37] Early ventricular diastolic filling may be less rapid in restrictive cardiomyopathy, though this is not always so.[32,38]

Summary

Constrictive pericarditis is a disorder in which diastolic filling of the heart is impeded by a pericardial disease process that results in a pericardial scar that abnormally restricts the volume of the heart. This abnormality significantly reduces the volumes and increases the filling pressures of the cardiac chambers, causing severe systemic and pulmonary congestion and, secondarily, tissue hypoperfusion. The pericardial process is a generalized one; it involves all cardiac chambers equally, causing equilibration of the filling pressures of both sides of the heart.

Constriction is minimal during systole and early diastole and maximal during the latter two-thirds of diastole. Ventricular filling is therefore abnormal, being confined to early diastole. This abnormality gives rise to the characteristic Y descent of venous pressure and the early diastolic dip and late diastolic plateau of ventricular pressure. The clinical picture is dominated by severe congestion, particularly of the liver. The clinician must also be alert to the possibility of mild constriction manifest solely by moderate elevation of the jugular venous pressure.

References

1. Holt JP, Rhode EA, Kines H: Pericardial and ventricular pressure. Circ Res 8:1171, 1960
2. Metcalfe J, Woodbury JW, Richards V, et al: Studies in experimental pericardial tamponade: Effects on intravascular pressures and cardiac output. Circulation 5:518, 1952

3. Reddy PS, Curtiss EI, O'Toole JD, et al: Cardiac tamponade: Hemodynamic observations in man. Circulation 58:265, 1978
4. Beck CS: Two cardiac compression triads. JAMA 104:714, 1935
5. Guberman BA, Fowler NO, Engel PJ, et al: Cardiac tamponade in medical patients. Circulation 64:633, 1981
6. Shabetai R: The Pericardium, p 231. New York, Grune and Stratton, 1981
7. Hancock EW: Subacute effusive constrictive pericarditis. Circulation 43:183, 1971
8. Banchero N, Rutishauser WJ, Tsakiris AG, et al: Pericardial pressure during transverse acceleration in dogs without thoracotomy. Circ Res 20:65, 1967
9. Roberts WC, Spray TL: Pericardial heart disease: A study of its causes, consequences and morphologic features. In Spodick DH (ed): Pericardial Diseases. Philadelphia, FA Davis, 1976
10. Hort W, Braun H: Untersuchungen an normalen und pathologisch veranderten Herzbeuteln. Verh Deutsche Ges Path 45:271, 1961
11. Rabkin SW, Ping Hwa Hsu: Mathematical and mechanical modeling of stress strain relationship of pericardium. Am J Physiol 229 (4):896, 1975
12. Ishihara T, Ferrans VJ, Jones M, et al: Histologic and ultrastructural features of normal human parietal pericardium. Am J Cardiol 46:744, 1980
13. Ferrans VJ, Ishimara T, Roberts WC: Anatomy of the Pericardium. In Reddy PS, Leon, DF, and SHavers JA (eds:) Pericardial Diseases. New York, Raven Press, 1982
14. Morgan BC, Guntheroth WC, Dillard DH: The relationship of pericardial to pleural pressure during quiet respiration and cardiac tamponade. Circ Res 16:493, 1965
15. Shabetai R: The Pericardium, p 74. New York, Grune and Stratton, 1981
16. Shabetai R: The Pericardium, p 241. New York, Grune and Stratton, 1981
17. Fowler NO, Shabetai R, Braunstein JR: Transmural ventricular pressures in experimental cardiac tamponade. Circ Res 7:733, 1959
18. Katz LN, Gauchat HW: Observations of pulsus paradoxus (with special reference to pericardial effusions). Arch Intern Med 33:371, 1924
19. Shabetai R, Fowler NO, Fenton JC, et al: Pulsus paradoxus. J Clin Invest 44:1882, 1965
20. Shabetai R: The Pericardium, p 73. New York, Grune and Stratton, 1981
21. Constant J: Bedside Cardiology, 2nd ed. Boston, Little Brown, 1976
22. Cassidy SS, Robertson CH Jr, Pierce AK, et al: Cardiovascular effects of positive end-expiratory pressure in dogs. J Appl Physiol 44(5):743, 1978
23. De Cristofaro D, Liu CK: The haemodynamics of cardiac tamponade and blood volume overload in dogs. Cardiovasc Res 3:292, 1969
24. Sharp JT, Bunnell IL, Holland JF, et al: Hemodynamics during induced cardiac tamponade in man. Am J Med 29:640, 1960
25. Swanton RH, Brooksby IAB, Davies MJ, et al: Systolic and diastolic ventricular function in cardiac amyloidosis: Studies in six cases diagnosed with endomyocardial biopsy. Am J Cardiol 39:658, 1977
26. Shabetai R, Mangiardi L, Bhargava V, et al: The pericardium and cardiac function. Prog Cardiovasc Dis 22:107, 1979
27. Bove AA, Santamore WP: Ventricular interdependence. Prog Cardiovasc Dis 23:365, 1981
28. Dock W: Inspiratory traction on the pericardium. Arch Intern Med 108:837, 1961
29. Craig RJ, Whalen RE, Behar VS, et al: Pressure and volume changes of the left ventricle in acute pericardial tamponade. Am J Cardiol 22:65, 1968
30. Ditchey R, Engler R, LeWinter M, et al: The role of the right heart in acute cardiac tamponade in dogs. Circ Res 48:701, 1981

31. Schiller NB, Botvinick EH: Right ventricular compression as a sign of cardiac tamponade: An analysis of echocardiographic ventricular dimensions and their clinical implications. Circ 56:774, 1977
32. Tyberg TI, Goodyer AVN, Hurst VW, et al: Left ventricular filling in differentiating restrictive amyloid cardiomyopathy and constrictive pericarditis. Am J Cardiol 47:791, 1981
33. Hansen AT, Eskildsen P, Gotzche H: Pressure curves from the right auricle and the right ventricle in chronic constrictive pericarditis. Circulation 3:881, 1951
34. Gaasch WH, Peterson KL, Shabetai R: Left ventricular function in chronic constrictive pericarditis. Am J Cardiol 34:107, 1974
35. Levine HD: Myocardial fibrosis in constrictive pericarditis: electrocardiographic and pathologic observations. Circulation 48:1268, 1973
36. Dines DE, Edwards JE, Burchell HB: Myocardial atrophy in constrictive pericarditis. Proceedings of the Staff Meetings of the Mayo Clinic 33:93, 1958
37. Lewis BS, Gotsman MS: Left ventricular function in systole and diastole in constrictive pericarditis. Am Heart J 86:23, 1973
38. Wood P: Chronic constrictive pericarditis. Am J Cardiol 7:48, 1961
39. Meaney E, Shabetai R, Bhargava V, et al: Cardiac amyloidosis, constrictive pericarditis and restrictive cardiomyopathy. Am J Cardiol 38:547, 1976
40. Swanton RH, Brooksby IAB, Davies MJ, et al: Systolic and diastolic ventricular function in cardiac amyloidosis. Studies in six cases diagnosed with endomyocardial biopsy. Am J Cardiol 39:658, 1977

14

SYSTEMIC HYPERTENSION

Suzanne Oparil, M.D.

Definition

Systemic hypertension is defined as elevated arterial blood pressure. Since blood pressure in the general population falls on a Gaussian curve of normal distribution, it is not possible to define with precision the limits of "normal" blood pressure. In addition, the pressure of any given normal individual varies widely over time, depending on a large number of variables, including sympathetic activity, posture, state of hydration, and skeletal muscle tone (Fig.14-1). Accordingly, any definition of hypertension must be arbitrary. The World Health Organization defined hypertension as a single casual (sitting or recumbent) blood pressure greater than 160/95 mm Hg.[1] Pressures less than 140/90 mm Hg were classed as normotensive, and values between 140/90 mm Hg and 160/95 mm Hg were not classified but were regarded as potentially abnormal, particularly when they occurred in young people (<30 years of age).[2] Subsequent investigation has shown that individuals within this blood pressure range have borderline hypertension, that their blood pressure rise with age is steeper than that of normotensive subjects, that their mortality and cardiovascular morbidity rates are greater than those in the normotensive population, and that they show evidence of abnormal circulatory regulation.[3]

In Western populations, blood pressure increases with age, so normal ranges for blood pressure must take age into account. A given level of blood pressure elevation has to be taken more seriously when it occurs in a younger person, since the related cardiovascular morbidity and mortality are greater in hypertension of early onset. Procedures recommended by the Joint National Committee on Detection, Evaluation and Treatment of High Blood Pressure

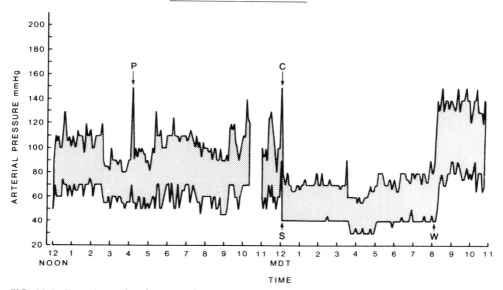

FIG. 14-1. Five-minute plots from a 24-hour continuous arterial pressure record in a healthy 31-year-old man during a normal day's activity and a night of sleep in his own house. *P*=painful stimulus (4.05 P.M.). *C*=coitus (midnight). S–W=sleep–waking (12.05–8.05 A.M.). (Pickering G: High Blood Pressure, p 56. London, J and A Churchill, 1968)

for evaluation of hypertension in adults are summarized in Figure 14-2.[4] Blood pressure in children is so heavily dependent on age that a nomogram of blood pressure versus age must be used to define the normal range.[5]

Essential or primary hypertension is systemic arterial hypertension of unknown cause. Over 95% of all cases of systemic hypertension are in this category. A multitude of pathophysiologic factors has been implicated in the genesis of the syndrome. No single cause has been found to account for even a fraction of the cases. It is likely that essential hypertension represents a collection of diseases or syndromes with distinct pathophysiologic features. The "mosaic theory" of hypertension, in which multiple interrelated abnormalities have been invoked as predisposing to blood pressure elevation, has found wide support.[6]

Secondary hypertension is systemic arterial hypertension of known cause. Fewer than 5% of all cases of systemic hypertension are in this category. The importance of identifying patients with secondary hypertension is that the disorder is sometimes curable by surgery and can easily be controlled by specific medical treatment. The most common causes of secondary hypertension are: oral contraceptives, renal parenchymal and renal vascular disease, pregnancy, the syndromes of mineralocorticoid excess, pheochromocytoma, and Cushing's syndrome.

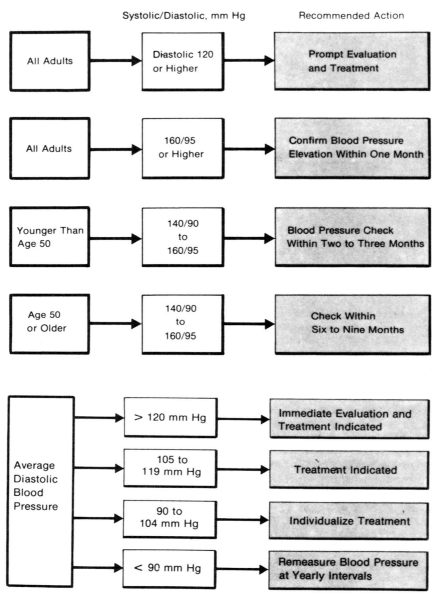

Systolic/Diastolic, mm Hg   Recommended Action

| All Adults | Diastolic 120 or Higher | Prompt Evaluation and Treatment |

| All Adults | 160/95 or Higher | Confirm Blood Pressure Elevation Within One Month |

| Younger Than Age 50 | 140/90 to 160/95 | Blood Pressure Check Within Two to Three Months |

| Age 50 or Older | 140/90 to 160/95 | Check Within Six to Nine Months |

Average Diastolic Blood Pressure	> 120 mm Hg	Immediate Evaluation and Treatment Indicated
	105 to 119 mm Hg	Treatment Indicated
	90 to 104 mm Hg	Individualize Treatment
	< 90 mm Hg	Remeasure Blood Pressure at Yearly Intervals

FIG. 14-2. Recommended action after blood pressure measurement. (*Top*) Recommended action after initial blood pressure measurement. (*Bottom*) Recommended action after repeated or confirmation blood pressure measurements. (Moser M: Report of the Joint National Committee on Detection, Evaluation and Treatment of High Blood Pressure: A Cooperative Study. JAMA 237:255, 1977)

Benign hypertension is a descriptive term for uncomplicated hypertension, usually hypertension of long duration and mild to moderate severity. Benign hypertension may be primary or secondary.

Malignant hypertension is the syndrome of accelerated hypertension associated with widespread degenerative changes in the walls of resistance vessels. It is usually characterized by extreme blood pressure elevations, sudden onset, a fulminant course, and evidence of severe generalized vascular damage, including papilledema, hypertensive encephalopathy, hematuria, and renal dysfunction. Malignant hypertension is usually fatal unless treated promptly and vigorously. Prognosis depends on the state of renal function and the ability to control the blood pressure.

Complicated hypertension is the descriptive term for systemic hypertension of any etiology in which there is evidence of cardiovascular damage related to the blood pressure elevation. Hypertensive complications commonly include stroke, congestive heart failure, renal failure, myocardial infarction, and arterial aneurysm.

Labile hypertension, sometimes referred to as prehypertension, borderline hypertension, or the hyperkinetic heart syndrome, is intermittent hypertension in which some blood pressures are elevated (> 90 mm Hg diastolic) and some are normal in the untreated patient. Patients with labile hypertension tend to maintain pressures that are above average for the general population, and they are at greater risk from increased cardiovascular morbidity and mortality.[7,8] These patients tend to manifest higher cardiac outputs, more rapid heart rates, and higher left ventricular (LV) ejection rates than either the normotensive population or the population of patients with stable hypertension.[9,10] The natural history of the syndrome is variable. The proportion of such patients who go on to develop sustained hypertension and secondary vascular damage varies from 10% to 70% in published series.[11-13] It has been suggested that the true incidence of progression of labile to sustained hypertension is in the range of 10% to 25% and that the reports of higher percentages are biased by the presence of mild hypertension in the study group at the beginning of the study.[14]

Physiology

Although it is not possible to identify a primary cause or set of causes of essential hypertension, factors that have been implicated in the pathogenesis of the syndrome include disorders of hemodynamics and vasomotor regulation, of autonomic nervous system function, of humoral control of pressure and volume, and of renal sodium handling, among others.

DISORDERS OF HEMODYNAMICS
AND VASOMOTOR REGULATION

Elevation of blood pressure may result from any disturbance of the circulation that leads to an increase in cardiac output or total peripheral resistance, or both. Increases in total peripheral resistance elevate both systolic and diastolic pressures, and both systolic and diastolic hypertension reflect elevated peripheral vascular resistance.[15] The pulse pressure is a function of stroke volume and of arterial capacitance, with LV ejection rate playing a minor part. Arterial capacitance is defined as the slope (dv/dp) of the curve relating volume to pressure in the large arteries.

A transient elevation in cardiac output has been demonstrated early in the course of several forms of experimentally induced hypertension in animals. It has been suggested that this evanescent elevation in cardiac output causes secondary increases in peripheral resistance that are responsible for the maintenance of hypertension.[16-18] The concept of total body autoregulation has been used to explain the adaptation of resistance vessels to such increases in cardiac output. According to the theory of autoregulation, systemic resistance vessels respond to an increased cardiac output and increased intravascular volume by constricting in order to reduce blood flow to normal.[16-18] As a result, blood pressure rises.

There is evidence that elevations in cardiac output may be involved early in the course of essential hypertension in man. Patients with labile hypertension of recent onset show a pattern of increased cardiac output, tachycardia, increased dp/dt, and venoconstriction, with normal or even low peripheral vascular resistance at rest.[19-21] In contrast, patients with long-standing established hypertension usually have a slightly decreased cardiac output and increased peripheral and renal vascular resistance.[19-21] These observations are compatible with the notion that increases in cardiac output play a role in the initiation of essential hypertension and that peripheral resistance rises later and is more important in the maintenance of hypertension. Longitudinal studies of untreated hypertensive patients have documented a fall in cardiac output, due mainly to a decrease in stroke volume and an increase in total peripheral resistance over time.[22,23]

The elevation in cardiac output seen in labile hypertensives has been related to increased sympathetic nervous function with enhanced venoconstrictor tone and a resultant redistribution of blood volume from the periphery to the cardiopulmonary segments (central redistribution of blood volume).[24] Central blood volume, the volume of blood in the heart and lungs, is generally normal or increased in the presence of decreased total blood volume in these patients.[21,25] Further, forearm venous distensibility has been found to be diminished in untreated essential hypertensives, indicating that venoconstrictor tone is increased.[26]

DISORDERS OF AUTONOMIC FUNCTION

Animal studies have implicated both peripheral and central catecholaminergic systems in the pathogenesis of hypertension. Increased activity of the sympathetic nervous system produced by continuous electrical stimulation of the renal nerves, splanchnic nerves, or stellate ganglion in conscious dogs leads to a sustained rise of arterial blood pressure.[27,28] Increased splanchnic nerve traffic has been recorded in the young, ("prehypertensive") spontaneously hypertensive rat, suggesting that neural pressor stimuli are increased in the developmental phase of hypertension.[29] As hypertension develops in this model, sympathetic nervous system activity correlates directly with the increase in blood pressure.[30] In rats made hypertensive with DOCA (desoxy-corticosterone acetate) and salt, there is biochemical evidence for increased activity of the peripheral sympathetic fibers and of the adrenal medulla.[31,32] Further, chemical destruction of central monoaminergic pathways has prevented the development of DOCA–salt hypertension, renovascular hypertension, and spontaneous genetic hypertension in the rat.[33,34] Thus, it appears that activation of the sympathetic nervous system is required for the development of hypertension in these experimental models.

Evidence for involvement of the sympathetic nervous system in the pathogenesis of essential hypertension in man is less direct, having been limited by the lack of availability of noninvasive techniques for assessing sympathetic function and by the heterogeneity of the hypertensive population. Measurement of plasma norepinephrine levels is the only generally accepted method of assessing sympathetic neural activity in man.[35] Most studies comparing circulating norepinephrine in patients with essential hypertension and normotensive controls have reported higher mean levels in the hypertensive subjects, but differences between groups have attained statistical significance in only a minority of studies[36] Such confounding factors as choice of assay method, age of the study subjects (plasma norepinephrine tends to increase with age), thyroid function, level of activation of the renin-angiotensin-aldosterone system, plasma volume, sodium balance, alpha- and beta-adrenergic receptor sensitivity, and psychological stress tend to complicate the relationship between plasma norepinephrine and blood pressure.[36] Elucidation of the role of the sympathetic nervous system in essential hypertension will require both a better assessment of these factors and the development of independent means of quantifying sympathetic activity in patients.

In patients with labile hypertension, both parasympathetic and sympathetic control mechanisms may be abnormal. The increased cardiac output characteristic of these patients may, in part, be due to the combination of elevated resting heart rate and increased myocardial contractility.[37,38] These hemodynamic abnormalities have been related to both diminished resting parasympathetic inhibition and enhanced sympathetic stimulation.[39] The increase in heart rate in response to atropine is less in these patients than in normotensive individuals, evidence that vagal inhibition is diminished. When autonomic blockade is achieved by administration of atropine and propranolol, resting heart rate and cardiac output fall to levels found in normal subjects under comparable conditions, indicating that increased beta-adrenergic stimulation as well as reduced vagal inhibition participates in the control of the circulation.[40,41]

The "inappropriately" elevated (within the normal range rather than decreased in the face of an elevated cardiac output) peripheral resistance seen in patients with labile hypertension has been attributed to increased sympathetic tone.[42,43] Exercise studies demonstrate less decrease in peripheral resistance in response to a given increase in cardiac output in these patients than in normotensive subjects, thus supporting the hypothesis that sympathetic tone is increased.[44]

The exaggerated pressor effect of stress in patients with essential hypertension has been interpreted as indirect evidence in favor of the importance of neurogenic control of blood pressure. For example, blood pressure falls during sleep, transcendental meditation, and other states of relaxation and rises during isometric exercise and the stress of mental arithmetic in most hypertensive patients.[45,46] Further, extremely stressful events have been shown to be followed by a high incidence of elevated blood pressure in a population.[47] The impressive fall in blood pressure that is frequently seen when a hypertensive patient is removed from his home environment and brought into the hospital suggests that environmental stress exacerbates hypertension. The increased prevalence of hypertension in urban populations compared to rural groups and the occurrence of age-related rises in blood pressure in societies with changing value systems but not in those with a stable social structure give evidence for a psychogenic contribution to essential hypertension.[48] Stress presumably mediates its pressor effect through the sympathetic nervous system.

DISORDERS OF HUMORAL CONTROL OF PRESSURE AND VOLUME

Humoral factors that influence pressure and volume homeostasis include the renin-angiotensin-aldosterone system, the kallikrein-kinin system, the prostaglandins, and arginine vasopressin. Other sodium-retaining adrenal cortical hormones and a number of vasodepressor lipids of renal origin have been described and partly characterized but are of uncertain physiologic significance.[49,50]

Renin is a proteolytic enzyme that is synthesized, stored, and secreted mainly in the kidney.[51] The physiologic consequences of renin release result from a sequence of enzymatic reactions that lead to the generation of an active polypeptide hormone, angiotensin II (Fig. 14-3). Angiotensin-converting enzyme,

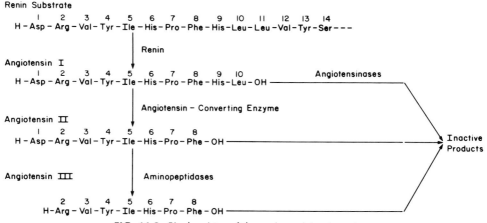

FIG. 14-3. Biochemistry of the renin-angiotensin system.

a dipeptidylcarboxypeptidase found mainly in lung but also in circulating plasma, kidney, and a variety of other organ beds, acts on angiotensin I to produce the octapeptide angiotensin II, a potent vasoconstrictor and a stimulator of aldosterone production.[51] Angiotensin II can be cleaved readily by aminopeptidases to yield (Des-aspartyl[1])-angiotensin II, or angiotensin III. Angiotensin III may be an important mediator of aldosterone synthesis and release.[52]

Renin release is the rate-limiting step in angiotensin production. It is subject to feedback control by angiotensin II and III directly and indirectly, through the effects of the angiotensins on blood volume, blood pressure, sodium balance, and the brain (Fig. 14-4).[51] The juxtaglomerular apparatus functions as a baroreceptor that stimulates renin release when local intra-arterial pressure falls. The macula densa, a specifically modified portion of the distal tubule, functions as a chemoreceptor sensitive to changes in sodium or chloride load or concentration in distal tubular fluid. It communicates with the renin-producing cells. An increase in renin release by any mechanism stimulates production of the angiotensins and aldosterone, which tend to cause increased

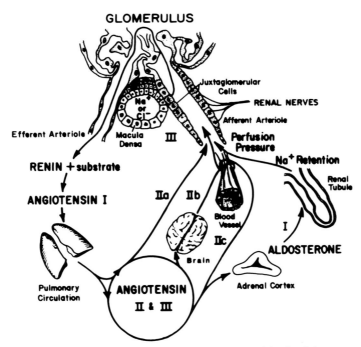

FIG. 14-4. Feedback regulation of renin release. Several feedback loops are shown. An increase in concentration in angiotensin II or III results in decreased renin secretion by: (*I*) Increased sodium retention resulting in increased extracellular fluid volume. (*IIa*) A direct negative feedback. (*IIb*) Increased blood pressure through the CNS. (*IIc*) Increased blood pressure through direct systemic vasoconstriction. (*III*) Direct sodium effects on the macula densa. (After Oparil S, Haber E: The renin-angiotensin system. N Engl J Med 291:389, 1974)

blood pressure and expanded extracellular fluid volume, thereby suppressing renin production and restoring pressure and volume to normal.[51]

Feedback regulation of renin release is defective in renovascular hypertension and in the syndromes of mineralocorticoid excess (Fig. 14-5). In renovascular hypertension, fixed obstruction to juxtaglomerular cell perfusion results in sustained elevation of renin and, secondarily, aldosterone. In the syndromes of mineralocorticoid excess, autonomous production of adrenal cortical hormone causes salt and water retention and suppression of renin release.[51]

The sympathetic nervous system interacts with the renin-angiotensin system and other determinants of volume homeostasis in the regulation of blood pressure. All of the components of the renin-angiotensin-aldosterone system have been extracted from brain and from brain cells in tissue culture. It is not yet known whether the endogenous brain angiotensins have a physiologic role in the genesis or maintenance of hypertension, but it has been shown that exogenous angiotensin II in pharmacological doses evokes a pressor response by central nervous system pathways.[53]

RENOVASCULAR DISEASE

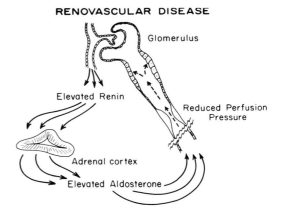

MINERALOCORTICOID EXCESS

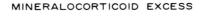

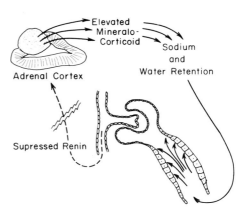

FIG. 14-5. Defective feedback regulation of renin release in secondary hypertension. (Oparil S: Plasma renin activity in hypertension. Compr Ther 1, No. 8: 63, 1975, courtesy The Laux Company, Inc., Publishers)

The kallikrein-kinin system may be involved in the maintenance of blood pressure by control of local blood flow and water and electrolyte excretion. Kinins are potent vasodilator and natriuretic peptides released from inactive precursors, the kininogens, by a group of serine proteases, the kininogenases, which includes the plasma and glandular kallikreins (Fig. 14-6).[54] Plasma kallikrein (Fletcher factor), which has a molecular weight of approximately 100,000 daltons and differs from glandular kallikrein in its biochemical, immunologic, and functional characteristics, releases bradykinin from the high molecular weight form of kininogen. Bradykinin released in this fashion is probably not involved in cardiovascular regulation. The plasma kallikrein-kinin system is, however, involved in coagulation, fibrinolysis, and, perhaps, the activation of the complement system. Glandular kallikreins found in kidney, pancreas, and salivary and sweat glands catalyze the release of the decapeptide Lys-bradykinin from both high and low molecular weight forms of kininogen. Lys-bradykinin is then converted to bradykinin by an aminopeptidase. The kinins are rapidly inactivated in plasma and in the pulmonary capillary bed by a family of proteolytic enzymes, the kininases, that includes the dipeptidylcarboxypeptidase referred to as kininase II or angiotensin-converting enzyme. The rapid inactivation of the kinins in the circulation suggests that, rather than producing systemic vasodilatation, their dominant physiologic role is to locally maintain regional blood flow and, in the case of the kidney, to influence sodium excretion.

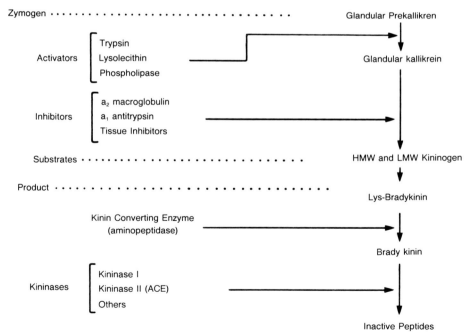

FIG. 14-6. Generation of kinins by glandular kallikrein. (Carretero OA, Scicli AG: Possible role of kinins in circulatory homeostasis. Hypertension 3:I–4, 1981. By permission of the American Heart Association, Inc.)

The renal kallikrein-kinin system has been implicated in the regulation of water and electrolyte transport by the distal nephron and in the control of renal vascular resistance. Kallikrein found in association with the luminal plasma membrane of the distal tubule catalyzes the formation of kinins that then effect a natriuresis by directly inhibiting sodium transport in the distal nephron, causing renal vasodilatation or alternations in the osmotic gradient of the renal medulla or both.[54] Further, the kallikrein-kinin system may alter renal blood flow and sodium handling by its effects on the renin-angiotensin-aldosterone system and on renal prostaglandins (Fig. 14-7).[55] Kallikrein stimulates renin releases and activates inactive renin. Further, kinins stimulate the synthesis of vasodilator prostaglandins, probably by activation of phospholipase A_2 and increased release of arachidonic acid.[56] Part of the vasodilator effect of kinins is mediated through the release of prostaglandins and can be inhibited by prostaglandin synthetase inhibitors such as indomethacin and meclofenamate. Conversely, angiotensin, aldosterone, and prostaglandins, as well as arginine vasopressin, can stimulate the release of renal kallikrein and perhaps the intrarenal formation of kinins.[57,58] The physiologic significance of these interactions is uncertain, but it is conceivable that renal kinins and prostaglandins function as local vasodilators to maintain tissue flow within the kidney in the face of angiotensin-induced vasoconstriction.[54]

Abnormalities in the renal kallikrein-kinin system have been described in many forms of experimental and clinical hypertension. Urinary kallikrein excretion is reduced in spontaneously hypertensive rats of the Okamoto, Bianchi, and New Zealand strains, in the Dahl-S (salt sensitive) rat, in rats with two-kidney, one-clip Goldblatt hypertension, and in rats with hypertension secondary to renal parenchymal disease.[55] In contrast, urinary kallikrein excretion is greatly increased in rats with DOCA–salt hypertension. It has not been shown that the alterations in kallikrein excretion seen in these models are related to changes in the intrarenal formation of kinins, nor has it been determined whether the abnormality in the kallikrein-kinin system precedes or follows the development of hypertension or whether it plays a role in the pathogenesis of hypertension. Indeed, in many of these models, the alterations in kallikrein

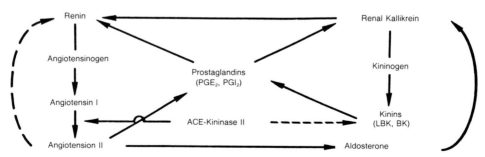

FIG. 14-7. A schematic representation of the interactions of the renal kallikrein-kinin, renin-angiotension, and prostaglandin systems. *Solid lines*=stimulation or conversion. *Dotted lines*=inactivation or inhibition. *LBK*=lysyl-bradykinin. *BK*=bradykinin. *ACE*=angiotensin converting enzyme. (Smith MC, Dunn MJ: Renal kallikrein, kinins and prostaglandins in hypertension. In Brenner BM, Stein JH (eds): Contemporary Issues in Nephrology, Vol 8. New York, Churchill and Livingstone, 1981)

excretion can be explained simply by reductions in renal mass or the stimulating effects of increased mineralocorticoid levels.

Reductions in basal urinary kallikrein excretion and blunting of responses to sodium deprivation and mineralocorticoid administration have been described in patients with essential hypertension or hypertension secondary to renal parenchymal disease, renal vascular disease, and pregnancy. Elevations in kallikrein excretion have been described in patients with primary aldosteronism, juxtaglomerular cell tumor, and pheochromocytoma. Interpretation of clinical data in this area is complicated by the fact that both race and renal function are important determinants of urinary kallikrein; kallikrein excretion is lower in blacks than whites, and it varies directly with glomerular filtration rate.[55] When hypertensive subjects are classified according to race, renin activity, and creatinine clearance, urinary kallikrein has been shown to be reduced only in those subjects with mild renal insufficiency, compared to race-matched normotensive individuals.[59] Thus, in both experimental and clinical settings, it is unclear whether abnormalities in kallikrein excretion occur independently of decrements in renal function or alterations in mineralocorticoid production and whether these abnormalities are etiologically related to hypertension.[58] Further studies in which additional components of the renal kallikrein-kinin system are measured are needed to settle these issues.

Prostaglandins are present in virtually every tissue and mediate a wide variety of biological functions, including control of pressure and volume homeostasis. The prostaglandins are 20-carbon cyclical fatty acids with substitutions or unsaturations in both the cyclopentane ring and the aliphatic side chains (Fig. 14-8). Common to all these compounds is their generation from

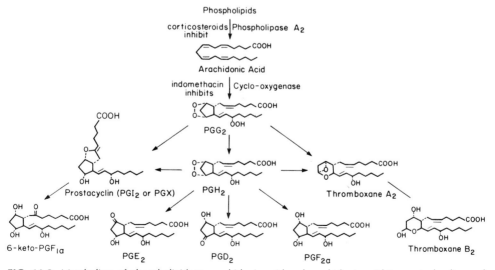

FIG. 14-8. Metabolism of phospholipids to arachidonic acid and arachidonic acid to prostaglandins and thromboxanes. PGG_2=endoperoxide. (Dunn MJ: Renal prostaglandins. In Klahr S, Massry SG, (eds): Contemporary Nephrology, Vol 1. New York, Plenum Publishing Corporation, 1981)

arachidonic acid by the enzyme cyclooxygenase (prostaglandin synthetase).[55] Arachidonic acid is stored in cells as phospholipid and is released by acyl hydrolyases, including phospholipase A_2. Acute stimulators of prostaglandin synthesis, such as bradykinin or angiotensin II, stimulate the deacylation of membrane phospholipids and thereby release arachidonic acid, which is then deoxygenated to the labile cyclic endoperoxides prostaglandins G_2 and H_2. The prostaglandin endoperoxides are rapidly transformed to prostaglandins E_2, $F_{2\alpha}$, D_2, and I_2, and thromboxane A_2. Prostaglandins are generated rapidly following an appropriate stimulus, exert their effects, and are quickly metabolized. They are not stored in cells. It is thought that prostaglandins act predominantly as autacoids rather than circulating hormones, but many of their functions are the consequences of their interactions with circulating hormones, including catecholamines and the angiotensins, in the target tissue.

Prostaglandins in kidney and blood vessel walls are thought to participate in blood pressure regulation through both their intrinsic effects and their interactions with other vasoregulatory systems. Prostaglandins stimulate both kallikrein-kinin and renin-angiotensin systems, and prostaglandin production is stimulated by both bradykinin and angiotensin II (see Fig. 14-7).[55] The cardiovascular and renal actions of prostaglandins that are responsible for their effects on blood pressure are summarized in Cardiovascular and Renal Actions of Prostaglandins and Blood Pressure.[55] The antihypertensive effects of the prostaglandins appear to predominate over their pressor effects, since intravenous administration of their precursor, arachidonic acid, generally lowers blood pressure, while indomethacin, which inhibits prostaglandin production, tends to exacerbate hypertension.

Prostaglandins oppose the vasoconstrictor effects of a number of humoral agents. Prostaglandins E_2 and I_2 have been shown to decrease the release of norepinephrine during sympathetic nerve stimulation and to reduce the vasoconstrictor effect of infused norepinephrine.[61] Further, prostaglandins whose

---

CARDIOVASCULAR AND RENAL ACTIONS OF PROSTAGLANDINS AND BLOOD PRESSURE

Vascular resistance
Vasodilatory: PGE_2, PGI_2, PGD_2
Vasoconstrictor: TxA_2, $PGF_{2\alpha}$

Natriuresis: PGE_2, PGD_2

Renin release: PGI_2, PGE_2, PGD_2

Adrenergic effects
Antiadrenergic: PGE_2, PGI_2
Proadrenergic: $PGF_{2\alpha}$

Cardiac output
Negative chronotropic: PGE_2, PGI_2
Positive inotropic: PGE_2

---

synthesis is stimulated by angiotensin II attenuate the effects of the octapeptide on vascular resistance and glomerular filtration rate.[62,63] Enhancement of vascular and renal synthesis of vasodilator prostaglandins has been described in several models of genetically mediated and experimentally induced hypertension in the rat.[55] Indomethacin exacerbates hypertension in these models. These data suggest that the synthesis of vasodilator prostaglandins is increased in response to chronic elevations in blood pressure and that the prostaglandins then play a homeostatic role to modulate the hypertension.

Prostaglandins, principally prostaglandin E (PGE), which are found in high concentrations in the renal medulla, act both as local vasodilators and as powerful natriuretic agents.[64] It has been proposed that the prostaglandins operate in concert with the kallikrein-kinin system to maintain renal blood flow and facilitate natriuresis, thus opposing those factors that elevate blood pressure through intrarenal mechanisms.[64]

There is evidence that prostaglandin metabolism may be altered in patients with essential hypertension. Urinary excretion of PGE_2 has been observed to be depressed in essential hypertension but not in hypertension secondary to aldosterone excess or renovascular disease, suggesting that reduction of renal PGE_2 synthesis in essential hypertension may be a primary abnormality rather than a secondary response to the elevated blood pressure.[55] These data, coupled with the observation that renal kallikrein-kinin activity is often reduced in essential hypertension, are consistent with the interpretation that these local renal hormones regulate systemic blood pressure and vascular resistance through control of renal blood flow and sodium excretion. Further studies in which additional prostaglandins in the kidney and systemic vasculature are measured and in which the developmental stage of hypertension is examined are needed to define the role of prostaglandins in the pathogenesis of essential hypertension.

Arginine vasopressin, the mammalian antidiuretic hormone, has recently been implicated in the pathogenesis of various forms of genetic and experimentally induced hypertension in animals.[65] It appears to act as a pressor hormone in these models, but its role is controversial. Increased pressor responsiveness to vasopressin, as well as an increase in its plasma concentration, are required in order for vasopressin to elevate blood pressure. Very little is known about the role of arginine vasopressin in human essential hypertension. Further study is needed to define the contribution of arginine vasopressin to various forms of systemic hypertension.

DISORDERS OF RENAL SODIUM HANDLING

The kidney plays an important role in the maintenance of intravascular volume and arterial blood pressure. It responds to increments in perfusion pressure by increasing the rate of sodium and water excretion (pressure natriuresis), thus reducing intravascular volume and restoring arterial pressure to normal levels. Normally, sodium intake and output are balanced at a mean perfusion pressure of 100 mm Hg. An alteration in this relationship such that higher perfusion pressures are needed to produce a natriuresis would tend to facilitate the development and maintenance of hypertension

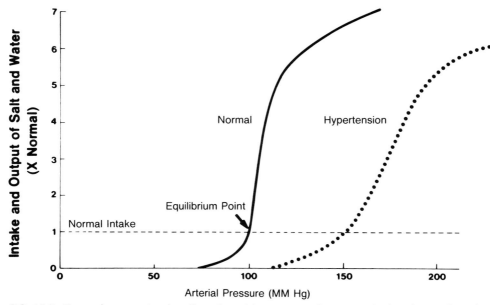

FIG. 14-9. Curves demonstrating the effect of arterial pressure on the output of salt and water from the normal kidney and hypertensive kidney. With hypertension there is a shift to the right of the renal function curve such that the pressure natriuresis occurs at a higher level of blood pressure. (Adapted from the work of Dr. Arthur C. Guyton and associates.)

(Fig. 14-9).[66] A variety of neurohumoral factors intrinsic and extrinsic to the kidney can influence the relationship between perfusion pressure and sodium excretion. Intrinsic factors include angiotensin II, prostaglandins, and kinins; extrinsic factors include circulating catecholamines, arginine vasopressin, aldosterone, and the sympathetic nervous activity. In addition, a kidney that is subjected to elevated pressure over time develops structural changes that limit its ability to excrete sodium and water in response to increases in pressure.

A defect in the excretion of salt and water may be central to the pathogenesis of many, if not all, forms of hypertension. Animal models have provided evidence that changes in the renal circulation due to increased sympathetic nervous system activity favor salt and water retention and the genesis of hypertension. The sustained hypertension produced by chronic intrarenal norepinephrine infusion in the one-kidney conscious dog is an example.[67] In this model, intrarenal norepinephrine infusions shift the pressure–sodium excretion relationship to the right, resulting in a positive sodium balance and a blunted pressure natriuresis. There is also evidence of abnormal sympathetic neural influence on the kidney in the spontaneous hypertensive rat of the Okamoto strain, the DOCA–salt hypertensive rat, and the one- and two-kidney renal hypertensive rat models.[68,69] In each of these models, renal denervation delays the development or attenuates the severity of hypertension (Fig. 14-10). Whether the antihypertensive effect of renal denervation results from altered excretory function of the kidney, interruption of renal afferent nerve

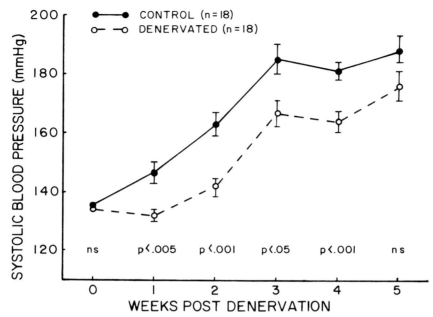

FIG. 14-10. Systolic blood pressures of spontaneously hypertensive male rats of the Okamoto strain subjected to renal denervation or sham operation at age 7 weeks. P values refer to comparison between groups using Student's *t* test for unpaired data.

traffic with secondary resetting of central pressor mechanisms, or a combination of these and other influences remains to be determined.

Renal abnormalities have been demonstrated in patients with essential hypertension.[70] In patients with uncomplicated essential hypertension, renal blood flow tends to be reduced in the presence of a normal or slightly reduced glomerular filtration rate. Alterations in renal blood flow and tubular function usually result from reversible arteriolar vasoconstriction rather than fixed structural changes. Two-thirds of patients with established essential hypertension have enhanced renal sympathetic tone.[70] Alpha-adrenergic blockade with phentolamine increases renal blood flow in patients with essential hypertension but not in normal subjects. The intrarenal administration of propranolol in low doses results in decreased renal blood flow in patients with essential hypertension but not in normotensive control subjects, suggesting that beta-adrenergic blockade in the renal vascular bed unmasks increased sympathetic vasoconstrictor activity.[71] Thus, increased sympathetic tone in patients with established essential hypertension could facilitate the renal retention of sodium and blunt a pressure natriuresis by increasing vascular resistance or by directly stimulating renal tubular reabsorption of sodium.[72] Renal blood flow and glomerular filtration rate fall progressively as the severity and duration of hypertension increase. These functional changes are consequences of longstanding elevations in pressure and can be related to structural alterations in resistance vessels of the kidney.

OBESITY AND HYPERTENSION

Several lines of evidence have established an association between obesity and hypertension, but the mechanisms by which obesity predisposes to hypertension are not known.[73] Whether hypertension is related to increased body weight or only to excess body fat is uncertain. It is clear, however, that weight reduction independent of sodium intake reduces arterial pressure in both normotensive and hypertensive subjects.[74] Decreases in plasma renin activity and aldosterone concentration, plasma catecholamines, and serum insulin may be involved in the blood pressure reduction associated with weight loss, suggesting indirectly that these factors contribute to the pathogenesis of obesity-related hypertension.[75] Further study is needed to assess the relative roles of these and other factors in mediating the hypertension.

DIETARY SODIUM AND HYPERTENSION

Increased dietary sodium may predispose to hypertension. It has been shown that populations with very high salt intakes have a high incidence of hypertension.[76,77] In contrast, in populations in which salt intake is low (less than 4 g daily), the incidence of hypertension is low, and blood pressure does not rise with advancing years. These epidemiologic studies, provocative as they are, fail to take into account other characteristics of the generally primitive "low-salt" societies that could affect arterial pressure, including high potassium intake, increased physical activity, small stature, and a low prevalence of obesity.[78] Recent studies have shown that not all normotensive people become hypertensive in response to a high sodium intake.[79,80] Increased dietary sodium has been shown to exacerbate established hypertension and to precipitate clinical hypertension in people who have a genetic predisposition to hypertension.[81] The nature of factor(s) other than heredity that must be present in order for increased dietary sodium to produce hypertension remains unknown. Conversely, dietary sodium restriction can both lower arterial pressure and reverse signs of progressive arteriolar disease in some hypertensive patients.[82,83] There is no simple way to predict which patients will respond to sodium restriction, but, in general, those whose hypertension is relatively mild respond better than those with high diastolic pressures.

The mechanism by which sodium predisposes to hypertension is not fully understood. A favored theory is that sodium and water accumulate in arteriolar walls, causing increased peripheral resistance and, for a given cardiac output, increased arterial pressure.[84] Water, cations (sodium, potassium, magnesium, and calcium), collagen, mucopolysaccharides, and elastin are increased in arterial tissue of hypertensive subjects. Whether or not these biochemical changes contribute to the initiation or maintenance of hypertension is unknown, but it is clear that resistance vessels develop increasing stiffness and show increased reactivity to neural and humoral stimuli.[85] This adaptive change in vascular reactivity could explain pressor-dependent hypertension in the presence of normal circulating levels of pressor agents.

POTASSIUM AND HYPERTENSION

Alterations in serum potassium concentration or total body potassium content produce hemodynamic effects that influence the control of blood pressure.[86] Acute administration of potassium has a direct vasodilatory effect that appears to result from stimulation of membrane Na-K-ATPase activity with resultant membrane hyperpolarization and vascular smooth muscle relaxation. In addition, oral potassium loading lowers blood pressure by causing natriuresis and diuresis and suppressing renin release. This hypotensive effect of potassium administration has been clearly demonstrated in animal models of hypertension but not in hypertensive man. Chronic potassium deficiency also causes vasodilatation in normotensive animals and may have an antihypertensive effect. The mechanism of this vasodilatory response appears to be a direct effect on vascular smooth muscle, since it occurs despite increases in total body sodium, renin, and arginine vasopressin. It is at present uncertain whether altering potassium levels by dietary or pharmacologic means is useful in the treatment of clinical hypertension.[86]

DIET AND HYPERTENSION

Many nutritional factors other than total calories, sodium, and potassium have been implicated in the pathogenesis of hypertension.[87] Prominent among these are calcium, carbohydrates, lipids, alcohol, vitamins, and trace elements, particularly cadmium, lead, vanadium, and copper. Further study is needed to assess the importance of diet in the development of hypertension and to test the potential of dietary manipulation in its prevention or treatment.

GENETICS AND HYPERTENSION

Although environmental factors influence the development of hypertension, there is also evidence that heredity may be important.[88] Several strains of rat with a polygenically inherited primary hypertension have been developed. These include the Dahl salt-sensitive rat and the Okamoto, New Zealand, and Bianchi strains of spontaneously hypertensive rat. Population studies that have examined the role of heredity in determining blood pressure in man have shown a direct quantitative relationship between the arterial pressure of the subjects under study and that of their first-degree relatives. For example, a monozygotic twin has a much greater risk of having borderline or sustained hypertension if his twin has either condition. To date, no specific set of blood pressure regulating genes has been identified, nor have genetic markers been characterized that would allow us to detect those individuals who are at risk for developing hypertension.[88] The current interest in measuring cellular ion fluxes and carrying out HLA typing studies in hypertensives and their families is an example of the effort to identify genetic risk factors for hypertension.[88]

In summary, the control of blood pressure is a dynamic process involving the complex interdependence of many factors. The stability of this system depends on appropriately sensitive negative feedback mechanisms. No single primary abnormality has been found to account for even a portion of cases of essential hypertension in man, but it is evident that alterations at many points in the control loop could account for elevated blood pressure. Therefore, essential hypertension in man is probably a complex syndrome made up of many different diseases.

PATHOPHYSIOLOGY OF SECONDARY HYPERTENSION

Renovascular Hypertension

Activation of the renin-angiotensin system is central to the initiation and maintenance of renovascular hypertension. Hypertension has been produced experimentally in a variety of species by renal artery constriction and has been attributed to the release of a pressor substance from the involved kidney(s).[89] Experiments in which circulating renin or angiotensin have been measured directly or in which the renin-angiotensin system has been pharmacologically blocked have shown that experimental renovascular hypertension is initially angiotensin-dependent. Later, hypertension is maintained primarily by sodium retention and volume expansion and perhaps also by a nonrenin renal pressor mechanism and the sympathetic nervous system. Deficiencies of antihypertensive factors, such as prostaglandins and renomedullary neutral lipid, have also been cited as contributing to these forms of hypertension.[90] Thus, multiple neural and humoral factors outside the renin-angiotensin system may be involved in the pathogenesis of experimentally induced renovascular hypertension. Cases of renovascular hypertension in man without demonstrable overactivity of the renin-angiotensin system have been reported, but these are unusual and generally occur in association with renal dysfunction and secondary volume expansion.[91,92] The clinical corollary of these experimental observations is that the diagnosis of renovascular hypertension requires documentation of increased renin production from the affected kidney(s) as well as anatomical demonstration of an obstructive arterial lesion.

Any lesion that gives rise to obstruction of either large or small renal arteries can cause renovascular hypertension in man. Of these lesions, the most common and clinically important are intrinsic lesions of the large vessels, because they can be surgically removed and the hypertension either cured or ameliorated. Atherosclerosis and fibrous and fibromuscular disease together account for 95% of such lesions in the North American population. Atherosclerotic disease is found in two-thirds of patients with renovascular hypertension; fibrous or fibromuscular disease, in one-third.[93] Patients with atherosclerotic renal artery lesions tend to be older and to have higher systolic blood pressures and more frequent extrarenal arterial disease than patients with essential hypertension and are more likely to develop target organ damage. In contrast, patients with fibromuscular hyperplasia tend to be younger and predominantly female, and they are less likely to have a family history of hypertension or to develop cardiovascular complications.[93] There are several anatomical types of fibrous and fibromuscular lesions of the renal artery that are thought to have distinct clinical courses.[94] The natural history of renal artery stenosis in untreated patients is poorly understood, but available information indicates a worse prognosis in atherosclerotic disease than in fibromuscular disease.[95] It is not possible to predict which lesions will progress either from angiography or from the clinical characteristics of the patient.

Less common causes of renovascular hypertension include renal vasculitis of any etiology; solitary renal cysts (which can cause hypertension by compressing intrarenal blood vessels); intrarenal, subcapsular, or perirenal hematomas; renal artery aneurysms; blunt trauma with secondary renal artery occlusion; renal vein thrombosis; radiation nephritis; neurofibromatosis; thromboembolic disease; congenital segmental renal hypoplasia (Ask–Upmark kidney); and arteriovenous fistula.[14] Such extrinsic lesions as congenital fibrous bands, retroperitoneal fibrosis, tumor, and ptosis cause renovascular hypertension by compressing the renal arteries. Ureteral obstruction can lead to a form of renovascular hypertension, presumably due to impingement on the intrarenal vessels by the engorged collecting system and interstitium. Stenosis of the celiac axis with "steal" of renal blood flow has been reported as a rare cause of hypertension.

Renal Parenchymal Disease

Patients with mild chronic renal insufficiency of any cause often develop a volume-dependent form of hypertension secondary to sodium and water retention that results from loss of functional renal mass.[96] Hypertension can often be prevented or controlled in these subjects by preventing volume excess from developing.

Chronic Renal Failure

Chronic renal failure of any etiology frequently causes hypertension. Approximately 90% of such patients have a predominantly volume-dependent form of hypertension in which exchangeable sodium, extracellular fluid volume, and plasma volume are increased in parallel with blood pressure levels.[97] In these patients circulating renin and angiotensin II levels are normal or slightly elevated, which is inappropriate in the face of the increased extracellular fluid volume.[98] The hypertension responds to sodium and water depletion by dialysis[97] but also to bilateral nephrectomy or infusion of saralasin, an angiotensin II antagonist, suggesting that the renin-angiotensin system participates in its maintenance.

A small percentage of patients with renal failure manifest a predominantly renin-dependent form of hypertension that fails to respond to sodium and volume depletion and may even be exacerbated by dialysis.[99] Renin, angiotensin, and aldosterone levels tend to be elevated in the renin-dependent group and are made still higher by the volume depletion of dialysis.[100] These patients tend to have decreased exchangeable sodium, extracellular fluid volume, plasma volume, and cardiac output and elevated peripheral vascular resistance.[101]

In other hypertensive patients with chronic renal failure and in anephric patients, neither increased volume nor increased renin seems adequate to explain the blood pressure elevation.[102] Mechanisms that have been suggested to account for hypertension in these patients include an excess of unidentified pressor factors and a deficiency of such renal vasodepressors as prostaglandins, kallikrein, and the medullary neutral lipid.

Renal Transplantation

Hypertension is a well-recognized complication of renal transplantation. Elevated blood pressure has been reported in up to 60% of patients with a functional transplant 6 to 12 months after surgery.[103] Possible mechanisms of chronic post-transplant hypertension include renal artery stenosis in the transplanted kidney, chronic rejection, recurrent glomerulonephritis, increased renin production in the recipient's own diseased kidney(s), the use of high-dose steroids, and volume expansion.[103] Renal angiography is useful in distinguishing among these possibilities.

Acute Renal Failure

Acute renal failure of any cause frequently results in hypertension associated with oliguria and salt and water retention. Both volume overload and increased function of the renin-angiotensin-aldosterone system have been implicated in the pathogenesis of the syndrome, and comparisons have been made with volume-dependent hypertension in chronic renal disease.[14]

Renin-secreting Tumors

Renin-secreting tumors are an uncommon but potentially curable cause of hypertension. Histologic types include the renal hemangiopericytoma, or juxtaglomerular cell tumor; the Wilms tumor, or nephroblastoma; clear cell carcinoma of the kidney; and some extrarenal neoplasms. All of the reported patients with juxtaglomerular cell tumors have had severe diastolic hypertension and hypokalemia, and most have had hyperaldosteronism. The hypertension has generally been related to overproduction of angiotensin II. It generally responds to measures that either prevent formation of angiotensin II or block its action.

Syndromes of Mineralocorticoid Excess

The syndromes of mineralocorticoid excess are characterized by hypertension, excessive mineralocorticoid production, sodium retention, potassium wasting, and renin suppression. Patients whose hypertension is secondary to overproduction of a known mineralocorticoid, such as aldosterone, desoxycorticosterone (DOC), 18-hydroxy-11-desoxycorticosterone (18-OH DOC), 16α,18-dihydroxy-11-desoxycorticosterone (16α,18-di OH DOC), 16β-hydroxydehydroepiandrosterone (16β-OH-DHEA), or dehydroepiandrosterone sulfate (DHEA-S), make up less than one percent of the hypertensive population.[104] It is possible, however, that overproduction of unidentified mineralocorticoids may be responsible for the syndrome of "low-renin essential hypertension," which accounts for 7% to 10% of all hypertensive patients. To further evaluate that hypothesis, many laboratories are actively engaged in an attempt to identify, quantify, and characterize new mineralocorticoids in patients with low-renin hypertension.

PRIMARY ALDOSTERONISM. Primary aldosteronism is the most common of the syndromes of mineralocorticoid excess and will be considered as the prototype. Despite its low prevalence in hypertensive populations, the syndrome of primary aldosteronism has received much attention because it can be easily identified by the finding of depressed serum potassium and can frequently be cured by surgery.

Primary aldosteronism is a syndrome of hypertension associated with hypokalemia, suppressed plasma renin activity, and increased aldosterone production in which the other abnormalities result from the autonomous or relatively autonomous secretion of aldosterone.[105,106] Autonomous production of aldosterone is associated with excessive salt and water retention, which leads to an increase in effective blood volume and suppression of renin release. Since mineralocorticoid production is not angiotensin-dependent, the feedback loop (see Fig. 14-4) is interrupted, and excessive mineralocorticoid production continues. In the syndromes of mineralocorticoid excess, renin is therefore suppressed and levels of aldosterone or mineralocorticoid are elevated. The use of peripheral plasma renin activity in screening for these syndromes is an accepted clinical practice. The electrolyte abnormalities are direct consequences of the effects of aldosterone on the renal tubule, but the pathogenesis of the hypertension remains poorly understood. While an increase in plasma volume has been described, it is an inconstant finding.[107,108] Hemodynamic studies suggest that increased peripheral resistance is important in maintaining the hypertension.[109] The syndrome of primary aldosteronism can be related to four kinds of adrenal disease: aldosterone-producing adenoma (APA); idiopathic hyperaldosteronism (IHA), a form of adrenocortical hyperplasia in which circulating aldosterone levels cannot be suppressed by exogenous mineralocorticoid; indeterminate hyperaldosteronism (Ind HA), a form of adrenocortical hyperplasia in which circulating aldosterone levels can be suppressed by exogenous mineralocorticoid; and glucocorticoid-remediable hyperaldosteronism, a form of adrenocortical hyperplasia in which the metabolic abnormalities and hypertension can be corrected by exogenous glucocorticoid.[106] Adrenal cortical carcinoma and extra-adrenal tumors are rare causes of primary aldosteronism. The different forms of the syndrome require specific treatment, so it is important to make a specific diagnosis.

CONGENITAL ADRENAL HYPERPLASIA. A number of inborn enzymatic defects in adrenal steroidogenesis lead to overproduction of mineralocorticoids and hypertension. A common denominator of these syndromes is deficient cortisol production, which, in turn, results in increased secretion of ACTH and secondary increases in synthesis of steroids proximal to the block. Two of the less common forms of congenital adrenal hyperplasia, C-11 hydroxylase deficiency and C-17 hydroxylase deficiency, are associated with hypertension secondary to overproduction of DOC and 11-desoxycortisol or corticosterone.

LICORICE INGESTION. Licorice contains glycyrrhetinic acid, a compound that has mineralocorticoid activity. Chronic excessive ingestion of licorice leads to a syndrome of hypertension, hypokalemia and sodium retention with or without edema, and congestive heart failure in which both plasma renin activity and aldosterone secretion rate are suppressed.[110] The hypertension and hypokalemia generally improve when licorice ingestion is decreased or discontinued, and the sodium-retaining and kaliuretic effects of licorice can be reversed by administration of spironolactone.

Pheochromocytoma

Pheochromocytoma is a rare but important cause of surgically curable hypertension. Although it accounts for less than 0.5% of all cases of hypertension,[111] diagnosis is critical because pheochromocytomas may be malignant, because the hypertension may be severe and refractory to conventional antihypertensive treatment, and because patients with unrecognized pheochromocytoma are subject to hypertensive crises during anesthesia and angiography and following administration of drugs such as guanethidine and the ganglion blockers.

Pheochromocytoma is a tumor of neural crest origin that produces sustained or paroxysmal hypertension by releasing catecholamines into the circulation. Most pheochromocytomas secrete a combination of norepinephrine and epinephrine. Less frequently, tumors secrete either norepinephrine or epinephrine exclusively or, rarely, dopamine, dopa, or serotonin. Ninety percent of pheochromocytomas are located in the adrenal medulla, and 10% of these are bilateral. The remaining 10% are scattered in the distribution of autonomic tissue. Fifteen percent of all pheochromocytomas are malignant. These are generally slow-growing and resistant to radiation therapy. They usually metastasize to lymph nodes, liver, lung, and bone. Malignant pheochromocytomas and their metastases may or may not be functional. Pheochromocytomas are common in patients with neurocutaneous syndromes such as Recklinghausen's disease and in families with the syndromes of multiple endocrine adenomatosis. Patients with pheochromocytoma have an increased incidence of neuroectodermal tumors, including brain tumors.

Oral Contraceptive–induced Hypertension

Oral contraceptive pill ingestion is associated with a threefold increase in risk of death from cardiovascular disease, including hypertension, thromboembolic disease, myocardial infarction, and cerebral vascular disease. Oral contraceptive–induced hypertension may be the most common form of secondary hypertension in adults.[112,113] Data from the study of the Royal College of General Practitioners of England showed that 5% of women who were maintained on oral contraceptives for 5 years developed hypertension, a risk 2.6 times greater than that of women who did not use oral contraceptives.[114] When hypertension develops in a patient on oral contraceptives, it usually appears within the first 6 months of treatment but is occasionally delayed for as much as 6 years. The factors that determine individual susceptibility to the hypertension-stimulating effects of oral contraceptives are largely unknown, but a number of possible risk factors, including heredity (family history of hypertension), pre-existing or occult renal disease, age, and obesity have been cited.[115] Women over 40 years of age have five times the risk of developing oral contraceptive–induced hypertension of those aged 30 to 34 and ten times the risk of those aged 25 to 29.[115]

The mechanisms by which oral contraceptives cause increases in blood pressure are obscure, but it appears that the estrogenic component of the preparation is responsible.[116] Changes in the renin-angiotensin-aldosterone system have been described, but these develop in all contraceptive users independently of hypertension.[117] Patients with oral contraceptive–induced hypertension respond to the hypotensive effects of saralasin, indicating that the hypertension is, at least in part, angiotensin II–dependent. Alterations in renal sodium and water handling have been proposed as an additional mechanism.[118] Estrogen is known to suppress urinary sodium excretion in normal women by causing enhanced aldosterone secretion and by direct effects on the kidney. Reductions in renal blood flow in association with increased levels of circulating renin and angiotensin II have been demonstrated in normotensive young women ingesting a variety of estrogen- and progestin-containing oral contraceptive agents.[119] Renal vasoconstriction secondary to increased circulating angiotensin II may contribute to the genesis of sodium retention and hypertension in oral contraceptive users. The hemodynamic effects of the oral contraceptives, which include increases in cardiac output, stroke volume, and plasma volume without accompanying alterations in heart rate or peripheral resistance, may also contribute to the hypertension.[120] Further study is needed before the relative contributions of the renin-angiotensin-aldosterone system, renal sodium and water retention, and increased cardiac output to the syndrome of oral contraceptive–induced hypertension can be assessed.

Hypertension in Pregnancy

Approximately 6% of pregnancies are complicated by hypertension, which may antedate conception or arise during gestation or in the early puerperium.[121] Such hypertension is often accompanied by edema or proteinuria and occasionally by seizures and coma. The hypertensive disorders of pregnancy account for approximately 20% of cases of maternal death and for increased perinatal mortality due to premature delivery, either spontaneous or induced for therapeutic reasons.[121] The pathophysiology of hypertension in pregnancy is a complex and controversial area that is beyond the scope of this chapter but that has recently been discussed in several excellent reviews.[122,123]

Coarctation of the Aorta

Coarctation of the aorta causes a form of surgically curable hypertension that usually presents in childhood. The lesion is congenital narrowing of the aorta that can occur anywhere along the length of the vessel but most commonly just beyond the origin of the left subclavian artery at or below the insertion of the ligamentum arteriosium. The hypertension associated with coarctation of the aorta is due to a combination of mechanical factors, increased plasma volume, activation of the renin-angiotensin system, and perhaps enhanced sympathetic nervous system activity. Dogs with surgically produced coarctation show initial increases in plasma renin activity that disappear when the hypertension becomes established.[124] Patients with coarctation hypertension may have normal or suppressed plasma renin activity when recumbent yet show an exaggerated renin response to postural change and to exercise compared to their own responses after surgical correction of the coarctation.[125,126] Patients with coarctation hypertension also show a significant reduction in blood pressure and increase in plasma renin activity in response to infusion of saralasin.[127] Further, plasma volume is increased in hypertensive patients with coarctation, and there is evidence that the renin-angiotensin system is hyperreactive to the stimulus of volume depletion, so that the "normal" plasma renin activity found in coarctation is, in fact, abnormal when related to an expanded plasma volume.[128,129] The abnormalities of renin release in coarctation may reflect dampening of pulsatile flow and lowering of perfusion pressure in the renal arteries.[130] Recent evidence suggests that increased activity of the sympathetic nervous system contributes to the maintenance of chronic coarctation hypertension and to the genesis of the paradoxical hypertension that sometimes develops immediately following coarctation repair.[131,132] Further study is needed to explore the interactions of the various mechanisms involved in the initiation and maintenance of coarctation hypertension and to determine why hypertension so often (31% in one series) persists following coarctation repair.

Cushing's Syndrome

Cushing's syndrome, a rare cause of systemic hypertension, is accompanied by blood pressure elevation in 85% of cases. The hypertension can be severe and, if left untreated, is frequently associated with cardiovascular complications, particularly congestive heart failure.[133] Mechanisms that have been invoked to explain the hypertension include the salt-retaining action of high levels of circulating cortisol, increased activity of the renin-angiotensin system secondary to stimulation of renin substrate synthesis by elevated levels of circulating cortisol, increased vascular reactivity to pressor substances, and, in some patients, increased production of a mineralocorticoid such as DOC or aldosterone. A hypotensive response to infusion of saralasin has been reported in Cushing's syndrome, supporting a role for the renin-angiotensin system in the pathogenesis of the hypertension.[134]

Rare Endocrine Causes of Hypertension

Primary hyperparathyroidism is accompanied by hypertension in 20% to 50% of patients. The hypertension, which frequently disappears following parathyroidectomy, has been attributed to stimulation of renin release by hypercalcemia.[135] Hypertension occurs in approximately 25% of patients with hypothyroidism and frequently disappears when thyroid replacement is given.[136] Hypertension that sometimes disappears with successful treatment of the primary disease has also been reported in 18% to 43% of acromegalic patients.[137] The mechanism of hypertension in acromegaly has been attributed to inappropriately elevated plasma renin activity and aldosterone concentration in the face of volume expansion. Growth hormone may act as a direct stimulus to renin release in such patients.

Systolic Hypertension

Isolated systolic hypertension occurs commonly in the elderly due to loss of compliance in the resistance vessels and less often in younger patients due to conditions in which cardiac output is increased in relation to decreased peripheral vascular resistance, as in arteriovenous shunts, Paget's disease of bone, or beriberi, or to increased inotropic activity of the heart, as in anemia, thyrotoxicosis, or aortic valvular insufficiency. Epidemiologic studies have shown that the occurrence of stroke and other cardiovascular complications of hypertension is as directly related to the systolic as to the diastolic pressure, and a two- to threefold increase in the incidence of cardiovascular complications has been demonstrated in elderly patients with isolated systolic hypertension compared to age-matched normotensive subjects.[138] The appearance of systolic hypertension in the elderly should not, then, be regarded as a normal consequence of aging.

Hypertension Following Cardiopulmonary Bypass

Systemic hypertension characterized by elevated peripheral vascular resistance is frequently encountered in the first few hours after open heart surgery in patients undergoing coronary artery bypass or valve replacement.[139] This form of hypertension is a particular problem in patients who have had coronary artery bypass surgery, in whom its estimated incidence is 33%. Neither history nor coronary artery anatomy is predictive of the development of hypertension after surgery. Increases in circulating catecholamines, renin, and angiotensin II have been reported in patients who develop hypertension, but the humoral changes have not been clearly related to the elevation in peripheral vascular resistance.[140] Although this form of hypertension is self-limited, it may contribute to the morbidity and mortality of cardiac surgery, and thus it merits further study and vigorous attempts at prevention and specific treatment.

Clinical Presentation

INITIAL DIAGNOSTIC PRESENTATION

The initial evaluation of the hypertensive patient is designed to establish the diagnosis of systemic hypertension, to grade its severity, to determine the need for treatment, and to assess the likelihood of a secondary cause for the hypertension. The Joint National Committee on Detection, Evaluation and Treatment of High Blood Pressure has published guidelines for the detection, followup, and stepped-care therapy of hypertensive patients.[4]

The accurate and reproducible measurement of blood pressure by the cuff technique is the most critical part of the diagnostic evaluation. On the initial visit, the blood pressure should be taken in both arms and one leg (to rule out coarctation of the aorta) after the patient has been supine for five minutes and again in one arm immediately after and two minutes after standing[141]; on followup visits, blood pressure measurements made with the patient in the sitting position are sufficient unless orthostatic hypotension is being looked for specifically. Two or three pressures should be taken at each visit, and at least two minutes should be allowed between readings to avoid false depressions in systolic pressure and false elevations in diastolic pressure due to venous congestion and partial filling of the vascular bed. Proper cuff size is critical to accurate blood pressure measurement.[141] The width should be about two-thirds the width of the arm (15 cm in most adults), and, more important, the bladder cuff should be long enough to circle the arm. Falsely elevated readings can be obtained when the bladder is too short, and the error is magnified if the cuff is also too narrow. Mercury manometers are preferred, but aneroid manometers can be used if they are standardized frequently against a mercury manometer.

To obtain an accurate systolic pressure, the cuff should be inflated rapidly to at least 30 mm Hg above the systolic pressure as determined by palpation of the radial artery. This is necessary to avoid underestimating the pressure because of the ausculatory gap, an unexplained disappearance of Korotkoff sounds for some interval between systole and diastole. The cuff should be deflated at a rate of 2 mm Hg to 3 mm Hg/sec. The systolic reading is taken at the level of pressure at which clear Korotkoff sounds are heard with each heartbeat. The diastolic reading is taken both at the level when sounds become muffled (Korotkoff phase IV) and when the sounds disappear (phase V). Both readings should be recorded. The hemodynamic significance of muffling is not well understood. Further, in patients with hyperkinetic circulations, and in situations in which the stethoscope is held too tightly over the artery, muffling is heard well below the expected diastolic pressure. For this reason the disappearance of sound is generally a more reliable and reproducible endpoint. It is not known whether the level of muffling or the level of disappearance is the more accurate reflection of the intra-arterial diastolic pressure, so selection of one over the other as a clinical measurement is a matter of convenience and reproducibility.

The use of home blood pressure recordings by either the patient or another person in the household is particularly useful in monitoring patients with labile hypertension, in anxious patients whose blood pressures tend to be falsely elevated in the doctor's office, and in patients whose doses of antihypertensive medication need to be adjusted. Home recordings should be taken at various times of the day, in various positions, and during periods of stress and relaxation in order to assess the effects of diurnal variations in hormones, posture, and emotional state on blood pressure. Standard sphygmomanometers and stethoscopes are appropriate for this purpose. The patient's skills at blood pressure measurement should be tested at frequent intervals by a professional.

Once a diagnosis of stable hypertension has been established, the need for antihypertensive treatment should be assessed and, where indicated, diagnostic evaluation for secondary causes of hypertension should be undertaken. In view of the rarity of secondary causes of hypertension and the high cost and risk of elaborate diagnostic studies, it is recommended that the routine pretreatment workup be limited to defining the severity of the hypertension and to identifying its complications and associated cardiovascular risk factors.[4,142] All of the secondary causes combined account for less than 10% of the adult hypertensive population, but since some patients with secondary hypertension are potentially curable, diagnostic evaluation is warranted in selected patients.[143,144] These include those in whom routine history, physical examination, or the recommended laboratory findings suggest a specific secondary cause; those who are younger than 30 years of age, since they have the greatest prevalence of correctable secondary hypertension; those in whom drug therapy is inadequate or unsatisfactory; and those whose blood pressure has suddenly worsened.[4] A careful, complete history should be obtained and physical examination should be performed in all hypertensive patients prior to the initiation of therapy.

The medical history should include:

1. Any previous history of hypertension, including prior and current antihypertensive treatment
2. A history of factors that are regarded as predisposing to hypertension, including excessive salt intake, use of oral contraceptives or other estrogen preparations, occupational stress, and family history of hypertension and its complications
3. Evidence of hypertensive complications, including congestive heart failure, coronary artery disease, renal dysfunction, and stroke
4. A history of other cardiovascular risk factors, including diabetes, obesity, cigarette smoking, and lipid abnormalities

A history of weakness, muscle cramps, and polyuria suggests hypokalemia and the possibility of hyperaldosteronism; a history of the triad of headaches, palpitations, and hyperhidrosis suggests pheochromocytoma. Nocturia is often found in hypertensive patients and may reflect a loss of urinary concentrating ability. Headache, epistaxis, tinnitus, dizziness, and syncope are commonly taken to be symptoms of hypertension. However, an analysis of symptoms present at the time of discovery of hypertension, using the findings of the U.S. national survey of 1960–1962, showed that these symptoms were no more common among previously unrecognized hypertensives than among normotensive subjects.[145] In a separate study it was shown that only 18% of patients unaware of their hypertension complained of headache, but most of these developed the symptoms once informed of their diagnosis.[146] It should be remembered that most patients with uncomplicated hypertension have no symptoms referable to their disease.

The physical examination should include two or more blood pressure measurements, at least one of which is obtained in the standing position; funduscopic examination of the eyes for hypertensive retinopathy; careful examination of the cardiovascular system for evidence of congestive heart failure, cardiomegaly, myocardial dysfunction, and peripheral vascular disease; examination of the abdomen for bruits; auscultation over all scars for evidence of arteriovenous fistulae and a careful neurologic examination for the stigmata of stroke.

Pretreatment laboratory tests can be restricted to those generally performed as part of a routine medical checkup: hematocrit, urinalysis, serum creatinine or blood urea nitrogen, serum potassium, chest film, and electrocardiogram. Other tests that can be obtained as part of most automated blood chemistry batteries, such as the blood glucose, serum cholesterol, and serum uric acid tests, are helpful in assessing other cardiovascular risk factors and can be used as a baseline for monitoring the effects of antihypertensive treatment. Serial chest films, electrocardiograms, and echocardiograms may be helpful in assessing the effects of hypertension and antihypertensive treatment on the heart.

HYPERTENSIVE CRISIS

Approximately 1% of hypertensive patients enter an accelerated phase characterized by severe hypertension and necrotizing arteriolitis that leads to progressive end-organ damage. Hypertensive crisis is a medical emergency; left untreated, the 5-year mortality rate is 100%.[14] This syndrome can result from essential hypertension or from hypertension secondary to any cause except coarctation of the aorta. The triggering mechanism for the development of arteriolar lesions has been related to absolute level or rate of rise of arterial pressure, to the presence of disseminated intravascular clotting in association with microangiopathic hemolytic anemia, and to activation of the renin-angiotensin system. Whatever the initiating mechanism, the syndrome is perpetuated by deposition of fibrin in arteriolar walls, which, in turn, leads to retinopathy, renal damage, and increased renin release.[147]

Patients with accelerated hypertension usually present with hypertensive encephalopathy, rapidly progressive renal insufficiency, or acute LV failure. Hypertensive encephalopathy is characterized by the rapid onset of confusion, headache, visual disturbances, seizures, and, in severe cases, somnolence and even coma. Increased intracranial pressure with papilledema occurs, presumably due to failure of autoregulation of cerebral blood flow with breakthrough vasodilatation and secondary extravasation of intravascular contents. Death from a cerebrovascular accident frequently occurs if the hypertension is untreated, but the encephalopathy usually clears rapidly following successful antihypertensive treatment. Renal damage secondary to necrotizing arteriolitis results in proteinuria, hematuria, and azotemia. Assuming that the blood pressure can be controlled, the presence of renal damage at the time of diagnosis has prognostic significance. The 5-year survival of treated patients with grade IV retinopathy and azotemia is 23%; of nonazotemic patients, 64%.[148]

EVALUATION OF PATIENTS FOR SECONDARY CAUSES OF HYPERTENSION

Renovascular Hypertension

Renal arterial disease is the most common cause of surgically curable hypertension. The clinical characteristics of patients most likely to have renovascular hypertension are, in summary:

Abrupt onset, especially in the young or in late middle age
Sudden acceleration of benign hypertension
Abdominal bruit
Fixed diastolic hypertension, moderately severe to severe
Refractory to conventional medical therapy
More common in malignant hypertension
Abnormal rapid-sequence intravenous pyelogram (IVP)
Responsive to saralasin and converting enzyme inhibitors

Both hypertension of abrupt onset, especially when it appears in the young or in late middle age and the sudden acceleration of benign hypertension are frequently secondary to renal artery stenosis. On physical examination, the presence of an upper abdominal bruit, particularly one that is high-pitched, systolic-diastolic or continuous in timing, and radiates laterally from the mid-epigastrium, is strongly suggestive of functionally significant renal artery stenosis. Such bruits have been described in one-half to two-thirds of cases of surgically proved renovascular hypertension, and their significance has been confirmed by palpation of a renal artery thrill at the time of surgery.[149] Because of the cost and morbidity of the diagnostic evaluation for renovascular hypertension, it is recommended that diagnostic study be reserved for patients with one or more of the characteristics listed above and not be used indiscriminately as part of the routine hypertension workup. Only patients with moderate to severe hypertension, patients whose hypertension is refractory to medical treatment, and patients whose renal function deteriorates on medical treatment are surgical candidates, and aggressive diagnostic evaluation should be reserved for these groups.

The rapid-sequence or hypertensive IVP is a commonly used screening test for renovascular hypertension.[150] Major features of renal artery stenosis on IVP include: delayed (> 1 minute) appearance time of contrast medium; differences (> 1.5 cm) in renal size; and delayed clearance of contrast medium.[151] Minor features include a scalloped appearance of the ureter, decreased volume of the collecting system, evidence of parenchymal atrophy, and renal ptosis.[151] In the large Cooperative Study of Renovascular Hypertension, in which two-thirds of the patients studied had atherosclerotic disease, the rapid-sequence IVP was abnormal in 78% of patients with high-grade (> 50% narrowing) unilateral renal artery stenosis and in 70.5% of patients with bilateral disease and high-grade stenosis on at least one side.[152] Of patients with either unilateral or bilateral disease who responded favorably to renal artery surgery, 83% had

had abnormal screening IVPs. Further, the IVP was useful in identifying the side of the predominant lesion in patients with bilateral disease. Unilateral surgery produced favorable results in 80% of such patients with abnormal IVPs but in only 18% of those with normal studies. Thus, the IVP may be useful in selecting the appropriate surgical procedure for patients with bilateral renal artery stenosis.

False negative IVPs have been reported in 7% to 48% of patients with functionally significant renal artery stenosis, perhaps due to the development of collateral vessels to the affected kidney.[149,153] False negative results are particularly common in fibromuscular hyperplasia: in one large series only 52% of patients with unilateral and 44% with bilateral lesions had abnormal rapid-sequence IVPs.[153] False positive studies have been reported in 8% to 30% of patients without functionally significant renal artery stenosis due to minor differences in renal mass of any cause, congenital abnormalities such as hypoplasia or a bifid vascular or collecting system, or parenchymal renal disease.[149,154] For all of these reasons, and because of its high cost and morbidity, the rapid-sequence IVP is a less-than-optimal screening test for renovascular hypertension.

Pharmacologic screening with the angiotensin II antagonist saralasin (sarenin) or the converting enzyme inhibitors captopril and teprotide has been used to assess the functional significance of renal artery stenosis. A fall in blood pressure immediately following the administration of one of these agents is taken as evidence that the hypertension is angiotensin-mediated, and the test is interpreted as positive. A potential difficulty with this interpretation is that the converting enzyme inhibitors also block the inactivation of bradykinin, a vasodilator peptide, and may stimulate synthesis of vasodilator prostaglandins or cause a generalized diminution in vascular reactivity to pressor agents. The latter effects, rather than inhibition of angiotensin II production, may be responsible for the drop in blood pressure in some patients.

Various pitfalls have been described in the use of the saralasin infusion test in screening for renovascular hypertension. The test has not been adequately standardized under conditions of known sodium balance. This is critical, since the blood pressure response to saralasin clearly depends on the pre-existing renin level. False positive responses to saralasin have been reported in sodium-depleted patients with essential hypertension; false negative responses, in patients who have functionally significant renal artery stenosis, particularly if they are volume expanded.[155,156] Further, hazardous hypotensive and hypertensive responses to saralasin have been described. Hypotension has been reported following saralasin administration to patients who are being maintained on antihypertensive therapy or who are volume depleted. Transient hypertension, which may relate to the agonistic effect of the agent on angiotensin II receptors or to the release of catecholamines from an unexpected pheochromocytoma, can occur up to several hours following saralasin infusion.[157] The agonistic effect of saralasin is most often seen in patients who have low levels of endogenous angiotensin II.[158]

Converting enzyme inhibitors are superior to angiotensin II antagonists for use in hypertension screening in that they lack intrinsic pressor activity. The depressor response that they induce lacks specificity, however. It is also seen in patients with malignant hypertension unrelated to renal vascular disease and in patients with high-renin and normal-renin essential hypertension. Converting enzyme inhibitors share with the angiotensin II antagonists the hazard of inducing profound hypotension in patients who are receiving other antihypertensive treatment or who have been volume depleted. Preliminary data thus suggest that captopril and other converting enzyme inhibitors may be useful in association with other diagnostic procedures in the preliminary identification of patients with surgically curable renovascular hypertension but do not permit differentiation of this syndrome from high-renin essential hypertension.[159]

Definitive diagnosis of functionally significant renal artery stenosis is made by a combination of selective renal angiography and differential renal vein renin measurement. Anatomic demonstration of renal artery stenosis in a hypertensive patient does not establish a renal vascular etiology for the hypertension, since high-grade renal artery stenosis is a common autopsy finding in normotensive people, particularly those over the age of 50.[160] Documentation of the functional significance of an anatomic lesion requires the demonstration of increased renin production by the involved kidney. When renin activity in the venous effluent from the involved kidney is 1.5 or more times that of the uninvolved side and when the uninvolved side can be shown not to produce renin, the probability of improvement in blood pressure after surgery is approximately 90%.[161] To demonstrate that the uninvolved kidney produces no renin it is necessary to show either that there is no arterial-venous difference in renin activity across the renal vascular bed or that there is no stepup in renin activity from vena caval to renal venous blood. Prior stimulation of renin release with provocative maneuvers such as tilting, salt deprivation, or administration of vasodilators, diuretics, or converting enzyme inhibitors has been shown to enhance selectively renin release from the affected kidney.[162,163] The diagnosis of surgically remediable renal artery stenosis can be missed when renal vein sampling is performed in the unstimulated state or when renin-suppressing antihypertensive drugs have not been discontinued prior to study, masking lateralization in patients with functionally significant unilateral renal artery stenosis.

The following antihypertensive drugs inhibit renin release:

> Alpha methyldopa
> Beta blockers
>> Atenolol
>> Metoprolol
>> Nadolol
>> Pindolol
>> Propranolol
>> Timolol
> Clonidine
> Ganglionic blockers
> Reserpine

It has been documented that increased renin release is restricted to that portion of the kidney distal to a segmental lesion, and that renin is suppressed in the remaining portion of the affected kidney, so the diagnosis of surgically remediable disease can be missed when samples are obtained only from the main renal veins in patients with segmental renal lesions.[164] Mixing of blood from the suppressed normal portion of the kidney with blood from the affected area can obscure the source of elevated renin. Thus, segmental renal vein sampling is used to define indications for partial nephrectomy in hypertensive patients with branch renal artery stenoses and other localized renal abnormalities such as renal infarction, renal cysts, or renin-secreting tumors.[164]

Measurement of plasma renin activity in peripheral veins is not generally useful in screening patients for renovascular hypertension or in predicting the outcome of renal vascular surgery.[161] Renin activity in peripheral venous blood has often been in the "normal range" in patients who were subsequently shown to have surgically remediable renal artery stenosis. Somewhat better correlations have been reported when sodium intake was rigorously controlled[165] and when renin activity was related to 24-hour sodium excretion,[166] but these standardization maneuvers make the procedure too cumbersome for screening purposes.

Renal Parenchymal Disease and Chronic Renal Failure

Renal damage can be either the cause or the effect of systemic hypertension. On the one hand, nephrosclerosis and secondary renal dysfunction are common complications of uncontrolled essential hypertension. Most patients with hypertension of greater than 5 years duration have been shown to have radiographically demonstrable nephrosclerosis, even in the presence of normal renal function. On the other hand, systemic hypertension can occur secondary to renal parenchymal disease of any etiology, with or without renal failure. If one excludes oral contraceptive–induced hypertension, more than half of all adults with secondary hypertension have renal parenchymal disease.[142,143] Moreover, up to 80% of cases of chronic hypertension in prepubertal children may be secondary to renal disease.[14]

Chronic renal disease can usually be detected from the history and physical examination, urinalysis, blood urea nitrogen, and serum creatinine. More sophisticated tests, including renal biopsy, are sometimes required to make a specific diagnosis, but etiologic diagnoses are seldom required for the hypertension evaluation per se.

Renal Transplantation

Renal angiography is the most useful procedure for distinguishing among the various causes of chronic post-transplant hypertension. Post-transplant renal artery stenosis is diagnosed by angiography, as is acute rejection. Renal rejection is characterized by prolongation of arterial clearance time, renal enlargement with diffuse edema, and progressive deterioration of the nephrogram. Peripheral vein renin measurements are not useful in the evaluation of patients with post-transplant hypertension.

Renin-secreting Tumors

Differential renal vein renin measurements, coupled with the finding of elevations in plasma renin activity in peripheral veins, have been shown to be useful in making the diagnosis of renin-secreting tumor. Plasma renin activity in the main renal vein on the side of the tumor has not uniformly been elevated, so segmental sampling has been needed for tumor localization.[165] The renin-secreting tumors reported to date have generally been small, ranging in size from the dimensions of a rice kernel to 4 cm in diameter. They frequently could not be visualized on angiography.[167]

Syndromes of Mineralocorticoid Excess

PRIMARY ALDOSTERONISM. The simplest screening test for primary aldosteronism is the determination of serum potassium. Approximately 50% of hypertensives with unprovoked hypokalemia have primary aldosteronism, whereas fewer than 0.5% of those with normal plasma potassium have the syndrome.[168] However, many patients with primary aldosteronism have intermittently normal plasma potassium values, particularly if dietary sodium is restricted or potassium supplementation is given, and hypertensives without adrenal disease often develop hypokalemia during diuretic therapy.[169] When hypokalemia is observed, the concomitant measurement of urinary potassium excretion when the patient is off diuretics is valuable in distinguishing primary aldosteronism from other causes.[168] Inappropriate potassium wastage (<40 mEq/24 hrs) is seen in primary aldosteronism with hypokalemia but not in hypokalemia of other causes. If plasma potassium is restored to normal, this test is not useful.

Measurement of plasma renin activity is useful in screening for primary aldosteronism. The observation of suppressed renin rules out the syndromes of secondary aldosteronism. A single determination of plasma aldosterone has limited usefulness in screening for primary aldosteronism, however, because circulating aldosterone levels oscillate rapidly in both normal subjects and patients with primary aldosteronism.[170] Urinary aldosterone measurements are not adequate to make a diagnosis of primary aldosteronism because of the substantial overlap with essential hypertension and secondary aldosteronism. One reason for this phenomenon is that hypokalemia inhibits aldosterone production, so that plasma and urinary aldosterone in severely hypokalemic subjects with untreated primary aldosteronism may be in the normal range for potassium-replete normal subjects.[171] To improve the diagnostic usefulness of aldosterone measurement in primary aldosteronism, the aldosterone response to volume expansion can be observed. This can be accomplished by administering DOCA, 10 mg IM every 12 hours for 3 days;[172] 9α-fluorohydrocortisone, 400 μg qd for 3 days;[173,174] or by intravenous sodium loading (normal saline, 2 liters over 2 hours).[175] Failure of aldosterone to suppress following these maneuvers is a consistent feature of aldosterone-producing adenoma, and it distinguishes adenoma from the syndromes of adrenal hyperplasia and secondary aldosteronism.

ALDOSTERONE-PRODUCING ADENOMA. A solitary adrenal cortical adenoma is the cause of primary aldosteronism in 75% to 85% of cases. The diagnosis and localization of such tumors is important, since patients whose hyperaldosteronism can be completely corrected by unilateral adrenalectomy generally have a remission of hypertension, whereas those who have bilateral hyperplasia often remain hypertensive even after both adrenals are removed.[173] A number of techniques are available for localizing aldosterone-producing adenomas. Direct adrenal vein sampling by percutaneous catheterization and measurement of adrenal venous aldosterone levels is the most accurate method of diagnosing adrenal pathology in primary aldosteronism and of localizing the site of the tumor, if one is present.[105] Simultaneous cortisol determinations are used to confirm that adrenal vein sampling has been achieved. Adrenal vein aldosterone concentrations range from 500 ng/100 ml to 1200 ng/100 ml in primary aldosteronism (versus 100 ng/100 ml to 400 ng/100 ml in normal subjects). Elevated values with a less than twofold difference between sides suggest bilateral hyperplasia; aldosterone-producing adenomas generally result in a greater than tenfold difference between sides[176]. [131]I-19-iodocholesterol scintiscans can be used to visualize adenomas greater than 0.9 cm in diameter.[177] Suppression of the remainder of the adrenal tissue with dexamethasone, 0.5 mg to 1.0 mg every 6 hours for 24 hours prior to the administration of iodocholesterol, improves the resolution of the technique. Adrenal venography is a reliable means of localizing aldosterone-producing adenomas but is no longer in general use because of the high incidence (5%–10%) of retroperitoneal and intra-adrenal hemorrhage.[178]

IDIOPATHIC HYPERALDOSTERONISM. Idiopathic hyperaldosteronism is generally associated with less severe hypertension, less extreme aldosterone elevation and renin suppression, and less marked electrolyte imbalance than aldosterone-producing adenoma.[172] However, overlap between the two syndromes is so great as to make differential diagnosis based on resting values of aldosterone, renin, and electrolytes impossible. Indirect methods of distinguishing primary aldosteronism secondary to adenoma from bilateral hyperplasia include the use of computer-assisted quadric analysis of multiple parameters (aldosterone, renin, sodium, potassium, and bicarbonate) and observation of the circadian rhythm of plasma aldosterone and the response of aldosterone to postural stimulation.[179] Plasma aldosterone rises in response to assumption of the upright posture in patients with essential hypertension or adrenal cortical hyperplasia but falls or remains unchanged in patients with aldosterone-producing adenomas. The fixed diurnal pattern of plasma aldosterone in patients with aldosterone-producing adenomas, which is not interrupted by alterations in posture, is thought to reflect a dependence on ACTH that is not found in adrenal cortical hyperplasia.[179] This difference in the control of aldosterone secretion in the two syndromes may thus reflect a difference in pathophysiology. Volume overload suppression and postural stimulation tests are useful, as previously discussed. Differential adrenal vein aldosterone determinations fail to lateralize, and ^{131}I-iodocholesterol scanning shows no adrenal abnormality.

INDETERMINATE HYPERALDOSTERONISM. Indeterminate hyperaldosteronism is less common than aldosterone-producing adenoma or idiopathic hyperaldosteronism and is generally associated with less severe hypertension and humoral and electrolyte abnormalities than the other two syndromes. In indeterminate hyperaldosteronism, plasma renin activity responds normally to upright posture, differential adrenal vein aldosterone determinations fail to lateralize, and ^{131}I-iodocholesterol scanning shows no adrenal abnormality. Diagnosis is made by the administration of exogenous mineralocorticoid, which lowers aldosterone levels into the normal range but, as is not the case in normal subjects, does not totally suppress them.[106]

GLUCOCORTICOID-REMEDIABLE HYPERALDOSTERONISM. Glucocorticoid-remediable hyperaldosteronism is a rare disorder that usually presents at an early age and occurs in kindreds. The hypertension and metabolic abnormalities are milder than those in the other syndromes of aldosterone excess and can be corrected by replacement doses of glucocorticoid hormones (*e.g.,* dexamethasone 0.5–1.0 mg QD or BID). A 2- to 3-week trial of such a regimen is adequate to make the diagnosis. ACTH secretion does not appear to be abnormal, but the glucocorticoid responsiveness suggests the existence in this syndrome of an aldosterone stimulating factor that is glucocorticoid-sensitive.[172]

CONGENITAL ADRENAL HYPERPLASIA. In C-11 hydroxylase deficiency, the formation of cortisol from 11-desoxycortisol and the conversion of DOC to corticosterone are blocked, resulting in excesses of DOC and 11-desoxycortisol and a deficiency of cortisol.[180] These patients have the stigmata of mineralocorticoid excess, hypertension, and hypokalemia, and are virilized because excess adrenal androgens are produced. In 17-hydroxylase deficiency, the formation of androgens and estrogens from pregnenolone and the synthesis of cortisol are blocked, causing deficiencies of the sex steroids and cortisol and excesses of the ACTH-stimulated steroids DOC and corticosterone.[181] A syndrome of hypogonadism and mineralocorticoid excess with hypertension and hypokalemia results. In both of these syndromes, diagnosis is made by a combination of inspection and steroid analysis.

Pheochromocytoma

Most patients with pheochromocytoma have signs and symptoms of the disease, so it is legitimate to use symptoms and physical signs in screening patients for pheochromocytoma. Biochemical tests then need to be performed only in patients who have clinical evidence of the disorder. The most common signs and symptoms are summarized in Common Signs and Symptoms of Pheochromocytoma. Tumors may produce intermittent or sustained hypertension. Patients with intermittent hypertension are thought to have tumors that secrete episodically, and the appearance of symptoms frequently coincides with a paroxysm of hypertension and presumably with an episode of secretory activity. Many patients with sustained hypertension secondary to pheochromo-

---

COMMON SIGNS AND SYMPTOMS OF PHEOCHROMOCYTOMA

Symptoms	Signs
Headache*	Postural hypotension
Excessive sweating*	Labile hypertension
Palpitations*	Weight loss
Pain in chest or abdomen	Diabetes mellitus
Pallor	Appearance of hypermetabolic state
Anxiety	Paradoxic response of blood pressure to
Tremor	ganglion blocking drugs and guanethi-
Nausea	dine
	Severe pressor response during induction
	of anesthesia

*One of these is almost invariably present.

---

cytoma also develop symptoms, so the presence or absence of symptoms alone does not provide a reliable clue to the secretory function of the tumor.[111]

Definitive diagnosis of pheochromocytoma requires the demonstration of increased concentrations of catecholamines or their metabolites in plasma or urine and the localization of tumor by computerized axial tomography (CT scan), radionuclide techniques, or angiography. Measurements of 24-hour urinary excretion of VMA (3-methoxy, 4-hydroxymandelic acid)[182] and of metanephrine and normetanephrine[183] are frequently used as screening tests for pheochromocytoma because VMA and the other 3-methoxy derivatives of catecholamines and their conjugates are the predominant forms in which catecholamines are excreted. These metabolites are excreted slowly, so diagnosis is sometimes possible even in patients with intermittently secreting tumors when urine is collected during a symptom-free period. Free catecholamines in plasma or urine can be measured directly by radioenzymatic techniques[184] or high-performance liquid chromatography[185]. Measurement of plasma catecholamines offers advantages over measurement of urinary catecholamines and metabolites in that it eliminates the variability inherent in 24-hour urine collections and permits sampling at the time that the patient has symptoms and paroxysms of hypertension, which are presumed to be related to episodes of secretory activity. Further, differential venous catheterization and measurement of regional plasma catecholamines are helpful in localizing pheochromocytomas.

CT scan is now regarded as the method of choice for localization of pheochromocytomas that reside in the adrenal gland.[186] It can reliably detect tumors 2 cm in diameter within the adrenal. For the 10% of pheochromocytomas that are smaller than the resolving power of the CT scan or are located outside the adrenal, other means of localization may be required. Differential venous catheterization and measurement of regional plasma catecholamines are helpful in localizing such tumors. Angiography can also be helpful, but frequently the arteries supplying extra-adrenal tumors cannot be found. Further, both arteriography and venography are associated with appreciable risks to the patient. Recently the guanethidine analog [^{131}I] meta-iodobenzylguanide (^{131}I-MIBG) has been shown to be useful in imaging pheochromocytomas that are undetectable by CT scan.[187] Tumors detected by ^{131}I-MIBG scanning include both benign and malignant and intra- and extra-adrenal pheochromocytomas that have different patterns of hormone secretion.

Pharmacologic screening for pheochromocytoma with the alpha-adrenergic blocking (Regitine) test or with provocative tests in which tyramine, glucagon, or histamine is administered has largely been abandoned because biochemical testing is more specific and safer.

Oral Contraceptive–Induced Hypertension

The diagnosis of oral contraceptive–induced hypertension can be made by documenting the onset of hypertension *de novo* during contraceptive therapy and the resolution of the hypertension upon drug withdrawal. Establishment of a cause-effect relationship between oral contraceptive administration and hypertension is made difficult by the occurrence of the delayed (up to 6 years) onset of hypertension following initiation of contraceptive therapy and the delayed (3 months or more) disappearance of hypertension following drug withdrawal.[188,189] Further, it may be difficult to separate oral contraceptive–induced hypertension from coincident, naturally occurring hypertension, since estrogen may unmask an underlying hypertensive diathesis.

Oral contraceptive–induced hypertension can, in part, be prevented by judicious use of these agents in women who are at high risk. Prior to prescribing an oral contraceptive, a careful history should be taken, and a detailed physical examination should be performed with particular attention to the cardiovascular system. Multiple blood pressure measurements should be made, and routine laboratory studies should be obtained. Evidence of thromboembolic disease or chronic hypertension of any cause is an absolute contraindication to oral contraceptives because of the risk of exacerbating the underlying disease.[190,191] A family history of hypertension and a personal history of pre-existing or occult renal disease or of pregnancy complicated by excessive weight gain, proteinuria, or hypertension are relative contraindications to oral contraceptive use. Women over 40 years of age, particularly if they are obese, should be cautioned about the increased risk of developing hypertension while ingesting oral contraceptives. Close observation of such patients should be planned, and they should be instructed to take and record home blood pressures and watch for excessive weight gain, edema, headaches, and blurred vision. Blood pressure measurement and a funduscopic examination should be performed and an interval history obtained on several occasions during the first year of treatment and at yearly intervals thereafter.

There is no evidence that the prevalence of subsequent hypertension can be reduced by choosing a particular oral contraceptive preparation. No relationship between magnitude of the increment in blood pressure and formulation or dose of estrogen has been found.[192] A relationship to dose and formulation of progestogen has been reported.[144,193] The incidence of thromboembolic complications, however, is related to the dose of estrogen in the contraceptive.[194] For this reason, it is preferable to start with a preparation of relatively low estrogen content.

All patients who become hypertensive while on oral contraceptive treatment should have the oral contraceptive withdrawn immediately. For those who are asymptomatic and have uncomplicated mild hypertension (blood pressure < 160/105), this is sufficient treatment. If blood pressure returns to normal within 6 months, no specific diagnostic studies are necessary. If, on the other hand, hypertension persists for more than 6 months after stopping the oral contraceptive, antihypertensive therapy should be started and a complete evaluation for underlying hypertension undertaken. For those who have symptoms referable to hypertension or who have moderate to severe disease (blood pressure > 160/105), antihypertensive therapy should be instituted immediately. Because of the relative infrequency of severe or symptomatic hypertension in association with oral contraceptive therapy, these patients should be evaluated for an underlying cause of hypertension.

Coarctation of the Aorta

The classic clinical feature of coarctation is elevated blood pressure in the upper extremities with reduced or absent pressure in the lower extremities. Diagnosis is made on physical examination on the basis of the blood pressure differential, weak pulses in the lower extremities, and a radial–femoral pulse delay. The typical systolic ejection murmur of coarctation is often heard most clearly on the back, and bruits due to the formation of collateral vessels are often heard over the ribs. The chest film supports the diagnosis when rib notching and the "3 sign" produced by dilatation of the aorta above and below the constriction are seen. Aortography is needed to make a definitive diagnosis and to localize the lesion before surgical correction can be attempted.

Summary

Systemic hypertension is the most common remediable cause of cardiovascular morbidity and mortality in the world. Hypertension leads to excess mortality and decreased life expectancy. The magnitude of the reduction in life expectancy increases with each increment in blood pressure but decreases with age, so that death rates for a given level of blood pressure elevation are greater in hypertension of early onset. The excess mortality associated with hypertension is related mainly to cardiovascular disease and cerebral hemorrhage. The cardiovascular complications of hypertension include stroke secondary to cerebral hemorrhage or thrombosis, coronary artery disease with associated angina pectoris and acute myocardial infarction, LV hypertrophy and congestive heart failure, aortic dissection, renal insufficiency, and peripheral vascular disease with intermittent claudication. Natural history studies performed in the era prior to the development of antihypertensive therapy revealed that the mean age of onset of hypertension was the early 30s and the mean survival was 20 years.[195,196] Thus life expectancy was shortened by 15 to 20 years on the average. Survival was shorter for men (20% 20 years) than for women (50% 20 years).[196] The prognosis for women was thought to be better because of their lesser incidence of coronary artery disease and accelerated hypertension. Despite the variable rate of progression of hypertensive vascular disease, the average hypertensive patient was free of symptoms and of vascular complications for most of the duration of the syndrome.[195]

Controlled studies have demonstrated that antihypertensive treatment that is effective in lowering diastolic blood pressure into the normal range reduces the incidence of cardiovascular complications. The most often quoted of these is the Veterans Administration Cooperative Study, a randomized, double-blind prospective clinical trial in 523 male patients whose initial diastolic pressures ranged from 90 mm Hg to 129 mm Hg.[197,198] Treatment with a combination of hydrochlorothiazide, reserpine, and hydralazine caused a sharp reduction in the incidence of stroke, congestive heart failure, accelerated hypertension, and renal failure. The benefits of antihypertensive therapy are less well defined in certain subclasses of patients, including those with mild hypertension, isolated systolic hypertension, or labile hypertension, and in all female hypertensives. Nevertheless, the evidence that drug treatment is useful in preventing the complications of hypertension is so compelling that the aggressive approach to evaluation and treatment outlined in Figure 14-2 has been espoused for all adults.[4]

Increased awareness of the importance of hypertension detection and treatment on the part of both physicians and patients has contributed to major improvements in the adequacy of antihypertensive treatment. Currently about three-quarters of hypertensive patients have been diagnosed; over half are under treatment and 38% to 45% are adequately controlled.[199,200] This contrasts with 10% to 15% control in the 1960s.[201,202]

Further refinements in our understanding of the pathophysiology of hypertension may lead to the development of better methods of detecting and treating hypertensive disease. These advances, coupled with more sophisticated and effective patient and physician education, are needed before systemic hypertension can be dismissed as a major health problem.

References

1. Hypertension and coronary heart disease: Classification and criteria for epidemiological studies. Technical report series No. 168. Geneva, World Health Organization, 1959.
2. Arterial hypertension and ischaemic heart disease: preventive aspects. Technical report series No. 231. Geneva, World Health Organization, 1962.
3. Julius S, Schork MA: Borderline hypertension: A critical review. J Chronic Dis 23:723, 1971
4. Moser M, Guyther JR, Finnerty F, et al: Report of the joint national committee on detection, evaluation and treatment of high blood pressure. A cooperative study. JAMA 237:255, 1977
5. Blumenthal S: Report of the task force on blood pressure control in children. Pediatrics 59:797, 1977

6. Page IH: The nature of arterial hypertension. The Eduardo Braun-Menendez Memorial Lecture. Arch Intern Med 111:103, 1963
7. Kannel WB, Gordon T, Castelli WP, et al: Electrocardiographic left ventricular hypertrophy and risk of coronary heart disease. Ann Intern Med 72:813, 1970
8. Society of Actuaries: Build and blood pressure study, Vol 1. Chicago, Society of Actuaries, 1959
9. Finkielman S, Worcel M, Agrest A. Hemodynamic patterns in essential hypertension. Circulation 31:356, 1965
10. Julius S, Conway J. Hemodynamic studies in patients with borderline blood pressure elevation. Circulation 38:282, 1968
11. Madsen PER, Buch J: Long-term prognosis of transient hypertension in young male adults. Aerospace Medicine 42:752, 1971
12. Hines EA Jr: Range of normal blood pressure and subsequent development of hypertension: a follow-up study of 1,522 patients. JAMA 115:271, 1940
13. Paffenbarger RS Jr, Thorne MC, Wing AL: Chronic disease in former college students. VIII. Characteristics in youth predisposing to hypertension in later years. Am J Epidemiol 88:25, 1968
14. Kaplan NM: Clinical Hypertension, 2nd ed. Baltimore, Md, Williams & Wilkins, 1978
15. Koch-Weser J: The therapeutic challenge of systolic hypertension. N Engl J Med 289:481, 1973
16. Coleman TG, Granger HJ, Guyton AC: Whole-body circulatory autoregulation and hypertension. Circ Res (Suppl 2)28:76, 1971
17. Guyton AC, Granger HJ, Coleman TG: Autoregulation of the total systemic circulation and its relation to control of cardiac output and arterial pressure. Circ Res (Suppl 1)28:93, 1971
18. Granger HJ, Guyton AC: Autoregulation of the total systemic circulation following destruction of the central nervous system in the dog. Circ Res 25:379, 1969
19. Eich RH, Cuddy RP, Smulyna H, Lyons RH: Hemodynamics in labile hypertension. Circulation 34:299, 1966
20. Frohlich ED, Tarazi RC, Dustan HP: Reexamination of the hemodynamics of hypertension. Am J Med Sci 257:9, 1969
21. Bello CT, Sevy RW, Harakal C: Varying hemodynamic patterns in essential hypertension. Am J Med Sci 250:24, 1965
22. Lund–Johansen P: Haemodynamic observations in mild hypertension. In Gross F, Strasser T (eds): Mild Hypertension: Natural History and Management, pp 102–115. Chicago, Year Book Medical Publishers, 1979
23. Julius S, Quadir H, Gajendragadkar S: Hyperkinetic state: A precursor of hypertension? A longitudinal study of borderline hypertension. In Gross F, Strasser T (eds): Mild Hypertension: Natural History and management, pp 116–126. Chicago, Year Book Medical Publishers, 1979
24. Ulrych M, Frohlich ED, Tarazi RC, et al: Cardiac output and distribution of blood volume in central and peripheral circulations in hypertensive and normotensive man. Br Heart J 31:570, 1969
25. Tarazi RC, Ibnahim MM, Dustan HP, et al: Cardiac factors in hypertension. Circ Res (Suppl 1)34:213, 1974
26. Wallace JM: Hemodynamic lesions in hypertension. Am J Cardiol 36:670, 1975
27. Liard J–F, Tarazi RC, Ferrario CM, et al: Hemodynamic and humoral characteristics of hypertension induced by prolonged stellate ganglion stimulation in conscious dogs. Circ Res 36:455, 1975
28. Kottke FJ, Kubicek WG, Visscher MB: The production of arterial hypertension by chronic renal artery-nerve stimulation. Am J Physiol 145:38, 1945

29. Okamoto K, Nosaka S, Yamori Y, et al: Participation of neural factor in the pathogenesis of hypertension in the spontaneously hypertensive rat. Jap Heart J 8:168, 1967
30. Okamoto K: Spontaneous Hypertension. Tokyo, Igaku Shoin, 1972
31. DeChamplain J, Krakoff L, Axelrod J: Interrelationships of sodium intake, hypertension and norepinephrine storage in the rat. Circ Res (Suppl 1)24:75, 1969
32. Reid JL, Zivin JA, Kopin IJ: Central peripheral adrenergic mechanisms in the development of deoxycorticosterone-saline hypertension in rats. Circ Res 37:569, 1975
33. Haeusler G, Gerold M, Thoenen H: Cardiovascular effects of 6-hydroxydopamine injected into a lateral brain ventricle of the rat. Naunyn Schmiedebergs Arch Pharmacol 274:211, 1972
34. Cutilletta AF, Erinoff L, Heller A, et al: Development of left ventricular hypertrophy in young spontaneously hypertensive rats after peripheral sympathectomy. Circ Res 40:428, 1977
35. Lake CR, Ziegler MG, Kopin IJ: Use of plasma norepinephrine for evaluation of sympathetic neuronal function in man. Life Sci 18:1315, 1976
36. Goldstein DS: Plasma norepinephrine in essential hypertension. A study of the studies. Hypertension 3:48, 1981
37. Ibrahim MM, Tarazi RC, Dustan HP, et al: Cardioadrenergic factor in essential hypertension. Am Heart J 88:724, 1974
38. Sannerstedt R, Julius S, Conway J: Hemodynamic responses to tilt and beta-adrenergic blockade in young patients with borderline hypertension. Circulation 42:1057, 1970
39. Wallace JM: Hemodynamic lesions in hypertension. Am J Cardiol 36:670, 1975
40. Julius S, Pascual AV, London R: Role of parasympathetic inhibition in the hyperkinetic type of borderline hypertension. Circulation 44:413, 1971
41. Korner PI, Shaw J, Uther JB, et al: Autonomic and non-autonomic circulation components in essential hypertension in man. Circulation 48:107, 1973
42. Frohlich ED: Clinical significance of hemodynamic findings in hypertension. Chest 64:94, 1973
43. Julius S, Esler MD, Randall OS: Role of autonomic nervous system in mild human hypertension. Clin Sci Mol Med 48:243s, 1975
44. Sannerstedt R: Hemodynamic findings at rest and during exercise in mild arterial hypertension. Am J Med Sci 258:70, 1969
45. Littler WA, Honour AJ, Carter RD, et al: Sleep and blood pressure. Br Med J 3:346, 1975
46. Patel C, North WRS: Randomized controlled trial of yoga and bio-feedback in management of hypertension. Lancet 2:93, 1975
47. Ruskin A, Beard OW, Schaffer RL: Blast hypertension: Elevated arterial pressures in the victims of the Texas City disaster. Am J Med 4:228, 1948
48. Cassel J: Hypertension and cardiovascular disease in migrants: A potential source of clues? Int J Epidemiol 3:204, 1974
49. Melby JC, Dale SL: New mineralocorticoids and adrenocorticosteroids in hypertension. Am J Cardiol 38:805, 1976
50. Prewitt RL, Leach BE, Byers LW, et al: Antihypertensive polar renomedullary lipid, a semisynthetic vasodilator. Hypertension 1:299, 1979
51. Oparil S, Haber E: The renin-angiotensin system. N Engl J Med 291:389, 446, 1974
52. Goodfriend TL, Peach MJ: Angiotensin III: (Des-Aspartic Acid-1)-Angiotensin II. Evidence and speculation for its role as an important agonist in the renin-angiotensin system. Circ Res 36:38, 1975

53. Ganten D: Studies on the existence of an independent brain renin-angiotensin system. In A Model for Extrarenal Tissue Renin. Ph.D. Dissertation. McGill University, Department of Experimental Medicine, Montreal, Canada, 1972

54. Carretero OA, Scicli AG: Possible role of kinins in circulatory homeostasis. Hypertension 3:I-4, 1981

55. Smith MC, Dunn MJ: Renal kallikrein, kinins and prostaglandins in hypertension. In Brenner BM, Stein JH (eds): Contemporary Issues in Nephrology, p 168. New York, Churchill & Livingstone, 1981

56. Nasjletti A, Malik KU: Relationships between the kallikeren-kinin and prostaglandin system. Life Sci 25:99, 1979

57. Mills IH: Kallikrein, kininogen and kinins in control of blood pressure. Nephron 23:61, 1979

58. Fejes-Toth G, Zahajszky T, Filep J: Effect of vasopressin on renal kallikrein excretion. Am J Physiol 239:F388, 1980

59. Holland OB, Chud JM, Braunstein H: Urinary kallikrein excretion in essential and mineralocorticoid hypertension. J Clin Invest 65:347, 1980

60. McGiff JC: Prostaglandins, prostacyclin and thromboxanes. Annu Rev Pharmacol Toxicol 21:479, 1981

61. Hedqvist P: Prostaglandin mediated control of sympathetic neuroeffector transmission. In Bergstrom S, Bernhard S (eds): Advances in the Biosciences, International Conference on Prostaglandins, Vol 9, p 461. Vienna, Pergamon Press, 1972

62. McGiff JC, Crowshaw K, Terregno NA, et al: Prostaglandin-like substances appearing in canine renal venous blood during renal ischemia: Their partial characterization by pharmacologic and chromatographic procedures. Circ Res 27:765, 1970

63. Aiken JW, Vane JR: Intrarenal prostaglandin release attenuates the renal vasoconstrictor activity of angiotensin. J Pharmacol Exp Ther 184:678, 1973

64. McGiff JC, Wong PYK: Compartmentalization of prostaglandins and prostacyclin within the kidney: Implications for renal function. Fed Proc 38:89, 1979

65. Share L, Crofton JT: The contribution of vasopressin to hypertension. Hypertension Vol. 4, no 3, p 85, 1982

66. Guyton AC, Coleman TG, Cowley AW Jr, et al: Arterial pressure regulation: Overriding dominance of the kidneys in long-term regulation and in hypertension. Am J Med 52:584, 1972

67. Katholi RE, Carey RM, Ayers CR, et al: Production of sustained hypertension by chronic intrarenal norepinephrine infusion in conscious dogs. Circ Res 40:1–118, 1977

68. Liard JF: Renal denervation delays blood pressure increase in the spontaneously hypertensive rat. Experientia 33:339, 1977

69. Kline RL, Kelton PM, Mercer PF: Effect of renal denervation on the development of hypertension in spontaneously hypertensive rats. Can J Physiol Pharmacol 56:818, 1978

70. Hollenberg NK, Adams DF: The renal circulation in hypertensive disease. Am J Med 60:773, 1976

71. Sullivan JM, Adams DF, Hollenberg NK: Beta-adrenergic blockade in essential hypertension: Reduced renin release despite renal vasoconstriction. Circ Res 39:532, 1976

72. DiBona GF: The functions of the renal nerves. Rev Physiol Biochem Pharmacol 94:76, 1982

73. Berchtold P, Jorgens V, Kemmer M, et al: Obesity and hypertension: Cardiovascular response to weight reduction. A review. Hypertension Vol 4, no 3, p 50, 1982

74. Reisin E, Abel R, Modan M, et al: Effect of weight loss without salt restriction on the reduction of blood pressure in overweight hypertensive patients. N Engl J Med 298:1, 1978
75. Jung RT, Shelty PS, Barrand M, et al: Role of catecholamines in hypertensive response to dieting. Br Med J 1:12, 1979
76. Page LB, Damon A, Moellering RC Jr: Antecedents of cardiovascular disease in six Solomon Islands societies. Circulation 49:1132, 1974
77. Prior IAM, Evans JG, Harvey HPB, et al: Sodium intake and blood pressure in two Polynesian populations. N Engl J Med 279:515, 1968
78. Dustan HP: Salt and hypertension. Cardiology Update, p 285, 1983
79. Kirkendall WM, Connor WE, Abboud F, et al: The effect of dietary sodium chloride on blood pressure, body fluids, electrolytes, renal function, and serum lipids of normotensive man. J Lab Clin Med 87:418, 1976
80. Luft FC, Rankin LI, Bloch R, et al: Cardiovascular and humoral responses to extremes of sodium intake in normal black and white men. Circulation 60:697, 1979
81. Page LB: Epidemiologic evidence on the etiology of human hypertension and its possible prevention. Am Heart J 91:527, 1976
82. Kempner W: Treatment of hypertensive vascular disease with rice diet. Am J Med 4:545, 1948
83. Corcoran AC, Taylor RD, Page IH: Controlled observations on the effect of low sodium dietotherapy in essential hypertension. Circulation 3:1, 1951
84. Tobian L Jr, Binion JT: Tissue cations and water in arterial hypertension. Circulation 5:754, 1952
85. Holloway ET, Bohr DF: Reactivity of vascular smooth muscle in hypertensive rats. Circ Res 33:678, 1973
86. Paller MS, Linas SL: Hemodynamic effects of alterations in potassium. Hypertension 4:III-20, 1982
87. McCarron DA, Henry HJ, Morris CD: Human nutrition and blood pressure regulation: An integrated approach. Hypertension Vol 4, no 3, p 27, 1982
88. Havlic RJ, Feinleib M: Epidemiology and genetics of hypertension. Hypertension Vol 4, no 3, p 27, 1982
89. Goldblatt H, Lunch J, Hanzal RF, et al: Studies on experimental hypertension. I. The production of persistent elevation of systolic blood pressure by means of renal ischemia. J Exp Med 59:347, 1934
90. Davis JO: The pathogenesis of chronic renovascular hypertension. Circ Res 40:439, 1977
91. Kurtzman NA, Pillay VKG, Rogers PW, et al: Renal vascular hypertension and low plasma renin activity. Interrelationship of volume and renin in the pathogenesis of hypertension. Arch Intern Med 133:195, 1974
92. Marks LS, Maxwell MH, Kaufmann JJ: Non-renin-mediated renovascular hypertension: A new syndrome? Lancet 1:615, 1977
93. Simon N, Franklin SS, Bleifer KH, et al: Clinical characteristic of renovascular hypertension. JAMA 220:1209, 1972
94. Harrison EG, McCormack LJ: Pathologic classification of renal arterial disease in renovascular hypertension. Mayo Clin Proc 46:161, 1971
95. Meaney TF, Dustan HP, McCormack LJ: Natural history of renal arterial disease. Radiology 91:881, 1968
96. Berretta-Piccoli C, Weidmann P, DeChatel R, et al: Hypertension associated with early stage kidney disease. Complementary roles of circulating renin, the body sodium/volume state and duration of hypertension. Am J Med 61:739, 1976
97. Blumberg A, Nelp WB, Hegstrom RM, et al: Extracellular volume in patients with

chronic renal disease treated for hypertension by sodium restriction. Lancet 2:69, 1967

98. Gutkin M, Levinson GE, King AS, et al: Plasma renin activity in end-stage kidney disease. Circulation 40:563, 1969
99. Vertes V, Cangiano JL, Berman LB, et al: Hypertension in end-stage renal disease. New Engl J Med 280:978, 1969
100. Brown JJ, Dusterdieck G, Fraser R, et al: Hypertension and chronic renal failure. Br Med Bull 27:128, 1971
101. Weidmann P, Maxwell MH: The renin-angiotensin-aldosterone system in terminal renal failure. Kidney International 8:S-219, 1975
102. Cannella G, Castellani A, Mioni G, et al: Blood pressure control in end-stage renal disease in man: Indirect evidence of a complex pathogenic mechanism besides renin or blood volume. Clin Sci Mol Med 52:19, 1977
103. Grunfeld JP, Kleinknect D, Moreau JF, et al: Permanent hypertension after renal homotransplantation in man. Clin Sci Mol Med 48:391, 1975
104. Melby JC, Dale SL: New mineralocorticoids and adrenocorticosteroids in hypertension. Am J Cardiol 38:805, 1976
105. McGuffin WL Jr, Gunnels JC Jr: Primary aldosteronism. Urol Clin North Am 4:227, 1977
106. Biglieri EG, Stockigt JR, Schambelan M: Adrenal mineralocorticoids causing hypertension. Am J Med 52:623, 1972
107. Biglieri EG, Forsham PH: Studies on the expanded extracellular fluid and the responses to various stimuli in primary aldosteronism. Am J Med 30:564, 1961
108. Chobanian AV, Burrows BA, Hollander W: Body fluid and electrolyte composition in arterial hypertension. II. Studies in mineralocorticoid hypertension. J Clin Invest 40:416, 1961
109. Tarazi RC, Ibrahim M, Bravo EL, et al: Hemodynamic characteristics of primary aldosteronism. N Engl J Med 289:1330, 1973
110. Conn JW, Rovner DR, Cohen EL: Licorice-induced pseudoaldosteronism. JAMA 205:492, 1968
111. Manger WM, Gifford RW Jr: Pheochromocytoma. New York, Springer-Verlag, 1977
112. Kaplan NM: Cardiovascular complications of oral contraceptives. Annu Rev Med 29:31, 1978
113. Beral V: Cardiovascular-disease mortality trends and oral-contraceptive use in young women. Lancet 2:1047, 1976
114. The Royal College of General Practitioners: Oral Contraceptives and Health, an Interim Report from the Oral Contraceptive Study of the Royal College of General Practitioners. New York, Pitman, 1974
115. Ramcharan S, Pellegrin FA, Hoag E: The occurrence and course of hypertensive disease in users and nonusers of oral contraceptive drugs. In Fregly MJ, Fregly MS (eds): Oral Contraceptives and High Blood Pressure, p 1. Gainesville, Fla, Dolphin Press, 1974
116. Spellacy WN, Birk SA: The effect of intrauterine devices, oral contraceptives, estrogens and progestogens on blood pressure. Am J Obstet Gyn 112:912, 1972
117. Beckerhoff R, Luetscher JA, Beckerhoff I, et al: Effects of oral contraceptives on the renin-angiotensin system and on blood pressure of normal young women. Johns Hopkins Med J 132:80, 1973
118. Laragh JH, Sealey JE, Ledingham JGG, et al: Oral contraceptives: Renin, aldosterone and high blood pressure. JAMA 201:918, 1967
119. Hollenberg NK, Williams GH, Burger B, et al: Renal blood flow and its response to angiotensin II. An interaction between oral contraceptive agents, sodium

intake and the renin-angiotensin system in healthy young women. Circ Res 38:35, 1976

120. Walters WAW, Cain D: Haemodynamic effects of low doses of female sex steroids. Aust NZ J Obstet Gyn 13:213, 1973

121. Chesley LC: Hypertensive Diseases in Pregnancy. New York, Appleton-Century-Crofts, 1978

122. Lindheimer MD, Katz AI: Pathophysiology of preeclampsia. Annu Rev Med 32:273, 1981

123. Lindheimer MD, Katz AI: Hypertension and pregnancy. In International Textbook on Hypertension: Physiopathology and Treatment, New York, McGraw-Hill, 1982

124. Yagi S, Kramsch DM, Madoff IM, et al: Plasma renin activity in hypertension associated with coarctation of the aorta. Am J Physiol 215:605, 1968

125. Markiewicz A, Wojczuk D, Kokot F, et al: Plasma renin activity in coarctation of aorta before and after surgery. Br Heart J 37:721, 1975

126. Van Way CW III, Michelakis AM, Anderson WJ, et al: Studies of plasma renin activity in coarctation of the aorta. Ann Surg 183:229, 1976

127. Ribeiro AB, Krakoff LR: Angiotensin blockade in coarctation of the aorta. N Engl J Med 295:148, 1976

128. Alpert BS, Bain HH, Balfe JW, et al: Role of the renin-angiotensin-aldosterone system in hypertensive children with coarctation of the aorta. Am J Cardiol 43:828, 1979

129. Bagby SP, Mass RD: Abnormality of the renin/body-fluid-volume relationship in serially-studied inbred dogs with neonatally-induced coarctation hypertension. Hypertension 2:631, 1980

130. Timmis GC, Gordon S: A renal factor in hypertension due to coarctation of the aorta. N Eng J Med 270:814, 1964

131. Whitlow PL, Katholi RE: Neuro humoral activity and the role of the renal nerves in canine coarctation of the aorta. Am J Cardiol 49:888, 1982

132. Rocchini AP, Rosenthal A, Barger AC, et al: Pathogenesis of paradoxical hypertension after coarctation resection. Circulation 54:382, 1976

133. Ross EJ, Marshall–Jones P, Friedman M: Cushing's syndrome: diagnostic criteria. Q J Med 35:149, 1966

134. Dalakos TG, Elias AN, Anderson GH Jr, et al: Evidence for an angiotensinogenic mechanism of the hypertension of Cushing's syndrome. J Clin Endocrin Metabol 46:114, 1978

135. Blum M, Kirsten M, Worth MH Jr: Reversible hypertension. JAMA 237:262, 1977

136. Fuller H Jr, Spittell JA Jr, McConahey WM, et al: Myxedema and hypertension. Postgrad Med 40:425, 1966

137. Taylor AA, Bartter FC: Hypertension in licorice intoxication, acromegaly and Cushing's syndrome. In Genest J, Koiw E, Kuchel O (eds): Hypertension, p 755. New York, McGraw-Hill 1977

138. Colandrea MA, Friedman GD, Nichaman MZ, et al: Systolic hypertension in the elderly: An epidemiologic assessment. Circulation 41:239, 1970

139. Wallach R, Karp RB, Reves JG, et al: Pathogenesis of paroxysmal hypertension developing during and after coronary bypass surgery: A study of hemodynamic and humoral factors. Am J Cardiol 46:559, 1980

140. Reves JG, Karp RB, Buttner EE, et al: Neuronal and adrenomedullary catecholamine release in response to cardiopulmonary bypass in man. Circulation 66:49, 1982

141. Kirkendall WM, Burton AC, Epstein FH, et al: Recommendations for human blood pressure determination by sphygmomanometers. Circulation 36:980, 1967

142. Ferguson RK: Cost and yield of the hypertensive evaluation. Ann Intern Med 82:761, 1975

143. Bech K, Hilden T: The frequency of secondary hypertension. Acta Medica Scand 197:65, 1975
144. Gifford RW Jr: Evaluation of the hypertensive patient with emphasis on detecting curable causes. Milbank Mem Fund Q 47:170, 1969
145. Weiss NS: Relation of high blood pressure to headache, epistaxis and selected other symptoms: The United States Health Examination Survey of Adults. N Engl J Med 287:631, 1972
146. Stewart I McD G: Headache and hypertension. Lancet 1:1261, 1953
147. Kincaid–Smith P, McMichael J, Murphy EA: The clinical course and pathology of hypertension with papilloedema (malignant hypertension). Q J Med 27:117, 1958
148. Breckenridge A, Dollery CT, Parry EHO: Prognosis of treated hypertension. Q J Med 39:411, 1970
149. Hunt JC, Strong CG, Sheps SG, et al: Diagnosis and management of renovascular hypertension. Am J Cardiol 23:434, 1969
150. Maxwell MH, Gonick HC, Wiita R, et al: Use of the rapid-sequence intravenous pyelogram in the diagnosis of renovascular hypertension. N Engl J Med 270:213, 1964
151. Bookstein JJ, Abrams HL, Buenger RE, et al: Radiologic aspects of renovascular disease: Part 2. The role of urography in unilateral renovascular disease (Co-operative Study of Renovascular Hypertension). JAMA 220:1225, 1972
152. Bookstein JJ, Maxwell MH, Abrams HL, et al: Cooperative study of radiologic aspects of renovascular hypertension: Bilateral renovascular disease. JAMA 237:1706, 1977
153. Stanley JC, Fry WJ: Renovascular hypertension secondary to arterial fibrodysplasia in adults: Criteria for operation and results of surgical therapy. Arch Surg 110:922, 1975
154. Foster JH, Oates JA, Rhamy RK, et al: Detection and treatment of patients with renovascular hypertension. Surgery 60:240, 1966
155. Geyskes GG, Boer P, Vos J, et al: Renin dependency of blood-pressure analysis by AII antagonist P113 in hypertensive patients treated with salt depletion and propranolol. Lancet 1:1049, 1976
156. Case DB, Wallace JM, Keim HJ, et al: Usefulness limitations of saralasin, a partial competitive agonist of angiotensin II for evaluating the renin and sodium factors in hypertensive patients. Am J Med 60:825, 1976
157. Dunn FG, DeCarvalho JGR, Kem DC, et al: Pheochromocytoma crisis induced by saralasin. Relation of angiotensin analogue to catecholamine release. N Engl J Med 295:605, 1976
158. Anderson GH Jr, Streeten DHP, Dalakos TG: Pressor response to 1-Sar-8-Ala-angiotensin II (saralasin) in hypertensive subjects. Circ Res 40:243, 1977
159. Case DB, Wallace JM, Keim HJ, et al: Possible role of renin in hypertension as suggested by renin-sodium profiling and inhibition of converting enzyme. N Engl J Med 296:641, 1977
160. Holley KE, Hunt JC, Brown AL Jr, et al: Renal artery stenosis: a clinical-pathologic study in normotensive and hypertensive patients. Am J Med 37:14, 1964
161. Oparil S, Haber E: The renin-angiotensin system. N Engl J Med 291:389, 446, 1974
162. Strong CG, Hung JC, Sheps SG, et al: Renal venous renin activity: Enhancement of sensitivity of lateralization by sodium depletion. Am J Cardiol 27:602, 1971
163. Re R, Novelline R, Escourrou MT, et al: Inhibition of angiotensin-converting enzyme for diagnosis of renal-artery stenosis. N Engl J Med 298:582, 1978
164. Schambelan M, Glickman M, Stockigt JR, et al: Selective renal-vein renin sampling in hypertensive patients with segmental renal lesions. N Engl J Med 290:1153, 1974

165. Gunnels JC Jr, McGuffin WL Jr, Johnsrude I, et al: Peripheral and renal venous plasma renin activity in hypertension. Ann Intern Med 71:555, 1969
166. Vaughan ED Jr, Buhler FR, Laragh JH, et al: Renovascular hypertension: Renin measurements to indicate hypersecretion and contralateral suppression, estimate renal plasma flow and score for surgical curability. Am J Med 55:402, 1973
167. Conn JW: Primary reninism, a new syndrome. Verhandlungen der Deutschen Gesellschaft fur Innere Medizin 80:171, 1974
168. Kaplan NM: Hypokalemia in the hypertensive patient. Ann Intern Med 66:1079, 1967
169. Brown JJ, Davies DL, Fraser R, et al: Plasma electrolytes, renin, and aldosterone in the diagnosis of primary hyperaldosteronism. Lancet 2:55, 1968
170. Horton R: Aldosterone: Review of its physiology and diagnostic aspects of primary aldosteronism. Metabolism 22:1525, 1973
171. Slaton PE Jr, Schambelan M, Biglieri EG: Stimulation and suppression of aldosterone secretion in patients with an aldosterone-producing adenoma. J Clin Endocrin Metabol 29:239, 1969
172. Biglieri EG: A perspective on aldosterone abnormalities. Clin Endocrinol 5:399, 1976
173. Biglieri EG, Stockigt JR, Schambelan M: A preliminary evaluation for primary aldosteronism. Arch Intern Med 126:1004, 1970
174. Dunn PJ, Espiner EA: Outpatient screening tests for primary aldosteronism. Aust NZ J Med 6:131, 1976
175. Espiner EA, Christlieb AR, Amsterdam EA, et al: The pattern of plasma renin activity and aldosterone secretion in normal and hypertensive subjects before and after saline infusions. Am J Cardiol 27:585, 1971
176. Melby JC, Spark RF, Dale SL, et al: Diagnosis and localization of aldosterone-producing adenomas by adrenal-vein catheterization. N Engl J Med 277:1050, 1967
177. Hogan MJ, McRae J, Schambelan M, et al: Location of aldosterone-producing adenomas with [131]I-19-iodocholesterol. N Engl J Med 294:410, 1976
178. Bayliss RIS, Edwards OM, Starer F: Complications of adrenal venography. Br J Radiol 43:531, 1970
179. Luetscher JA, Ganguly A, Melada GA, et al: Preoperative differentiation of adrenal ademona from idiopathic adrenal hyperplasia in primary aldosteronism. Circ Res 34:175, 1974
180. New MI, Seaman MP: Secretion rates of cortisol and aldosterone precursors in various forms of congenital adrenal hyperplasia. J Clin Endocrin 30:361, 1979
181. Biglieri EG, Herron MA, Brust N: 17-hydroxylation deficiency in man. J Clin Invest 45:1946, 1966
182. Armstrong MD, McMillan A, Shaw KNF: 3-Methoxy-4-hydroxy-D-mandelic acid, a urinary metabolite of norepinephrine. Biochim Biophys Acta 25:422, 1957
183. Pisano JJ: A simple analysis for normetanephrine and metanephrine in urine. Clin Chim Acta 5:406, 1960
184. Peuler JD, Johnson GA: Simultaneous single radioenzymatic assay of plasma norepinephrine, epinephrine and dopamine. Life Sci 21:625, 1977
185. Hallman H, Farnebo LO, Hamberger B, et al: A selective method for the determination of plasma catecholamines using liquid chromatography with electrochemical detection. Life Sci 23:1049, 1978
186. Stewart BH, Brown EL, Haaga J, et al: Localization of pheochromocytoma by computed tomography. N Engl J Med 299:460, 1978
187. Sisson JC, Frager MS, Valk TW, et al: Scintigraphic localization of pheochromocytoma. N Engl J Med 305:12, 1981
188. Beckerhoff R, Luetscher JA, Wilkinson R, et al: Plasma renin concentration, ac-

tivity and substrate in hypertension induced by oral contraceptives. J Clin Endocrin Metab 34:1067, 1972

189. Laragh JH: Oral contraceptives, female hormones, the renin axis and high blood pressure. In Fregly MJ, Fregly MS (eds): Oral Contraceptives and High Blood Pressure, p 50. Gainesville, Fla, Dolphin Press, 1974

190. Weinberger MH, Collins RD, Dowdy AJ, et al: Hypertension induced by oral contraceptives containing estrogen and gestagen. Ann Intern Med 71:891, 1969

191. Newton MA, Sealey JE, Ledingham JGG, et al: High blood pressure and oral contraceptives. Am J Obstet Gyn 101:1037, 1968

192. Fisch IR, Freedman SH, Myatt AV: Oral contraceptives, pregnancy and blood pressure. JAMA 222:1507, 1972

193. Meade TW, Chakrabarth R, Haines AP, et al: Haemostatic, lipid, and blood-pressure profiles of women on oral contraceptives containing 50 μg or 30 μg oestrogen. Lancet 2:948, 1977

194. Inman WHW, Vessey MP, Westerholm B, et al: Thromboembolic disease and the steroidal content of oral contraceptives. Br Med J 2:203, 1970

195. Perera GA: Hypertensive vascular disease: Description and natural history. J Chronic Dis 1:33, 1955

196. Bechgaard P: The natural history of benign hypertension—one thousand hypertensive patients followed from 26 to 32 years. In Stamler J, Stamler R, Pullmon TN (eds): The Epidemiology of Hypertension, p 357. New York, Grune & Stratton, 1967

197. Veterans Administration Cooperative Study Group of Antihypertensive Agents: Effects of treatment on morbidity in hypertension: I. Results in patients with diastolic blood pressures averaging 115 through 129 mmHg. JAMA 202:1028, 1967

198. Veterans Administration Cooperative Study Group on Antihypertensive Agents: Effects of treatment on morbidity in hypertension. II. Results in patients with diastolic blood pressure averaging 90 through 114 mmHg. JAMA 213:1143, 1970

199. Stamler J, Stamler R, Riedlinger WF, et al: Hypertension screening of 1 million Americans: CHEC Program, 1973–1975. JAMA 235:2299, 1976

200. Hypertension Detection and Follow-Up Program Cooperative Group: Blood pressure studies in 14 communities: A two-stage screen for hypertension. JAMA 237:2385, 1977

201. Wilber JA, Barrow JG: Hypertension—a community problem. Am J Med 52:653, 1972

202. Schoenberger JA, Stamler J, Shekelle RB, et al: Current status of hypertension control in an industrial population. JAMA 222:559, 1972

15

PULMONARY HYPERTENSION

Bertron M. Groves, M.D., and John T. Reeves, M.D.

Definition

In utero the pulmonary and systemic circulations function with equal pressures. Since intrauterine pulmonary blood flow represents only a small percentage of total cardiac output, the pulmonary resistance is much higher than the systemic resistance. Shortly after birth, pulmonary vascular resistance falls precipitously and the ductus arteriosus closes, resulting in a marked drop in pulmonary arterial pressure to a level less than 20% of the systemic arterial pressure.[1]

A recent review of published pressure measurements indicates that after about 10 days of age the normal mean pulmonary arterial pressure remains remarkably constant throughout life.[2] Thus, after the neonatal adjustments have occurred, the normal value is 15 ± 3 (standard deviation) mm Hg. In this chapter, we will adopt a frequently used clinical definition for persons beyond the immediate newborn period that indicates that pulmonary hypertension is present when mean pulmonary arterial pressure is 25 mm Hg or more. In one sense, this definition is conservative because 25 mm Hg is more than three standard deviations above the normal mean. In another sense, the definition is incomplete because it focuses on pulmonary arterial pressure alone and ignores important variables, including flow and left atrial (LA) pressure. Pulmonary blood flow at rest and during exercise decreases with advancing age in normal humans. In healthy subjects over 60 years of age, an increase in wedge pressure during exercise reflects an increase in LA pressure from altered left ventricular (LV) compliance. Thus, an abnormality of the pulmonary circulation may be indicated when pulmonary arterial pressure, pulmonary blood flow, wedge or LA pressure, or some combination of these is abnormal considering the patient's age and metabolic state.

The severity of pulmonary hypertension cannot be established without direct pressure measurement by invasive heart catheterization. Recent reports indicate that empiric methods may allow a noninvasive estimate of pulmonary arterial pressure.[3,4] Currently we view these noninvasive methods as screening procedures that must be verified by direct measurement of intrapulmonary arterial pressure.

Physiology and Pathogenetic Mechanisms

The pathogenetic mechanisms of pulmonary hypertension are:

Passive venous distention
   LA hypertension
Reactive disease of smooth muscle
Pulmonary vascular obstruction
   Pulmonary embolism
   Parenchymal lung disease
   Chronic endothelial damage
Increased pulmonary blood flow
Increased blood viscosity

PASSIVE VENOUS DISTENTION

When LA pressure is raised in experimental animals, passive and extensive recruitment of the microvasculature quickly follows.[5] The pulmonary veins and the pulmonary venules in many species, including the canine and human, but probably not the bovine species, contain little smooth muscle and, being very compliant, dilate readily when the pressure in their lumina is increased. The opening of the lung capillaries to their largest diameter is solely determined by this intraluminal pressure.[6] Thus, when pressure in a venule rises, the capillaries supplying that venule will become fully dilated. This simple concept is extremely important because in the lung (unlike the systemic circulation) only about one-third of the vascular resistance is in the arterioles and the remaining two-thirds is in the capillary net and the venules.[7] Thus, when the downstream (LA) pressure is raised, with subsequent dilatation of venules and recruitment of capillaries, the resistance to flow through these segments becomes very low. This concept is supported by experiments that show that pulmonary venous pressure, when acutely raised, closely approximates the pulmonary arterial pressure.[8] The consequence is that with acute pulmonary venous hypertension, the rise in pulmonary arterial pressure is slightly less than the rise in venous pressure.

Although increased LA pressure (lasting for minutes, days, or, perhaps, weeks) is a common clinical problem, such acute or subacute pressure elevation does not usually lead to right heart failure. The explanation for this is that pulmonary edema will develop at pressures below those that cause acute right heart failure. The evidence may be summarized as follows:

1. With elevated pulmonary venous pressure, the capillaries become fully recruited, maximizing the surface area for fluid filtration.[5]
2. Because pulmonary venous pressure is nearly equal to pulmonary arterial pressure, the capillary pressure must also be elevated nearly to the level of pulmonary arterial pressure.[8]
3. In a healthy lung, fluid filtration from capillary to interstitium increases rapidly at capillary pressures above 20 mm Hg, that is, at pressures usually well tolerated by the right ventricle.[9]
4. During acute hydrostatic stresses, the pulmonary lymphatics are capable of removing only a few ml of fluid per hour (*i.e.*, less than can be filtered at high capillary pressures), causing fluid to accumulate in the lung. Thus, the major threat to the patient with acute (or subacute) elevation of LA pressure is pulmonary edema rather than right ventricular (RV) failure from pulmonary hypertension.

REACTIVE DISEASE OF SMOOTH MUSCLE

The effect of chronic elevation of LA pressure is quite different from that of elevation of short duration. When LA pressure is elevated for many months or years (particularly in young people), as occurs in mitral stenosis, lung microvascular changes occur that protect the patient from pulmonary edema.[10] A recent review indicated that the evidence for such changes is primarily morphological.[10] By electron microscopy, the capillaries showed impressive thickening of the basement membrane, subendothelial hyalinization, swelling of the endothelial cells, and alteration of the adjacent adventitial cells. In the larger vessels, including arteries, arterioles, and venules, there were changes in the intima, media, and adventitia. The media showed increased numbers of smooth muscle layers, and there were fibrotic changes in the media and thickened adventitia. Capillary thickening possibly retards filtration of water from lumen to interstitium. One might also speculate that interstitial fibrosis would decrease the compliance of the interstitial compartment. If so, the interstitium might withstand higher pressures, which would, in effect, decrease the driving pressure across the capillary wall and thereby reduce filtration. High interstitial pressures also could provide a more favorable pressure gradient for removal of fluid by lymphatics. If so, capillary thickening, interstitial fibrosis, and augmented lymphatic transport developing over months or years might allow patients to live with high capillary pressures without developing alveolar edema.

One negative effect of the capillary thickening and interstitial fibrosis is that oxygen transport from alveolus to capillary blood is less effective, as indicated by a widened alveolar-to-arterial O_2 gradient and a reduced O_2 diffusing capacity. The other effect pertinent to this chapter is the development of pulmonary hypertension. With increased LA pressure of prolonged duration, there is an increased pressure gradient from pulmonary artery to pulmonary vein.[11]

(This is in contrast to the narrowed pressure gradient seen when LA pressure is acutely raised, as discussed above). How much of the increased pressure drop can be attributed to hypertrophied and reactive arterioles and how much to an increased resistance in capillaries and veins is not clear. There is evidence that at least part of the drop is across the precapillary segment:[11]

1. The arterioles have a thickened smooth muscle coat.[10]
2. With relief of mitral stenosis and a decrease in LA pressure, the pulmonary vascular resistance falls immediately and the decrease continues for days, indicating that at least part of the fall is a result of vasodilatation.[11]
3. Acute administration of vasodilators or alpha adrenergic blocking agents is accompanied by a decrease in the pressure gradient from artery to vein (and occasionally by the development of pulmonary edema).[11]

With chronic elevation of LA pressure, pulmonary hypertension may become extreme, reaching suprasystemic levels. In such cases, the right ventricle becomes hypertrophied and ultimately fails. It is a paradox that with chronic elevation of LA pressure the threat to the patient is RV failure whereas with acute elevation the greater threat is pulmonary edema.

The mechanisms that produce reactive pulmonary hypertension and hyperplastic changes in the vessels and interstitium secondary to chronic LA pressure elevation are unknown.[5] However, it has been shown that a nonfatal episode of pulmonary edema that lasts only a few hours stimulates an increase in lung protein synthesis that reaches a peak in 24 hours and persists for up to 8 days.[12] Further, in the rat monocrotaline model of pulmonary hypertension, the increase in protein synthesis and dry lung weight accompanies and is closely related to the development of the pulmonary hypertension.[13] In this model of lung injury, vascular leak occurs early and persists. Although cause and effect are not clear, we suspect that an important relationship exists among vessel leak, hyperplasia, and pulmonary hypertension. Possibly a persistent leak stimulates a cellular reaction in lung vessel walls and interstitium. Such a sequence could be a mechanism for pulmonary hypertension with chronic elevation of LA pressure.

A well-known form of vasospastic or reactive pulmonary hypertension is that due to chronic hypoxia. Hypoxia is considered to cause arteriolar vasoconstriction in the lung, and, indeed, recent micropuncture studies have shown that the arteriolar site is the major locus for the constriction.[7] What is less clear is the mechanism of hypoxic vasoconstriction. Evidence has continued to accumulate to support two complementary concepts. First, calcium entry into some crucial lung cell, possibly the smooth muscle cell, is essential in the vasoconstriction. Second, hypoxic vasoconstriction is closely linked to metabolism; that is, hypoxia, as well as other forms of metabolic inhibition, appears to induce the constriction.[15] Recently, a suggestion has been made that leukotrienes may be involved in the response.[16] Although these substances may act as calcium ionophores, their role in hypoxic vasoconstriction requires further study. Clearly, we do not yet know whether hypoxia acts directly on the smooth muscle cell to induce the constriction or on some trigger cell (endothelium, mast cell, etc.) that then releases a chemical mediator of the constriction.

The magnitude of the pulmonary hypertension resulting from chronic hypoxia is variable between species and is also variable within a species (including man).[17] In addition, chronic hypoxia as at high altitude may interact unfavorably with other forms of pulmonary hypertension.

PULMONARY VASCULAR OBSTRUCTION

Pulmonary Embolism

One might expect that of all the mechanisms of pulmonary hypertension, the most clearly understood might be those involved in hypertension from pulmonary embolism. Perhaps this is so in massive embolism in which an old fibrotic clot blocks the main pulmonary artery or its main branches. Since the embolus is an organized clot, it is relatively impervious to endogenous and exogenous lytic agents.[18] When patients with such a diagnosis survive, RV hypertension may persist. Even so, the lung distal to the obstructed vessels may remain functional for years. The evidence is (1) histologically, the arteries distal to the obstruction are thin walled;[19] (2) collateral circulation from the bronchial arteries becomes gently increased and may provide nutrient support for the parenchyma; (3) rather heroic surgery to remove chronic massive clot apparently yields impressive benefit.[20]

However, with smaller emboli or thromboses *in situ* and with large embolism when the clot is fresh, the mechanisms are not as clearly understood. For example, in experimental animals, embolism with either blood clots or plastic beads must be induced repeatedly over many months before sustained pulmonary hypertension appears. In the case of fresh autologous blood clots, that the cumulative burden required to cause pulmonary hypertension in experimental animals is huge may be due to the body's prodigious capacity for clot lysis. However, with materials that are not lysed, such as plastic beads, repeated embolism is also required before pulmonary hypertension becomes sustained. When embolic episodes are distributed over many weeks, the cumulative dose of the beads is many times what would be a fatal single dose.[21] The peripheral lung vessels have mechanisms for adaptation to repeated emboli that at present are not understood. Even though we do not understand the mechanisms, it is clear that the ability of the body to recover repeatedly from pulmonary embolic episodes has important implications for recognizing the initial episodes and preventing their recurrence.

Parenchymal Lung Disease

Because the pulmonary vessels are located within the lung, alterations in lung parenchyma necessarily involve the vessels. When the pulmonary involvement is extensive, pulmonary hypertension results. The mechanisms of pulmonary vascular involvement in parenchymal diseases are complex and include destruction of pulmonary vessels, as in emphysema; vasoconstriction from alveolar hypoxia, as may occur particularly in chronic inflammation of the airways; obliteration of vessels, as in pulmonary fibrosis; and vascular and perivascular inflammation, as in systemic lupus erythematosus or scleroderma.

Any patient with pulmonary parenchymal disease will likely show some combination of these mechanisms.

Several paradoxes in these mechanisms are apparent. For example, although there is clear destruction of alveolar walls in centrilobular emphysema, there is no relation between the proportion of abnormal air space and the degree of RV hypertrophy.[10,22] Even in panacinar emphysema, which displays more extensive lung destruction, up to 70% of the lung must be involved before RV hypertrophy occurs.[10,22] Thus, lung destruction must be extensive before there is evidence of hypertrophy of the right heart. The picture is no less confusing with regard to hypoxic vasoconstriction in lung disease. The paradox here is that even though hypoxemia may be present in chronic bronchitis and emphysema, chronic oxygen therapy causes little, if any, relief of the pulmonary hypertension, according to a large multicenter trial.[23] In patients with chronic lung disease, breathing oxygen acutely caused less vasodilatation than did administration of the vasodilator prostaglandin E_1 (PGE_1). The PGE_1 effect showed that vasoconstriction was present and was probably not entirely due to hypoxia. Residence at high altitude increases the incidence of cor pulmonale in patients with chronic lung disease. Thus, although we have classified pulmonary hypertension secondary to lung disease under the category of vascular obstruction, it is clear that pulmonary hypertension probably results from the interaction of multiple causes.

Chronic Endothelial Damage

One could easily take the position that the lung vascular endothelium must remain healthy for the pulmonary arterial pressure to maintain its normal low values. When the endothelium is denuded, platelets are deposited on the exposed collagen. Two factors may combine to facilitate activation and adherence of platelets. First, normal endothelium is known to produce prostacyclin, one of the most potent known inhibitors of platelet activation.[24] When the endothelium is denuded or damaged, the normal prostacyclin production may be inhibited. Second, collagen, in particular, stimulates platelet deposition and activation.[25] Once activated, platelets liberate factors that act as mitogens and chemotaxins. Smooth muscle cells migrate to the area of endothelial damage, where they participate in the fibrotic response leading to irreversible plaque formation. Further loss of the endothelium will facilitate vascular leak, which, as discussed above, may have adverse effects of its own.

Two forms of chronic endothelial damage are known to occur in the dog. One is that caused by a chronic high flow state created when a systemic artery is anastomosed to a lung lobe. The lobe is thus exposed to systemic arterial pressure, resulting in a high blood flow to the lobe. The endothelium lining the vessels is thus subjected to high shear stress, the shear force being directly related to the pressure drop within a vessel segment and inversely proportional to the length of the vessel. Endothelium may be rather sensitive to high shear forces and, thus, be susceptible to damage. In the shunted dogs, high vascular resistance develops in the lobe several months after the anastomosis is made.[26] In this model, pulmonary endothelial sclerosis develops particularly at points of vascular branching, where the shear forces are expected to be maximal.

Scanning electron microscopy has confirmed the endothelial damage. More recently, platelet inhibitors have been shown to reduce the rise in vascular resistance that follows creation of the shunt.

A second form of chronic endothelial damage is that which accompanies heart worm infestation in dogs living in the Gulf coast states of the United States.[27] Adult worms live in the right ventricle, whence eggs and worm fragments embolize to lodge in the lung. The immunologic reaction to these foreign proteins apparently induces endothelial damage followed by platelet deposition that contributes to the subsequent pulmonary hypertension. Here, again, antiplatelet drugs are able to modify favorably the early stages of this pathogenetic sequence.

These dissimilar experimental models provide hints that endothelial damage, platelet deposition, and subsequent cellular and humoral events may be of importance in some forms of pulmonary hypertension.

INCREASED PULMONARY BLOOD FLOW

The pulmonary circulation, being normally rather passive, shows a rise in pressure gradient from artery to vein with increases in flow.[28] For example, with muscular exercise, a tripling of flow brings about nearly a tripling of the pressure gradient. Two opposing influences apparently account for this result. With an increase in pressure (as flow increases) new channels are recruited, tending to lower exercise resistance. Some other mechanism, possibly hypoxic vasoconstriction in the lung bases acting to defend arterial oxygenation, acts to raise resistance.[29] Normally, the net result is that pulmonary vascular resistance is not significantly changed with exercise.

In pulmonary hypertension, exercise fails to lower pulmonary vascular resistance, probably because the lung circulation at rest is already fully recruited in the hypertensive state. In chronic lung disease, the resistance usually rises with exercise, possibly reflecting alveolar hypoxia in some lung segments.[2] The important point is that muscular exercise, or, indeed, any cause of increased lung blood flow, acts to increase pulmonary hypertension further. Conversely, reducing flow, as, for example, the chronically elevated flow in a patient with a congenital left-to-right shunt, will reduce pressure. To the extent that the pressure gradient is reduced, shear stress on the endothelium will be reduced, and, thus, one might expect that the progression of vascular disease might be ameliorated. Thus, flow measurements are essential, not only when assessing the pulmonary vascular disease but also when contemplating therapy.

INCREASED BLOOD VISCOSITY

Like increased blood flow, increased blood viscosity unfavorably affects pulmonary hypertension of any etiology. This straightforward concept does not imply that viscosity of blood is a simple matter; it is not. First of all, we cannot directly measure relevant values for viscosity in man. For example, at a constant hematocrit, the effective viscosity of blood decreases as blood flows through smaller and smaller vessels to diameters approaching those of the capillary.[30] Thus, viscosity of blood varies, depending on the vascular segment under consideration. The various devices that measure the viscosity of blood after it is removed from the body yield values that may or may not be relevant to the vascular bed. Second, blood is a complex tissue, only one component of which is water. Viscosity can be dramatically increased *in vivo* by altering the state of the proteins (*i.e.*, by clotting) or of the cells (*i.e.*, by clumping or by decreasing the ease of erythrocyte deformation). Third, increasing the hematocrit, the most common cause of increased viscosity, lowers cardiac output, possibly by providing for increased oxygen transport.[31] Thus, increased hematocrit, while acting to raise resistance by increasing viscosity, also limits the rise in pressure by lowering pulmonary blood flow. Fourth, the increase in vascular resistance is not linear with increasing hematocrit but is hyperbolic, with resistance rising rapidly for hematocrits above 55% to 60%[32].

Despite these difficulties, some experimental evidence is available for the lung circulation. For example, in acute dog experiments, increasing the hematocrit to double the normoxic pulmonary vascular resistance also doubles the pulmonary pressor response to acute hypoxia.[33] Further, during chronic high-altitude exposure, certain species (such as the rabbit, whose hematopoetic response to prolonged hypoxia is marked) developed RV hypertrophy and dilatation that related directly to the increased hematocrit.[34] In humans at high altitude with chronic lung disease or with hypoventilation in the presence of normal lungs, excessive polycythemia is an important indicator of chronic mountain sickness. We lack direct measurements of pulmonary arterial pressure and resistance before and after phlebotomy in these patients. However, reducing their excessive polycythemia improves arterial oxygenation and decreases symptoms[35].

Clinical Presentation

ETIOLOGIES OF PULMONARY HYPERTENSION

The clinical etiologies of pulmonary hypertension can be grouped as follows:

PASSIVE PULMONARY HYPERTENSION

Left ventricular outflow obstruction
    Systemic hypertension
    Coarctation of the aorta
    Supravalvular aortic stenosis
    Valvular aortic stenosis
    Subvalvular aortic stenosis
        Discrete, membranous subvalvular aortic stenosis
        Muscular, idiopathic hypertrophic subaortic stenosis
Left ventricular cardiomyopathy
    Hypertrophic, nonobstructive cardiomyopathy
    Congestive cardiomyopathy

Idiopathic cardiomyopathy
Coronary artery disease
Restrictive cardiomyopathy
Left ventricular inflow obstruction
Mitral valve stenosis
Left atrial obstruction
Congenital cor triatriatum
Myxoma
Thrombus
Pulmonary vein stenosis
Pericardial effusion or constriction
Idiopathic
Radiation
Traumatic
Neoplastic
Infectious
Chronic renal failure

REACTIVE PULMONARY HYPERTENSION
Mitral valve stenosis
Alveolar hypoxia
High-altitude exposure
Alveolar hypoventilation
Obesity (Pickwickian syndrome)
Adenoid hyperplasia
Sleep apnea

OBSTRUCTIVE PULMONARY HYPERTENSION
Thromboembolic disease
Pulmonary parenchymal disease
Chronic obstructive pulmonary disease
Interstitial fibrosis
Peripheral pulmonary arterial stenosis
Congenital
Acquired mediastinal fibrosis
Veno-occlusive disease
Collagen vascular disease
Scleroderma (CREST syndrome)
Rheumatoid arthritis
Eisenmenger's syndrome
Atrial septal defect
Ventricular septal defect
Patent ductus arteriosus
Chronic liver disease
Drug or chemical
Aminorex
Toxic rapeseed cooking oil
Primary or unexplained pulmonary hypertension

Passive Pulmonary Hypertension

The most common etiology of pulmonary hypertension is left-sided heart disease. When LV diastolic pressure is elevated, the LA mean pressure rises as a compensatory mechanism for maintaining adequate LV filling and forward flow. The elevated LA mean pressure is then transmitted retrograde through the pulmonary veins and results in elevation of the pulmonary arterial wedge pressure. The mean pulmonary arterial pressure then becomes elevated to ensure forward flow. In most circumstances, elevation of the pulmonary arterial wedge mean pressure above 25 mm Hg to 30 mm Hg is sufficient to produce not only pulmonary venous congestion but alveolar pulmonary edema. If the condition accounting for elevation of the pulmonary arterial wedge mean pressure is of sufficient chronicity, such as rheumatic mitral valve stenosis, the mean wedge pressure may rise to more than 25 mm Hg without producing overt clinical pulmonary edema.

Any condition that causes an increased resistance or afterload against which the left ventricle must contract is capable of producing LV systolic and diastolic hypertension, hypertrophy, or failure (decompensation) that secondarily leads to passive elevation of the pulmonary arterial pressure. A common condition that, if uncontrolled, can produce pulmonary hypertension by this mechanism is chronic, severe, systemic hypertension. Mechanical LV outflow tract obstruction occurring at any of four levels can similarly produce pulmonary hypertension. The most distal level of fixed obstruction to LV outflow is coarctation of the descending thoracic aorta. Supravalvular aortic stenosis is analogous to coarctation of the ascending aorta with the constriction located at, or slightly above, the level of the coronary ostia. In adults the most common form of LV outflow tract obstruction is valvular aortic stenosis, which, in most circumstances, is due to a congenital bicuspid aortic valve that produces symptoms during the fifth and sixth decades of life. Calcification of a congenital bicuspid aortic valve appears to be a significant factor contributing to the progressive obstruction that occurs in later life. When isolated calcific aortic stenosis presents in the seventh and eighth decades of life, it is more likely that a tricuspid aortic valve has degenerated and calcified to become immobile and stenotic, without the commissural fusion that would be expected if the underlying disease process were valvular rheumatic heart disease. Coexistent coronary arterial and mitral valve annular calcification occur frequently in elderly patients with degenerative calcific aortic stenosis. Subvalvular aortic stenosis occurs as a congenital form of LV outflow tract obstruction and can be due to either a discrete membrane or, in the condition which has been described as hypertrophic obstructive cardiomyopathy (HOCM) or idiopathic hypertrophic subaortic stenosis (IHSS), a dynamic muscular obstruction.

Left heart disease primarily involving the LV myocardium has been designated as LV cardiomyopathy. The three types of LV cardiomyopathy are: hypertrophic—obstructive (IHSS) or nonobstructive, indicating the absence of a resting or provocable pressure gradient between the body of the left ventricle and the ascending aorta; congestive, which may be idiopathic or secondary to ischemic coronary artery disease; and restrictive, which clinically presents with signs and symptoms mimicking constrictive pericarditis.

The most common cause of LV inflow obstruction is mitral stenosis as a manifestation of valvular rheumatic heart disease. Rarely, obstruction within the left atrium is due to congenital cor triatriatum, LA myxoma, or thrombus. The least common form of obstruction to flow between the pulmonary artery and left ventricle is pulmonary vein stenosis.

Patients with pericardial constriction may present with mild or moderate pulmonary hypertension and peripheral signs of ascites and edema. The etiology of constrictive pericarditis in the past was commonly tuberculous, but currently it is more likely to be idiopathic or due to radiation therapy or trauma (including cardiac surgery). Occasionally, patients with neoplastic heart disease or chronic renal failure may present with effusive-constrictive pericardial disease. Pericardial effusion is usually associated with only mild pulmonary hypertension, even when cardiac tamponade is present.

Reactive Pulmonary Hypertension

If the pulmonary artery diastolic pressure exceeds the pulmonary artery wedge mean pressure by more than 5 mm Hg to 10 mm Hg, a *reactive component* of pulmonary hypertension may be present. A common circumstance in which reactive pulmonary hypertension is clinically encountered is rheumatic mitral valvular stenosis. Patients with mitral stenosis frequently have pulmonary hypertension significantly out of proportion to the severity of their wedge pressure elevation.[36–38] It has been hypothesized that pulmonary vasoconstriction in patients with mitral stenosis may be a protective mechanism that reduces pulmonary capillary pressure and prevents alveolar fluid transudation when pulmonary venous pressure exceeds plasma colloidal pressure.[39] Fortunately, most patients with severe pulmonary hypertension due to mitral stenosis experience a substantial reduction in their pulmonary artery pressure following mitral valve surgery regardless of the degree of reactive pulmonary hypertension. On the other hand, it is not uncommon for such patients to be left with mild residual pulmonary hypertension following successful mitral valve surgery.

Another circumstance in which reactive pulmonary hypertension is prominent is alveolar hypoxia. Due to the fact that our laboratory is located in Denver, Colorado, at 5,280 feet, it is not uncommon for us to encounter patients who dwell at altitudes with a chronically low concentration of oxygen in the inspired air (FIO_2). Residents in Leadville, Colorado (10,150 feet altitude) are known to have a higher hemoglobin concentration and higher pulmonary arterial pressure than lower-altitude residents. However, a small percentage of this population dwelling at high altitude appear to have a more dramatic response to the lower FIO_2.[17,40,41] These patients have pulmonary hypertension that may be significantly improved by an increase in the FIO_2 by moving to sea level.[42] Other varieties of alveolar hypoxia include syndromes of hypoventilation associated with obesity (Pickwickian syndrome),[43] airway obstruction due to enlarged adenoids,[44] and sleep apnea.[45] A potentially malignant combination is high altitude and sleep apnea, in which the combined effects produce significant pulmonary hypertension.[46]

Obstructive Pulmonary Hypertension

The hallmark of pulmonary hypertension due to pulmonary vascular obstructive disease is the presence of a normal pulmonary arterial wedge pressure in association with significant elevation of the pulmonary arterial pressure. Pulmonary hypertension secondary to pulmonary emboli is suggested by the finding of multiple segmental perfusion abnormalities in association with a normal pulmonary ventilation scan. In patients with no prior cardiopulmonary disease, acute thromboemboli rarely produce a mean pulmonary artery pressure in excess of 40 mm Hg.[47] Confirmation of this diagnosis may require pulmonary angiography to delineate pathognomonic intravascular clots[48]. Establishing the diagnosis of thromboembolic disease is especially important in view of the fact that many patients will have improved perfusion following thrombolytic (streptokinase or urokinase) or anticoagulant (intravenous heparin) therapy. If significant improvement is not accomplished acutely, preventing a further embolus with chronic coumadin therapy may be lifesaving in a patient with pulmonary hypertension and limited cardiac output reserve.

Many different etiologies of pulmonary parenchymal disease can be associated with pulmonary hypertension once a substantial amount of the pulmonary vascular bed has been destroyed by the underlying disease process. Examples of this type of pulmonary hypertension include chronic obstructive pulmonary disease and interstitial pulmonary fibrosis.

Anatomical pulmonary vascular obstructive disease may be congenital, as in patients with congenital absence of one pulmonary artery or peripheral pulmonary artery branch stenoses, or acquired, as in mediastinal fibrosis or the rare entity of pulmonary veno-occlusive disease.[49–57] In the latter condition there is widespread, unexplained thrombosis and destruction of the microscopic venules of the lung, which may or may not produce radiographic pulmonary venous congestion and elevation of the pulmonary arterial wedge pressure. Therefore, this diagnosis can only be confirmed by histopathology. Pulmonary vascular disease accounting for the development of pulmonary hypertension can be due to collagen vascular disease (scleroderma [CREST syndrome],[58–61] systemic lupus erythematosus,[62,63] rheumatoid lung disease), Eisenmenger's syndrome (ventricular septal defect, patent ductus arteriosus, or atrial septal defect),[64–68] chronic liver disease,[69–74] drug induction (aminorex an amphetaminelike appetite suppressant),[75,100] and, as recently reported from Spain, the ingestion of toxic rapeseed cooking oil.[76]

Once the above etiologies of pulmonary vascular disease have been excluded, there is a subset of patients with *primary* or *unexplained* pulmonary hypertension who present with a pathologic picture of medial hypertrophy of the pulmonary arterioles that progresses to more advanced stages of pulmonary arteriopathy and that ultimately becomes irreversible with plexiform lesions associated with a relentless clinical syndrome of severe pulmonary hypertension, chronic right heart failure, and sudden death.[77–79]

SYMPTOMS OF PULMONARY HYPERTENSION

The symptoms of pulmonary hypertension are:

Dyspnea
Fatigue
Dizziness

Syncope
Edema
Nausea
Cyanosis
Hoarseness
Hemoptysis
Chest pain
Sudden death

The most common symptom occurring in the early stages of pulmonary hypertension is exertional dyspnea that is progressive in nature and is associated with the subtle onset of easy fatigability due to limited cardiac output reserve. As pulmonary hypertension becomes more severe, patients will frequently complain of dizziness with exertion. As the disease progresses, syncope with effort may occur. Long-standing, severe pulmonary hypertension usually leads to symptoms of RV failure manifested initially as peripheral edema that is frequently complicated by associated right upper quadrant tenderness, loss of appetite, and nausea due to hepatic and gastrointestinal venous congestion. A small percentage of patients will develop cyanosis due to right-to-left shunting through a patent foramen ovale that is stretched open by elevated pressure in the right atrium. This physiologic right-to-left shunt at atrial level accounts for the rare occurrence of a paradoxic systemic arterial embolus originating in the venous system. Hoarseness, due to vocal cord paralysis, occurs in a small percentage of patients with severe pulmonary hypertension due to stretching of the left recurrent laryngeal nerve as it courses around the enlarged pulmonary artery. Severe pulmonary hypertension may also present as recurrent hemoptysis in the absence of thromboembolic disease and pulmonary infarction.

Exertional chest pain, occurring in patients with severe pulmonary hypertension and normal coronary cineangiography is assumed to be due to RV ischemia reflecting an imbalance between myocardial oxygen supply and demand. The end-stage of severe pulmonary hypertension is often terminated by sudden death. The mechanism of sudden death is not clear but is thought to reflect a progressively deteriorating contractility of the right ventricle, which ultimately is unable to sustain adequate forward flow in the presence of severe elevation of the pulmonary vascular resistance. Death may be precipitated by a vasovagal reaction that produces the lethal combination of bradycardia (which severely reduces cardiac output) and peripheral vasodilatation (which further drops the systemic arterial pressure).

CLINICAL SIGNS OF PULMONARY HYPERTENSION

Physical Examination

Clinical signs of pulmonary hypertension on physical examination are as follows:

VITAL SIGNS

Brachial arterial pressure
Low systolic pressure

Narrow pulse pressure
Mild sinus tachycardia
Tachypnea

INSPECTION

Nailbeds
  Cyanosis
  Clubbing
Lower extremities
  Varicose veins
  Deep vein thrombosis
  Edema
Jugular venous pulsation
  Prominent A wave
  Elevated mean pressure
  Kussmaul's sign
Left parasternal impulse

PALPATION

Pulmonary artery impulse
RV lift
Hepatomegaly

AUSCULTATION

Pulmonary ejection sound
Prominent pulmonary valve closure sound (P_2)
Right-sided third (S_3) and fourth (S_4) heart sounds
Murmur of tricuspid regurgitation (Carvallo's sign)
Murmur of pulmonary regurgitation

In patients with significant pulmonary hypertension, it is not uncommon to find a relatively low brachial arterial systolic blood pressure—in the range of 90 mm Hg to 105 mm Hg—with a reduced pulse pressure. The carotid arterial pulse is usually normal on palpation but may reflect a decrease in stroke volume in advanced stages of pulmonary hypertension. Orthostatic changes in blood pressure or heart rate should be carefully noted, especially if the patient is being treated with a vasodilator. The resting heart rate may or may not be mildly elevated. An increased resting respiratory rate (tachypnea) may be observed in the patient who has dyspnea on exertion due to pulmonary hypertension.

INSPECTION of the patient who is suspected of having pulmonary hypertension should include looking for the presence of cyanosis of the fingernails and toenails with or without associated clubbing (Fig. 15-1). Familial, nonpathologic "spooning" of the nails may be present and mimic clubbing. The most reliable method of detecting clubbed nails is to palpate the base of the nail to determine whether or not an abnormal sponginess of the nailbed is present. Pathologic clubbing, reflecting chronic systemic arterial desaturation, is usually associated with this type of spongy nailbed.

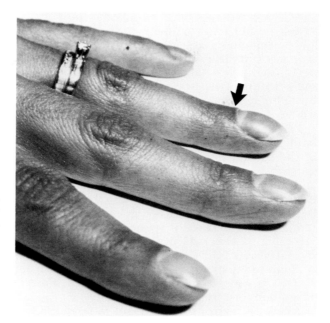

FIG. 15-1. Hand photograph of 32-year-old woman with ventricular septal defect and Eisenmenger's syndrome (PA pressure, 120/60 mean 84 mm Hg) who developed cyanosis with effort from right-to-left shunting. Note the clubbing of fingernails. Palpation revealed sponginess at the base of the nails (*arrow*).

Examination of the jugular venous pulse usually reveals predominance of the A wave, which reflects the need for a forceful atrial contraction to fill the hypertensive, hypertrophic, relatively noncompliant right ventricle (see Fig. 15-20d). The mean jugular venous pressure does not become elevated until the early stages of RV failure. A positive Kussmaul's sign (a paradoxic increase in the mean jugular venous pressure with inspiration) reflects significant reduction in RV compliance. RA or jugular venous mean pressure may or may not be elevated with quiet respiration, but a deeper inspiratory effort may bring out the inability of the right ventricle to accept increased venous return without elevating the venous pressure. When evaluating Kussmaul's sign, make sure that the Valsalva maneuver is not being performed during exaggerated inspiration, since it causes spurious elevation of the venous pressure. Only in patients with far advanced RV decompensation should one expect to find the prominent V wave in the jugular venous pulse that reflects hemodynamically significant tricuspid regurgitation.

PRECORDIAL PALPATION frequently reveals a sustained RV lift along the lower left sternal border. In addition, there may be visible and palpable distention of the pulmonary artery in the second or third left intercostal space along the sternal border due to forceful expansion of the hypertensive pulmonary artery during systole. In the absence of parenchymal lung disease, auscultation of the lungs usually reveals clear breath sounds with no rales.

CARDIAC AUSCULTATION may be very helpful in evaluating a patient suspected of having pulmonary hypertension. The first heart sound (S_1) is usually normal. In significant pulmonary hypertension, it is not uncommon to hear an early systolic ejection sound that represents sudden distention of the hypertensive pulmonary artery (see Fig. 15-20a).[80] This high-frequency ejection sound is usually best heard with the stethoscopic diaphragm in the second and third left intercostal spaces but may be difficult to differentiate from a widely split S_1.

The auscultatory hallmark of pulmonary hypertension is the presence of a loud pulmonary valve closure sound (P_2) that may also be palpable. Splitting of the second heart sound (S_2) is usually physiologic. As the severity of pulmonary hypertension progresses, the inspiratory separation of the aortic (A_2) and pulmonic (P_2) components of S_2 is reduced. The explanation for this phenomenon relates to the fact that the "hangout time," which is the interval between the decreasing RV pressure curve and the dicrotic notch of the pulmonary arterial trace, is reduced as the vascular impedance of the pulmonary arterial bed becomes progressively increased with long-standing pulmonary hypertension.[49,50,81,82] In severe pulmonary hypertension, the loud P_2 may be difficult to separate from the normal intensity A_2. The presence of a prominent P_2 that is widely and persistently split from A_2 suggests the possibility of an Eisenmenger atrial septal defect.

As RV hypertrophy progresses in response to chronic pulmonary hypertension, an audible fourth heart sound (S_4) may be heard along the lower left sternal border as a presystolic low-frequency sound that increases with inspiration and is best heard with the bell of the stethoscope. The presence of a right-sided S_4 indicates decreased compliance of the right ventricle but does not imply RV failure. On the other hand, the presence of an early diastolic RV filling sound (S_3) is indicative of RV decompensation and a more advanced stage of the disease. The right-sided S_3 is also best heard along the lower left sternal border and can be augmented with exaggerated inspiration. This observation allows one to separate RV and LV filling sounds with confidence. It should be noted that RV dilatation may cause the cardiac apical impulse to be occupied by the right ventricle. Therefore, an S_3 heard at the cardiac apex in patients with severe pulmonary hypertension and RV failure may, indeed, be a "right-sided" phenomenon. In such circumstances, LV events are displaced posteriorly and may not be appreciated by palpation or auscultation.

The murmur of tricuspid regurgitation is usually best heard along the lower left sternal border during inspiration. Characteristically, tricuspid regurgitation produces a pansystolic high-frequency murmur. However, at times this murmur may have a crescendo-decrescendo ejection quality that may be difficult to interpret clinically unless it is noted that inspiration increases its intensity (Carvallo's sign).[83] Less commonly, the murmur of tricuspid regurgitation may be a late systolic murmur suggesting prolapse of the tricuspid valve. There have been reports of precordial "whoops" or "honks" being produced by tricuspid regurgitation secondary to pulmonary hypertension.[84,85]

The murmur of valvular pulmonary regurgitation due to pulmonary hypertension that dilates the pulmonary valve annulus is a high-frequency, diastolic, decrescendo, blowing murmur that is initiated by a loud P_2 and is best heard along the left parasternal region in the third intercostal space. Less frequently, the murmur of pulmonary regurgitation may also be augmented by inspiration. At the bedside, it may be very difficult to differentiate the murmur of aortic regurgitation from that of pulmonary regurgitation.

The murmur of tricuspid regurgitation or pulmonary regurgitation may not be significantly altered by inspiration. A recent report describes the use of manual pressure below the liver to augment venous return to the right heart and thereby accentuate right-sided ausculatory events.[86] We have found manual compression of the central abdominal contents to accomplish the same increase in venous return without causing hepatic discomfort.

The mechanism of tricuspid regurgitation in patients with pulmonary hypertension is dysfunction of the tricuspid valve papillary muscles due to dilatation and abnormal contractility of the hypertensive right ventricle. In one patient with primary pulmonary hypertension, fatal tricuspid regurgitation was proven to be caused by spontaneous rupture of the septal papillary muscle.[87] Rarely, a right-sided Austin Flint diastolic rumble may be heard in the presence of hemodynamically significant pulmonary regurgitation that creates a relative tricuspid stenosis rumble (see Fig. 15-22).[88]

Examination of the abdomen may reveal tender hepatomegaly. Manual compression of the abdomen can be used to increase venous return to the right heart in patients with borderline elevation of the jugular venous pressure. An increase in the jugular venous pressure in response to abdominal compression reflects the inability of the noncompliant right ventricle to receive increased venous return without elevating the RA mean pressure (*i.e.*, positive hepatojugular reflux). Examination of the lower extremities should include a search for varicose veins or evidence of deep vein thrombosis that might suggest the presence of thromboembolic disease. Ankle or presacral edema may provide confirmatory evidence of RV failure.

Laboratory Studies

Laboratory studies relating to pulmonary hypertension include:

HEMATOLOGY

Polycythemia
Thrombocytopenia
Abnormal liver function tests

CHEST X-RAY

Prominent pulmonary arteries
  Distal tapering
  Shunt vascularity
RV enlargement
Pulmonary parenchymal disease

VENTILATION/PERFUSION SCAN

Multiple segmental perfusion defects
Nonspecific, patchy, perfusion abnormalities
Matched ventilation/perfusion defects

PULMONARY ARTERIOGRAPHY

Intraluminal filling defect
Peripheral branch stenoses
Tapering or "pruning" of distal branches

ELECTROCARDIOGRAPHY

RV hypertrophy
RA abnormality

ECHOCARDIOGRAPHY

RV enlargement/hypertrophy
RA enlargement
Pulmonary valve abnormalities
  Flattened diastolic slope
  Decreased A dip
  Systolic anterior notching ("flying W")
Flattened ventricular septum
Compressed LV cavity
  Pseudo mitral stenosis
Saline bubble study (right-to-left shunt detection)

PULMONARY FUNCTION TESTS

Flow/volume measurements
Carbon monoxide diffusing capacity (DLCO)
Arterial blood gas determination
Treadmill exercise test with ear oximetry

HEMATOLOGY frequently reveals evidence of polycythemia in patients with pulmonary hypertension associated with chronic hypoxia. The platelet count may be reduced in patients with severe pulmonary hypertension. It is speculated that there may be platelet consumption in the diseased pulmonary vasculature. We have studied several patients with cirrhosis associated with severe pulmonary hypertension who had marked thrombocytopenia that appeared to be out of proportion to any other evidence for hypersplenism. Renal function is normal until the cardiac output falls sufficiently to produce prerenal azotemia. In patients with no hepatocellular disease, liver function tests frequently reveal mild abnormalities caused by chronic hepatic congestion. As a result of such abnormalities, alkaline phosphatase, SGOT, LDH, serum bilirubin, and prothrombin time may be elevated.

CHEST ROENTGENOGRAMS are a very useful noninvasive test for evaluating patients suspected of having pulmonary hypertension. Figures 15-2 to 15-5 demonstrate the spectrum of radiographic findings we have seen in patients with primary pulmonary hypertension. The early finding in patients with significant pulmonary hypertension is prominence of the main pulmonary artery and enlargement of the proximal right and left pulmonary arteries. The heart size remains normal until RV enlargement occurs. We have found it useful to compare serial chest x-rays for the purpose of trying to identify specific pulmonary arteries that might have "dropped out" during an interval between

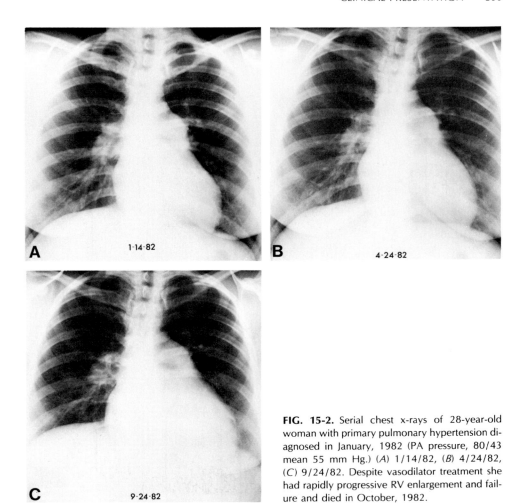

FIG. 15-2. Serial chest x-rays of 28-year-old woman with primary pulmonary hypertension diagnosed in January, 1982 (PA pressure, 80/43 mean 55 mm Hg.) (*A*) 1/14/82, (*B*) 4/24/82, (*C*) 9/24/82. Despite vasodilator treatment she had rapidly progressive RV enlargement and failure and died in October, 1982.

serial films. The loss of such vessels may provide an important clue to the presence of thromboembolic disease with destruction of large pulmonary branches. The chest x-ray in thromboembolic pulmonary hypertension may mimic that seen in primary pulmonary hypertension (Figs. 15-6, 15-7). Patients with Eisenmenger's syndrome due to an atrial septal defect tend to have marked cardiomegaly from extreme RV enlargement (Fig. 15-8). When pulmonary hypertension is associated with chronic liver disease the chest x-ray may reveal prominent vascularity and mimic an Eisenmenger's atrial septal defect (Fig. 15-9). This may be due to the tendency for such patients to have pulmonary hypertension in association with high cardiac output. The chest x-ray of patients with Eisenmenger's syndrome from a ventricular septal defect

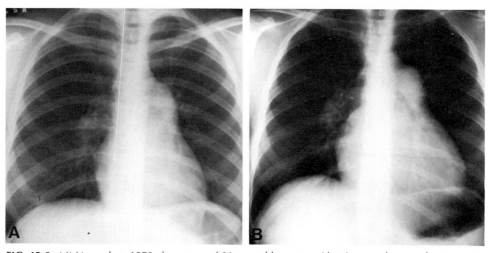

FIG. 15-3. (*A*) November, 1973 chest x-ray of 21-year-old woman with primary pulmonary hypertension (PA pressure, 75/43 mean 55 mm Hg; cardiac output 4.9 liters/min). (*B*) Same patient in January, 1981 (PA pressure, 70/40 mean 50 mm Hg; cardiac output 2.3 liters/min). Note progressive cardiac enlargement (right ventricle and right atrium) during the eight-year interval. The most significant hemodynamic change was a marked reduction in cardiac output due to deterioration of RV function, which also explains the slight reduction in pulmonary artery pressure.

is more likely to reveal less cardiomegaly and more marked tapering of the pulmonary arteries (Fig. 15-10).

Careful assessment of the pulmonary venous pattern and LA size provides important clues that help in ruling out underlying left-sided heart disease. Similarly, careful examination of the film for evidence of chronic obstructive or interstitial lung disease may provide important information about the underlying etiology of pulmonary hypertension (Figs. 15-11 and 15-12). Once RV failure occurs, enlargement of the right ventricle is usually evident. Pleural effusion may also be detected in patients with isolated RV decompensation. In patients with severe pulmonary hypertension, aneurysmal dilatation of pulmonary arteries is frequently misinterpreted as a nonvascular mediastinal mass. Figure 15-5 shows such an x-ray that led to the request for a computed tomographic (CT) scan to rule out a tumor mass. The contrast-enhanced CT scan revealed unequivocal evidence of pulmonary arterial enlargement.

VENTILATION/PERFUSION LUNG SCANS (V/Q scans) are very helpful in distinguishing patients, whose severe pulmonary hypertension is secondary to thromboembolic disease.[89] A properly performed and interpreted V/Q scan that reveals a low probability or thromboembolic disease in a patient with severe pulmonary hypertension may be used to exclude thromboembolic disease without subjecting the patient to the risk of pulmonary angiography. Figure 15-7 illustrates the classic multiple segmental perfusion abnormalities that are characteristic of recurrent pulmonary emboli. This patient presented

(text continues on p. 407)

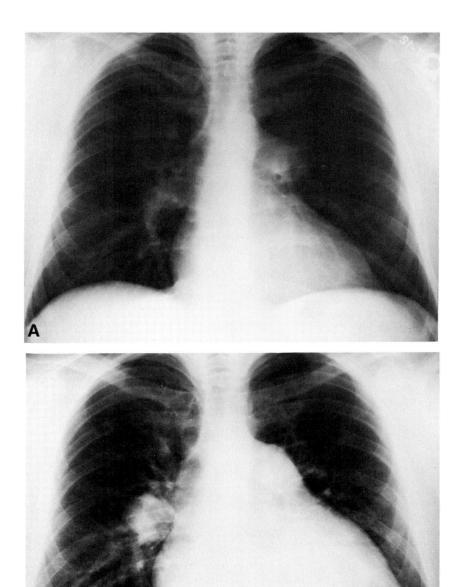

FIG. 15-4. (*A*) Chest x-ray of 32-year-old man when the diagnosis of primary pulmonary hypertension was made in May, 1979 (PA pressure, 140/74 mean 92 mm Hg). (*B*) Same patient in September, 1981 (PA pressure, 180/85 mean 115 mm Hg) when he was hospitalized for recurrent syncopal episodes. Significant right ventricular enlargement and development of an aneurysm of the right pulmonary artery occurred during the 28-month interval. The patient died in October, 1982 fifteen years after his first episode of syncope.

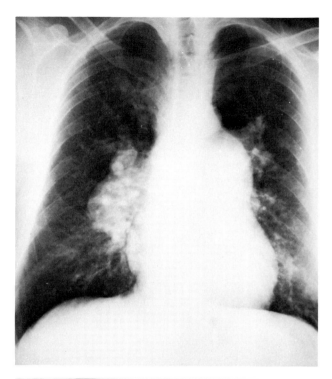

FIG. 15-5. Chest x-ray of 53-year-old mentally retarded man, taken in October, 1982 (PA pressure, 80/40 mean 55 mm Hg). Primary pulmonary hypertension had been diagnosed in our laboratory in April, 1964 (PA pressure, 78/40 mean 54 mm Hg). The 1964 chest x-ray had been discarded but was described as showing "right ventricular enlargement" and "huge pulmonary vasculature." This patient with documented severe pulmonary hypertension remained hemodynamically and clinically stable for 18 years without treatment. His ECG in October, 1982 revealed minimal evidence of RV hypertrophy (see Fig. 15-18).

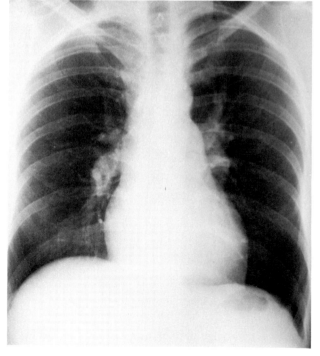

FIG. 15-6. May, 1981 chest x-ray of 36-year-old man who was admitted with syncope complicated by a skull fracture. Cardiac catheterization revealed pulmonary hypertension (PA pressure, 100/38 mean 65 mmHg) and normal wedge pressure. He was presumed to have primary pulmonary hypertension until a ventilation/perfusion lung scan (see Fig. 15-7) revealed normal ventilation with multiple segmental perfusion abnormalities consistent with multiple pulmonary emboli. After 11 months of coumadin treatment, repeat cardiac catheterization documented that his pulmonary artery pressure had improved dramatically (resting PA pressure, 32/24 mean 20 mm Hg; maximum supine exercise PA pressure rose to 60/30 mean 43 mm Hg).

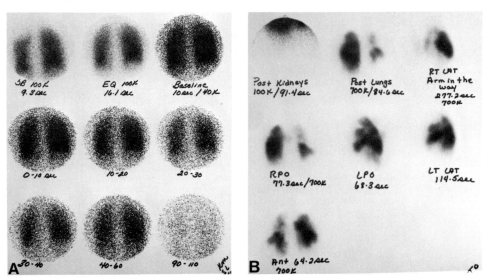

FIG. 15-7. Ventilation/perfusion lung scan of patient in Figure 15-6. (*A*) Ventilation scan: The single breath (*SB*), equilibrium (*EQ*) and 0–110 second "washout" images of ^{133}xenon represent a normal posterior ventilation study. (*B*) Perfusion scan: Multiple segmental defects are evident in all projections, with right lung perfusion more reduced than the left. The V/Q scan is characteristic of multiple pulmonary emboli. No renal activity was detected on the posterior scan over the region of the kidneys, which precluded significant right-to-left shunt. *Post* = posterior. *Ant* = anterior. *Rt* = right. *Lt* = left. *Lat* = lateral. *RPO* = right posterior oblique. *LPO* = left posterior oblique.

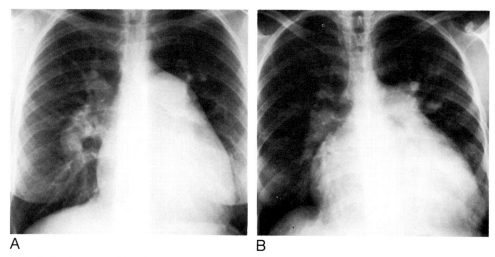

A   B

FIG. 15-8. Chest x-ray films from two adults with atrial septal defect and pulmonary hypertension. (*A*) A 28-year-old woman who presented with severe dyspnea on exertion and fatigue due to pulmonary hypertensive secundum atrial septal defect (PA pressure, 87/30 mean 47 mm Hg; 1.7 to 1, left-to-right shunt). Note very large right ventricle and aneurysmal dilation of the main and proximal pulmonary arteries with prominent vascularity in the mid lung fields. (*B*) A 34-year-old woman with ostium primum atrial septal defect and severe pulmonary hypertension (PA pressure, 128/48 mean 80 mm Hg; 1.9 to 1, left-to-right shunt). Echocardiography revealed that her right ventricle was massively enlarged and compressed the left ventricle. This film demonstrates marked enlargement of the right ventricle (which occupies the cardiac apex and almost touches the lateral chest wall) and right atrium (RA mean pressure, 9 mm Hg).

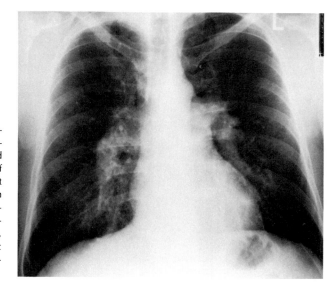

FIG. 15-9. Chest x-ray of a 38-year-old man with alcoholic cirrhosis who presented with syncope and findings on physical examination of pulmonary hypertension. The chest x-ray was felt to be consistent with left-to-right shunt vascularity. Cardiac catheterization revealed pulmonary hypertension (PA pressure, 80/43 mean 55 mm Hg; cardiac output 7.2 liters/min) with no evidence of a shunt.

FIG. 15-10. Chest x-ray, taken in January, 1982, of a 32-year-old woman with ventricular septal defect and Eisenmenger's syndrome (PA pressure, 120/60 mean 84 mm Hg). Note the absence of significant ventricular enlargement in this adult, who had equal systolic pressures in the pulmonary artery and aorta at the time of her first catheterization in 1969. She delivered normal full-term infants in 1971 and 1973 without significant cardiopulmonary complications. Currently she performs all of her housework and leads an active life avoiding only strenuous physical activities such as mowing the lawn and playing volleyball. She has clubbing and becomes cyanotic with physical exertion (see Fig. 15-1).

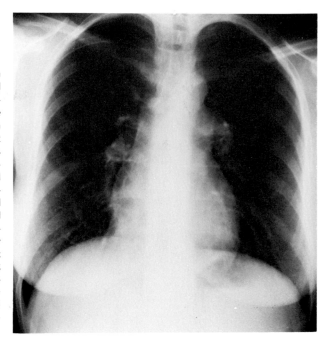

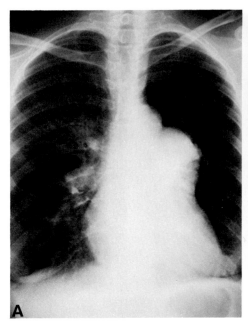

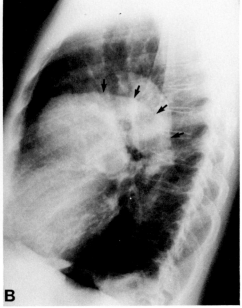

FIG. 15-11. (*A*) Posteroanterior chest x-ray in 64-year-old woman with severe chronic obstructive lung disease and marked pulmonary hypertension (PA pressure, 105/45 mean 68 mm Hg). Note the left upper lung field, avascular due to large bullae. Pulmonary function tests revealed severe chronic obstructive lung disease and marked hypoxemia, which was treated with home oxygen therapy. (*B*) Lateral chest x-ray demonstrates superimposition of a main and left pulmonary artery aneurysm (*arrows*) on the thoracic aorta.

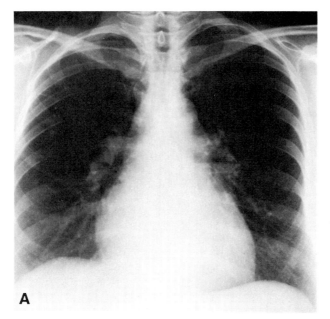

FIG. 15-12. (A) Chest x-ray of 47-year-old woman with scleroderma and pulmonary hypertension (PA pressure, 90/40 mean 55 mg Hg) associated with the CREST syndrome (*C*alcinosis, *R*aynaud's phenomenon, *E*sophageal motility dysfunction, *S*clerodactyly, and *T*elangiectases). Note increased interstitial markings in both lower lung fields. (B) Hand x-rays of this patient reveal subtle evidence of subcutaneous calcification at the tip of the left ring finger and right thumb (*arrows*).

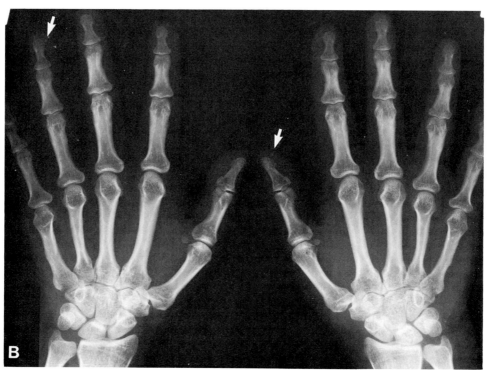

with an episode of syncope that was complicated by a skull fracture and sub-dural hematoma when the patient fell to the floor. Cardiac catheterization revealed a normal wedge pressure and severe pulmonary arterial hypertension, which was initially interpreted as primary pulmonary hypertension. Once the V/Q scan was obtained, it became clear that the patient's pulmonary hypertension was due to recurrent pulmonary emboli secondary to trauma sustained in a vehicular accident ten months before admission to the hospital. On the other hand, patchy defects in the perfusion scan have been reported in patients with primary pulmonary hypertension (Fig. 15-13)[90] It is not clear what produces these patchy defects. The V/Q scan in patients with chronic obstructive lung disease reveals matched abnormalities of ventilation and perfusion.

Following completion of the pulmonary perfusion images, we acquire a single image of the abdomen posteriorly. This image is used to screen for the presence of a right-to-left shunt through a patent foramen ovale or septal defect. If a right-to-left shunt is present, radiolabeled microaggregates will enter the systemic arterial circulation and allow visualization of the kidneys.

PULMONARY ARTERIOGRAPHY in patients with primary pulmonary hypertension usually demonstrates dilatated proximal arteries that taper more abruptly than normal, as in Figure 15-14. Figure 15-15 demonstrates an unusual pattern of arteriopathy in a patient with postpartum primary pulmonary hypertension. Pulmonary emboli are represented by discrete intraluminal filling defects or abrupt arterial occlusion or cutoff.[89,91] In patients with severe pulmonary hypertension of any etiology, multiple selective injections of smaller amounts of contrast material into lobar pulmonary arteries are safer than one large bolus into the main pulmonary artery. The use of superselective magnification pulmonary arteriograms viewed in oblique projections is recommended.[92]

ELECTROCARDIOGRAMS have been useful in confirming the presence of severe, long-standing, pulmonary hypertension. Figure 15-16 illustrates RV hypertrophy characteristic of patients with primary pulmonary hypertension. In an adult, a monophasic R wave in lead V_1 (*i.e.*, no S wave in V_1) associated with ST depression and T wave inversion in the right precordial leads (frequently called the *RV strain* pattern), appears to be highly specific for severe elevation of RV systolic pressure (approaching LV systolic pressure). RA abnormality may be more evident than RV hypertrophy (RVH) (Fig. 15-17). However, the absence of marked RV hypertrophy and RV strain does not preclude the presence of severe RV hypertension (Fig. 15-18). Patients with mild to moderate pulmonary hypertension may have minimal or no electrocardiographic changes indicative of RVH or RA abnormality. Serial electrocardiograms are useful in following the progression or regression of pulmonary hypertension. Figure 15-19 demonstrates the preoperative and postoperative electrocardiograms in a patient with pulmonary hypertension due to a secundum atrial septal defect. As noted, 20 months postoperatively, RV hypertrophy was markedly improved.

ECHOCARDIOGRAMS provide a noninvasive method of following the RV dimensions over time. The characteristic echocardiographic pattern of the

(text continues on p. 415)

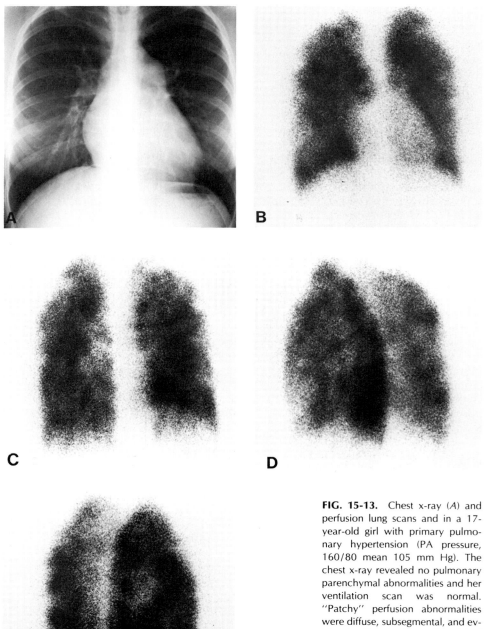

FIG. 15-13. Chest x-ray (*A*) and perfusion lung scans and in a 17-year-old girl with primary pulmonary hypertension (PA pressure, 160/80 mean 105 mm Hg). The chest x-ray revealed no pulmonary parenchymal abnormalities and her ventilation scan was normal. "Patchy" perfusion abnormalities were diffuse, subsegmental, and evident in all projections. The clinical interpretation that these defects were not due to segmental pulmonary emboli was confirmed by autopsy. *B* = anterior. *C* = posterior. *D* = left posterior oblique. *E* = right posterior oblique projections.

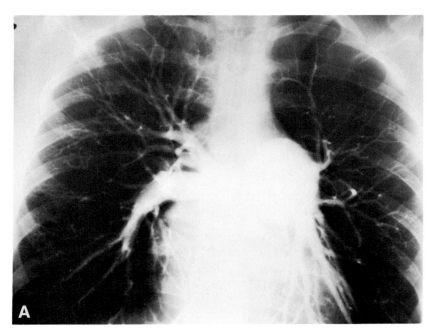

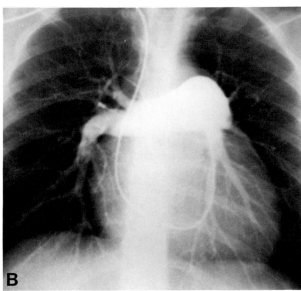

FIG. 15-14. Pulmonary arteriograms in patients with primary pulmonary hypertension. (*A*) A 16-year-old girl with PA pressure 78/34 mean 51 mm Hg. (*B*) A 21-year-old woman with PA pressure 75/43 mean 55 mm Hg. In both patients there is dilation of the main and proximal pulmonary arteries, with distal tapering. No intraluminal defects or arterial "cutoffs" were found to suggest thromboembolic disease.

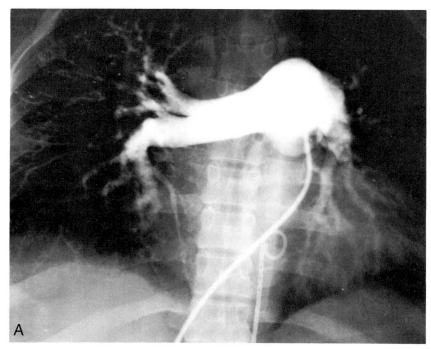

FIG. 15-15. Pulmonary arteriogram. (*A*) Early, (*B*) mid and (*C*) late frames of a 26-year-old woman with primary pulmonary hypertension that presented clinically as fulminant pulmonary hypertension with RV decompensation in the immediate postpartum period. There is a bizarre pattern of branching in the mid and distal third of the lung fields, giving a "honeycomb" appearance to the pulmonary vasculature that was presumed to represent an unusual arteriopathy.

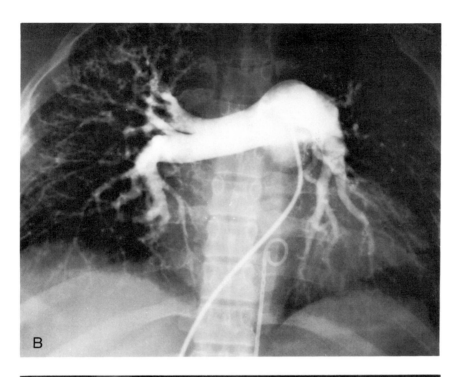

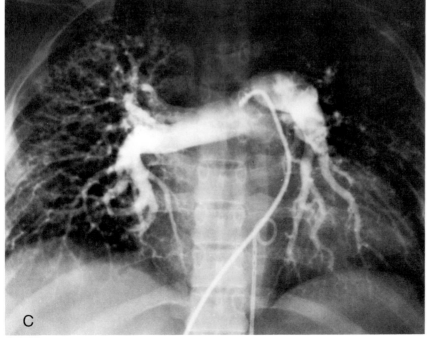

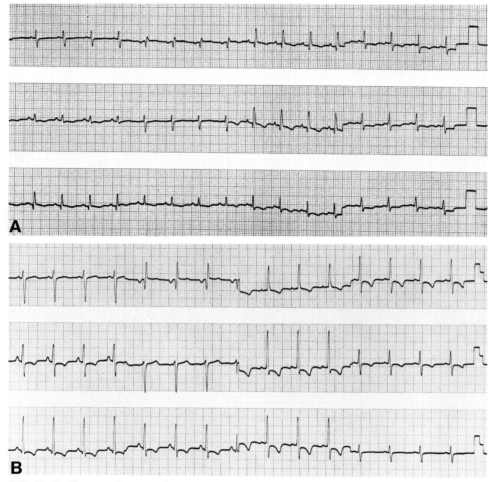

FIG. 15-16. Electrocardiograms illustrating RV hypertrophy with "strain" (ST depression with T wave inversion in V_1–V_6 probably reflecting RV ischemia) in patients with primary pulmonary hypertension. (*A*) A 26-year-old woman (PA pressure, 65/35 mean 43 mm Hg). (*B*) A 17-year-old girl (PA pressure, 160/80 mean 105 mm Hg). Leads V_1–V_6 were recorded at ½ standard amplitude.

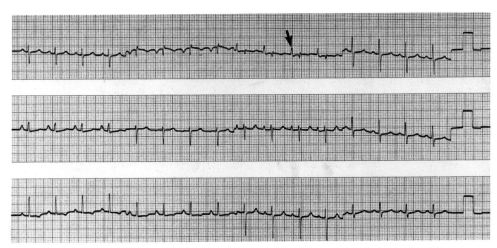

FIG. 15-17. Electrocardiogram from a 44-year-old woman with pulmonary hypertension (PA pressure, 95/35 mean 62 mm Hg) secondary to interstitial fibrosis. This ECG demonstrates right axis deviation (mean QRS axis = +110°), small R′ in V_1–V_2, and persistent S in V_6 as features of mild RVH. The most impressive finding is a 3.0 mm P wave in V_1 indicative of RA abnormality (*arrow*).

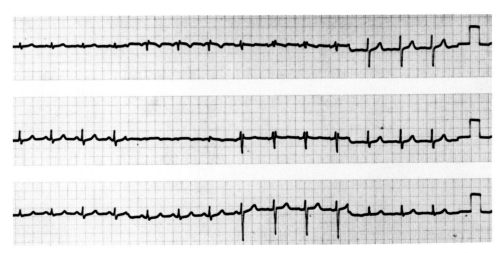

FIG. 15-18. October, 1982 electrocardiogram from the patient in Figure 15-5. Despite documentation in this patient of severe, unexplained pulmonary hypertension (PA pressure, 80/40 mean 55 mmHg, with no intracardiac shunt) for 18 years, the only ECG abnormality is R = S in V_1 with an RSR′ that is minimal evidence for RVH.

413

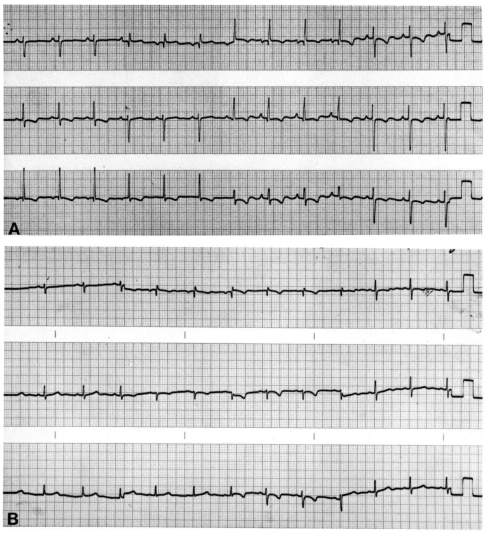

FIG. 15-19. Serial electrocardiograms in a 28-year-old woman who had surgical closure of secundum atrial septal defect in September, 1981. (Patient's preop chest x-ray is shown in Figure 15-8A.) (*A*) Preoperative ECG August, 1981 (PA pressure, 87/30 mean 47 mm Hg). (*B*) Postoperative ECG May, 1983 (PA pressure, 23/11 mean 14 mm Hg). Note the dramatic resolution of the pattern of RVH during the 20-month interval since closure of her ASD.

pulmonary valve ECHO in patients with severe pulmonary hypertension has been described as a flat diastolic E to F slope, loss of the A wave, and anterior systolic notching of the pulmonary valve (also referred to as a "flying W") (Fig. 15-20).[93-98] We have found anterior systolic notching to be highly specific for severe pulmonary hypertension in adults. On the other hand, we have frequently noted preservation of the pulmonary valve A wave in patients with severe pulmonary hypertension. Likewise, the degree of flattening of the E to F slope of the pulmonary valve motion has not been as sensitive an indicator in our experience for estimating pulmonary artery pressure.

The two-dimensional echocardiographic features of severe pulmonary hypertension include enlargement of the right ventricle and right atrium (which can only be evaluated with the two-dimensional echocardiogram). Flattening or "pancaking" of the ventricular septum is seen frequently in patients with severe RV hypertension. Compression of the LV chamber by a bulging ventricular septum is relatively common in patients with severe pulmonary hypertension. In addition, the E to F slope of the mitral valve anterior leaflet may be reduced enough to mimic the echocardiographic features of mitral valve stenosis (Fig. 15-21). Attention to the pattern of the posterior mitral valve leaflet, which moves posteriorly during diastole, allows one to differentiate this pattern of "pseudomitral stenosis" in patients with pulmonary hypertension. The presence of a B notch on the tricuspid valve echocardiogram is an indication of significant elevation of the RV end-diastolic pressure (Fig. 15-22).[101]

We have found it useful to perform a peripheral venous saline injection while viewing the four-chamber, two-dimensional echocardiographic image to detect right-to-left shunting at the atrial level in patients with severe pulmonary hypertension and a patent foramen ovale. Saline "bubble studies" can also help to confirm the presence of tricuspid regurgitation or pulmonary regurgitation by demonstrating a to-and-fro movement of bubbles that do not clear promptly from the right heart.

COMPLETE PULMONARY FUNCTION TESTS including measurements of flow, lung volume, and carbon monoxide diffusing capacity (DLCO), are useful in establishing whether parenchymal lung disease is a primary or contributing cause to pulmonary hypertension. Arterial blood gas determination is needed to confirm the presence of arterial hypoxia at rest. Treadmill exercise testing with ear oximetry is an excellent method to screen for exercise-induced arterial desaturation. Patients with primary pulmonary hypertension frequently have mild to moderate reduction of DLCO. These patients may also have mild abnormalities of ventilation but can readily be distinguished from patients whose major problem is parenchymal lung disease. Significant alteration in gas exchange may occur in patients with pulmonary hypertension who are treated with a vasodilator. It has been hypothesized that some areas of the lung may be successfully vasodilated with increased pulmonary blood flow but may have persistent abnormal gas exchange. Therefore, vasodilator therapy may create intrapulmonary right-to-left shunting and decreased arterial oxygen tension.

(text continues on p. 420)

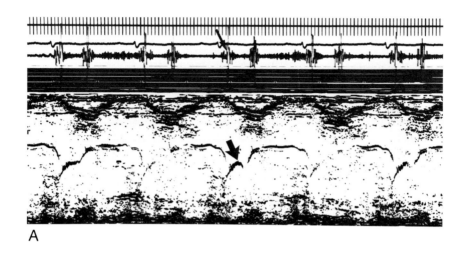

A

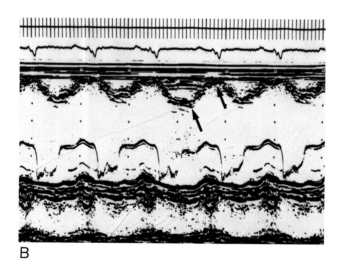

B

FIG. 15-20. Echocardiographic abnormalities of pulmonary valve motion in patients with pulmonary hypertension. (*A*) A 28-year-old woman with secundum atrial septal defect (PA pressure, 87/30 mean 47 mm Hg). Systolic ejection sound was documented by phonocardiography from the 2nd left intercostal space (*top arrow*). Anterior systolic notch ("flying W") of the pulmonary valve ECHO is indicated by the lower arrow. Also note flat diastolic slope and preserved "a" dip of the pulmonary valve ECHO. (*B*) A 34-year-old woman with ostium primum atrial septal defect (PA pressure, 128/48 mean 80 mm Hg). "Flying W" pulmonary valve motion is prominent. Note the unusual anterior motion of the pulmonary valve during diastole, which parallels the hyperdynamic motion (*arrows*) of the anterior cardiac structure (RV outflow tract or main PA) in this patient with atrial septal defect and left-to-right shunt.

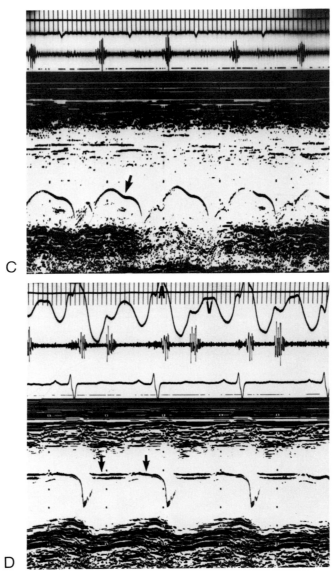

C

D

(C) A 26-year-old woman with primary pulmonary hypertension (PA pressure, 65/35 mean 43 mm Hg). Anterior systolic notch varies in its appearance from beat to beat. Note the presence of an "a" dip (arrow) and normal diastolic slope. (D) A 16-year-old girl with primary pulmonary hypertension (PA pressure, 78/34 mean 51 mm Hg). The jugular venous pulse tracing at the top demonstrates persistent dominance of the "a" wave in this patient, despite the presence of tricuspid regurgitation. The pulmonary valve ECHO shows a flat diastolic slope (arrows), absence of the "a" dip, and visualization of the valve during systole but no apparent anterior systolic notch.

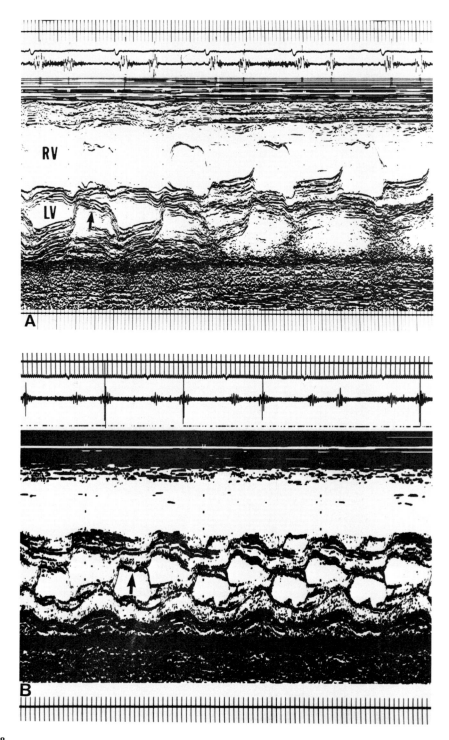

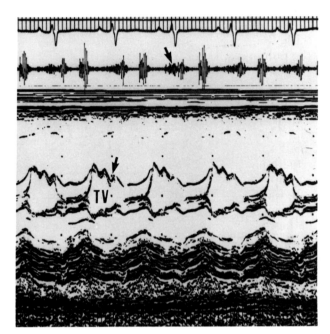

FIG. 15-22. Phonocardiogram from left lower sternal border and tricuspid valve ECHO from same patient as Figure 15-20D. Note the presystolic right-sided Austin Flint murmur (*upper arrow*) recorded in this young woman with pulmonary valvular regurgitation. A prominent "B" notch (*lower arrow*) on the tricuspid valve ECHO (*TV*) reflects significant RV dysfunction, with elevation of the RV end-diastolic pressure (RVEDP = 10 mm Hg; C.O. = 2.0 liters/min).

FIG. 15-21. Echocardiographic recordings of mitral valve motion, depicting "psuedo mitral stenosis" from compression of the LV cavity by a hypertensive, enlarged right ventricle that functions as the dominant ventricle. (*A*) A 28-year-old woman with atrial septal defect (PA pressure, 87/30 mean 47 mm Hg). Note RV larger than LV and flattened EF slope of anterior leaflet of mitral valve (*arrow*). (*B*) A 41-year-old man with primary pulmonary hypertension (PA pressure, 88/40 mean 56 mm Hg). The anterior leaflet of the mitral valve is making contact with the bulging ventricular septum throughout diastole with a flat EF slope. However, the posterior mitral valve leaflet moves posteriorly as a mirror image to the anterior leaflet. Thus, the mitral valve pattern is designated as "pseudo mitral stenosis," reflecting altered compliance of the left ventricle rather than mitral valve stenosis.

Hemodynamic Evaluation

After noninvasive testing is completed in patients with significant pulmonary hypertension, cardiac catheterization is usually required to establish a specific diagnosis and quantify the severity of the pulmonary hypertension and its effect on RV function. We routinely record a pulmonary artery hydrogen curve to test for a small residual left-to-right shunt that might indicate the presence of Eisenmenger's syndrome from a congenital heart defect. The hydrogen curve method is a much more sensitive indicator of trivial left-to-right shunting than any other method available.[102] If a left-to-right shunt is detected and localized by hydrogen curves, an oximetry series is performed to quantify its size.

In patients with severe pulmonary hypertension, the balloon-tipped flotation Swan-Ganz type of thermodilution catheter has proved to be far superior to the stiffer end-hole catheters used in the past. Not uncommonly, however difficulties are encountered placing a balloon-tipped Swan-Ganz catheter in the pulmonary artery and in obtaining a satisfactory wedge pressure in patients with severe pulmonary hypertension, enlarged right hearts, and associated tricuspid or pulmonary regurgitation. This frustration stimulated us to collaborate with American Edwards Laboratories, Inc., in developing a "guidewire thermodilution Swan-Ganz catheter" (American Edwards Laboratories catheter Model 93A-821H-7.5F) that provides a separate lumen for insertion of a 0.028-in teflon-coated guidewire that does not come in contact with the bloodstream and that, therefore, can be left in place during prolonged monitoring to improve catheter stability and prevent the catheter from prolapsing back into the right ventricle. Our preliminary experience with the use of this catheter documented its efficacy and safety. A multicenter clinical trial using this catheter is in progress. The guidewire Swan-Ganz catheter is especially beneficial if patients with severe pulmonary hypertension are being studied using the percutaneous femoral vein approach. A normal wedge pressure precludes all of the etiologies listed above in the section on Clinical Presentation under the passive pulmonary hypertension category.

The thermodilution cardiac output method is very useful when serial cardiac output determinations are required to assess pulmonary vasoreactivity during cardiac catheterization or during prolonged periods of monitoring in the intensive care unit. To confirm the validity of the baseline thermodilution cardiac output, we routinely measure baseline resting cardiac output by the Fick method. Our studies have demonstrated that the thermodilution method overestimates cardiac output when the measured Fick cardiac output is less than 3.5 liter/min.[103] We presume that heat loss in low flow states accounts for this discrepancy. An indocyanine green dye dilution curve obtained by injecting the right atrium and withdrawing from a peripheral arterial site tests for the presence of a right-to-left shunt. A patent foramen ovale may be tested for by repeating the RA indocyanine green dye dilution curve immediately after a Valsalva maneuver is released, at which time the patent foramen ovale is stretched open in response to the surge of increased venous return. This has been proposed as the mechanism of paradoxic systemic arterial embolization in patients with a patent foramen ovale, which may be opened by an activity producing a Valsalva maneuver, such as straining during a bowel movement. In the presence of significant tricuspid valve regurgitation or a right-to-left shunt at atrial or ventricular levels, cardiac output measurement using the indocyanine green dye dilution method with injection into the pulmonary artery is theoretically superior to the thermodilution method.

During cardiac catheterization, the response of the patient's pulmonary artery pressure and cardiac output to vasodilator agents may be assessed. Agents that have been used in evaluating and treating patients with pulmonary hypertension include oxygen,[104] tolazoline,[105,106] isoproterenol,[107–109] hydralazine,[110–114] nifedipine,[115,119,120] diltiazem,[116,117] verapamil,[118] phentolamine,[115,121,122] diazoxide,[123–127] captopril,[128,129] nitroprusside,[130] isosorbide dinitrate,[131] nitroglycerin,[132] and multiple drugs in comparison.[133–135] Experience with the use of intravenous prostacyclin suggests to us that it is an ideal pharmacologic agent to determine the degree to which the pulmonary vascular resistance can be altered by acute drug administration.[136–138] It is our current impression that patients who do not respond to intravenous prostacyclin will not respond to other vasodilators. If a significant response to intravenous prostacyclin is observed, we feel it is appropriate to pursue the administration of other vasodilators in search of an oral agent that might benefit the patient during long-term therapy.

Our experience has convinced us that patients with primary pulmonary hypertension do not respond in a significant way to either hypoxia (FIO$_2$ 16%, which is equivalent to 11,500 feet altitude) or hyperoxia (FIO$_2$ greater than 96%). It is worth mentioning that we have evaluated several patients with primary pulmonary hypertension who had been previously challenged with 100% oxygen inhalation and were said to have improved on the basis of an observed lowering of their pulmonary artery pressure during exposure to hyperoxia. However, when we measured the cardiac output during hyperoxia in these patients, we found the characteristic response to be a reduced cardiac output, which accounted for the fall in pulmonary artery pressure. Therefore, the calculated pulmonary vascular resistance may actually increase in such patients who have a modest fall in mean pulmonary artery pressure, thus leading to an entirely different conclusion regarding the patient's response to oxygen inhalation.

In our laboratory, isoproterenol infusions have revealed the characteristic response of patients with primary pulmonary hypertension to be an increase in cardiac output and heart rate that frequently increases mean pulmonary artery pressure despite a calculated fall in pulmonary vascular resistance. In addition, we have noted in several patients during isoproterenol infusion the development of ischemic chest pain that appears to be a manifestation of RV ischemia. Therefore, it is our current practice not to use intravenous infusions of isoproterenol to challenge patients with primary pulmonary hypertension.

Patients who show a favorable response to intravenous prostacyclin in our laboratory are currently placed on an 8-week trial of diltiazem, nifedipine, or hydralazine. It is our impression that patients who respond to prostacyclin with significant increases in cardiac output and drops in pulmonary artery pressure will respond to one or more other vasodilators. Patients with severe primary pulmonary hypertension frequently will not have an impressive change in their resting hemodynamics when restudied on vasodilator therapy. However, we have noted that patients who suffer from exertional syncope from primary pulmonary hypertension have usually stopped having syncope when treated with either diltiazem or nifedipine. In addition, it is common for a patient with primary pulmonary hypertension who shows no substantial alteration in resting hemodynamics to relate clinically an improvement in exercise tolerance and functional capacity that seems to improve the quality of life for the patient. Therefore, it is our practice to continue vasodilator therapy in a patient who has control of syncope or significant improvement in functional capacity unless there is an objective deterioration of measured hemodynamics.

When possible, it is desirable to measure the patient's hemodynamic response to therapy at rest and with exercise. Exercise studies, which add an additional risk to the procedure, may confirm hemodynamic benefit from vasodilator therapy when the resting hemodynamics are unchanged from control values.

Because noninvasive techniques do not adequately assess the effect of vasodilator therapy, serial right heart catheterizations are needed to document patients' response to therapy. We and others are working on improved noninvasive methodologies to allow estimation of pulmonary artery pressure and blood flow without cardiac catheterization.[99] A preliminary Doppler study in our laboratory has shown that measurement of RV relaxation time (the interval between pulmonary valve closure and tricuspid valve opening) allows estimation of RV systolic pressure.[4] It is anticipated that technological advances will allow earlier detection of pulmonary hypertension and accurate outpatient assessment of pulmonary artery pressure and flow with less cost and risk to the patient.

Cardiopulmonary Transplantation

Recently, surgical and immunologic advancements have allowed the development of cardiopulmonary transplantation as a therapeutic modality for patients in whom medical therapy fails to improve RV function and exercise tolerance. Pioneered at the Stanford Medical Center under the leadership of Dr. Norman Shumway, cardiopulmonary transplantation has now been performed in approximately 25 patients worldwide, with an overall mortality rate of approximately 50%. The availability of cyclosporin immunosuppressive therapy in combination with prednisone is credited as being a major factor in this successful transplantation experience. Patients with primary pulmonary hypertension are particularly good candidates for this procedure since they characteristically are young and without associated systemic disease. Seven out of the first ten patients receiving cardiopulmonary transplantation at Stanford Medical Center survived.[139] The first Stanford patient received cardiopulmonary transplantation in March, 1981 and was recatheterized two years later with the finding of normal resting hemodynamics. Each of the survivors is living a productive life with excellent exercise tolerance. The use of percutaneous transvenous RV endomyocardial biopsy has allowed the detection and treatment of early pulmonary rejection episodes in these patients. The availability of RV biopsy for this purpose has been credited as being a major factor in allowing successful cardiopulmonary transplantation. Isolated pulmonary transplantation was uniformly unsuccessful in the past when no method was available for obtaining serial tissue biopsies to detect graft rejection.

Summary

The normal adult mean pulmonary artery pressure is less than 25 mm Hg. Pulmonary hypertension can be classified into three clinical etiologic categories: passive, reactive, and obstructive. The most common symptoms of severe pulmonary hypertension are dyspnea, fatigue, chest pain, syncope, and sudden death. Signs of pulmonary hypertension include prominent A waves in the jugular venous pulse, RV lift, increased P_2, and the murmur of tricuspid regurgitation. Noninvasive studies include electrocardiographic evidence of RVH, roentgenographic prominence of the main and proximal pulmonary arteries, and echocardiographic pulmonary valve motion characterized by a flattened diastolic slope associated with anterior systolic notching ("flying W"). In patients with pulmonary arterial disease, cardiac catheterization usually reveals an elevated pulmonary artery pressure, a normal wedge pressure, and a reduced resting cardiac output. With progression of pulmonary hypertensive disease, RV failure is reflected by elevation of the venous pressure, edema, right-sided S_3, and hypoxemia associated with roentgenographic evidence of RV enlargement. In some patients, the functional and hemodynamic status can be improved by treatment with a vasodilator. The eventual outcome for patients with severe fixed pulmonary vascular obstructive disease may be refractory RV failure and death unless cardiopulmonary transplantation can be accomplished.

References

1. Nadas AS, Flyer DC: The fetal circulation and its adjustment after birth. In Nadas AS, Flyer DC (eds): Pediatric Cardiology. Philadelphia, WB Saunders, 1972
2. Reeves JT, Groves BM: Approach to the patient with pulmonary hypertension. In Weir EK, Reeves JT (eds): Pulmonary Hypertension. New York, Futura Press, 1984
3. Hatle L, Anglesen BAJ, Troms A, et al: Non-invasive estimation of pulmonary artery systolic pressure with doppler ultrasound. Br Heart J 45:157, 1981
4. Reeves JT, Groves BM, Micco AJ, et al: Valid measurement by Doppler of right ventricular isovolumic relaxation time: A non-invasive estimate of systolic pressure. Circulation 68:404, 1983
5. Wagner WW: Personal communication
6. Wagner WW, Latham LP, Capen RL: Capillary recruitment during airway hypoxia: Role of pulmonary artery pressure. J Appl Physiol 47:383, 1979
7. Nagasaka Y, Bhattacharya J, Cropper MA, et al: Micropuncture measurement of lung microvascular pressure profile during hypoxia in cats. Fed Proc 42:595, 1983

8. Benumof JL, Wahrenbrock EA: Blunted hypoxic pulmonary vasoconstriction by increased lung vascular pressures. J Appl Physiol 38:846, 1975

9. Staub NC: Pulmonary edema. Physiol Rev 54:678, 1979

10. Harris P, Heath D: Human Pulmonary Circulation, Edinburgh, Churchill Livingstone, 1977

11. Dexter L: Pulmonary vascular disease in acquired heart disease. In Lenfant C (series ed): Lung Biology in Health and Disease, Vol 14, Moser KM (ed): Pulmonary Vascular Diseases, pp 427–484. New York, Marcel Dekker, 1979

12. Fricke RF, Secker–Walker RH: Recovery from ethchlorvynol-induced pulmonary edema in the rat. Clin Res 28:425A, 1980

13. Sugita T, Hyers TM, Dauber IM, et al: Lung vessel leak precedes right ventricular hypertrophy in monocrotaline-treated rats. J Appl Physiol 54:371, 1983

14. McMurtry IF, Davidson AB, Reeves JT, et al: Inhibition of hypoxic pulmonary vasoconstriction by calcium antagonists in isolated rat lungs. Circ Res 38:99, 1976

15. Stanbrook HS, McMurtry IF: Inhibition of glycolosis potentiates hypoxic vasoconstriction in rat lungs. J Appl Physiol 55:1467, 1983

16. Morganroth ML, Murphy RC, Voelkel NF: Diethylcarbamazine (DEC), a leukotriene synthesis blocker, blocks hypoxic pulmonary vasoconstriction. Fed Proc 42:303, 1983

17. Grover RF, Vogel JHK, Averill KH, et al: Pulmonary hypertension. Individual and species variability relative to vascular reactivity. Am Heart J 66:1, 1963

18. Moser KM: Pulmonary vascular obstruction due to embolism and thrombosis. In Lenfant C (series ed): Lung Biology in Health and Disease, Vol 14, Moser KM (ed): Pulmonary Vascular Diseases, pp 341–386. New York, Marcel Dekker, 1979

19. Wagenvoort CA: Lung biopsies and pulmonary vascular disease. In Weir EK, Reeves JT (eds): Pulmonary Hypertension. New York, Futura Press, 1984

20. Moser KM, Spragg RG, Long WB, et al: Chronic thrombotic obstruction of major pulmonary arteries: Results of thromboendarterectomy in 15 patients. Am Rev Resp Dis 125:87, 1982

21. Shellub I, van Grondelle A, McCullough R, et al: A model of embolic pulmonary hypertension in the dog. J Appl Physiol 56:810, 1984

22. Heath D, Smith P: Pulmonary vascular disease secondary to lung disease. In Lenfant C (series ed): Lung Biology in Health and Disease, Vol 14, Moser KM (ed): Pulmonary Vascular Disease, pp 387–426. New York, Marcel Dekker, 1979

23. Nocturnal oxygen therapy trial group: Continuous nocturnal oxygen therapy in hypoxemic chronic obstructive lung disease. Ann Intern Med 93:391, 1980

24. Marcus AJ: The role of prostaglandins in platelet function. In Brown EB (ed): Progress in Hematology, Vol 2, pp 147–171. New York, Grune and Stratton, 1979

25. Greglewski, Korbut R, Ocetkiewicz AC: Generation of prostacyclin by lungs in vivo and its release into the arterial circulation. Nature 273:765, 1978

26. Van Benthuysen KM, Hammon JW, Mitchener JS, et al: Electron microscopic alterations in experimental pulmonary hypertension. J Surg Res 22:398, 1977

27. Shaub RG, Rawlings CA, Keith JC: Platelet adhesion and myointimal proliferation in canine pulmonary arteries. Am J Pathol 104:13, 1981

28. Grover RF, Wagner WW, McMurtry IF, et al: Pulmonary circulation. In Shepherd JT, Abboud FM (eds): Handbook of Physiology, vol 3, The Cardiovascular System. Bethesda, American Physiological Society, 1983

29. Lindenfeld J, Reeves JT, Horwitz LD: Active vasoconstriction occurs in the pulmonary vascular bed during exercise in dogs. Clin Res 31:72A, 1983

30. Haynes RH: Physical basis of the dependence of blood viscosity on tube radius. Am J Physiol 198:1193, 1960
31. Lindenfeld J, Weil JV, Horwitz LD: Oxygen content, not viscosity, regulates cardiac output during induced polycythemia in dogs. Clin Res 31:72A, 1983
32. Burton AC: Physiology and Biophysics of the Circulation, pp 50–57. Chicago, Yearbook Publishers, 1965
33. McGrath RL, Weil JV: Adverse effects of normovolemic polycythemia and hypoxia on hemodynamics in the dog. Circ Res 43:793, 1978
34. Reeves JT, Grover EB, Grover RF: Circulatory responses to high altitude in the cat and the rabbit. J Appl Physiol 18:575, 1963
35. Cruz JC, Diaz C, Marticonena, et al: Phlebotomy improves pulmonary gas exchange in chronic mountain sickness. Respiration 38:305, 1979
36. Braunwald E, Braunwald NS, Ross J Jr, et al: Effects of mitral valve replacement on the pulmonary vascular dynamics of patients with pulmonary hypertension. N Engl J Med 273:509, 1965
37. Dalen JE, Matloff JM, Evans GL, et al: Early reduction of pulmonary vascular resistance after mitral valve replacement. N Engl J Med 277:387, 1967
38. Zener JC, Hancock EW, Shumway NG, et al: Regression of extreme pulmonary hypertension after mitral valve surgery. Am J Cardiol 30:820, 1972
39. Walston A, Peter RH, Morris JJ, et al: Clinical implications of pulmonary hypertension in mitral stenosis. Am J Cardiol 32:650, 1973
40. Vogel JHK, Weaver WF, Rose RL, et al: Pulmonary hypertension on exertion in normal man living at 10,150 feet. Med Thorac 19:461, 1962
41. Vogel JHK, Pryor R, Blount SG Jr: The cardiovascular system in children from high altitude. J Pediatrics 64:315, 1964
42. Grover RF, Vogel JHK, Voigt GC, et al: Reversal of high altitude pulmonary hypertension. Am J Cardiol 18:928, 1966
43. Semerano A, Bevilacqua M, Battistin L: Blood gas analysis and polygraphic observations in the Pickwickian syndrome. Bull Physiol Pathol Respir 8:1193, 1972
44. Levy A, Tabakin B, Hanson J: Hypertrophied adenoids causing pulmonary hypertension and severe congestive heart failure. N Engl J Med 177:506, 1967
45. Schroeder J, Motta J, Guilleminault C: Hemodynamic studies in sleep apnea, In Guilleminault C, Dement W (eds): Sleep Apnea Syndromes, pp 177–196. New York, Alan R Liss, 1978
46. Weil JV, Kryger M, Scoggin C: Sleep and breathing at high altitude In Guilleminault C, Dement W (eds): Sleep Apnea Syndromes, pp 119–136. New York, Alan R. Liss Inc, 1978
47. McIntyre KM, Sasahara AA: The hemodynamic response to pulmonary embolism in patients without prior cardiopulmonary disease. Am J Cardiol 28:288, 1971
48. Sasahara AA, Stein M, Simon M, et al: Pulmonary angiography in the diagnosis of thromboembolic disease. N Engl J Med 270:1075, 1964
49. Pool PE, Vogel JHK, Blount SG Jr: Congenital unilateral absence of a pulmonary artery: The importance of flow in pulmonary hypertension. Am J Cardiol 10:705, 1962
50. Eldredge WJ, Tingelstad JB, Robertson LW, et al: Observations on the natural history of pulmonary artery coarctations. Circulation 45:404, 1972
51. Cosio FG, Gobel FL, Harrington DP, et al: Pulmonary arterial stenosis with wide splitting of the second heart sound due to mediastinal fibrosis. Am J Cardiol 31:372, 1973
52. Heath D, Segel N, Bishop J: Pulmonary veno-occlusive disease. Circulation 34:242, 1966

53. Edwards HD, Edwards JE: Clinical primary pulmonary hypertension: Three pathologic types. Circulation 56:884, 1977

54. Rosenthal A, Vawter G, Wagenvoort CA: Intrapulmonary veno-occlusive disease. Am J Cardiol 31:78, 1973

55. Anderson JL, Durnin RE, Ledbetter MK, et al: Clinical pathologic conference. Am Heart J 97:233, 1979

56. Scully RE (ed): Case records of the Massachusetts General Hospital, Weekly clinicopathological exercises. Case 14-1983. New Engl J Med 308:823, 1983

57. Massumi A, Woods L, Mullins CE, et al: Pulmonary venous dilation in pulmonary veno-occlusive disease. Am J Cardiol 48:585, 1981

58. Trell E, Lindstrom C: Pulmonary hypertension in systemic sclerosis. Ann Rheum Dis 30:390, 1971

59. Salerni R, Rodnan GP, Leon DF, et al: Pulmonary hypertension in the CREST syndrome variant of progressive systemic sclerosis (scleroderma). Ann Intern Med 86:394, 1977

60. Naslund MJ, Pearson TA, Ritter JM: A documented episode of pulmonary vasoconstriction in systemic sclerosis. Johns Hopkins Med J 148:78, 1981

61. Scully RE (ed): Case records of the Massachusetts General Hospital, Weekly clinicopathological exercises. Case 43:1979. New Engl J Med 301:929, 1979

62. Santini D, Fox D, Kloner RA, et al: Pulmonary hypertension in systemic lupus erythematosus: Hemodynamics and effects of vasodilator therapy. Clin Cardiol 3:406, 1980

63. Perez HD, Kramer N: Pulmonary hypertension in systemic lupus erythematosus: Report of four cases and review of the literature. Semin Arthritis Rheum 11:177, 1981

64. Brammell HL, Vogel JHK, Pryor R, et al: The Eisenmenger syndrome: A clinical and physiological reappraisal. Am J Cardiol 28:679, 1971

65. Young P, Mark H: Fate of the patient with the Eisenmenger syndrome. Am J Cardiol 28:658, 1971

66. Disesa VJ, Cohn LH, Grossman L: Management of adults with congenital bidirectional cardiac shunts, cyanosis, and pulmonary vascular obstruction: Successful operative repair in 3 patients. Am J Cardiol 51:1495, 1983

67. Wagenvoort CA, Wagenvoort N: Pathology of the Eisenmenger syndrome and primary pulmonary hypertension. Adv Cardiol 11:123, 1974

68. Haworth SG: Pulmonary vascular disease in secundum atrial septal defect in childhood. Am J Cardiol 51:265, 1983

69. Naeye RL: Primary pulmonary hypertension with coexisting portal hypertension. Circulation 22:376, 1960

70. Cohen N, Mendelow H: Concurrent active juvenile cirrhosis and primary pulmonary hypertension. Am J Med 39:127, 1965

71. Segel N, Kay JM, Bayley TJ, et al: Pulmonary hypertension with hepatic cirrhosis. Br Heart J 30:575, 1968

72. Lal S, Fletcher E: Pulmonary hypertension and portal venous system thrombosis. Br Heart J 30:723, 1968

73. Senior RM, Britton RC, Turino GM, et al: Pulmonary hypertension associated with cirrhosis of the liver and with portocaval shunts. Circulation 37:88, 1968

74. Cryer PE, Kissane J (eds): Clinicopathologic conference. Chronic active hepatitis and pulmonary hypertension. Am J Med 63:604, 1977

75. Fishman AP: Dietary pulmonary hypertension. Circ Res 35:657, 1974

76. Garcia–Dorado D, Miller DD, Garcia EJ, et al: An epidemic of pulmonary hypertension after toxic rapeseed oil ingestion in Spain. J Am Coll Cardiol 1:1216, 1983

77. Kuida H, Dammin GJ, Haynes FW, et al: Clinical studies. Primary pulmonary hypertension. Am J Med 23:166, 1957
78. Blount SG Jr: Primary pulmonary hypertension. Mod Concepts Cardiovasc Dis 36:67, 1967
79. Voelkel NF, Reeves JT: Primary pulmonary hypertension. In Lenfant C (series ed): Lung Biology in Health and Disease, Vol 14, Moser KM (ed): Pulmonary Vascular Diseases, pp 573–628. New York, Marcel Dekker, 1979
80. Martin CE, Shaver JA, O'Toole JD, et al: Ejection sounds of right-sided origin. In Leon DF, Shaver JA (eds): Physiologic Principles of Heart Sounds and Murmurs. American Heart Association Monograph 46, pp 35–44. Dallas, American Heart Association, 1975
81. Murgo JP, Altobelli SA, Dorethy JF, et al: Normal ventricular ejection dynamics in man during rest and exercise. In Leon DF, Shaver JA (eds): Physiologic Principles of Heart Sounds and Murmurs, American Heart Association Monograph 46, pp 92–101. Dallas, American Heart Association, 1975
82. Shaver JA, Nadolny RA, O'Toole JD, et al: Sound pressure correlates of the second heart sound: An intracardiac study. Circulation 39:316, 1974
83. Cha SD, Gooch AS, Maranhao V: Intracardiac phonocardiography in tricuspid regurgitation: Relation to clinical and angiographic findings. Am J Cardiol 48:578, 1981
84. Keenan TJ, Schwartz MJ: Tricuspid whoop. Am J Cardiol 31:642, 1973
85. Upshaw CB: Precordial honk due to tricuspid regurgitation. Am J Cardiol 35:85, 1975
86. Gooch AS, Cha SD, Maranhao V: The use of the hepatic pressure maneuver to identify the murmur of tricuspid regurgitation. Clin Cardiol 6:277, 1983
87. Kunhali K, Cherian G, Bakthavizian A, et al: Rupture of a papillary muscle of the tricuspid valve in primary pulmonary hypertension. Am Heart J 99:225, 1980
88. Green EW, Agruss NS, Adolph RJ: Right-sided Austin Flint murmur. Documentation by intracardiac phonocardiography, echocardiography and postmortem findings. Am J Cardiol 32:370, 1973
89. McIntyre KM, Sasahara AA: Angiography, scanning, and hemodynamics in pulmonary embolism: Critical review and correlations. CRC Crit Rev Radiol Sci 3:489, 1972
90. Wilson AG, Harris CN, Lavender JP, et al: Perfusion lung scanning in obliterative pulmonary hypertension. Br Heart J 35:917, 1973
91. Dalen JE, Brooks HL, Johnson LW, et al: Pulmonary angiography in acute pulmonary embolism: Indications, techniques, and results in 367 patients. Am Heart J 81:175, 1971
92. Novelline RA, Baltarowich OH, Athanasoulis CA, et al: The clinical course of patients with suspected pulmonary embolism and a negative pulmonary arteriogram. Radiology 126:561, 1978
93. Weyman AE, Dillon JC, Feigenbaum H: Echocardiographic patterns of pulmonic valve motion with pulmonary hypertension. Circulation 50:905, 1974
94. Nanda NC, Gramiak R, Robinson TI, et al: Echocardiographic evaluation of pulmonary hypertension. Circulation 50:575, 1974
95. Lew W, Karliner JS: Assessment of pulmonary valve echogram in normal subjects and in patients with pulmonary arterial hypertension. Br Heart J 42:147, 1979
96. Tahara M, Tanaka H, Nakao S, et al: Hemodynamic determinants of pulmonary valve motion during systole in experimental pulmonary hypertension. Circulation 64:1249, 1981
97. Acquatella H, Schiller NB, Sharpe DN, et al: Lack of correlation between echo-

cardiographic pulmonary valve morphology and simultaneous pulmonary artery pressure. Am J Cardiol 43:946, 1979

98. Goodman DJ, Harrison DC, Popp RL: Echocardiographic features of primary pulmonary hypertension. Am J Cardiol 33:438, 1974

99. Kitabatake A, Inoue M, Asao M, et al: Noninvasive evaluation of pulmonary hypertension by a pulsed Doppler technique. Circulation 68:302, 1983

100. Gurtner HP: Hypertensive pulmonary vascular disease. Some remarks on its incidence and etiology. In Baker SB (ed): Proceedings of the 12th Meeting of the European Society for the Study of Drug Toxicity, Uppsala, 1970, pp 81–88 Amsterdam, Excerpta Medica, 1971

101. Starling MR, Crawford MH, Walsh RD, et al: Value of the tricuspid valve echogram for estimating right ventricular end-diastolic pressure during vasodilator therapy. Am J Cardiol 45:966, 1980

102. Vogel JHK, Grover RF, Blount SG Jr: Detection of the small intracardiac shunt with the hydrogen electrode: A highly sensitive and simple technique. Am Heart J 64:13, 1962

103. van Grondelle A, Ditchey RV, Groves BM, et al: Thermodilution method overestimates low cardiac output in humans. Am J Physiol 14:H690, 1983

104. Krongrad E, Helmholz HF, Ritter DC: Effect of breathing oxygen in patients with severe pulmonary vascular obsructive disease. Circulation 47:94, 1973

105. Rudolph AM, Paul AM, Sommer LS, et al: Effects of tolazoline hydrochloride (Priscoline) on circulatory dynamics of patients with pulmonary hypertension. Am Heart J 55:424, 1958

106. Grover RF, Reeves JT, Blount SG Jr: Tolazoline hydrochloride (Priscoline): An effective pulmonary vasodilator. Am Heart J 61:5, 1961

107. Shettigar UR, Hultgren HN, Specter M, et al: Primary pulmonary hypertension Favorable effect of isoproterenol. N Engl J Med 295:1414, 1976

108. Daoud FS, Reeves JT, Kelly DB: Isoproterenol as a potential pulmonary vasodilator in primary hypertension. Am J Cardiol 42:817, 1978

109. Elkayam U, Frishman WH, Yoran C, et al: Unfavorable hemodynamic and clinical effects of isoproterenol in primary pulmonary hypertension. Cardiovasc Med 3:1177, 1978

110. Rubin LJ, Peter RH: Oral hydralazine therapy for primary pulmonary hypertension. N Engl J Med 302:69, 1980

111. Rubin LJ, Peter RH: Hemodynamics at rest and during exercise after oral hydralazine in patients with cor pulmonale. Am J Cardiol 47:116, 1981

112. Fripp RP, Gewitz MH, Werner JC, et al: Oral hydralazine in patients with pulmonary vascular disease secondary to congenital heart disease. Am J Cardiol 48:380, 1981

113. Lupi–Herrera E, Sandoval J, Seoane M, et al: The role of hydralazine therapy for pulmonary arterial hypertension of unknown cause. Circulation 65:645, 1982

114. Packer M, Greenberg B, Massie B, et al: Deleterious effects of hydralazine in patients with pulmonary hypertension. N Engl J Med 306:1326, 1982

115. Pickering TG, Ritter S, Devereux RB: Beneficial effects of phentolamine and nifedipine in primary pulmonary hypertension. Cardiovascular Reviews and Reports 3:303, 1982

116. Kambara H, Fukimoto K, Wakabayashi A, et al: Primary pulmonary hypertension: Beneficial therapy with dilitiazem. Am Heart J 101:230, 1981

117. Crevey BJ, Dantzker DR, Bower JS, et al: Hemodynamic and gas exchange effects of intravenous diltiazem in patients with pulmonary hypertension. Am J Cardiol 49:578, 1982

118. Landmark K, Refsum AM, Simonsen S, et al: Verapamil and pulmonary hypertension. Acta Med Scand 204:299, 1978

119. Camerini F, Alberti E, Klugman S, et al: Primary pulmonary hypertension: Effects of nifedipine. Brit Heart J 44:352, 1980
120. Rubin LJ, Nicod P, Hillis LD, et al: Treatment of primary pulmonary hypertension with nifedipine. Ann Intern Med 99:433, 1983
121. Gould L, Zahir M, DeMartino A, et al: Hemodynamic effects of phentolamine in chronic obstructive pulmonary disease. Br Heart J 33:445, 1971
122. Ruskin JN, Hutter AM: Primary pulmonary hypertension treated with oral phentolamine. Ann Intern Med 90:772, 1979
123. Klinke WP, Gilbert JAL: Diazoxide in primary pulmonary hypertension. N Engl J Med 302:91, 1980
124. Hall DR, Petch MC: Remission of primary pulmonary hypertension during treatment with diazoxide. Br Med J 282:1118, 1981
125. Want SWS, Pohl JEF, Rowlands DJ, et al: Diazoxide in treatment of primary pulmonary hypertension. Brit Heart J 40:532, 1978
126. Rubino JM, Schroeder JS: Diazoxide in treatment of primary pulmonary hypertension. Br Heart J 42:362, 1979
127. Honey M, Cotter L, Davies N, et al: Clinical and hemodynamic effects of diazoxide in primary pulmonary hypertension. Thorax 35:269, 1980
128. Niarchos AP, Whitman HH, Goldstein JE, et al: Hemodynamic effects of captopril in pulmonary hypertension of collagen vascular disease. Am Heart J 104:834, 1982
129. Leier CV, Bambach D, Nelson S, et al: Captopril in primary pulmonary hypertension. Circulation 67:155, 1983
130. Knapp E, Gmeiner R: Reduction of pulmonary hypertension by nitroprusside. Int J Clin Pharmacol Biopharmacol 15:75, 1977
131. Danahy DT, Tobis JM, Aronow WS, et al: Effects of isosorbide dinitrate on pulmonary hypertension in chronic obstructive pulmonary disease. Clin Pharmacol Ther 25:541, 1979
132. Pearl RG, Rosenthal MH, Schroeder JS, et al: Acute hemodynamic effects of nitroglycerin in pulmonary hypertension. Ann Intern Med 99:9, 1983
133. Person B, Proctor R: Primary pulmonary hypertension response to indomethacin, terbutaline and isoproterenol. Chest 76:60, 1979
134. Hermiller JB, Bambach D, Thompson MJ, et al: Vasodilators and prostaglandin inhibitors in primary pulmonary hypertension. Ann Intern Med 97:480, 1982
135. Rich S, Martinez J, Lam W, et al: Reassessment of the effects of vasodilator drugs in primary pulmonary hypertension: Guidelines for determining a pulmonary vasodilator response. Am Heart J 105:119, 1983
136. Watkins WD, Peterson MB, Crone RK, et al: Prostacyclin and prostaglandin E₁ for severe idiopathic pulmonary artery hypertension. Lancet 1:1083, 1980
137. Guadagni DN, Ikram H, Maslowski AH: Hemodynamic effects of prostacyclin (PGI₂) in pulmonary hypertension. Br Heart J 45:385, 1981
138. Rubin LJ, Groves BM, Reeves JT, et al: Prostacyclin-induced acute pulmonary vasodilation in primary pulmonary hypertension. Circulation 66:334, 1982
139. Jamieson SW, Baldwin J, Reitz BA, et al: Combined heart and lung transplantation. Lancet 1:1130, 1983

16

QUANTITATIVE AND QUALITATIVE NUCLEAR IMAGING OF CARDIAC PATHOLOGY

Dennis L. Kirch, M.S.E.E., and Peter P. Steele, M.D.

Definition

Radionuclide-based methods of cardiac diagnosis permit qualitative and quantitative assessment of ischemic or infarcted regions of the myocardium. To make such diagnostic determinations accurately, it is necessary to understand the technical characteristics of scintigraphic instrumentation, the biochemical and physical properties of the radiopharmaceutical compounds used, the conceptual models required in quantitative imaging, and the pathophysiology of myocardial ischemia and infarction. Methods are currently available to study regional myocardial blood flow, mechanical performance of ventricular muscle, and biochemical alterations in damaged myocardial cells. Although the different types of radionuclide studies provide quite varied information, all the studies are based on the same principles.

In every application of scintigraphic imaging systems to clinical cardiac studies, a compromise between resolution and other factors must be made. Most notably, the need to limit patient exposure to radiation and, on occasion, radiopharmaceutical cost requires limitation of radionuclide doses to levels that are often less than optimum for the technical aspects of the tests being performed. In most cases, the quality and quantity of detectable photons from gamma-ray-emitting tracers is the major determinant of the adequacy of the diagnostic information provided.

There are both similarities and differences between radionuclide and x-ray imaging methods. Both involve the projection of a two-dimensional image generated by detection of the distribution of ionizing radiation. On the most fundamental level, mapping of the *in vivo* radionuclide distribution is an emissive imaging modality, whereas x-ray images are created by detection of a planar wave of radiation that has been transmitted through the body. That is, scintigraphic images display the quantity and distribution of a gamma-ray-emitting material inside the body, and x-ray films are a representation of the variations in absorption of rays from an external radiation source. Since radionuclides are distributed in the body by physiologic mechanisms, their detection is sometimes termed *functional imaging*. Because x-rays provide information that is related to anatomical configurations, their use is sometimes described as *structural imaging*. Since structure and function are inevitably related, information derived from scintigraphic images and x-rays is often usefully combined to reach diagnostic conclusions.

Physiology and Methods

RADIONUCLIDE TRACERS

Among the most important determinants of the quality and reliability of scintigraphic imaging are the physical and biochemical characteristics of the radionuclide compounds used. Ideal isotopes do not emit alpha or beta particles, which are highly attenuated by tissues, increase radiation exposure, and cannot be imaged adequately. Most clinically useful radionuclides are gamma-ray emitters. The usable energy range for current imaging devices is 80keV to 300 keV. The three types of cardiovascular imaging tests for which radionuclides are employed are blood pool studies, myocardial perfusion studies, and acute myocardial infarct studies. All require different radiopharmaceuticals.

Technetium-99m (^{99m}Tc) is the most commonly used agent for blood pool studies, including both first pass and equilibrium gated cardiac exams. It provides monoenergetic gamma rays at 140 keV, has a short half-life of 6 hours and is conveniently available in an inexpensive generator form. It can be used to label either red blood cells or serum albumin for blood pool studies.

Thallium-201 (^{201}Tl) is used for myocardial perfusion studies. It is taken up intracellularly in a manner similar to potassium and has energy characteristics more suitable for imaging than other radionuclides taken up by myocardial cells. It has a physical half-life of 73.1 hours, more prolonged than other intracellular agents but still requiring frequent shipment at higher cost.

Agents for imaging myocardial infarcts have been less satisfactory than those developed for other types of cardiac studies. Agents that will localize selectively in freshly infarcted myocardial tissue and permit imaging include ^{99m}Tc-labeled pyrophosphate and tetracycline. Tetracycline accumulates in other soft tissues and pyrophosphate accumulates in bone, both factors that may interfere with accurate myocardial infarct imaging.

All of the above agents and their available alternatives have some less-than-ideal physiologic properties that limit their diagnostic use. Blood pool tracers do not exclusively reside in the blood pool. Myocardial perfusion agents are not taken up in exact proportion to the reduced blood flow rates that exist during ischemia. Radionuclide compounds that have an affinity for infarcts are also extracted by other tissues with a variety of inflammatory or myopathic conditions. These factors present considerable challenges for successful diagnostic radionuclide imaging.

INSTRUMENTATION

State-of-the-art, computer-based gamma camera imaging systems are essential for performing nuclear cardiac diagnostic tests. The complexity of these systems makes it necessary to take their characteristics and limitations into account as part of the interpretive process.[1] A functional block diagram of a typical radionuclide imaging system is shown in Figure 16-1. Single-crystal (Anger-type) gamma scintillation cameras are the most commonly used detectors. The signals from the camera are processed by a digital computer system that displays the image and performs quantitative analyses of the data. A convenient way to discuss the functional characteristics of a scintigraphic imaging system is to describe the components in sequence from the point of gamma ray emission (within the patient) to the final repository of the data as images, curves, and other quantitative determinations.

Gamma rays are emitted from loci within the patient in all directions with equal probability. The gamma radiation is selectively passed through a lead collimator and projected onto the scintillation crystal in the gamma camera detector. The projection process creates a two-dimensional mapping of the three-dimensional distribution of activity within the patient. A single image generated in this fashion does not permit determination of the depth within the patient at which a gamma ray originated. Thus, activity that overlies or is beneath the heart also contributes counts to the cardiac region of the image. In addition, gamma rays undergo scattering when photons interact with nonradioactive tissue in a manner that changes their direction of travel. As a result, scattered gamma events can pass through the collimator, appearing to come from the heart even though they originated elsewhere. Analytic functions built into the camera/computer system can eliminate some but not all of the contaminating effects due to gamma rays originating outside the heart.

The scintillation detector consists of a circular sodium iodide crystal that is between 6.35 cm and 12.7 cm in thickness and between 25 cm and 38 cm in diameter. When gamma rays hit the crystal their energy is converted to light, which in turn is detected by photomultiplier tubes. The output from the detection circuitry is described as a temporal series of coordinates in an x, y cartesian system. The total amount of energy represented by each detected gamma ray event is measured so that events associated with highly scattered gamma rays can be discarded. Because of the desirability of performing this event-by-event analysis of photon energy, gamma camera operation is inherently a serial process that can process only one photon at a time. Herein lies the mechanism that fundamentally limits the gamma camera to operation at photon acceptance rates of 200,000 counts per second or less. Above this count rate, the probability of two events occurring simultaneously becomes significant. Events that overlap one another in time can either paralyze the camera

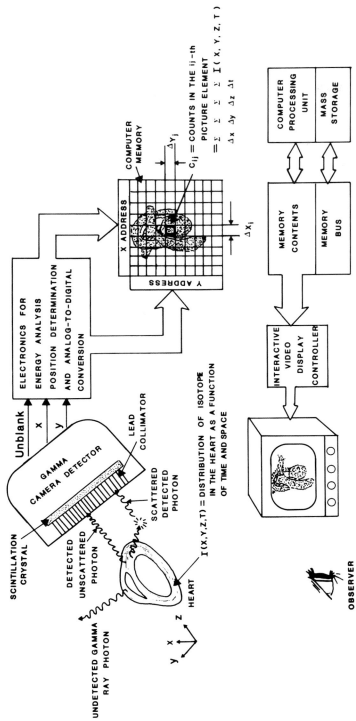

FIG. 16-1. Block diagram of the functional components of a computer-based gamma camera imaging system. The gamma camera detector locates the x, y coordinate of each photon and then adds a one count to the corresponding location in the computer memory, where the image is accumulated. Images are then written out to mass storage, analyzed by programs executed by the computer processing unit, and displayed on the video terminal for visual and quantitative evaluation.

circuitry, causing an erroneous drop in the observed count rate or, alternatively, can falsely localize the gamma ray at some site near the mean coordinate of the multiply detected events.

Collimators are single-pinhole or multihole honeycomb lead devices placed between the patient and the scintillation crystal of the gamma camera. Their purpose is to project gamma rays traveling along essentially straight lines onto the detector in a manner that is analogous to the lens in an optical imaging system. The resolution and sensitivity characteristics of collimators are traded off: the heart must be viewed with sufficient resolution to observe small features of diagnostic importance while at the same time enough photons must be detected to generate images with sufficient statistical accuracy. The most frequently used collimators emphasize sensitivity and achieve intermediate spatial resolution. This is appropriate because the heart is not stationary within the chest (a result of both heart beats and respiration) and because we are often interested in obtaining images in the shortest possible time (immediately following or during exercise or prior to the resolution of ischemia). The use of high-resolution collimation for cardiac studies provides no advantage because the heart motion that is always a factor in clinical studies causes blurring.

Figure 16-2 is a depiction of the transformation of an ideal point source of radiation into an observed distribution that is stored as discrete samples in computer memory. The basis for qualitative and quantitative interpretation of radionuclide studies is the count proportionality that exists between the source and the stored sample. The contaminant effects of background noise

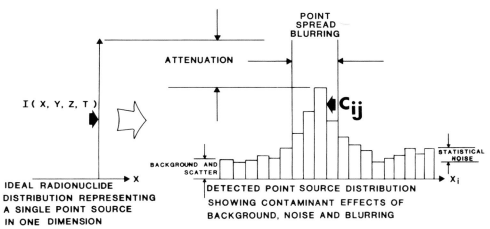

FIG. 16-2. One-dimensional plots illustrating the transformation between an ideal point-source radionuclide distribution and the detected distribution. C_{ij} represents the counts in the ij pixel element as in Fig. 16-1. The background and scattered activity create a bias for the data. The statistical fluctuations are due to the Poisson nature of the radionuclide decay process. The blurring of the point source is a result of the point spread transfer function of the collimation device. Attenuation occurs when photons are absorbed before leaving the body. The detected radionuclide distribution is shown as an incrementally sampled function, which is the way in which it would be stored in computer memory.

and blurring adversely affect this relationship. Image processing or filtering helps in analyzing the stored data but may also introduce error affecting the reproducibility of the diagnostic analysis.

Limitations on radiation dosage place an upper bound on the amounts of radioactivity that can be used in clinical studies, making the detection efficiency of the collimator one of the principle factors determining the quality of these studies. Detection efficiency can be increased to some extent without further sacrificing resolution through the use of converging and multiple-view methods of collimation, such as the seven-pinhole tomographic device.[2,3] These techniques allow the total detector surface to be visualized more efficiently than does projecting only a single image at one time. Since these techniques also furnish multiple projections of the radionuclide distribution taken from different directions, they also form the basis for developing a form of tomographic data that eliminates much of the contamination due to extracardiac activity.

The traditional way to interpret radionuclide scintigraphic images has been visually to assess abnormalities based on the presence of hot or cold lesions, depending on the type of radiopharmacutical employed. This is a highly subjective method of interpretation that requires a high degree of observer training, is subject to considerable variability between observers, and is further complicated by the presence of spatial and temporal variations in background activity and in the contrast and gray scale latitudes of the display device. These factors and the availability of digital computers make it advantageous to develop quantitative modalities for image interpretation that provide more exact and reproducible information. In each instance in which quantitative diagnosis of radionuclide studies is applied to the heart, a conceptual basis for performing the analysis has been formulated and tested in control groups of patients, with the diagnosis being separately determined by other methods. This arduous and time-consuming approach to validation of radionuclide techniques for cardiac studies is absolutely necessary to establish and ensure that these methods are correctly applied in a manner that contributes to the overall management of patients with heart disease.

Establishing which methodology is optimal from reports in the medical literature is often difficult. The disparities in reported results are most often attributable to differences in study protocols, variations in the equipment used, and the selection of patient populations. The imaging system and the study protocol must be appropriate for the diagnostic problem under investigation.

PHYSIOLOGY OF MYOCARDIAL PERFUSION SCINTIGRAPHY

Generally, radiopharmaceuticals for the study of myocardial perfusion have been capable of entering one of the cellular metabolic pathways. For this reason, isotopes of potassium were originally investigated. Undesirable energy levels, however, made them unsuitable for use with the standard gamma camera. Isotopes of cesium and rubidium were also used, but problems of cost, energy, and half-life impeded clinical use. Thallium has biologic similarities to potassium, but the lack of practical methods for its production limited availability until 1975, when the technical problems were overcome, leading to production of a single, pure isotope. [201]Tl has more suitable physical characteristics for gamma camera imaging than the isotopes that preceded it, with 95% photon abundance in the 68 keV to 80 keV range and 8% abundance at 165 keV. Just as important, however, is its half-life of 73.1 hours, which allows widespread availability by air shipment of precalibrated vials.

To understand the methodology underlying ^{201}Tl utilization in clinical studies, it is necessary to know how ^{201}Tl is transported to and taken up by myocardial cells.[4] It is injected as a *p*H-compatible solution of thallous chloride in saline solution. In less than a minute, about half of the available ^{201}Tl circulating in the blood has been taken up in the cells of the metabolically active organ systems throughout the body. The extraction of ^{201}Tl in lung tissue and secretion by the gastric mucosa present some interference problems for cardiac imaging, but this can be dealt with by injecting the patient in the upright position and withholding solid food for 2 hours prior to injection. The extraction efficiency of the myocardium is very high (85%), and about 5% of the injected dose is localized in the myocardium. The injection of ^{201}Tl during a graded treadmill exercise test has the twofold benefit of maximizing the percentage of cardiac output supplied to the myocardium and establishing the flow-deficient conditions indicative of transient ischemia associated with coronary artery disease. Beta blocking drugs, and, possibly, nitrites or calcium blockers, may limit diagnostic information related to ischemic myocardium. Submaximal exercise performance also can reduce the ability of this technique to demonstrate perfusion deficits.

The initial uptake of ^{201}Tl immediately after exercise reflects the distribution of myocardial blood flow during the stress and, thus, favors normal over ischemic regions of the myocardium. [201]Tl crosses the cell membrane rapidly because its valence and ionic radius are compatible with the active transport mechanisms of the cell. Once inside the cell, however, it seems to function more in character with its nature as a heavy metal. Intracellularly, it is retained by enzymatic binding in the mitochondria. This binding seems to be more pronounced in ischemic tissue, and, following the initial low uptake, its concentration in ischemic tissue remains essentially constant for 4 to 5 hours following injection. Normal myocardium, on the other hand, will typically give up 20% to 30% of its ^{201}Tl in the same period, depending on the rate at which the concentration decreases in the circulating blood. The biologic half-life of [210]Tl in humans is approximately 50 hours. In some cases, redistribution imaging can be satisfactorily performed as long as 24 hours after injection.

From this description of the biodynamics of ^{201}Tl, we can comprehend the rationale for using it in the study of ischemic heart disease. The initial imaging is performed as soon after the termination of graded treadmill stress as possible, so that perfusion defects will be maximally demonstrated. It is desirable to wait for 3 to 4 hours before reimaging so that ischemic regions can be identified by quantification of dynamic changes occurring between the two studies. Redistributional changes do not occur in scars left by myocardial infarctions, and perfusion defects are similar in exercise and rest images. Examples of ^{201}Tl stress and redistribution images in patients with normal, ischemic, and infarct patterns are shown in Figure 16-3. [201]Tl studies can be interpreted on two

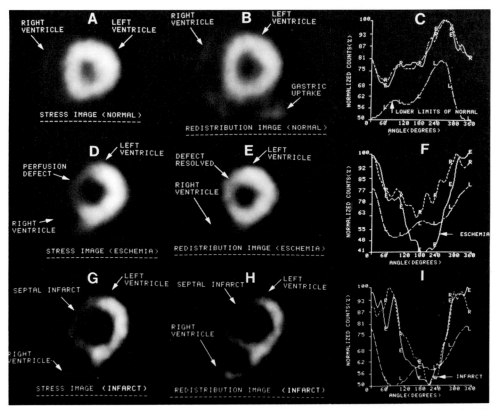

FIG. 16-3. Stress and redistribution images of the distribution of ²⁰¹thallium uptake in myocardium for (A–C) a normal study, (D–F) an abnormal study demonstrating marked ischemic changes, and (G–I) a septal infarct. The heart is shown in the left anterior oblique (LAO) or short axis view. The circumferential profile plots quantify the maximum wall counts for stress and redistribution (curves labeled E and R, respectively). The curves are developed from maximum wall counts beginning at 3 o'clock and proceeding clockwise through 360° in 6° increments. Note the lack of redistributional changes in the infarcted region. Curves labeled L show lower limit of normal range.

levels. First, group standards for the lower limits of normal for perfusion can be applied to the stress images alone. Then, when they become available, delayed redistribution images can be analyzed in comparison with the stress images for differences that reflect alterations in perfusion patterns. If these results are still inconclusive, further delay and reimaging can be helpful. The quantitative circumferential profile approach to analyzing these studies enhances diagnostic accuracy.[5–7]

While the most common application of ²⁰¹Tl is for the comparative stress/redistribution study of coronary artery disease, other useful applications have begun to emerge. The lack of a reliable method for labeling and imaging tissues in the early stages of infarction has prompted some to use ²⁰¹Tl as a tool for direct identification of the flow-deficient regions associated with infarction. Inability of the patient to exercise can be compensated for by the use of vasodilators such as dipyridamole. ^{201}Tl is also used as a tool for studying the results of therapeutic interventions.

PHYSIOLOGY OF HEMODYNAMIC BLOOD POOL SCINTIGRAPHY

Radionuclide studies of ventricular function can be classified into two general categories: first pass studies and equilibrium gated blood pool studies.[8-10] Virtually any ^{99m}Tc-labeled compound injected as a bolus can be used for first pass studies because the single-view data acquisition is completed before the injected material can leave the blood. Gated equilibrium studies, however, accumulate a limited sequence of images from several hundred heart beats synchronized to the R-wave of the electrocardiogram.Thus, the tracer must remain in the intravascular space long enough to allow data acquisition, a period of at least 30 minutes. Often, diagnosis can best be approached using both techniques. Initially, the first pass study is performed at frame rates of 15 to 25 frames per second. This is followed by the gated data acquisition, in which 16 to 32 frames are accumulated over approximately 90% of the R-to-R interval. When equilibrium gated studies are contemplated, the ^{99m}Tc can be retained in the blood pool by human serum albumin labeling or by *in vivo* or *in vitro* red cell labeling using stannous pyrophosphate as a chemical binding agent.

First pass techniques originally were developed for the study of hemodynamic events such as pulmonary transit time, cardiac output and inter- and intracardiac shunting. However, the availability of gamma camera/computer systems with the features described above makes it possible to examine ventricular function in both its global and its segmental aspects with gated studies. Of the possible viewing orientations, the anterior or left anterior oblique views are most often chosen because the atrial and ventricular separation is large enough to allow accurate ventricular ejection fractions to be computed and the important inferior portion of the left ventricular (LV) silhouette is delineated. While the right anterior oblique view fits the conventional cine angiographic area-length methodology for computation of ventricular volumes and total ejection fraction, the quantitative approach, which has proven most reliable and accurate for radionuclide data, is based on background corrected count proportionalities applied to the left anterior oblique view.

The gated blood pool ventriculogram is more useful than first pass studies in the clinical setting but is not without shortcomings. The right anterior oblique view that has been favored for cine ventriculography and first pass studies does not allow quantification of LV function in gated equilibrium studies because of overlap between the right and left ventricles. Instead, the left anterior oblique view is used for this purpose although the contaminating presence of the left atrium behind the ventricle can compromise results in conditions, such as mitral regurgitation, in which the atrium is enlarged. This difficulty can be moderated somewhat by using caudad angulation in an attempt to separate the four chambers of the heart. The four-chamber view, when achieved, is also useful for quantification of valvular regurgitation, once again using the concept that diastolic/systolic count changes are proportional to stroke volumes.

Equilibrium gated blood-pool studies allow visual as well as quantitative assessment of segmental wall motion abnormalities. Ventricular kinetics are usually studied in the left anterior oblique projection, which best reveals septal thickening, and the anterior or right anterior oblique projection, which more clearly reveals apical dynamics, is used to augment the study. Examples of a normal gated study and one demonstrating an apical LV aneurysm are shown in Figure 16-4. The visual and quantitative information developed by this technique must corroborate each another. Failure to reconcile these two aspects of the diagnostic information usually results in erroneous diagnostic findings.

The most important concept on which quantitative analysis of blood pool studies is based is the proportionality that exists among counts detected over a period in a single region of interest (*e.g.*, the left ventricle, as shown in Fig. 16-4 C and G). That is, volumetric changes in cardiac chamber size result in proportionate changes in the number of gamma photons detected in regions corresponding to the chambers. In spite of the problems previously described with background, scatter, attenuation, and the like, this concept provides measures of ventricular function that have proved both reliable and repeatable.

The ability to perform gated blood pool studies in serial sequences has stimulated interest in applying this technique under conditions of physiologic stress. The patient is positioned on a special ergometer table that immobilizes the upper torso to the degree necessary to allow image accumulation during bicycle ergometric exercise. A resting, baseline study is acquired in the left anterior oblique view and is followed by commencement of pedaling and data acquisition in 2 to 3 minute stages. Data accumulation ends about 6 minutes after termination of exercise but sometimes is followed by administration of nitroglycerin and one final acquisition.

PHYSIOLOGY OF MYOCARDIAL INFARCTION IMAGING

^{99m}Tc pyrophosphate is the most commonly used agent for imaging acute myocardial infarctions.[9] Examples of a normal pyrophosphate scan and of a transmural infarct are shown in Figure 16-5. Uptake of the radiopharmaceutical by the infarct depends on regional myocardial blood flow, the extent of tissue damage, and the calcium distribution in the infarct. The greater the reduction in blood flow to the infarct, the less the delivery of isotope to the site. In part because perfusion is lowest in the center of the infarct, the heaviest concentration of isotope is in the outer portions of the infarct.

The area of the isotope uptake correlates with the size of the infarct. However, the concentration of isotope in the infarct is not related to the extent of necrosis. Thus, the number of counts in the infarct does not give an indication of the degree of damage or of infarct size.

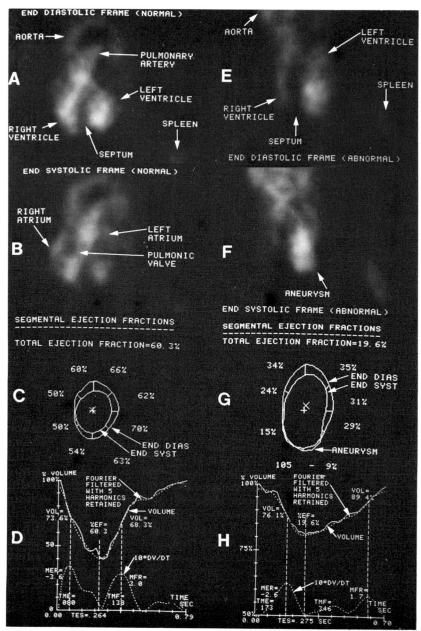

FIG. 16-4. End-diastolic and end-systolic frames from a gated blood pool study in the LAO view are shown from (A–D) a normal study and (E–H) a study demonstrating a dyskinetic aneurysm. The LV outlines are shown along with the 45° segmental ejection fractions in C and G. Note the negative ejection fraction, −9% for the inferior posterior segment corresponding to the aneurysm. The volume versus time plots (D and H) are labeled to show the maximum rates of ventricular emptying (MER) and filling (MFR). Both emptying and filling are substantially depressed in the patient with the aneurysm.

440

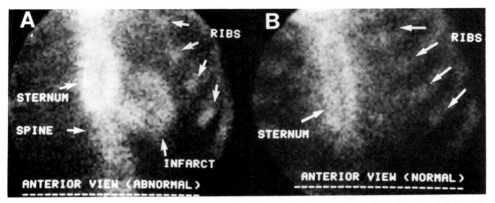

FIG. 16-5. ^{99m}Technetium pyrophosphate used in the demonstration of myocardial infarction. (*A*) A study showing marked uptake associated with transmural infarction. (*B*) A normal study with no myocardial uptake. Note the substantial uptake of pyrophosphate in the sternum, ribs and spine. Bone uptake, the inability to quantify the degree of affected myocardium, and poor sensitivity for subendocardial infarction has hampered the reliability of this test.

There appears to be a relationship between uptake of pyrophosphate and the presence of calcium. Approximately 50% of a dose of the radionuclide is taken up by bones (the agent is also used for bone scans). In necrotic myocardium, there is marked calcification of mitochrondria by 24 hours after damage begins. Presumably, accumulation of intracellular calcium causes chelation with pyrophosphate. The calcium concentration is higher in the outer edges of the infarct and this, together with the higher blood flow, is thought to account for the higher uptake of isotope in peripheral portions of the necrotic region. However, some studies have shown poor correlation between pyrophosphate uptake and concentration of calcium in the heart, and factors other than calcium binding may influence the localization of isotope in the infarct.

Clinical Presentation

CLINICAL USE OF THALLIUM MYOCARDIAL PERFUSION SCINTIGRAPHY

Myocardial ^{201}Tl imaging is useful for the detection of myocardial ischemia and for defining the effects of therapy on myocardial blood flow distribution in patients known to have coronary disease. When ^{201}Tl is injected during exercise and imaging is performed shortly after exercise, and is followed by delayed (redistribution) imaging, the sensitivity and specificity of conventional exercise test results are improved in such areas as clinical symptoms, heart rate, blood pressure, work-load, and ST changes.[4,6–9] ^{201}Tl imaging has the potential to detect multiple-vessel coronary disease, although the accuracy for single-vessel involvement is probably greater than that for multiple vessels.

Image quality can be enhanced and regional counts can be quantified by computer processing of ^{201}Tl scintigraphy. Background subtraction substantially improves image quality. Filtering techniques that limit high-frequency components reduce noise. Circumferential count profiles can be used to quantify regional count levels.[5-7] Anatomical features of the ventricle and distances from the camera cause variation in counts. However, these variations can be allowed for by use of values obtained from groups of normal patients (see Fig. 16-3 A, B, C). The most reliable method for detecting reversible ischemia by quantitative circumferential count profiles is to compare normalized exercise and rest (redistribution) circumferential count profile values. Regions in which normalized counts during exercise drop substantially below redistribution levels have stress-induced ischemia. Regions with low count levels on both the immediate postexercise and the redistribution curves are probably involved by scar from myocardial infarction (Fig. 16-3).

Use of tomographic techniques with computer processing of images from a seven-pinhole collimator offers the theoretical advantage of separating the myocardium into layers for analysis. The seven projections of the left ventricle are processed into 12 tomographic planes spaced 0.5 cm to 1.5 cm apart perpendicular to the long axis of the left ventricle. This method affords the capability to detect small lesions that are overlaid by normal myocardium. Great care must be taken in positioning the patient correctly or serious technical errors may be made. When proper technique is used, tomography enhances the sensitivity of ^{201}Tl imaging in comparison to planar imaging.[6,7]

Quantitative ^{201}Tl imaging procedures require the use of normalized count analysis. Counts from areas of myocardium are normalized to the area having the highest count density. For this reason, ^{201}Tl images represent the relative distribution of thallium within the myocardium rather than absolute flow values. Interpretations based on normal ranges are not entirely satisfactory due to the wide ranges in distribution sometimes observed in normal persons. Even with these problems, however, thallium imaging appears to be a useful adjunct to exercise testing for the diagnosis of myocardial ischemia.

For the patient with established coronary disease, ^{201}Tl imaging can be used to define the effects of therapy. Comparison of a control (or pretreatment) exercise image with an image obtained while the patient is being treated can be very useful in determining the results of therapy. This approach might be particularly useful following coronary bypass surgery to assess the situation early after surgery (2–3 months), a time when most vein graft occlusion has occurred.

Of the various procedures for defining short- to medium-term morbidity and mortality after myocardial infarction, submaximal exercise with ^{201}Tl imaging and measurement of LV ejection fraction at rest have been suggested as being of particular value. Submaximal exercise with normal ^{201}Tl images should exclude critical left system coronary disease.

[201]Tl imaging to quantify myocardial infarct size may also be useful. Images are obtained at rest and can be repeated at frequent intervals to define the effects of therapy and of time. The fact that radionuclide imaging can be undertaken in the coronary care unit or catheterization laboratory with portable camera/computer systems further enhances its value as a tool for monitoring the status and benefits of treatment in severely ill cardiac patients.

CLINICAL USE OF HEMODYNAMIC
BLOOD POOL SCINTIGRAPHY

Blood pool imaging is useful in that an accurate measurement of ventricular volume is obtained with very little trauma to the patient. Radioactive imaging of the blood pool is theoretically accurate, since chamber counts are a direct reflection of chamber volume irrespective of chamber geometry. Correlative studies have suggested that isotopically determined ventricular volumes are accurate in humans over a wide range of volumes.[11]

LV volume is measured using the patient's electrocardiogram as a gating reference to synchronize the summing of several hundred cardiac cycles from which an average cardiac cycle is then generated. Either electrocardiographic equilibrium gating after an intravenous injection or gating during first transit through the heart can be used. RV volume is best determined by the first transit method because the geometry of the ventricle is sufficiently complex that equilibrated imagery presents difficulties with RV boundary determination.

Ejection fraction is a convenient expression of ventricular performance and is determined as the ratio between two volumes, expressed as integrated, background-corrected counts from diastolic and systolic frames. It does not need to be corrected for image distortion. Blood pool imaging is useful when it is desirable to know the performance of either the right or the left ventricle. The reproducibility of the technique allows the results of therapy or passage of time to be rather precisely defined.

Gated blood pool imaging during exercise has been usefully applied to problems in patients with coronary disease and valvular heart disease.[10] The stress of exercise may induce a sudden decrease in LV performance due to ischemia. Exercise ejection fractions are less reliable than rest ejection fractions because of the short imaging time (2–3 min) and relatively low count rates obtained. Also, it appears that ejection fraction changes rapidly during exercise, perhaps more rapidly than minute-to-minute. Nevertheless, exercise ejection fractions are of clinical value. The technique would be improved if imaging times were shorter. This could be achieved by either supplemental injections of ^{99m}Tc or by the use of isotopes with very short half lives (*e.g.*, radioactive ^{195m}Au).

LV wall-motion studies can be undertaken with gated blood pool imaging. Segmental motion abnormalities at rest suggest infarction whereas motion abnormalities that develop during exercise suggest ischemia. Quantification of segmental wall-motion abnormalities would be useful but the technique is, as yet, poorly developed.

CLINICAL USE OF PYROPHOSPHATE MYOCARDIAL
INFARCT IMAGING

Myocardial infarct imaging is useful when other information (electrocardiogram, enzyme test) is unclear. Perhaps imaging of this kind is most helpful when a delay in diagnosis has been such that enzyme data are normal. In these circumstances, infarct imaging with pyrophosphate is useful because a positive accumulation may occur when electrocardiographic abnormalities (*e.g.,* left bundle branch block) obscure a diagnosis of infarction.

Infarct imaging has been suggested as a useful test to define a population at risk of death following infarction. Infarcts that show a pattern of persistently positive images for more than 2 or 3 weeks after infarction have been associated with a higher 6- to 12-month morbidity and mortality than have infarcts that are not persistently abnormal.[12] The first pattern, however, is almost always associated with more extensive infarctions, anterior myocardial involvement, and depressed LV ejection fraction. Ejection fractions are more readily quantifiable than infarction imaging and may be more useful for prognostic purposes.

Infarct imaging has not been useful in establishing a diagnosis in borderline cases, and particularly in subendocardial infarcts. Separating the diffuse myocardial pyrophosphate uptake in these infarctions from normal uptake has proved very difficult. Reimaging several hours after the initial image may help to clarify the situations in some patients in whom diffuse uptake persists on delayed imaging. A second problem with infarct imaging is the time needed for the image to become abnormal. A positive image may not occur until 48 to 72 hours after the event. Pericarditis, inflammation, or contusion of the heart may, on occasion, give positive pyrophosphate images.

Infarct imaging was developed as an aid to diagnosis and for its potential for quantifying myocardial injury. However, because of radioactivity in adjacent tissues (bones in particular) and because the count density in infarcted tissue depends on blood flow, which is very low in the central zones of infarction, radioactivity is not a simple expression of injury, so that quantitative analysis is difficult and quantification may never become a reality.

Summary

Both quantitative and qualitative assessments of cardiac function and myocardial ischemia can be obtained with current radionuclide methods. Myocardial perfusion scintigraphy, hemodynamic blood pool scintigraphy, and myocardial infarction imaging are the three most commonly employed tests.

Myocardial perfusion scintigraphy with ^{201}Tl for detection of ischemia is performed first with exercise or administration of a vasodilator and subsequently for redistribution under resting conditions. Regions that are ischemic during exercise or pharmacologic vasodilation can be identified quantitatively and qualitatively by a diminution in their uptake of isotope. Ischemic areas are differentiated from scar tissue by confirming redistribution of the isotope at rest. The technique can also be used to quantify acute myocardial infarction size.

Gated blood pool imaging with ^{99m}Tc allows the ventricular ejection fraction to be quantified and provides qualitative information about ventricular wall-motion abnormalities. Pyrophosphate myocardial infarct imaging is a sensitive qualitative technique for detecting recent acute myocardial damage.

References

1. Hine GJ, Sorenson JA (eds): Instrumentation in Nuclear Medicine. New York Academic Press, 1974
2. Brownell GL, Burnham CA, Chesler DA, et al. Transverse section imaging of radionuclide distributions in heart, lung and brain. In Ter-Pogossian MM (ed): Reconstruction Tomography in Diagnostic Radiology and Nuclear Medicine, pp 315–342. Baltimore, University Park Press, 1980
3. Price RR, Gilday GL, Croft BY (eds): Single Photon Emission Computed Tomography and Other Selected Computer Topics. New York, Society of Nuclear Medicine, 1980
4. Ritchie JL, Hamilton GW: Biologic properties of thallium In Ritchie JL, Hamilton GW, Wackers FJ (eds): Thallium-201 Myocardial Imaging. New York, Raven Press, 1978
5. Burow RD, Pond ML, Schafer WE, et al: Circumferential profiles: A new method for computer analysis of thallium-201 myocardial perfusion images. J Nucl Med 20:771, 1979
6. Bateman T, Garcia E, Maddahi J, et al: Clinical evaluation of seven-pinhole tomography for the detection and localization of coronary artery disease: Comparison with planar imaging using quantitative analysis of myocardial thallium-201 distribution and washout after exercise. Am Heart J 106:263, 1983
7. Rizi HR, Kline RC, et al: Thallium-201 myocardial scintigraphy: A critical comparison of seven-pinhole tomography and conventional planar imaging. J Nucl Med 22:493, 1981
8. Straus HW, Pitt B (eds): *Cardiovascular Nuclear Medicine*, 2nd ed. St. Louis, CV Mosby, 1979
9. Serafini AN, Gilson AJ, Smoak WM (eds): Nuclear Cardiology: Principles and Methods. New York, Plenum, 1977
10. Borer JS, Green MS, Bacarach SL: Realtime radionuclide cineangiography in the noninvasive evaluation of global and regional left ventricular function at rest and during exercise in patients with coronary artery disease. N Engl J Med 296:839, 1977
11. Steele PP, Kirch DL, LeFree M: Radionuclide angiocardiographic measurement of left ventricular volume and ejection fraction. Chest 69:672, 1976
12. Olson HG, Lyons KP, Aronow WS, et al: Follow-up technetium-99m stannous pyrophosphate myocardial scintigraphy after acute myocardial infarction. Circulation 56:181, 1977

17

ECHOCARDIOGRAPHIC EVIDENCE OF CARDIAC ABNORMALITIES

Nathaniel Reichek, M.D.

Echocardiography displays intracardiac valvular and myocardial structures in motion with excellent temporal and spatial resolution. Temporal and axial resolution (distance from the chest wall) are particularly good for M-mode strip chart recordings (1,000 samples per second, axial resolution 1 mm). Two-dimensional (2D) echocardiography (30 frames per second) complements M-mode by offering extensive tomographic images of cardiac structure. Consequently, echocardiography provides a wealth of physiologic information throughout the cardiac cycle in normal and diseased hearts. In this review we will confine our attention to selected echo phenomena that have dynamic pathophysiologic connotations and will not consider many other important morphologic abnormalities that are well covered in standard texts.[1]

Physiology and Clinical Manifestation of Valvular Abnormalities

THE AORTIC VALVE

Aortic valve motion in systole begins when left ventricular (LV) pressure rises to the level of end-diastolic aortic pressure. At that time, normal aortic valve leaflets move rapidly to full separation, which is maintained until LV ejection is complete (Fig. 17-1A). Within 10 msec to 20 msec after completion of forward flow across the aortic valve, isovolumic relaxation drops LV pressure sufficiently below aortic pressure to move the aortic leaflets rapidly back to their fully closed position. Leaflet position after the initial opening movement is heavily flow-dependent, and leaflet separation may be reduced whenever forward flow is impaired. This can occur early in systole in obstructive hypertrophic cardiomyopathy—idiopathic hypertrophic subaortic stenosis (IHSS) or obstructive asymmetric septal hypertrophy (ASH)—due to abrupt diminution or cessation of ejection flow at the onset of obstruction.[2] The result is a so-called spike and plateau pattern (Fig. 17-1B). The same pattern of leaflet motion is often found in fixed congenital subvalvular aortic stenosis due to a subvalve membrane or fibromuscular collar.[3] The mechanism of this leaflet motion abnormality must differ from that in hypertrophic cardiomyopathy with obstruction, since obstruction is presumably constant in fixed subvalvular stenosis, but detailed studies of LV outflow pressure and flow dynamics are lacking. In patients with severe myocardial dysfunction, the aortic leaflets may drift together in the latter part of systole, presumably due to a gradual decline in ejection velocity and flow (Fig. 17-1C).[4] This phenomenon is also common in severe mitral regurgitation.[5] In that setting, it is likely that the ratio of forward flow across the aortic valve to regurgitant flow back across the mitral valve becomes progressively lower during late systole. Regurgitant flow then continues after aortic valve closure, so that no real isovolumic relaxation period exists. All of these leaflet motion abnormalities are better appreciated on M-mode than on 2D echo studies.

In contrast, the systolic aortic valve motion abnormality produced by a congenitally bicuspid aortic valve is not readily appreciated on M-mode recordings because it occurs in a plane perpendicular to the M-mode beam, moving the valve leaflets superiorly in the aorta to produce a "doming" effect (Fig. 17-2).[6] This doming motion is readily identified on 2D long-axis images of the LV outflow tract and aorta, which can also roughly quantify the severity of stenosis, expressed as the leaflet separation at the valve orifice level.[7] The abrupt cessation of leaflet motion that occurs as the doming valve reaches its maximum superior excursion is responsible for generation of the ejection sound commonly produced by bicuspid valves. The wide excursion of the leaflets downward to a closed position at the time of aortic valve closure commonly leads to the preserved aortic second sound characteristic of noncalcified bicuspid stenotic valves. Other forms of aortic valve stenosis are associated with a marked diminution in leaflet motion that is readily identified by echo and that results in absence of an ejection sound and a soft or absent aortic closure sound. Calcific aortic stenosis in the elderly results from deposition on the aortic aspect of the valve leaflets of calcified atherosclerotic debris that, in severely stenotic valves, literally holds the leaflets in place. In milder instances, the process affects only the basal portions of the leaflets and results in a systolic murmur without obstruction (Fig. 17-3). A continuous spectrum of severity exists that is readily appreciated by 2D echo. Consequently, echo assessment of the aortic valve has become an essential part of the diagnostic assessment of the symptomatic older patient with a murmur suggestive of a diseased aortic valve.

Diastolic abnormalities of aortic leaflet motion are much less common than systolic abnormalities but are almost always associated with severe aortic regurgitation. Aortic valve prolapse can occur chronically in roughly 10% of subjects with myxomatous mitral valves and mitral prolapse.[8] This phenome-

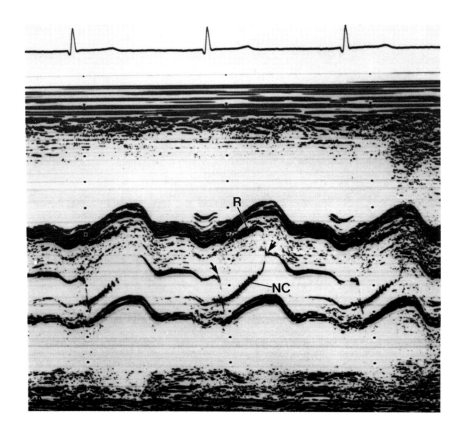

FIG. 17-1. M-mode echogram of normal aortic valve. The two leaflets seen are the right (*R*) and non-coronary (*NC*) cusps. The arrows denote the onset of valve opening and completion of valve closure respectively and thus represent the onset and end of left ventricular ejection. The aortic component of the second heart sound synchronizes with echographic valve closure. (*B*) Aortic valve motion from a patient with IHSS shows normal initial opening (*O*) followed by an abnormal systolic motion pattern with an early systolic reduction in leaflet separation (*arrow*), producing a "spike and plateau" pattern that closely parallels the systolic ejection pattern of rapid early ejection and diminished or absent mid- and late systolic ejection. (*C*) Normal aortic valve opening (*O*) is followed by late systolic drifting of the aortic leaflets toward each other (*arrow*) in this patient with mitral regurgitation.

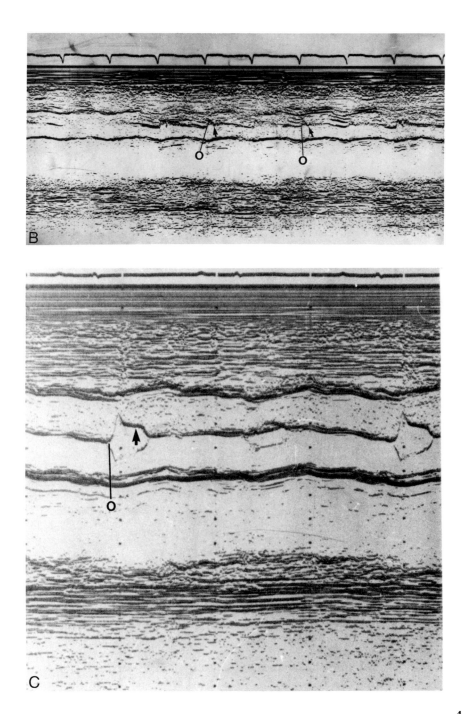

449

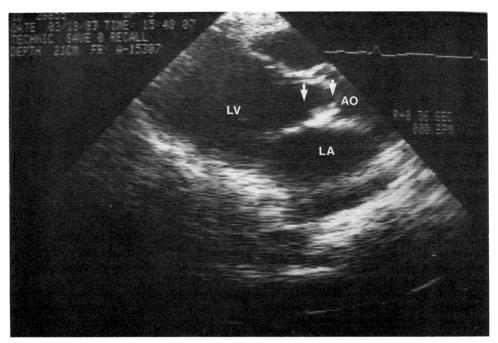

FIG. 17-2. Two-dimensional echo long-axis systolic image of the base of the aorta (*AO*), left atrium (*LA*) and left ventricle (*LV*) in a patient with a doming bicuspid aortic valve. Left arrow denotes the diastolic position of aortic leaflet echoes. Right arrow points to the more cephalad systolic position of the leaflet tips and valve orifice.

non is characterized by the appearance on M-mode recordings of leaflet echoes in diastole in the LV outflow tract without any gross distortion of the temporal pattern of coordination of aortic leaflet motion. In contrast, a "flail" aortic valve leaflet due to endocarditis or noninfective aortic leaflet rupture usually produces a pattern of diastolic flutter of the aortic valve due to the associated high-velocity jet of aortic regurgitation.[9] In the extreme form, the affected leaflet extends linearly into the LV outflow tract. Because of vegetations, the "flail" leaflet may have a lumpy appearance (Fig. 17-4). Other causes of aortic regurgitation are not associated with this finding.[10]

MITRAL VALVE

By far the most common systolic abnormality of mitral valve motion is mitral valve prolapse. M-mode and 2D echo have become valuable tools for recognition and assessment of this phenomenon, but they have also added significantly to the confusion surrounding it. If one compares auscultatory, ventriculographic, M-mode echo, and 2D echo findings in a large population, the two largest subgroups are, first, one that is normal by all parameters and,

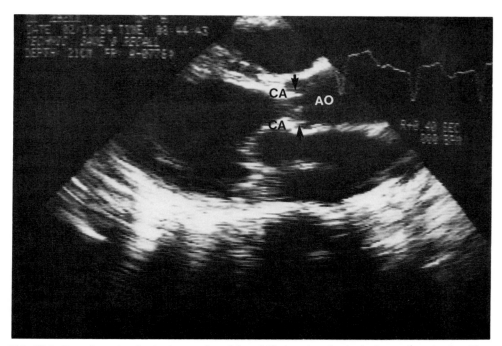

FIG. 17-3. Two-dimensional echo image of a mildly calcified aortic valve in the long-axis projection. The leaflets are denoted by arrows and show an increase in width and intensity due to calcification (*CA*) at their points of attachment to the walls of the aorta (*AO*).

second, one that is abnormal by all parameters. However, every possible combination of positive and negative findings appears in a significant proportion of the population. For this reason, among others, it may be best to regard mitral prolapse as a phenomenon rather than a disease.

On M-mode echocardiography, normal mitral valve motion during systole consists of a straight line sloping gradually anteriorly from the point of closure of the mitral leaflets (Fig. 17-5, point C) at the time of the first heart sound (S_1) to leaflet separation (Fig. 17-5, point D) at the end of isovolumic relaxation. Mitral valve prolapse produces a concave posterior displacement of the systolic valve plane that may begin with systole ("holosystolic sagging") or at any time thereafter, but always persists until point D is reached (Fig. 17-6). Posterior deflection of the valve must be at least 3 mm in magnitude to be called mitral prolapse, according to a commonly accepted convention.[11] If a single systolic click is present in a patient with mitral prolapse, it most commonly aligns with the point of maximal posterior deflection of the valve plane. A late systolic murmur, when present, generally begins following the point of maximal deflection. At times, however, clicks are multiple, a single click does not time with M-mode valve movement, or a click is present without M-mode prolapse. All of these phenomena probably reflect the multiplicity of potential sources of clicks in a prolapsing valve and the limitations on the M-mode method's

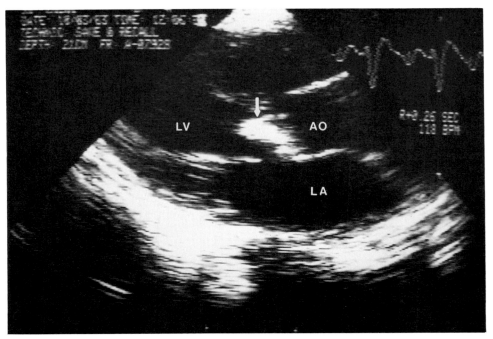

FIG. 17-4. Two-dimensional diastolic long-axis view of the aorta (*AO*), left atrium (*LA*), left ventricle (*LV*). Arrow points to a prolapsing aortic valve vegetation that lies in the LV outflow tract.

ability to sample the valve surface. Each segment of leaflet between chordal insertions comprises a potential source of prolapse, but only a few of these segments in the center of the leaflets are demonstrated on M-mode recording. Indeed, it is surprising that the M-mode method is at all useful in assessment of prolapse, since the principal direction of motion of prolapsing valve segments is actually not posterior, but superior, out of the M-mode beam. It is possible to demonstrate this superior motion on 2D echo images, particularly in the long-axis, four-chamber, and two-chamber views. However, the prolapse motion itself is relatively subtle and the patterns of motion possible are complex and variable. Surprisingly, the prominence of echocardiographic prolapse by either M-mode or 2D echo does not correlate well with the hemodynamic severity of valve dysfunction. Often, echo evidence of prolapse is minimal in subjects with severe mitral regurgitation but striking in subjects with little or no mitral regurgitation. Like other expressions of the prolapse phenomenon, echo prolapse is exquisitely sensitive to variations in LV volume. The prolapse phenomenon can occur only if the surface area of leaflet tissue available to obstruct the mitral orifice exceeds the area of that orifice. Since leaflet area is constant, reductions in LV volume increase the surplus of leaflet tissue and promote more marked prolapse or allow prolapse to occur earlier in the cardiac cycle. Consequently, echo manifestations of prolapse, like auscultatory manifestations, are exaggerated, or even elicited for the first time, by Valsalva's

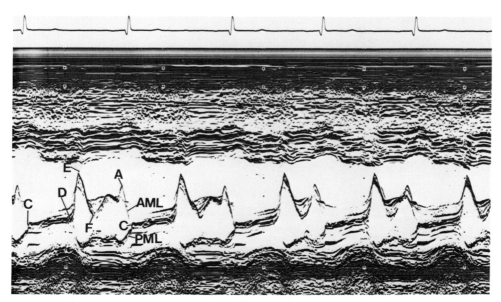

FIG. 17-5. M-mode echogram of a normal mitral valve. Point *C* indicates the time of systolic apposition of the anterior (*AML*) and posterior (*PML*) mitral leaflets. Point *D* denotes the time of early diastolic leaflet separation. Between points *C* and *D*, leaflet motion during systole is gradually anterior and roughly linear. Point *E* represents the time of peak separation of the leaflets during the early diastolic rapid filling phase. Point *F* represents the end of the rapid filling period. Point *A* represents the maximal reopening of the leaflets by atrial systole. The posterior mitral leaflet (*PML*) moves in a shallow mirror image of the anterior leaflet motion.

maneuver, upright posture, administration of amyl nitrite, or occurrence of hypovolemia of any cause.[12]

A second type of systolic motion abnormality of the mitral valve is that due to chordal rupture.[13] Although much less common than mitral prolapse, this finding is often of great clinical importance because it provides the commonest anatomical basis for the hemodynamics of acute severe mitral regurgitation. Chordal rupture often occurs in the setting of long-standing mitral prolapse with severe myxomatous leaflet changes, but it can also occur as a result of endocarditis or, occasionally, in the absence of any evident underlying cause. The motion pattern produced by chordal rupture actually includes both diastolic and systolic components. The systolic motion pattern includes a very dramatic asymmetric superior protrusion of a convex segment of one leaflet into the left atrium, which is well seen on 2D long-axis and apical four-chamber views. It may not be visible on M-mode, presumably because a posterior component to the motion is lacking. A second common feature on 2D views is linear protrusion of a portion of chordal and leaflet tissue into the left atrium. Diastolic motion abnormalities due to chordal rupture are better seen on M-mode because of their dynamic nature and short duration. When the posterior mitral leaflet is involved, the first abnormality seen is often abrupt anterior

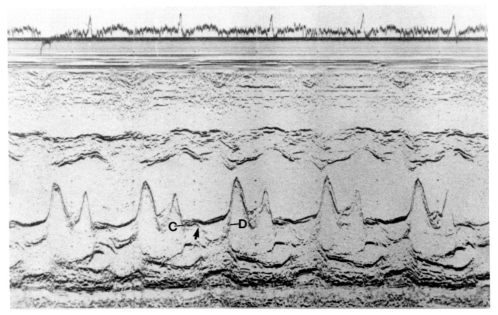

FIG. 17-6. Late systolic mitral valve prolapse (*arrow*) begins well after point *C*. The valve plane moves initially in the expected straight-line anterior motion of a normal valve but then moves posteriorly and remains posterior to that imaginary line until valve opening begins at point *D*.

early diastolic motion, followed by irregular oscillating motion of the unsupported tissue later in diastole (Fig. 17-7). The anterior motion occasionally may make differentiating chordal rupture from rheumatic disease difficult. Anterior leaflet chordal rupture produces a low-frequency flutter due to lack of leaflet tethering (Fig. 17-8). This can occasionally be difficult to distinguish from the coarse variety of leaflet flutter seen in a small proportion of patients with aortic regurgitation

Chordal rupture can produce acute severe mitral regurgitation with severe left atrial (LA) and pulmonary hypertension. In this disorder, clinical findings may be deceptively subtle: decrescendo systolic murmur, normal heart size, and tachycardia. Echo findings other than the abnormal mitral valve motion are also nonspecific. Thus, the echo feature can be decisive in clinical appraisal of the patient. Chordal rupture also occurs in a substantial proportion of patients with chronic severe mitral regurgitation due to myxomatous valves. In this setting, it usually has no specific clinical or physiologic correlates. Occasionally, there are clearcut, abrupt changes in auscultatory findings or symptoms that may be attributable to an episode of acute chordal rupture superimposed on chronic mitral regurgitation.

Systolic anterior motion of the anterior leaflet of the mitral valve (SAM) is the phenomenon that produces obstruction to the left ventricular outflow tract in IHSS, also commonly called obstructive ASH. Echocardiographic SAM

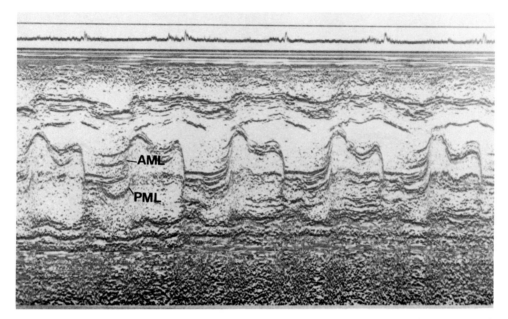

FIG. 17-7. Rupture of chordae tendineae to the posterior mitral leaflet (*PML*) results in disappearance of the normal mirror image pattern of PML relative to anterior mitral leaflet (*AML*) motion in diastole. Instead, the PML moves anteriorly in an erratic fashion.

(Fig. 17-9) correlates in severity with the degree of obstruction expressed as the pressure gradient across the outflow tract and is an essential diagnostic feature of obstructive ASH or IHSS.[14-16] The mechanism of SAM is thought to be a Bernoulli effect. In ASH, the small size of the LV cavity and the prominence of the septum narrow the LV outflow tract even without SAM. Ejection from the left ventricle in ASH is faster than normal in the absence of SAM or prior to the onset of SAM.[17] The combination of a narrow outflow tract and a high velocity of early ejection drops pressure in the outflow tract by the Bernoulli principle, creating a pressure gradient across the free edge of the anterior leaflet and its chordae that propels them into the outflow tract, resulting in SAM and consequent obstruction.

The presence and degree of SAM on echo can be used to subset patients with ASH into nonobstructive ASH, ASH with provocable obstruction, and obstructive ASH. In ASH with provocable obstruction, any intervention that reduces LV volume or increases ejection velocity (such as Valsalva's maneuver, administration of amyl nitrite, or isoproterenol) will increase the severity of SAM and, in parallel, elicit a pressure gradient across the LV outflow tract below the aortic valve. Conversely, interventions that increase LV volume or slow ejection reduce SAM and the intraventricular gradient. SAM is detected more readily on M-mode than on 2D echo, in most instances, because the relatively slow frame rate of 2D echo often does not capture the quick motion of the anterior leaflet tip and chordae toward the septum.

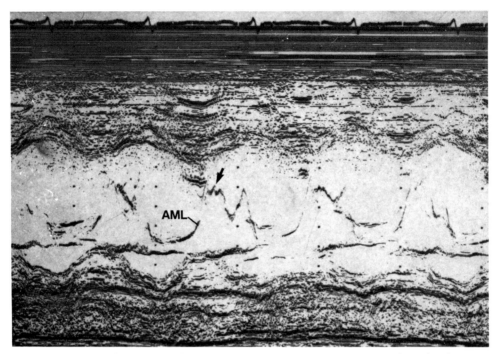

FIG. 17-8. Rupture of chordae tendineae to the anterior mitral leaflet (*AML*) results in low-frequency diastolic flutter (*arrow*) that is much slower than the high-frequency flutter produced by aortic regurgitation (see Fig. 17-11).

The timing and severity of SAM correlate well with the physical findings in obstructive ASH. The bifid systolic contour of both the arterial pulse contour and the LV impulse immediately follow the onset of SAM if the SAM is severely obstructive and brings the anterior leaflet tip and chordae close to the septum. Systolic murmur intensity and duration also correlate with the timing and severity of SAM, although the relative contribution to the murmur of mitral regurgitation, which is produced by abnormal anterior leaflet position, and ejection turbulance remains unclear. It is clear that the typical murmur can occur if SAM is marked in the absence of angiographic mitral regurgitation.

Normal diastolic mitral valve motion is entirely a passive phenomenon that directly reflects the volume and rate of transmitral flow and LV filling. The initial opening motion of the valve (see Fig. 17-5, D–E) occurs during the latter part of isovolumic relaxation, when LV pressure falls to a level below that present in the left atrium. Thus, the initial DE velocity is a function of the rate of fall of LV pressure, end-systolic LA pressure, and the minimal level of early diastolic LV pressure. Abnormally slow DE motion is usually seen in association with marked elevation of early diastolic LV pressure and extreme degrees of LV dysfunction.[18]

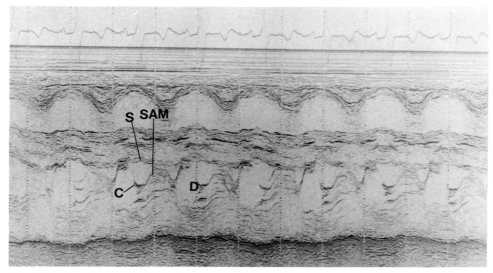

FIG. 17-9. M-mode mitral valve echogram, showing systolic anterior motion (*SAM*) due to idiopathic hypertrophic subaortic stenosis (IHSS). During systole (between points *C* and *D*), in contrast to the gradual linear anterior movement of the normal mitral valve, valve echoes in IHSS show prominent convex SAM toward the left side of the interventricular septum (*S*), producing a pressure gradient within the outflow tract of the left ventricle.

The position of the mitral anterior leaflet at point E (see Fig. 17-5) relative to the interventricular septum is a function of the size of the diastolic flow column from left atrium into left ventricle relative to the size of the ventricle. In normal left ventricles, the separation of the E point of the anterior leaflet from the septum is ordinarily 5 mm or less. However, when LV function is depressed significantly, the size of the diastolic flow stream is generally reduced and the E-point septal separation increases.[19] In the absence of severe aortic or mitral regurgitation, a separation or more than 1 cm is a reliable marker for a reduced systolic ejection fraction.

The early diastolic motion of the mitral valve from point E to point F (see Fig. 17-5) correlates well with the rate of filling of the left ventricle and is thought to be due to lifting of the leaflets toward a closed position by swirling eddy currents of inflowing blood.[20-22] In the early development of echocardiography, it was believed that reduction in the EF slope, or velocity , which was one of the few intracardiac phenomena readily identified in early studies, was specific for mitral stenosis. It is clear, however, that reduced rates of LV early diastolic filling of any cause can lessen the EF slope. As in many areas of echocardiography, there are several possible ways of determining the EF slope, so that it is advisable for each laboratory to develop its own range of normal values. The commonest cause of reduced EF velocity in most settings is actually reduced LV diastolic distensibility associated with elevated LV diastolic pressure and reduced stroke volume, or concentric hypertrophy with normal systolic function. However, pericardial disease, hypovolemia, and even primary right heart dysfunction can all cause this abnormality.

The mitral valve reopens from point F to point A (see Fig.17-5) following atrial systole, which not only raises LA and LV pressure, but propels roughly 20% of the normal stroke volume across the mitral valve. Although numerous efforts have been made to relate the magnitude of mitral valve opening due to atrial systole to diastolic left heart dynamics, no meaningful relationships have been defined. However, studies of the closing motion, from point A to point C, during atrial relaxation and the early portion of isovolumic LV contraction have been more fruitful. The normal closing motion of the valve is continuous and uninterrupted. However, when the hemodynamic A wave due to atrial systole is large (8 mm Hg or more) and LV end-diastolic pressure is elevated, a more complex multiphasic closing motion is found (Fig. 17-10).[18] The interruption or plateau in the middle of the closing motion of the valve has been given several names, including "AC shoulder" and "B bump." Efforts have been made also to generate a quantitative index of LV end-diastolic pressure by measuring the duration of the AC interval and subtracting it from the P–R interval on the electrocardiogram. In general, however, it is more reliable in the individual case to rely on the presence or absence of the contour

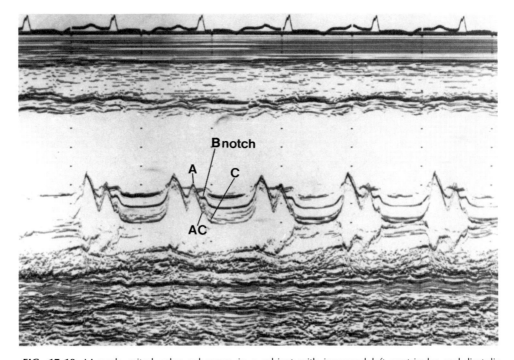

FIG. 17-10. M-mode mitral valve echogram in a subject with increased left ventricular end-diastolic pressure associated with a large atrial systolic pressure wave demonstrates an "AC shoulder" (*AC*). Between points *A* and *C*, the normal mitral valve closure (see Fig. 17-5) is a smooth continuous linear movement. Here, in contrast, the brief plateau of the AC shoulder (or "B notch") interrupts the *AC* line.

abnormality rather than on interval measurement. It is possible, however, to see relatively similar motion high up on the normal anterior leaflet, near the leaflet insertion into the aorta. Thus, it is necessary to look for the motion abnormality at the leaflet tips, or where both leaflets are seen and come together at point C on the M-mode echo. All of the hemodynamically determined mitral valve diastolic motion abnormalities can be found on 2D echo studies. However, it is generally much easier to evaluate them on the M-mode recording because of its better temporal display.

Diastolic mitral valve flutter is a high-frequency oscillating movement that can be seen in a variety of settings. The commonest is aortic regurgitation (Fig. 17-11).[23] In this setting, flutter of the anterior mitral leaflet and, in some instances, the left side of the interventricular septum is produced by the turbulent regurgitant jet of blood returning from the aorta to the left ventricle in diastole. At times, the posterior mitral leaflet may also flutter in aortic regurgitation. This abnormality can serve as a qualitative marker for aortic regurgitation but does not give an indication of the severity of the disorder. When the left side of the septum is also fluttering, the finding is specific for aortic regurgitation. However, as discussed above, flutter of the mitral anterior leaflet or both leaflets can be seen in ruptured chordae tendineae, where it is generally coarser in frequency than in aortic regurgitation. It is also found occasionally in other disorders that result in extremely high-velocity diastolic flow antegrade across the mitral valve, such as ventricular septal defect, chronic severe mitral regurgitation without ruptured chordae, and even severe anemia. The flutter in these settings, like that in aortic regurgitation, is generally high in frequency. In these disorders, the turbulence that produces mitral leaflet flutter also commonly results in a diastolic flow rumble. Because flutter is usually a high-frequency event, it is usually seen more readily on M-mode than on 2D echo images. It should also be stressed that the absence of diastolic

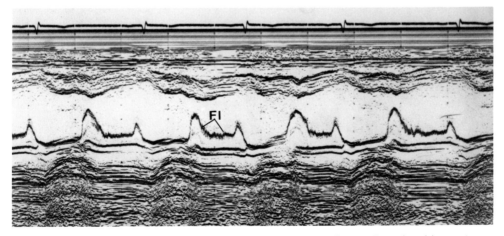

FIG. 17-11. Mitral valve echogram showing diastolic high-frequency flutter (*Fl*) produced by aortic regurgitation. Flutter is produced by the turbulent regurgitant jet striking the anterior leaflet. Contrast this fine, high-frequency flutter with the coarser flutter produced by anterior chordal rupture (see Fig. 17-8).

flutter does not exclude the presence of aortic regurgitation, since the regurgitant jet does not always impinge on the anterior leaflet.

Premature closure of the mitral valve, prior to the onset of ventricular contraction (Fig. 17-12) is an extremely important and specific abnormality. Virtually the only disorder that produces this finding is acute severe aortic regurgitation of the most hemodynamically severe type.[24] To obtain premature closure, LV diastolic pressure must exceed LA pressure. In acute severe aortic regurgitation, reflux of a large volume of blood into a left ventricle that is normal or near-normal in size can produce the rapid, marked elevation of LV pressure required. At times, LV diastolic pressure exceeds 45 mm Hg. This phenomenon is rare in chronic aortic regurgitation and not found in other disorders. The presence of premature closure in patients with acute severe aortic regurgitation identifies those who form a high-risk subset and is probably an adequate basis for determining that aortic valve replacement is required. This can be very helpful clinically, since the clinical manifestations of acute aortic regurgitation can be quite unimpressive, even in hemodynamically severe instances. Thus, as diastolic LV pressure becomes abnormal with worsening regurgitation, the murmur may get softer and shorter. The only other

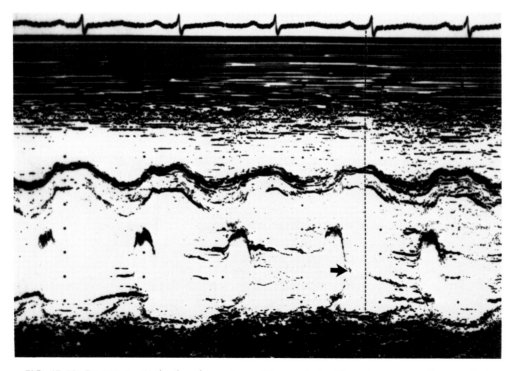

FIG. 17-12. Premature mitral valve closure (*arrow*) in a patient with acute severe aortic regurgitation. Valve closure normally follows the QRS onset (*dashed line*) by at least 50 msec. Here, in contrast, valve closure occurs well before the QRS onset.

bedside finding noted by the inexperienced examiner may be tachycardia and a third heart sound (S_3). More experienced observers, however, will usually note that S_1 is soft or absent when premature closure is noted echocardiographically, and that the S_3 actually introduces a mid-diastolic Austin Flint rumble. Echophonocardiographic studies have been helpful in elucidating the mechanism and physiologic significance of the Austin Flint diastolic murmur. It appears that the rumble is generated by continuing antegrade flow across the mitral valve, presumably as a result of inertial forces, at a time when pressure increase in the ventricle is closing the mitral orifice. Thus, a presystolic rumble is generally associated with mild or incomplete premature closure, which is associated with less severe hemodynamic changes, while a mid-diastolic Austin Flint rumble is associated with earlier, more complete premature closure and more severe hemodynamic abnormalities.

Rheumatic mitral valves generate a constellation of motion abnormalities, some of which are characteristic but not entirely specific. The only abnormalities that are specific relate to the effects of commissural fusion on mitral valve motion. Commissural fusion is a unique and characteristic feature of rheumatic valves, not found in other disorders. On M-mode echocardiography, commissural fusion results in reversal of the direction of posterior leaflet diastolic motion (Fig. 17-13).[25] It is believed that the reversal is due to the fact that the anterior leaflet is longer than the posterior leaflet. When the two are coupled, elevated LA pressure exerts rotational torque on both leaflets, but the greater length of the anterior leaflet results in a greater angular moment, which pulls the posterior leaflet along in the direction of anterior leaflet opening motion. Occasionally, this M-mode abnormality is mimicked by the chaotic diastolic motion produced by posterior chordal rupture or even by mitral prolapse without chordal rupture. The inexperienced echocardiographer may mistake the passive diastolic motion of a calcified mitral annulus for rheumatic posterior leaflet motion, particularly if the EF slope is also abnormal. On 2D echo, the abnormal direction of posterior leaflet motion is less readily appreciated. Commissural fusion, however, can be seen directly in the short-axis view (Fig. 17-14). On 2D echo in the long-axis view it is also possible to appreciate the way that commissural fusion turns the mitral apparatus into a truncated pyramid in diastole, with the narrow end at the mitral orifice. When the anterior leaflet is not greatly shortened and thickened, it billows anteriorly above the true rheumatic mitral orifice, which is at the leaflet tip level (Fig. 17-15). This bowed diastolic shape of the anterior leaflet is quite characteristic of the rheumatic valve. In contrast, reduced mitral leaflet excursion, abnormal EF slope, and leaflet thickening are nonspecific findings commonly observed in mitral stenosis. Recent studies have demonstrated convincingly that the EF slope is not a reliable indicator of the severity of mitral stenosis. This is hardly surprising in view of the hemodynamic determinants of the EF motion discussed above. Fortunately, 2D echo permits direct determination of the size of the mitral orifice in mitral stenosis, so that the unreliability of the EF slope is no longer of clinical consequence.[26]

M-mode and 2D echo can demonstrate many of the variations in mitral valve morphology and function that relate to physical findings and operative approach. A valve that shows echocardiographically that stenosis is due mainly

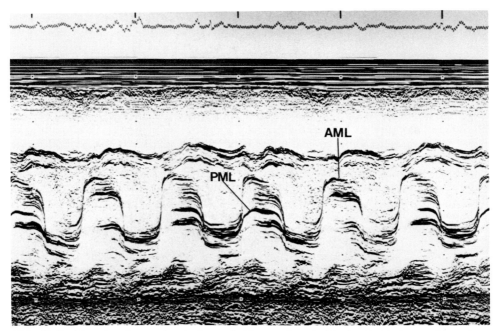

FIG. 17-13. M-mode echogram in mitral stenosis. The anterior mitral leaflet (*AML*) shows a flat EF slope, absence of an A wave despite persistence of normal sinus rhythm, and a multiplicity of echoes. The posterior mitral leaflet (*PML*) shows multiple dense echoes and moves in an anterior direction during diastole, in contrast to its normal mirror-image motion relative to the anterior leaflet (see Fig. 17-5).

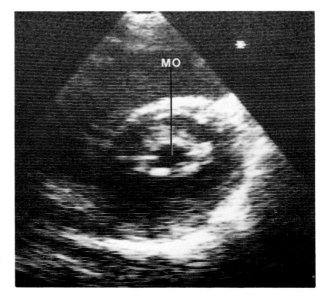

FIG. 17-14. Short-axis two-dimensional echogram showing the open mitral orifice (*MO*) in early diastole. The lateral edges of the mitral orifice are produced by fusion of the commissures of the mitral leaflets.

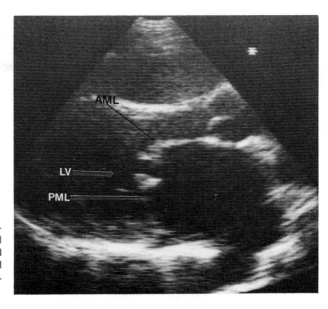

FIG. 17-15. Long-axis two-dimensional echo stop frame of the mitral valve in diastole. The anterior mitral leaflet (*AML*) and posterior mitral leaflet (*PML*) bow into the left ventricle (*LV*).

to commissural fusion, with little shortening of the anterior leaflet and thickening limited to the leaflet tips, will have a large excursion of the bowed body of the anterior leaflet in diastole. In turn, the abrupt checking of this large excursion produces a loud opening snap. Reversal of this excursion during mitral valve closure results in a loud S_1. In the absence of mitral regurgitation, such a valve is ideally suited to repair, by mitral valvotomy, rather than replacement. Since the perioperative risk and long-term outlook are somewhat more favorable for patients undergoing valvotomy than those undergoing valve replacement, the echo findings can play an important role in the decision-making process.

Conversely, echocardiographic findings of diffuse anterior leaflet and chordal thickening and markedly restricted motion in a rheumatic valve are associated with a soft opening snap and S_1 and a valve that is unsuited for valvotomy. Such valves are more likely to be incompetent as well as stenotic. Furthermore, since the opening snap is soft or absent, the clinician may fail to appreciate the presence of mitral stenosis in this setting, particularly if the patient presents in rapid atrial fibrillation and the diastolic murmur is difficult to hear.

TRICUSPID VALVE

The tricuspid valve can become myxomatous and prolapse, like the mitral valve. Because M-mode echo can sample only very limited portions of the tricuspid apparatus, 2D echo is far superior for demonstration of tricuspid prolapse.[27] Severe tricuspid regurgitation due to prolapse is uncommon in the absence of severe chronic mitral regurgitation. When severe chronic mitral regurgitation is present, determining the relative contributions of tricuspid prolapse and ordinary functional tricuspid regurgitation is quite difficult.

When RV diastolic pressure is elevated with an abnormally large A wave, the tricuspid valve also develops a "B bump" or "AC shoulder". Unfortunately, since this phenomenon is difficult to recognize on 2D, and M-mode shows only small portions of the tricuspid valve, this finding is often not demonstrated even in the presence of the appropriate physiologic abnormality. It is possible that M-mode data selected from a 2D apical image would be the best index of this phenomenon.

The rheumatic tricuspid valve shows leaflet thickening, reduction of the EF slope, and reduced excursion.[28] In some instances, abnormal diastolic motion of the septal leaflet, presumably analogous to abnormal mitral posterior leaflet motion, can be found. Two-dimensional echo gives a more complete image of the rheumatic tricuspid valve, but more specific descriptions have not been defined. However, since other causes of tricuspid valve thickening and reduced mobility are rare, and since tricuspid stenosis always occurs in the setting of mitral stenosis, the diagnosis can be made reliably. The echo findings in tricuspid stenosis are of great value to the clinician because, in most instances, the physical findings in patients with mitral and tricuspid stenosis provide few clues to the presence of tricuspid stenosis, particularly if atrial fibrillation is present. A second opening snap is rare and a tricuspid rumble is frequently obscured by the mitral diastolic rumble. Tricuspid regurgitation is usually present, but because most subjects have pulmonary hypertension due to mitral disease, the findings are usually indistinguishable from those of functional tricuspid regurgitation in mitral stenosis. Only a slow Y descent in the jugular venous pulse is commonly found. If the patient is in sinus rhythm, a large jugular venous A wave with unimpressive evidence of pulmonary hypertension in the RV impulse and pulmonic second sound can be of assistance.

It should also be pointed out that the cardiac catheterization laboratory can easily overlook tricuspid stenosis, particularly in atrial fibrillation, unless it is specifically sought. The gradient in diastole is small and can be unrecognized on pullback pressure recordings, particularly in atrial fibrillation, so that simultaneous RA and RV pressure recordings are required. Often, echo findings suggestive of tricuspid stenosis will be the clue that leads to this approach.

PULMONIC VALVE

The normal pulmonic valve in the adult is difficult to image, in many instances. On M-mode, only the posterior leaflet is usually recorded (Fig. 17-16). The characteristic normal pattern of motion consists of 1 mm to 5 mm of posterior motion in presystole due to the distention of the right ventricle by the RA A wave. The valve then opens quickly, and the posterior leaflet gradually drifts anteriorly during ejection and posteriorly in early diastole. In compensated pulmonary hypertension, the valve A wave is usually diminished or absent.[29] However, if RV filling pressure is markedly elevated and the RA A wave is large, the valve A wave can reappear. The opening velocity of the valve increases in pulmonary hypertension but is difficult to

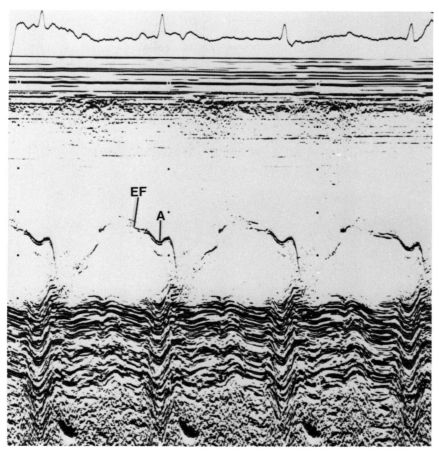

FIG. 17-16. M-mode echogram of normal pulmonic valve motion shows the EF slope (*EF*), A wave produced by right atrial contraction (*A*) and rapid systolic opening motion of the posterior valve leaflet.

measure accurately because of its short duration. In systole, the pulmonary hypertensive valve usually shows a W-shaped motion pattern, with midsystolic partial closure and late systolic reopening. The mechanism of the pattern is not well understood. In early diastole, the hypertensive pulmonic valve tends to drift posteriorly more slowly than normal. None of these findings are entirely specific or highly sensitive. However, the full constellation is a helpful guide to the presence of pulmonary hypertension.

M-mode pulmonic valve motion can provide additional useful information in congenital heart disease. In pulmonic stenosis, the valve A wave can be augmented, since the RA A wave increases in size. On 2D echo, doming of the stenotic valve, analogous to the doming of a stenotic bicuspid aortic valve, can be seen. This motion accounts for the characteristic pulmonic ejection sound. Its respiratory variation is due to the normal inspiratory increase in venous return, which, when combined with a vigorous RA systole, can move the valve to its domed position in presystole.

The pulmonic valve echogram can be used with a simultaneous electrocardiogram to determine RV systolic time intervals, and these can be helpful in assessing pulmonary hypertension in congenital heart disease.[30]

Alterations in Cardiac Chamber Size and Wall Thickness

LEFT VENTRICLE

Although the morphology of the left ventricle is generally treated as static, descriptive information, the morphology actually represents an extremely important pathophysiologic adaptive mechanism in many forms of chronic heart disease, including all forms of LV pressure and volume overload and congestive cardiomyopathy.

In chronic LV systolic pressure overload, whether due to systemic hypertension, aortic valve stenosis, or fixed subvalvular or supravalvular obstruction, the major long-term compensatory mechanism is concentric hypertrophy.[31] By keeping LV volume normal and increasing the thickness of the walls to the left ventricle, concentric hypertrophy permits each unit of myocardium to function under normal loading conditions for an extended period of time. In the compensated phase, which may last for years, there is a direct quantitative relationship between the ratio of LV myocardial mass to chamber volume and the ambient level of LV systolic presusre. The relationship can be simply assessed by examination either of the ratio of LV wall thickness to radius on M-mode echo (*relative wall thickness* or *h/r ratio*), or of the ratio of myocardial area to chamber area on 2D echo. In normal hearts, the relative wall thickness is closely regulated at both end-systole and end-diastole. When LV pressure rises, this ratio increases throughout the cardiac cycle (Fig. 17-17). Numerous studies have demonstrated that in congenital aortic stenosis, in which LV systolic function is generally excellent, the end-systolic or end-diastolic relative wall thickness is a good predictor of LV pressure.[32,33] In adults, the end-systolic relative wall thickness correlates less closely with LV systolic pressure, probably because the contractile state is more variable.[34] However, the end-diastolic relative wall thickness remains a useful rough guide to LV systolic pressure.[35] The mean normal value (calculated as posterior wall thickness divided by one-half the LV M-mode diameter) is 0.33 ± 0.06. A value of 0.45 is predictive of an LV pressure of 140 mm Hg or more, while a value of 0.50 generally correlates with a pressure of 180 mm Hg or more. Exceptions are due mainly to treated hypertension or to aortic regurgitation, which, even in its compensated stages, is often associated with mild afterload excess, resulting in a low relative wall thickness for any level of pressure.[36] It may seem odd that end-diastolic measurements relate so closely to a systolic

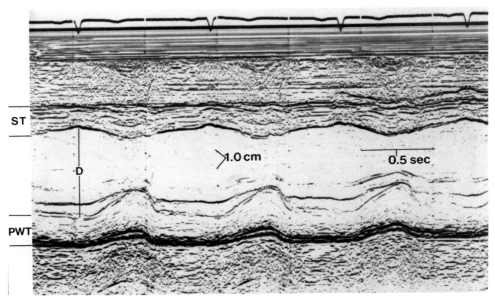

FIG. 17-17. Left ventricular echogram in a patient with aortic stenosis. The ventricular diameter (*D*) is normal in both systole and diastole, but both posterior wall thickness (*PWT*) and septal thickness (*ST*) are increased by concentric hypertrophy. Vertical calibration dots are separated by 1 cm. Horizontal separation of calibration dots is 0.5 sec.

load abnormality. However, the end-diastolic values of wall thickness and diameter are very close to those that occur at the time of peak wall stress, which occurs very early in systole and is believed to be a major regulator of concentric hypertrophy.[31] The concentric hypertrophy pattern also explains the characteristic findings on palpation and ausculation of the precordium in chronic pressure overload. The increase in relative wall thickness reduces the distensibility of the left ventricle, resulting in a compensatory increase in the forcefulness of atrial systole, which results in the palpable "A kick" and audible fourth heart sound. The increase in wall thickness with normal chamber volume in compensated pressure overload produces the characteristic systolic impulse, which is not displaced and is only slightly larger than normal, but which is much more forceful and sustained than normal.

When clinical manifestations of heart failure develop in LV pressure overload, examination of the LV size and relative wall thickness can provide important insights into the pathophysiology of the individual patient. In many instances, it is mainly diastolic failure that has occurred. The left ventricle is thick-walled, is normal in size, and shows normal systolic function. In this setting, afterload reduction in hypertensive heart disease may have relatively limited immediate benefits, since systolic function is normal.[37] In the long term, however, LV systolic pressure reduction can lead to a reduction in hypertrophy and, presumably, to restoration of more normal diastolic function. Conversely, cautious preload reduction may be immediately beneficial because it addresses the direct consequence of diastolic dysfunction, elevated pulmonary venous pressure. However, preload reduction must be used in such hearts with great caution, since it can easily result in excessively reduced LV systolic pressure if it is sufficient to actually reduce LV myocardial end-diastolic length.

A more marked stage of ventricular dysfunction in pressure overload occurs when the matching of relative wall thickness to pressure begins to fail. The ventricle then usually dilates and becomes inappropriately thin for its pressure and diameter. In this setting, the mechanical force generated by each unit of myocardium must increase dramatically, resulting in so-called afterload excess or, to express it another way, inadequate hypertrophy. In this setting, even if the contractile state of the myocardium remained normal, systolic function would be impaired. The clinical correlate is often more marked clinical heart failure, including, in many instances, right heart dysfunction, as a result of pulmonary hypertension. At the bedside, the patient with aortic stenosis in this phase will, as a result of reduced LV stroke volume, have obscured physical findings. The arterial pulse becomes so small in amplitude that the characteristic contour of aortic stenosis is not detectable. The apical impulse becomes enlarged and displaced. The reduced ejection velocity results in shortening of the systolic murmur, pulmonic closure becomes accentuated, and mitral regurgitation and even tricuspid regurgitation may appear. It is easy to mistake such a constellation of findings for a disorder other than aortic stenosis unless the presence of a calcified stenotic aortic valve is known from echo results. Another important clue is the increase in absolute wall thickness found on the ventricular echogram, even though the relative wall thickness is lower than would ordinarily result from the degree of pressure overload present if the patient had compensated LV function.

In contrast to pressure overload, LV volume overload, due, for example, to aortic or mitral regurgitation, invokes a chronic adaptive mechanism that relies on magnification of the size of the left ventricle. In the compensated phase, the result is an increased LV volume and normal LV relative wall thickness and systolic function. Thus, the size of the chronically volume-loaded left ventricle can be used as a guide to the severity of the volume load. As a rule, increases in LV diameter above 6.0 cm by M-mode (top of the normal range is 5.4 cm) are to be expected in severe mitral or aortic regurgitation, and clinical decompensation is uncommon unless diameter is roughly 6.5 cm or more (Fig. 17-18). The largest diameters likely to be encountered are 8.0 cm to 9.0 cm. The range of LV diameter variation seems small on first inspection. However, LV volume is a function of the cube of these values, so that a diameter increase from 5.4 cm to 6.0 cm can result in a 37% increase in volume if LV shape remains constant.

The details of the volume overload hypertrophy adaptive response are influenced importantly by the type and etiology of volume overload. In mitral regurgitation, the left ventricle tends to become spherical relatively early, whereas in aortic regurgitation, only a slight change in the ratio of ventricular length to short-axis radius is evident in the compensated phase. A particular exception to the general case is found in rheumatic disease with predominant mitral regurgitation. Here the increase in LV volume tends to be more modest than in other forms of mitral regurgitation at a comparable hemodynamic

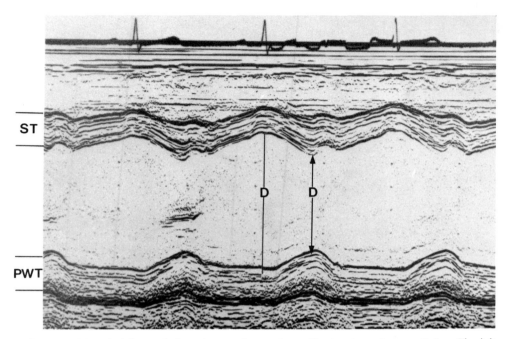

FIG. 17-18. M-mode left ventricular echogram in a patient with chronic aortic regurgitation. The left ventricular diameter (*D*) is markedly increased in diastole and systole and the percent systolic thicknesses (*PWT* and *ST*) are also increased, proportional to the increase in *D*. The result is "magnification hypertrophy".

phase. The reason for this lower increase is unclear, but it may in part result from the effect of scarring and fibrosis of the mitral apparatus and perhaps the ventricular endocardium itself in retarding dilatation. In any event, ventricular diameter rarely exceeds 6.0 cm in severe rheumatic mitral regurgitation. An alternative reason may be that even mild mitral stenosis raises LA pressure sufficiently so that the severity of mitral regurgitation required to produce a given degree of pulmonary hypertension and right heart dysfunction is much less than in mitral regurgitation due to myoxomatous mitral valve.

If the volume overload hypertrophy responses were perfectly adaptive, symptoms would never develop. However, the relative wall thickness begins to decline relatively early in the adaptive response, as has been found most clearly in aortic regurgitation.[36] The result is that hypertrophy is never fully adaptive and that afterload excess is built into the disorder. The degree of afterload excess, or, in other words, the inadequacy of hypertrophy, can be expressed as the relative wall thickness, but no quantitative guidelines are available for clinical application of the data as yet.

The volume overload adaptive response accounts for some of the principal physical findings, so that the echo data can predict the characteristic enlarged, displaced, dynamic, LA apical impulse that is the hallmark of severe LV volume overload at the bedside, as well as the dynamic filling pattern that results in a third heart sound and, often, the flow rumble of mitral regurgitation.

In congestive cardiomyopathy, LV enlargement and hypertrophy are important compensatory responses, but relative wall thickness falls to subnormal levels early in the disorder, resulting in marked increases in afterload, per unit of myocardium (Fig. 17-19). In contrast to volume overload, this more marked increase in afterload, combined with depressed contractile state, accounts for the fact that the enlarged, displaced, ventricular precordial impulse of congestive cardiomyopathy is hypodynamic.

Analysis of ventricular morphology is also of value in the recognition of restrictive cardiomyopathy when this is due to an infiltrative process, such as cardiac amyloidosis. In this setting, the infiltrative process results in an inappropriate increase in the relative wall thickness of the left ventricle in the absence of pressure overload and impaired diastolic wall thinning.[38] It can be distinguished from hypertrophic cardiomyopathy by the fact that ventricular systolic function, while often not markedly depressed, is not hyperdynamic as it often is in nonobstructive ASH.

Just as the presence of changes in LV size are important characteristics of chronic LV volume overload, the presence of a normal or minimally enlarged LV diameter is an important, albeit nonspecific, hallmark of acute aortic or mitral regurgitation. Because LV volume does not increase, cardiac output in acute volume overload cannot be maintained without tachycardia. Thus, the combination of normal or slightly increased LV diameter; normal or increased systolic function; persistent tachycardia; and specific echo features of either chordal rupture in mitral regurgitation or diastolic mitral and septal flutter, with or without premature closure, in aortic regurgitation, should lead to recognition of the acute volume overload syndrome.

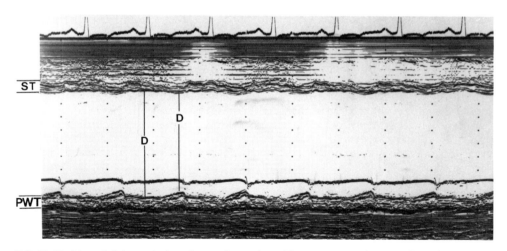

FIG. 17-19. M-mode left ventricular echogram in a patient with congestive cardiomyopathy. Left ventricular diameter (*D*) is increased at end-diastole and even more markedly increased at end-systole, so that percent systolic fractional shortening is quite depressed. PWT and ST are normal, so that they have not increased proportional to the increase in D.

LEFT ATRIUM

LA volume overload occurs as a result of either mitral regurgitation or an increase in pulmonary blood flow due to a central left-to-right shunt. In either instance, LA dilatation is likely to occur, usually more markedly in chronic mitral regurgitation. LA size has an important influence on pathophysiology, since, for a given degree of mitral regurgitation, for example, a smaller LA size will result in higher pulmonary venous and pulmonary arterial pressures. The extreme example of this occurs in acute severe mitral regurgitation, where LA V waves can approach the level of systemic arterial systolic pressure and extreme pulmonary arterial hypertension is the rule. In LA pressure overload, even in mitral stenosis, LA size tends to increase less than in volume overload, although extreme instances of LA enlargement can be seen occasionally. LA size can be readily assessed from the M-mode echo. However, it is important to realize that because LA shape can be quite asymmetric, multiple 2D image planes should be used to permit optimal assessment of LA size. LA volume determination appears to be feasible from biplane 2D echo, but most clinical studies to date have relied on the M-mode end-systolic LA diameter. LA size also influences the likelihood of atrial fibrillation and may be a predictor of the likelihood of restoring a given patient to sinus rhythm.

RIGHT VENTRICLE

In adults, three important constellations of RV morphologic change are relatively common. In compensated pulmonary hypertension, which is usually due to left heart disease, RV volume remains normal, but interventricular septal and RV free wall thickness increase as part of the concentric hypertrophy response. The increase in septal thickness can result in the echo appearance of nonobstructive ASH as a consequence of pulmonary hypertension. Adequate determination of RV free wall thickness from either parasternal M-mode or from 2D echo images is difficult and the finding is best demonstrated using a high frequency M-mode system (3.5 mHz–5 mHz) from the subcostal space.

Pulmonary hypertension often results in a more advanced stage of RV change that is characterized by dilatation of the chamber. This change can be associated with an obvious decrease in systolic function, as in the decompensated phase of aortic stenosis. RV decompensation also occurs in congestive cardiomyopathy, even with near-normal pulmonary artery pressure. It is also common for RV dilatation to result in tricuspid regurgitation. The low-pressure runoff available to the right ventricle in this setting can result in the echo pattern of a dilated right ventricle with normal percent ejection of RV volume. This RV volume overload pattern results in a reversal of normal interventricular septal curvature and systolic motion and can mask underlying ventricular dysfunction. The combination of RV dilatation and reversed septal motion, so that the septum moves anteriorly during systole, is quite specific for right heart volume overload and always requires a search for clinical correlates (Fig. 17-20).[39] If tricuspid regurgitation is absent, serious consideration should be given to the possibility of an unsuspected atrial septal defect or partial

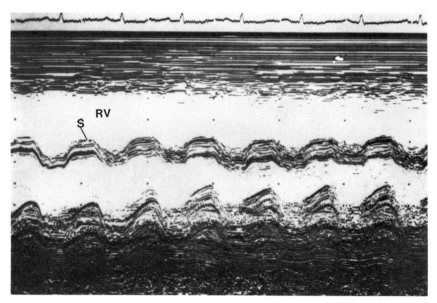

FIG. 17-20. M-mode echogram in a patient with right ventricular (*RV*) volume overload shows increased RV diameter and reversal of motion of the interventricular septum (*S*) so that it moves anteriorly during systole.

anomalous pulmonary venous return. The septal motion abnormality due to RV volume overload is actually the result of the abnormal diastolic position of the septum in this disorder, which causes loss of the normal septal curvature and displacement of the septum toward the left ventricle. In systole, the left ventricle regains a normal, circular cross-sectional shape, resulting in anterior displacement of the septum. Septal motion can become abnormal in ischemic heart disease because of intrinsic myocardial dysfunction,[40] which results in reduced systolic septal thickening; in RV volume overload, systolic thickening is normal. Another pattern of abnormal septal motion caused by a reversed excitation sequence in the septal myocardium, can be seen in left bundle branch block. The complex multiphasic pattern of leftward and posterior septal systolic motion produced by this abnormality, however, is readily distinguishable from that due to RV volume overload.[41] RV size and performance are best assessed echocardiographically by 2D imaging from the apical four-chamber or subcostal four-chamber projections. The M-mode does show an RV dimension, and it displays septal wall motion, but because of the complex shape of the right ventricle, it is not a good guide to overall RV size.

RIGHT ATRIUM

Increases in RA size occur early in compensated pulmonary hypertension, before RV enlargement.[42] RA volume overload due to either tricuspid regurgitation or atrial septal defect results in RA enlargement of more marked degree. The diagnosis of tricuspid regurgitation can be confirmed echocardiographically by contrast echo, with saline injection into an arm vein.[43] Microbubbles in the saline produce echoes that can be seen to fill the right atrium on 2D echo. If tricuspid regurgitation is present, some of the echoes will reflux into the inferior vena cava during systole. These can be imaged from the subcostal position with the transducer crossing the intrahepatic portion of the inferior vena cava. As always, use of M-mode information enhances the ability to time the appearance of contrast bubbles in the inferior vena cava. Since diastolic reflux can occur into the vena cava without tricuspid regurgitation, this is an important consideration.

Echo Indices of Global Ventricular Function

Echocardiographic indices of LV systolic function include M-mode percent reduction in LV diameter (%D), 2D echo ejection fraction, and M-mode mean and peak velocity of circumferential fiber shortening (VCF).[44–47] M-mode %D is analogous to ejection fraction, with certain important limitations. First, changes in the ratio of ventricular length to minor axis alter the relationship of %D to overall ejection fraction. Second, %D is determined from the diameter between the basal portions of the interventricular septum and the LV posterior wall. In settings that alter septal motion, such as RV volume overload, left bundle branch block, or prior cardiac surgery, %D is not a reliable index of ventricular function. In some disorders, such as aortic regurgitation, %D actually overestimates global function because the short-axis diameter between septum and posterior wall is shortened more than the diameter between the anterior and inferior walls of the ventricle. Finally, any segmental abnormality of myocardial function, such as those often present in ischemic heart disease, renders %D meaningless as an index of global function. Efforts to predict global ejection fraction from M-mode echo data have been generally discarded in favor of analysis of %D. In most laboratories, the lower limit of normal for %D is 26% to 28%.

In contrast to M-mode echo, 2D echo does permit estimation of LV ejection fraction with clinically useful results (Fig. 17-21). A variety of approaches have been devised that, in conjunction with biplane imaging and either Simpson's rule or area-length reconstruction, permit useful estimates of LV ejection fraction.[47–50] However, absolute LV chamber volume and mass can be assessed from 2D echo only after careful correction of systematic errors that result in reductions in the apparent ventricular cavity area and increases in the myocardial area.[51,52] Fortunately, correction can be done with simple calibration procedures.

VCF can be measured from either M-mode or 2D images and may be a more sensitive parameter of LV function than ejection fraction. Because of the relatively low frame rate, and the need for tedious manual image processing, 2D is less satisfactory than M-mode, which permits determination of both mean and peak instantaneous VCF values. It must be remembered that, like ejection fraction, VCF is an ejection phase index that is inherently load-dependent and is not a true "contractility" index. Thus, fluctuations in volume

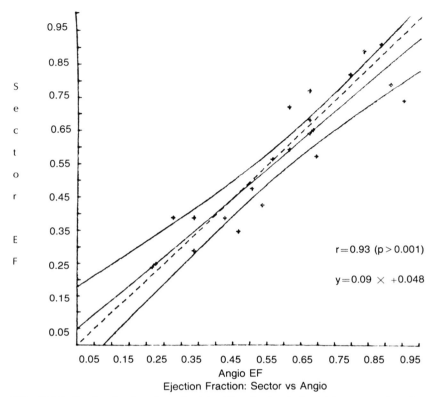

FIG. 17-21. Ejection fraction determined by 2D echo (vertical axis) is compared to that determined by left ventriculography at catheterization (horizontal axis). A good correlation is observed. (Carr KW, Engler RL, Forsythe JR, et al: Measurement of left ventricular ejection fraction by mechanical cross-sectional echocardiography. Circulation 59:116, 1979. Reprinted by permission of the American Heart Association, Inc.)

status and arterial pressure, and systematic changes in LV loading due to valve dysfunction must be taken into account in interpreting such data.

Recently, both M-mode and 2D echo have received wide attention as a means of estimating LV wall stress because they offer a more physiologic approach to studying abnormalities of LV loading and contractility.[53–58] LV wall stress is the force generated within the myocardium per unit cross-sectional area and thus represents the afterload actually experienced by the myocardium. At any moment in time, it is the product of ventricular pressure and the Laplace relationship, in which the other variables of interest are chamber radius and wall thickness. Using M-mode echo, stress in the meridional plane (long axis) of the ventricle can be estimated as:

$$\text{Stress} = 0.334PD/T(1 + T/D)$$

where P = LV pressure, T = posterior wall thickness, and D = LV diameter.[58] Analogous equations permit estimates of stress in both the meridional and circumferential planes with 2D data.[59]

Since LV pressure, diameter, and wall thickness all change progressively during systole, stress is not constant but changes continually (Fig. 17-22). In the earlier angiographic literature, much attention was focused on peak stress as a marker for LV afterload.[60] In recent years, however, end-systolic stress has appeared to be a more important single point value.[53-58] End-systolic stress is the limiting afterload that terminates LV ejection because it represents the greatest tension the myocardium can generate isometrically at that muscle length. Consequently, it is both an index of afterload and an index of isometric LV performance. Increases in afterload, expressed as end-systolic stress, have been found uniformly in ventricles with impaired systolic function studied in this fashion and in ventricles with compensated volume loading due to aortic regurgitation.[58] End-systolic stress can also be used to develop a load-independent index of contractility. The relationship between end-systolic stress and LV diameter is generally linear in a single heart with constant inotropic state. Therefore, administration of pharmacologic agents that alter load, such as nitroglycerin, nitroprusside, or phenylephrine, can permit development of an end-systolic stress-diameter plot, the slope and D intercept of which describe LV contractility in a load-independent way (Fig. 17-23).

The clinical utility of echo-based stress analysis would be quite limited if it required high-fidelity measurement of LV pressure for its calculation. Fortunately, several groups have shown that cuff blood pressure can be used instead

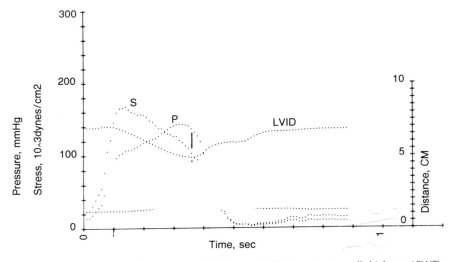

FIG. 17-22. Left ventricular pressure (*P*), diameter (*LVID*), posterior wall thickness (*PWT*) and calculated meridional stresses are plotted at 10 msec intervals through a single cardiac cycle. Vertical line indicates end of systole (*ES*). (Reichek N, Wilson J, St John Sutton M, et al: Noninvasive determination of left-ventricular end-systolic stress. Circulation 65:99, 1982. Reprinted by permission of the American Heart Association, Inc.)

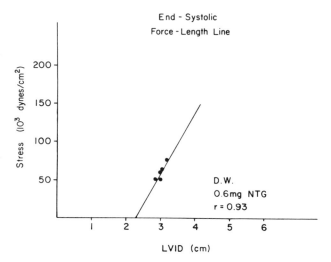

FIG. 17-23. Plot of end-systolic meridional stress (vertical axis) against end-systolic diameter (horizontal axis) in series of cardiac cycles before and after load manipulation in a single patient (D.W.) using sublingual nitroglycerin (*NTG*). The slope and intercept of the resultant line are related to contractile state. (LVID=left ventricular internal dimension.) Reichek N, Wilson J, St John Sutton M, et al: Noninvasive determination of left ventricular end-diastolic stress. Circulation 65:99, 1982. By permission of the American Heart Association, Inc.

of invasive LV pressure. Consequently, end-systolic stress can be used noninvasively both as an index of afterload and to develop stress-diameter plots.[58]

Another area of current interest is use of echo to identify LV filling abnormalities. The high sampling rate of M-mode makes it particularly suitable for this problem, but 2D data can be used as well, if lower temporal resolution is acceptable. Using M-mode, digitization of LV diameter at 5 msec to 10 msec intervals throughout diastole permits instantaneous examination of LV filling rate as well as assessment of the relative contributions of the rapid filling phase and atrial systole.[61,62] Additionally, the isovolumic relaxation time of the ventricle can be determined from the interval between development of minimal LV diameter and mitral valve opening. Impaired diastolic filling has been demonstrated in this fashion in mitral stenosis, hypertrophic cardiomyopathy, constrictive pericarditis, and restrictive cardiomyopathy.[38,61-63]

Segmental Myocardial Function

Because of its ability to sample myocardial thickness in many regions, and because changes in myocardial thickness directly parallel changes in segment length, echo can be used to evaluate segmental myocardial function. Systolic function has been most extensively explored. It is known that many disorders of wall motion, particularly those involving the interventricular septum, do not reflect impairment of intrinsic contractile function. Thus, in abnormal septal motion due to RV volume overload, left bundle branch block, or previous cardiac surgery, septal thickening is actually normal. Conversely, in acute ischemia, abnormal wall motion can be shown to be associated with reduced wall thickening or, in transmural ischemia, actual systolic wall thinning.[64-66] Wall thickening appears to be both more specific and more sensitive than endocardial motion as a means of identifying abnormalities in intrinsic myocardial function.

Digitized techniques have also been used to examine the relation of diastolic myocardial segmental function to wall thinning, in terms of both the absolute value of the change in wall thickness and the instantaneous rate of change.[61-63] Abnormal segmental diastolic myocardial function appears to be a particularly sensitive marker of myocardial abnormality, although its physiologic determinants remain to be characterized.

References

1. Feigenbaum H: Echocardiography, 3rd ed. Philadelphia, Lea & Febiger, 1981
2. Shah PM, Gramiak R, Adelman AG, et al: Role of echocardiography in diagnostic and hemodynamic assessment of hypertrophic subaortic stenosis. Circulation 44:891, 1971
3. Davis RH, Feigenbaum H, Chang S, et al: Echocardiographic manifestations of discrete subaortic stenosis. Am J Cardiol 33:277, 1974
4. Okumachi F, Komine Y, Yamaoka S, et al: Diagnostic significance of aortic valve motion. J Cardiogr 3:367, 1978
5. Feigenbaum H: Echocardiography, 3rd ed, p 199. Philadelphia, Lea & Febiger, 1981
6. Nanda NC, Gramiak R: Evaluation of bicuspid aortic valves by two-dimensional echocardiography. Am J Cardiol 41:372, 1978
7. Weyman AE, Feigenbaum H, Dillon JC, et al: Cross-sectional echocardiography in assessing the severity of valvular aortic stenosis. Circulation 52:828, 1975
8. Shiu MF, Coltart DJ, Braimbridge MV: Echocardiographic findings in prolapsed aortic cusp with vegetation. Br Heart J 41:118, 1979
9. Chandraratna PAN, Robinson MJ, Byrd C, et al: Significance of abnormal echoes in left ventricular outflow tract. Br Heart J 39:381, 1977
10. Mintz GS, Kotler MN, Segal BL, et al: Comparison of two-dimensional and M-mode echocardiography in the evaluation of patients with infective endocarditis. Am J Cardiol 43:738, 1979
11. Markiewicz W, Stoner J, London E, et al: Mitral valve prolapse in one hundred presumably healthy young females. Circulation 53:464, 1976
12. Devereux R, Perloff JK, Reichek N, et al: Mitral valve prolapse. Circulation 54:3, 1976
13. Mintz GS, Kotler MN, Parry WR, et al: Statistical comparison of M-mode and two-dimensional echocardiographic diagnosis of flail mitral leaflets. Am J Cardiol 45:253, 1980
14. Henry WL, Clark CE, Glancy DL, et al: Echocardiographic measurement of the left ventricular outflow gradient in idiopathic hypertrophic subaortic stenosis. N Engl J Med 288:989, 1973
15. Henry WL, Clark CE, Epstein SE: Asymmetric septal hypertrophy (ASH): The unifying link in the IHSS disease spectrum. Observations regarding its pathogenesis, pathophysiology, and course. Circulation 47:827, 1973
16. Henry WL, Clark CE, Griffith JM, et al: Mechanism of left ventricular outflow obstruction in patients with obstructive asymmetric septal hypertrophy (Idiopathic hypertrophic subaortic stenosis). Am J Cardiol 35:337, 1975

17. Murgo JP, Alter BR, Dorethy JF, et al: Dynamics of left ventricular ejection in obstructive and non-obstructive hypertrophic cardiomyopathy. J Clin Invest 66:1369, 1980
18. Konecke LL, Feigenbaum H, Chang S, et al: Abnormal mitral valve motion in patients with elevated left ventricular diastolic pressures. Circulation 47:989, 1973
19. Massie BM, Schiller NB, Ratshin RA, et al: Mitral-septal separation: New echocardiographic index of left ventricular function. Am J Cardiol 39:1008, 1977
20. Rubenstein JJ, Pohost GM, Dinsmore RE, et al: The echocardiographic determination of mitral valve opening and closure: Correlation with hemodynamic studies in man. Circulation 51:98, 1975
21. Pohost GM, Dinsmore RE, Rubenstein JJ, et al: The echocardiogram of the anterior leaflet of the mitral valve: correlation with hemodynamic and cineroentgenographic studies in dogs. Circulation 51:88, 1975
22. Laniado S, Yellin E, Kotler M, et al: A study of the dynamic relations between the mitral valve echogram and phasic mitral flow. Circulation 51:104, 1975
23. D'Cruz I, Cohen HC, Prabhu R, et al: Flutter of left ventricular structures in patients with aortic regurgitation, with special reference to patients with associated mitral stenosis. Am Heart J 92:684, 1976
24. Mann T, McLaurin L, Grossman W, et al: Assessing the hemodynamic severity of acute aortic regurgitation due to infective endocarditis. N Engl J Med 293:108, 1975
25. Duchak JM Jr, Chang S, Feigenbaum H: The posterior mitral valve echo and the echocardiographic diagnosis of mitral stenosis. Am J Cardiol 29:628, 1972
26. Henry WL, Griffith JM, Michaelis LL, et al: Measurement of mitral orifice area in patients with mitral valve disease by real-time, two-dimensional echocardiography. Circulation 51:827, 1975
27. Werner JA, Schiller NB, Prasquier R: Occurrence and significance of echocardiographically demonstrated tricuspid valve prolapse. Am Heart J 96:180, 1978
28. Joyner CR, Hey EB Jr, Johnson J, et al: Reflected ultrasound in the diagnosis of tricuspid stenosis. Am J Cardiol 19:66, 1967
29. Weyman AE: Pulmonary valve echo motion in clinical practice. Am J Med 62:843, 1977
30. Silverman NH, Snider AR, Rudolph AM: Evaluation of pulmonary hypertension by M-mode echocardiography in children with ventricular septal defect. Circulation 61:1125, 1980
31. Grossman W, Jones D, McLaurin LP: Wall stress and patterns of hypertrophy in the human left ventricle. J Clin Invest 56:56, 1975
32. Johnson GL, Meyer RA, Schwartz DC, et al: Echocardiographic evaluation of fixed left ventricular outlet obstruction in children. Pre- and post-op assessment of ventricular systolic pressures. Circulation 56:299, 1977
33. Aziz KU, van Grondelle A, Paul MH, et al: Echocardiographic assessment of the relation between left ventricular wall and cavity dimensions and peak systolic pressure in children with aortic stenosis. Am J Cardiol 40:775, 1977
34. Schwartz A, Vignola PA, Walker HJ, et al: Echocardiographic estimation of aortic-valve gradient in aortic stenosis. Ann Intern Med 89:329, 1978
35. Reichek N, Devereux RB: Reliable estimation of peak left ventricular systolic pressure by M-mode echographic-determined end-diastolic relative wall thickness: Identification of severe valvular aortic stenosis in adult patients. Am Heart J 103:202, 1982
36. Wilson JR, Reichek N, Hirshfeld J: Noninvasive assessment of load reduction in patients with asymptomatic aortic regurgitation. Am J Med 68:664, 1980

37. Wilson JR, Reichek N, Dunkman BW, et al: Ventricular geometry as a determinant of hemodynamic response to diuretic therapy in heart failure. Circulation (Suppl 2) 60:39, 1979

38. St. John Sutton MG, Reichek N, Kastor JA, et al: Computerized M-mode echocardiographic analysis of left ventricular dysfunction in cardiac amyloid. Circulation 66:790, 1982

39. Popp RL, Wolfe SB, Hirata T, et al: Estimation of right and left ventricular size by ultrasound. A study of the echoes from the inter-ventricular septum. Am J Cardiol 24:523, 1969

40. Feigenbaum H, Corya BC, Dillon JC, et al: Role of echocardiography in patients with coronary artery disease. Am J Cardiol 37:775, 1976

41. Dillon JC, Chang S, Feigenbaum H: Echocardiographic manifestations of left bundle branch block. Circulation 49:876, 1974

42. Kushner FG, Lam W, Morganroth J: Apex sector echocardiography in evaluation of the right atrium in patients with mitral stenosis and atrial septal defect. Am J Cardiol 42:733, 1978

43. Lieppe W, Behar VS, Scallion R, et al: Detection of tricuspid regurgitation with two-dimensional echocardiography and peripheral vein injections. Circulation 57:128, 1978

44. Quinones MA, Pickering E, Alexander JK: Percentage of shortening of the echocardiographic left ventricular dimension: Its use in determining ejection fraction and stroke volume. Chest 74:59, 1978

45. Cooper RH, O'Rourke RA, Karliner JS, et al: Comparison of ultrasound and cineangiographic measurements of the mean rate of circumferential fiber shortening in man. Circulation 46:914, 1972

46. Traill TA, Gibson DG, Brown DJ: Study of left ventricular wall thickness and dimension changes using echocardiography. Br Heart J 40:162, 1978

47. Schiller NB, Acquatella H, Ports TA, et al: Left ventricular volume from paired biplane two-dimensional echocardiography. Circulation 60:547, 1979

48. Carr KW, Engler RL, Forsythe JR, et al: Measurement of left ventricular ejection fraction by mechanical cross-sectional echocardiography. Circulation 59:1196, 1979

49. Bommer W, Chun T, Kwan OL, et al: Biplane apex echocardiography versus biplane cineangiography in the assessment of left ventricular volume and function: Validation by direct measurements. Am J Cardiol 45:471, 1980

50. Wyatt HL, Heng MK, Meerbaum S, et al: Cross-sectional echocardiography II: Analysis of mathematic models for quantifying volume of the formalin-fixed left ventricle. Circulation 61:1119, 1980

51. Helak JW, Reichek N: Quantitation of human left ventricular mass and volume by two-dimensional echocardiography: *In vitro* anatomic validation. Circulation 63:1398, 1981

52. Helak JW, Plappert T, Muhammad A, et al: Two-dimensional echocardiographic imaging of the left ventricle: Comparison of mechanical and phased-array systems in vitro. Am J Cardiol 48:728, 1981

53. Matsumoto M, Hanrath P, Kremer P, et al: A new method for the evaluation of left ventricular function by simultaneous recording of two-dimensional echocardiograms and left ventricular pressure. Circulation (Suppl 3) 62:258, 1980

54. Marsh JD, Green LH, Wynne J, et al: Left ventricular end-systolic pressure-dimension and stress-length relations in normal human subjects. Am J Cardiol 44:1311, 1979

55. Quinones MA, Mokotoff DM, Nouri S, et al: Noninvasive quantification of left

ventricular wall stress: Validation of method and application to assessment of chronic pressure overload. Am J Cardiol 45:782, 1980

56. Wilson JR, Reichek N, Hirshfeld JW: Noninvasive assessment of load reduction in patients with asymptomatic aortic regurgitation. Am J Med 68:664, 1980

57. Caraballo BA, Green LH, Grossman W, et al: Hemodynamic determinants of prognosis of aortic valve replacement in critical aortic stenosis and advanced congestive heart failure. Circulation 62:42, 1980

58. Reichek N, Wilson J, St. John Sutton M, et al: Noninvasive determination of left ventricular end-systolic stress: Validation of the method and initial applications. Circulation 65:99, 1982

59. St. John Sutton MG, Reichek N, Plappert T, et al: Efficacy of afterload reduction in aortic regurgitation: Assessment by two-dimensional echo. Am J Cardiol 47:413, 1981

60. Hood WP Jr, Rackley CE, Rolett EL: Wall stress in the normal and hypertrophied human left ventricle. Am J Cardiol 22:550, 1968

61. St. John Sutton MG, Tajik AJ, Gibson DG, et al: Echocardiographic assessment of left ventricular filling and septal and posterior wall dynamics in idiopathic hypertrophic subaortic stenosis. Circulation 57:512, 1978

62. St. John Sutton MG, Traill TA, Ghafour AS, et al: Echocardiographic assessment of left ventricular filling after mitral valve surgery. Br Heart J 39:1283, 1977

63. Friedman MJ, Sahn DJ, Burris HA, et al: Computerized echocardiographic analysis to detect abnormal systolic and diastolic left ventricular function in children with aortic stenosis. Am J Cardiol 44:478, 1979

64. Kerber RE, Marcus ML, Ehrhardt J, et al: Correlation between echocardiographically demonstrated segmental dyskinesis and regional myocardial perfusion. Circulation 52:1097, 1975

65. Heger JJ, Weyman AE, Wann LS, et al: Cross-sectional echocardiography in acute myocardial infarction: Detection and localization of regional left ventricular asynergy. Circulation 60:531, 1979

66. Likoff M, Reichek N, St. John Sutton M, et al: Epicardial mapping of segmental myocardial function: An echocardiographic method applicable to man. Circulation 66:1050, 1982

INDEX

An *f* following a page number indicates a figure; a *t* represents tabular material.